The Essential Guide to Prescription Drugs

JAMES W. LONG, M.D.

THE ESSENTIAL GUIDE TO
PRESCRIPTION DRUGS

FOURTH EDITION

1817
HARPER & ROW, PUBLISHERS, New York
Cambridge, Philadelphia, San Francisco, London
Mexico City, São Paulo, Singapore, Sydney

for Alice
who understood so well
and helped so much

Library of Congress Cataloging in Publication Data

Long, James W.
  The essential guide to prescription drugs.

  Bibliography: p.
  Includes index.
  1. Drugs—Side effects. 2. Drugs—Safety measures.
3. Drugs. I. Title. [DNLM: 1. Drugs—handbooks.
2. Drugs—popular works. QV 39 L848e]
RM302.5.L66 1985 615′.1 84-47973
ISBN 0-06-181551-9   85 86 87 88 10 9 8 7 6 5 4 3 2 1
ISBN 0-06-091193-X (pbk.) 85 86 87 88 10 9 8 7 6 5 4 3 2 1

Contents

Acknowledgments   vii

Author's Note for the Fourth Edition   xi

SECTION ONE

1. Drug Actions and Reactions in Perspective   3
2. The Patient's Guidelines for Safe Drug Use   14
3. How to Use This Book   17

SECTION TWO: Drug Profiles   27

Estrogen and the Menopause   337

SECTION THREE: Drug Classes   869

SECTION FOUR: Glossary of Drug-Related Terms   899

SECTION FIVE: Tables of Drug Information

1. A Checklist of Health Conditions That Can Influence the
   Choice of Drugs   929
2. Your Drugs, Your Anesthetic, and Your Surgery   931
3. Specific Diseases and the Drugs That Can Interfere with
   Their Management   932
4. Symptoms That May Warn of Serious Adverse Effects   939
5. Your Drugs and Alcohol   948
6. Photosensitivity: Your Drugs and the Sun   952

7. Drug Use During the First Trimester (First Three
   Months) of Pregnancy   954
8. Drug Use During the Second and Third Trimesters
   (Fourth Through Ninth Month) of Pregnancy   955
9. Drug Use While Nursing an Infant   957
10. Drug Use During Infancy (Birth to Two Years of Age)   958
11. Drug Use During Childhood (Two to Twelve Years of
    Age)   959
12. Drugs and the Elderly   960
13. Your Drugs and Sexual Activity   963
14. Your Drugs and Vision   965
15. Your Drugs and Hearing   969
16. Your Drugs and Sleep   970
17. Your Drugs and Your Mood (Emotions)   973
18. Your Drugs and Mental Function   975
19. Your Drugs and Personal Identification   977

SECTION SIX: Personal Drug Histories

1. Drugs Taken During Pregnancy   980
2. Drugs Taken During Infancy and Childhood   981
3. Drugs Taken by Adults   982
4. Medical Alert   983

Sources   985

Index of Brand and Generic Names   991

Acknowledgments

Many individuals in diverse professional settings have contributed in a variety of ways to the creation of this book. I wish to acknowledge with particular gratitude the helpful suggestions and tangible assistance provided by the following individuals:

Graeme S. Avery, Editor-in-Chief, Australasian Drug Information Services, ADIS Press Australasia Pty Limited, Auckland, New Zealand.

Jacob A. Brody, M.D., Associate Director for Epidemiology, Demography, and Biometry Program, National Institute on Aging, National Institutes of Health, Bethesda, Maryland.

James A. Donahue, Jr., Group Vice-President, Health Care Services, IMS America Ltd., Ambler, Pennsylvania.

S. B. Gusberg, M.D., D.Sc., Professor and Chairman, Department of Obstetrics and Gynecology, Mount Sinai School of Medicine, New York, New York.

S. Mitchell Harman, M.D., Ph.D., National Institute on Aging, Gerontology Research Center, Baltimore City Hospitals, Baltimore, Maryland.

J. Donald Harper, President, The Proprietary Association of Canada, Ottawa, Ontario, Canada.

Robert P. Heaney, M.D., Vice-President for Health Sciences, Creighton University, Omaha, Nebraska.

Barbara S. Hulka, M.D., M.P.H., Professor, Department of Epidemiology, The School of Public Health, University of North Carolina, Chapel Hill, North Carolina.

Nelson S. Irey, M.D., Chief, Division of Tissue Reactions to Drugs, Armed Forces Institute of Pathology, Washington, D.C.

Hershel Jick, M.D., Boston University Medical Center, Boston Collaborative Drug Surveillance Program, Waltham, Massachusetts.

Don Harper Mills, M.D., J.D., Clinical Professor of Pathology, University of Southern California School of Medicine, Los Angeles, California.

Lloyd G. Millstein, Ph.D., Deputy Director, Division of Drug Advertising and Labeling, Bureau of Drugs, Food and Drug Administration, Rockville, Maryland.*

Stanley R. Mohler, M.D., Professor and Vice-Chairman, Department of Community Medicine, and Director, Aerospace Medicine, Wright State University School of Medicine, Dayton, Ohio.

Gabriel G. Nahas, M.D., Ph.D., Professor of Anesthesiology, Department of Anesthesiology, College of Physicians and Surgeons of Columbia University, New York, New York.

Gerald N. Rotenberg, B.Sc.Phrm., F.A.C.A., Pharmaceutical Consultant, Drug Data Services, Thornhill, Ontario, Canada.

Isaac Schiff, M.D., Assistant Professor of Obstetrics and Gynecology, Boston Hospital for Women, Harvard Medical School, Boston, Massachusetts.

Thomas H. Shepard, M.D., Professor of Pediatrics, Head, Central Laboratory for Human Embryology, Department of Pediatrics, University of Washington School of Medicine, Seattle, Washington.

John E. Steinhaus, M.D., Ph.D., Chairman, Department of Anesthesiology, Emory University School of Medicine, Atlanta, Georgia.

Christopher Tietze, M.D., Senior Fellow, The Population Council, New York, New York.

Catherine Urbaitis, R.N., Staff Nurse, Norwell Knoll Long-Term Care Facility, Norwell, Massachusetts.

Wulf H. Utian, M.D., Ph.D., F.R.C.O.G., F.A.C.O.G., F.I.C.S., Director of Obstetrics and Gynecology, Mount Sinai Hospital of Cleveland; Associate Professor, Department of Reproductive Biology, Case Western Reserve University, Cleveland, Ohio.

Professor Owen L. Wade, M.A., M.D., F.R.C.P., (London) Hon. F.R.C.P.I., Department of Therapeutics and Clinical Pharmacology, The Medical School, The University of Birmingham, Birmingham, England.

Leonard A. Wisneski, M.D., Associate Clinical Professor of Medicine, Department of Medicine, George Washington University, Washington, D.C.

The helpful cooperation of many pharmaceutical manufacturers is greatly appreciated. In response to numerous inquiries they provided

*Dr. Millstein served exclusively as an editorial consultant in a private capacity for the compilation of information provided in the Pregnancy Category of the Drug Profiles. The information presented does not necessarily represent the official position of the Food and Drug Administration and does not have the endorsement of that agency.

much detailed and hard-to-find information needed to complete the Drug Profiles in Section Two.

   In addition, I wish to express my sincere thanks and appreciation to Carol Cohen, my editor at Harper & Row. Her wise counsel and competent guidance have made this collaboration a genuine pleasure.

Author's Note for the Fourth Edition

When the first edition of this guide was in preparation ten years ago, the issue of providing the patient with detailed and specific information about medicinal drugs was highly controversial. After ten years of open discussion and debate, a consensus is gradually emerging: the optimal use of therapeutic drugs requires an informed public. However, effective implementation of this recognition is just beginning. Recent surveys by the Food and Drug Administration reveal that half of the people in this country taking medicines are taking them improperly. A 1982 poll found that 70 percent of those responding were not given appropriate information regarding the proper use of the drugs prescribed for them, and that only 4 percent of patients questioned their physicians regarding drugs used in treatment. This traditional lack of physician-patient communication has greatly stimulated public interest and demand for other sources of practical drug information. The continued acceptance of this guide is gratifying evidence of its contribution to the growing sophistication of those among us who prescribe, dispense, and take medicinal drugs.

As with previous editions, the need to maintain the reasonable size and price of the guide has influenced the scope of its contents, especially the number of drugs included in Section Two, the Drug Profiles. To remain current, 13 Drug Profiles were deleted and 21 new Profiles were added to provide a total of 218 in this edition. The criteria for selection include the current (or anticipated) volume of a drug's use, the seriousness of the conditions for which it is prescribed, and its inherent complexity of actions and management. Any attempt to cover all or most available drugs that would seem to warrant inclusion would require a book of prohibitive size and cost.

Because of the ever-growing volume and ever-changing nature of drug information, it is obvious that *no claim can be made* that *all* known side-effects, adverse effects, interactions, precautions, etc., for a drug are included in the information provided in the Drug Profiles. While diligent care has been taken to ensure the accuracy of the information provided during the preparation of this revision, the continued accuracy and currentness are ever subject to change relative to the dissemination of new information in drug development and research.

The original purpose of this guide remains unchanged: to provide the reader with the knowledge and understanding needed to use medicinal drugs with maximal benefit and minimal risk.

SECTION ONE

1

DRUG ACTIONS AND REACTIONS IN PERSPECTIVE

2

THE PATIENT'S GUIDELINES FOR SAFE DRUG USE

3

HOW TO USE THIS BOOK

1

Drug Actions and Reactions in Perspective

Approximately two-thirds of the population of the United States use prescription drugs at one time or another. At present, an estimated 75 million Americans are taking one or more drugs on a regular basis. The annual volume of prescriptions and drug orders written in this country now approaches three billion—almost double the volume of ten years ago—and market analysts predict that drug sales will double again by the early 1980s. From 70 to 80 percent of the prescriptions written by private physicians are for drugs used by non-hospitalized patients—drugs that are self-administered, usually without direct supervision. Huge quantities of non-prescription drugs are consumed daily. Over 15 million people take aspirin or combination drugs containing aspirin regularly; more than 10 million people are taking drugs for high blood pressure; 10 million women are using oral contraceptives; and another 5 million citizens are taking mild tranquilizers. The magnitude of drug consumption in most western cultures has become a major scientific, social, and economic concern.

Increasing public debate repeatedly exposes the consumer to claims and counterclaims regarding the virtues and evils of drugs, both those prescribed in medical practice and the numerous over-the-counter drugs often taken without the physician's knowledge or approval. Spokesmen for the drug industry, medical professions and government agencies, lawmakers, consumer advocates, and even the world of entertainment have all provided us with distorted and conflicting accounts of the role of drugs in modern society. Understandably, many citizens are confused and frustrated about safety in drug therapy. To comprehend the full potential for benefit and for harm which today's medicines have to offer, we must sort fact from fiction and put the picture of rational drug use in reasonable perspective.

The Wanted and Intended Actions of Drugs

The human body is an intricate chemical system. Most medicinal drugs are chemicals which are alien to the natural body chemistry. They are useful in treatment, however, because a particular aspect of their chemical interactions within the body favorably modifies some tissue structure or function. This, in turn, assists natural mechanisms that heal and restore. Drug actions alone do not "cure" disease. They benefit the patient by making a significant contribution to the total scheme of processes needed to restore health. Many illnesses are normally self-limiting; recovery often occurs as a result of natural recuperative forces, without the use of drugs.

When drugs are advisable, the "drug of choice" is the one which, in the judgment of the physician, is most likely to produce those effects most desired in a given treatment situation. This selection—the best drug, in the right dose, for the right person, at the right time—is the crucial first step in the successful use of drugs. But this decision can never be made with complete assurance that the interactions of drug, patient, and disease will be exactly as intended or predicted. When a patient takes any prescribed drug for the first time, he or she is in fact participating in an experiment under the physician's direction. While the physician's knowledge of the patient's general condition, his current illness, and the actions of the drug make it possible to predict the probable (and certainly the desirable) course of the experiment, the full consequences can never be foreseen. There is always an inescapable element of uncertainty.

The reasons for this are clear. The first relates to the drug itself: All drugs have multiple actions. There is no such thing as a drug with a single action. If a drug is to have any usefulness in treatment, it must be active enough to alter body chemistry and function in a beneficial way and to a sufficient degree. The complex nature of the human body makes it impossible to design a drug that can selectively limit its action to produce *only* one desired effect at a precise location. In actual use, a drug is selected because of its *principal* action—that particular one of its several effects which is wanted and intended. Simultaneously, however, its other actions ("side-effects") will occur, some of them trivial and unimportant, others more significant and even serious, but all quite natural and unavoidable.

The second reason for unpredictability relates to the patient: All patients experience multiple responses, some of which may not be readily apparent. The body's reaction to a drug varies widely from person to person, and in the same person at different times and under different circumstances. Personal characteristics due to inherited sensitivities, allergies, variations in metabolism, etc., all influence the total drug experience. At the outset of drug therapy, individual variation in response to both the intended effects and the side-effects of a drug is always unknown.

A third factor in the unpredictability of drug therapy is encountered in treating the chronically ill and the elderly. In these situations vital body functions are often impaired, and a new and urgent illness of immediate concern may be superimposed on a state of chronic illness or general deterioration. All hazards of drug treatment are usually increased in the elderly, and it is difficult to predict either the favorable or the unfavorable consequences of drug action in such situations.

When one understands all of the possible variables that must be considered, one realizes how truly remarkable it is that modern medical practice has achieved a reasonable standardization in drug selection and use.

The Unwanted and Unintended Actions of Drugs

All drugs can produce both wanted and unwanted effects. Unwanted drug responses are of two kinds. The first is the "side-effect," a natural, expected, and predictable action of the drug, which accompanies its principal and intended action; it occurs *on the side.* Many patients experience side-effects in one form or another. When the antihistamine Benadryl (a brand of diphenhydramine) is given to reduce the nasal congestion and excessive flow of mucus caused by seasonal hayfever, the drying effect on the lining of the nose is its principal (wanted and intended) action. The drowsiness it produces is one of its side-effects. When the same drug is given to treat insomnia, drowsiness is its principal action, and dryness of the nose and throat are side-effects. And so it is with many drugs in common use; while the obvious goal of drug therapy is to obtain the greatest relief possible with the least unpleasantness, in many treatment situations it is necessary to accept the minor annoyance of side-effects in order to obtain the more important therapeutic effect. Many side-effects are transient, gradually disappearing as the body adjusts to the continued use of the drug. In many instances the intensity of side-effects can be reduced by adjusting the dosage schedule or by substituting another drug from the same drug family. The wide variation in the frequency and nature of side-effects is responsible, in part, for the large number of similar drugs available to treat the same condition; this sometimes enables the physician to choose a drug which will produce fewer side-effects in a particular patient.

A second kind of unwanted drug response is the "adverse reaction," an unusual, unexpected, and infrequent response that is clearly undesirable and potentially harmful. Adverse reactions can and do occur when the best drug is being used in the correct dosage to treat the right patient for the right condition. Most adverse reactions are unpredictable; some can be prevented (as described at length later in this chapter).

Many sources of drug information use the terms "side-effect," "adverse reaction," and "untoward effect" interchangeably. The failure to draw a distinction between an understandable and acceptable drug action (a side-effect) and an unexpected and unacceptable toxic response (an adverse reaction) is one reason for widespread popular apprehension and misunderstanding about drug effects and their proper management.

Over the past 20 years both professional and lay publications have given increasing attention to adverse drug reactions, often referring to them as "drug-induced illnesses." These are now generally accepted as a major health problem. The magnitude and seriousness of the problem justify concern and appropriate action, but it is important to remember that its true dimensions have not yet been established. Statistics of illness and death attributed to the adverse effects of drugs have been widely publicized, but these figures are crudely drawn estimates projected improperly from the results of a few studies limited in size and scope. When we analyze the studies, we find significant discrepancies of interpretation and representation. Some studies which collected "adverse reaction" data ignored the distinction between the natural consequences of overdose, which is a misuse of a drug, and truly unavoidable toxic effects. Reports of other studies have failed to include balanced consideration of the roles of advanced disease and fatal illness in cases of "drug-related" death. To attribute death in such cases primarily to drug effects is clearly inaccurate and misleading.

Another aspect of the problem which publicized reports have failed to explain is that the majority of drug-related illnesses and deaths involve *a small number* of highly potent drugs which are known to have narrow margins of safety. In most such instances, the life-threatening nature of the illness clearly justifies the hazards of treatment, even though the nature and severity of the underlying disease often render the patient more vulnerable to possible adverse effects of drugs, some of which are quite toxic by nature.

The distorted and exaggerated picture of drug-induced illness in this and other countries is a disservice to the best interests of the public. (Unfortunately, this critical field of public health lends itself to exploitation as "sensational" news.) Misrepresentation of the actual situation has a negative influence on both the health professional and the health consumer. A growing number of physicians are now more inclined to prescribe defensively, using a less effective drug which is "safer" rather than a more effective one reputed to be "less safe." Surveys of physicians have verified that fear of an adverse reaction (with the possibility of a resulting malpractice suit) is a major reason for not prescribing a particular drug. Many studies have also documented the frequency with which wary patients underutilize drugs prescribed for them. An example of this is the unusually high incidence of omitted doses and discontinued medications by individuals on drug treatment for high blood pressure. Thus fear deprives them of the best available treatment. This problem of patient noncompliance, already serious, can only worsen as public uncertainty and concern grow in response to heated debate that is lacking in balance and perspective.

Studies published to date have not been large enough, or adequately enough designed, to obtain an accurate assessment of the overall incidence of adverse drug reactions or the causative factors which characterize them. However, the few sober reviews available to this author support the following realistic conclusions

- Considered in the context of national drug consumption, serious adverse reactions are relatively uncommon.
- Most adverse reactions are transient and of a minor nature.
- The majority of life-threatening drug reactions occur in people who are already severely ill with advanced or known fatal disease.
- Most serious adverse reactions are caused by a small number of drugs which are quite hazardous by nature.
- The number of deaths properly attributed to drugs is quite small in relation to the number of lives saved by these same drugs.
- The reported high incidence of drug-induced illness and death reflects primarily the magnitude and extent of drug use rather than the inherent toxicity of drugs in general.

While this analysis suggests a positive and optimistic perspective of drug therapy, the individual who is about to begin a course of medication may be apprehensive about his or her chances of experiencing an unfavorable drug response. He or she is now aware of dual needs: the benefit to be derived from the proper drug *and* the protection to be sought through appropriate safeguards. Fortunately, both the health professions and spokesmen for the general public are devoting increased attention to meeting these needs more effectively.

The Balance of Benefit and Risk

The drug of choice in any treatment situation is the one that produces the most desirable combination of effects—the net worth of the drug's benefits, allowing for its hazards. This decision must be made in the context of the patient's overall condition and the natural history of his disease. The variables which require evaluation are many, and their possible interactions are often extremely complex. Rational drug therapy is not a simple exercise. The physician's responsibility is to devise a plan of treatment that tips the balance as far as possible in the direction of recovery and cure. He or she must ask simultaneously, How ill is the patient? How threatening is the disease? How dangerous is the drug? The more threatening the illness, the greater the potency (and consequently the toxic potential) of the drugs required to treat it. In serious illnesses, *every* appropriate drug may have some relative contraindication (see Glossary). Drug selection in these circumstances requires the most careful consideration of *all* pertinent factors—patient profile, disease profile, and drug profile.

Whenever possible the drug selected will have a wide margin of safety—a sizable spread between the helpful dose and the harmful dose. Fortunately, most drugs in general use today have a reasonable safety margin. However, a few drugs with uncomfortably narrow margins of safety are also in wide use. This is because they are often the only appropriate drugs available, they are highly effective, and the conditions requiring them are very common. The use of these drugs calls for an extra measure of vigilance by *both physician and patient* to maintain the delicate balance between benefit and harm. The patient should be sure that he fully understands the amount of variation in dosage he is permitted when he assumes the management of his medication. It is important that he realize that fluctuations in his living routines can temporarily alter his drug requirement and that from time to time he may experience indications of too much or too little of the drug. The well-informed patient will know what adjustments to make until he is able to consult his physician. He will also understand that the occasional annoyance and discomfort of incorrect dosage is a small price to pay for the long-run benefits which sustain his health and performance.

The use of highly potent and potentially toxic drugs in the treatment of life-threatening disease is another area which requires the closest cooperation between patient and physician. Here the trade-off between highly undesirable reactions and possible cure or control of the illness calls for much greater understanding and tolerance on the part of the patient. Close observation and periodic examinations to monitor the course of the disease and the effects of drugs on body functions are of utmost importance in achieving the best possible balance of benefit and risk.

Considered within the context of their proper use, the vast majority of drugs in use today offer benefits which significantly outweigh their hazards.

Preventing Adverse Drug Reactions

Our knowledge of the mechanisms of adverse reactions is very limited. For the most part, we cannot identify with certainty the person who is at greater risk of experiencing a true adverse effect. Available tests for the early detection of toxicity are of definite value, but they do not provide as full a measure of protection as we could wish.

As our understanding of drug actions and reactions expands, it becomes more apparent that there *is* a sizable proportion of adverse effects that are, to some extent, predictable and preventable. The exact percentage of preventable reactions is yet to be determined, but several contributing factors are now well recognized, and specific recommendations are available to guide both physician and patient. These fall into eleven categories of consideration.

PREVIOUS ADVERSE REACTION TO A DRUG

There is evidence to indicate that an individual who has experienced an adverse drug reaction in the past is more likely to have adverse reactions to other drugs, even though the drugs are unrelated. This suggests that some individuals may have a genetic (inborn) predisposition to unusual and abnormal drug responses. *The patient should inform the physician of any history of prior adverse drug experiences.*

ALLERGIES

Individuals who are allergic by nature (hayfever, asthma, eczema, hives) are more likely to develop allergies to drugs than are nonallergic individuals. The allergic patient must be observed very closely for the earliest indication of a developing hypersensitivity to any drug. Known drug allergies must be noted in the medical record. The patient must inform every physician and dentist he consults that he is allergic by nature and is allergic to specific drugs by name. *The patient should provide this information without waiting to be asked.* The physician will then be able to avoid those drugs which could provoke an allergic reaction, as well as those related drugs to which the patient may have developed a cross-sensitivity.

CONTRAINDICATIONS

Both patient and physician must strictly observe all known contraindications to any drug under consideration. *Absolute contraindications* include those conditions and situations which prohibit the use of the drug for any reason. *Relative contraindications* include those conditions which, in the judgment of the physician, do not preclude the use of the drug altogether, but make it essential that special considerations be given to its use to prevent the intensification of preexisting disease or the development of new disease. Such conditions and situations usually require adjustment of dosage, additional supportive measures, and close supervision.

PRECAUTIONS IN USE

The patient should know about any special precautions to observe while taking the drug. This includes the advisability of use during pregnancy or while nursing an infant; precautions regarding exposure to the sun (or ultraviolet lamps); the avoidance of extreme heat or cold, heavy physical exertion, etc.

DOSAGE

The patient must adhere to the prescribed dosage schedule as closely as possible. *This is most important with those drugs that have narrow margins of safety.* Circumstances which interfere with taking the drug as prescribed (nausea, vomiting, diarrhea) must be reported to the physician so that appropriate adjustments can be made.

INTERACTIONS

Much is known today about how some drugs can interact unfavorably with certain foods, alcohol, and other drugs to produce serious adverse effects. *The patient must be informed regarding all likely interactants* that could alter the action of the drug he is using. If, during the course of treatment, the patient has reason to feel he has discovered a new interaction of importance, he should inform the physician so that its full significance can be determined. (It is through such observations that much of our understanding of drug interactions has come.)

WARNING SYMPTOMS

Experience has shown that many drugs will produce symptoms that are actually early indications of a developing adverse effect. Examples include the appearance of severe headaches and visual disturbances *before* the onset of a stroke in a woman taking oral contraceptives; the development of acid indigestion and stomach distress *before* the activation of a bleeding peptic ulcer in a man taking phenylbutazone (Butazolidin) for shoulder bursitis. *It is imperative that the patient be familiar with those symptoms and signs that could be early indicators of impending adverse reactions.* With this knowledge he can act in his own behalf by discontinuing the drug and consulting the physician for additional guidance.

EXAMINATIONS TO MONITOR DRUG EFFECTS

Certain drugs (less than half of those in common use) are capable of damaging vital body tissues (bone marrow, liver, kidney, eye structures, etc.)—especially when these drugs are used over an extended period. Such adverse effects are relatively rare, and many of them are not discovered until the drug has been in wide use for a long time. As our knowledge of such effects accumulates, we learn which kinds of drugs (that is, which chemical structures) are most likely to produce such tissue reactions. Hence, we know those drugs which should be monitored periodically to detect as early as possible any evidence of tissue injury resulting from their use. *The patient should cooperate fully with the physician in the performance of periodic examinations for evidence of adverse drug effects.*

ADVANCED AGE AND DEBILITY

The altered functional capacity of vital organs that accompanies advancing age and debilitating disease can greatly influence the body's response to drugs. Such patients tend not to tolerate drugs with inherent toxic potential well; it is usually necessary for them to use smaller doses at longer intervals. *The effects of drugs on the elderly and severely ill are often unpredictable.* The frequent need for dosage adjustments or change in drug selection requires continuous observation of these patients if adverse effects are to be prevented or minimized.

POLYPHARMACY

This term refers to the concurrent use of many drugs during the course of treatment for a particular illness or condition. Several studies have demonstrated that the frequency of adverse reactions for any individual increases in proportion to the number of drugs he is taking. *In any situation requiring drug therapy, it is always best to use the fewest drugs possible.* The smaller the number of drugs in use, the smaller the chance for adverse reactions.

APPROPRIATE DRUG CHOICE

The drug(s) selected to treat any condition should be the most appropriate of those available. Many adverse reactions can be prevented if both physician and patient exercise good judgment and restraint. *The wise patient will not demand overtreatment.* He or she will cooperate with the physician's attempt to balance properly the seriousness of the illness and the hazard of the drug.

The Relativity of Risk

When we reflect on the changes in patterns of major disease that have been brought about over the past 60 years, we see that the remarkable contribution of modern drugs to our present health and well-being is most impressive. No one can reasonably deny the magnificent benefits that society derives from the intelligent use of today's medicines. Many serious illnesses regarded as incapacitating or fatal before the development of effective drugs now lend themselves to "routine" therapy and easy cure or control. Today we take for granted the large array of anti-infective drugs that change the course of many infectious diseases so dramatically that we refer to them as "miracle drugs." It is now the rule rather than the exception that, with appropriate drug therapy, we recover from typhoid fever, pneumonia, meningitis, and "blood poisoning" (septicemia). Families no longer experience the trauma and disruption of prolonged separation when a member contracts tuberculosis. The child with diabetes now grows to adulthood and often leads a full and vigorous life.

Such gains, however, have extracted their price, for there can be no progress without risk. Our present abundance of effective drugs has brought with it an increased potential for serious harm. This is a reasonable and unavoidable consequence and, indeed, not greatly different from any other of man's major endeavors. This year, for example, each of us has a greater than 2-in-10,000 chance of dying in an automobile accident, and a 1-in-500 chance of being seriously injured. Estimates of fatal reactions to the use of penicillin are 2 in 100,000, to mono-amine oxidase inhibitor drugs (antidepressants) from 1 in 10,000 to 1 in 100,000. The most carefully designed and evaluated study published to date found the rate of drug-attributed deaths per course of drug treatment in hospitals to be about 3 in 10,000. And over two-thirds of these drug-related deaths occurred in patients who were terminally ill or whose illness was judged to be fatal in the absence of drug therapy.

The concept of maximal benefit with minimal risk is the accepted basis for all rational drug use. The seriousness of the illness and the benefit sought must always justify the known risks of any drug to be used. A drug which is "completely safe for everyone" must also be weak and ineffective, for such a goal is not only unrealistic but unobtainable. To demand absolute protection against all possible injury from drugs is to ensure the unavailability of useful drugs for all.

The inherent complexities of drug development, regulation, and utilization in this country promote contention and unrest. Not until the health professions and the general public jointly acknowledge their *obligations* to communicate can we hope to achieve a system of drug therapy that provides the greatest possible benefit at the lowest cost in unavoidable injury and death. The process begins when patient and physician collaborate with candor, reason, and mutual concern—in shared responsibility.

2

The Patient's Guidelines for
Safe Drug Use

DO NOT

- pressure your physician to prescribe drugs which, in his or her judgment, you do not need.
- take prescription drugs on your own or on the advice of friends and neighbors because your symptoms are "just like theirs."
- offer drugs prescribed for you to anyone else without a physician's guidance.
- change the dose or timing of any drug without the advice of your physician (except when the drug appears to be causing adverse effects).
- continue to take a drug which you feel is causing adverse effects, until you are able to reach your physician for clarification.
- take *any* drug (prescription or non-prescription) while pregnant or nursing an infant until you are assured by your physician that no harmful effects will occur to either mother or child.
- take any more medicines than are absolutely necessary. (The greater the number of drugs taken simultaneously, the greater the likelihood of adverse effects.)
- withhold from your physician important information about previous drug experiences. He or she will want to know both beneficial and undesirable drug effects you have experienced in the past.
- take any drug in the dark. Identify every dose of medicine carefully in adequate light to be certain you are taking the drug intended.
- keep drugs on a bedside table. Drugs for emergency use, such as nitroglycerin, are an exception. It is advisable to have only one such drug at the bedside for use during the night.

DO

- know the name (and correct spelling) of the drug(s) you are taking. It is advisable to know both the brand name and the generic name.
- read the package labels of all non-prescription drugs to become familiar with the contents of the product.
- follow your physician's instructions regarding dosage schedules as closely as possible. Notify him if it becomes necessary to make major changes in your treatment routine.
- thoroughly shake all liquid suspensions of drugs to ensure uniform distribution of ingredients.
- use a standardized measuring device for giving liquid medications by mouth. The household "teaspoon" varies greatly in size.
- follow your physician's instruction on dietary and other treatment measures designed to augment the actions of the drugs prescribed. This makes it possible to achieve desired drug effects with smaller doses. (A familiar example is the reduction of salt intake during drug treatment for high blood pressure.)
- keep your personal physician informed of all drugs prescribed for you by someone else. Consult him regarding non-prescription drugs you intend to take on your own initiative at the same time that you are taking drugs prescribed by him.
- inform your anesthesiologist, surgeon, and dentist of *all* drugs you are taking, prior to any surgery.
- inform your physician if you become pregnant while you are taking any drugs from any source.
- keep a written record of *all* drugs (and vaccines) you take during your entire pregnancy—name, dose, dates taken, and reasons for use (see Section Six).
- keep a written record of *all* drugs (and vaccines) to which you become allergic or experience an adverse reaction. This should be done for each member of the family, especially the elderly and infirm (see Section Six).
- keep a written record of *all* drugs (and vaccines) to which *your children* become allergic or experience an adverse reaction (see Section Six).
- inform your physician of all known or suspected allergies, especially allergies to drugs. Be certain that this information is included in your medical record. (Allergic individuals are four times more prone to drug reactions than those who are free of allergy).
- inform your physician promptly if you think you are experiencing an overdose, a side-effect, or an adverse effect from a drug.

- determine if it is safe to drive a car, operate machinery, or engage in other hazardous activities while taking the drug(s) prescribed.
- determine if it is safe to drink alcoholic beverages while taking the drug(s) prescribed.
- determine if any particular foods, beverages, or other drugs should be avoided while taking the drug(s) prescribed.
- keep all appointments for follow-up examinations to determine the effects of the drugs and the course of your illness.
- ask for clarification of any point that is confusing or difficult to understand, at the time the drug(s) are prescribed or later if you have forgotten. Request information in writing if circumstances justify it.
- discard all outdated prescription drugs. This will prevent the use of drugs which have deteriorated with time.
- store all drugs to be retained for intermittent use out of the reach of children to prevent accidental poisoning.

How to Use This Book

Your physician has advised you to take a drug (or drugs), or you have been directed to administer a drug (or drugs) to someone under your care. The kind and amount of information you have been given about how to use these drugs, and what to expect from them, will vary tremendously. In many instances it will not be practical or possible for the physician to provide you with *all* the information that could be considered appropriate and useful, or it will be difficult for you to remember it. From time to time you will find it desirable—even necessary—to seek clarification and guidance about some aspect of drug action or drug use. The aim of this book is to give you the kind of information you may need to supplement the direction and guidance you receive from your physician.

The book consists of six sections. The first section will give you the orientation and insight necessary to appreciate the complexities of modern drug therapy and help you to make the best use of the information contained in Sections Two through Six.

Section Two is a compilation of Drug Profiles covering more than 200 prescription (and several non-prescription) drugs used widely in the United States and Canada. The selection of each drug was based upon three considerations: the extent of its use; the urgency of the conditions for which it is prescribed; the volume and complexity of the information essential to its proper utilization. The Drug Profiles are arranged alphabetically by generic name. (Some generic names have spellings similar to other generic names; be careful not to confuse one with another.)

The Profile of each drug is presented in a uniform sequence of information categories. (When you become familiar with the format, you will be able to find quickly specific items of information on any drug, without having to read the entire Profile.) The standard (complete) Drug Profile contains 36 separate categories of information. This edition of the guide introduces the Abbreviated Drug Profile which contains fewer information categories but still provides information that is essential for proper drug use. Because it requires less space, the Abbreviated Profile permits the inclusion of a larger number of important drugs in current use.

YEAR INTRODUCED

This tells you how long the drug has been in general use. The older the drug, the more likely its full spectrum of actions is known and the less likely its continued use will produce new surprises. Most dates represent the year the drug was introduced in the United States. Where a drug had been used widely in other countries for a significant time before it was marketed in the United States, the date of its earlier foreign introduction is given.

BRAND NAMES

These are provided to confirm that you are consulting the correct Drug Profile. They may also help you to recognize a brand name that identifies this drug as one that produced in you an unfavorable reaction on previous use. Brand names and their manufacturers are listed for the United States and for Canada. A combination drug (a drug product with more than one active ingredient) is identified by [CD] following the brand name.

In a few instances a particular brand name in current use in both the United States and Canada will represent entirely different generic drugs (in a single drug product), or a significantly different mixture of generic ingredients (in a combination drug product). The generic composition of such brand name products is identified by country in the index. Travelers between the two countries who obtain their medications by brand name in either country are advised to ascertain that they are being provided the intended generic drug(s) in every instance.

COMMON SYNONYMS ("STREET NAMES")

Because most generic drug names are derived from the chemical configuration of the drug, they are generally awkward, unfamiliar, and difficult for the average patient to recall. Many brand names—which *are* designed to facilitate recall—are often forgotten. Some individuals find it easier and adequate to identify a medication according to its assumed purpose—"water pills" (any diuretic), "heart pills" (usually a form of digitalis), "nerve pills" (a sedative or a tranquilizer). Such designations in common use are provided in this category.

The drug abuse culture has coined its own vocabulary of "street names" for many drug products that are used illicitly. As an aid to identification of the generic component(s) of the drugs classified under the Controlled Substances Act of 1970, widely used "street names" are also provided here.

DRUG CLASS

This identifies the principal therapeutic class(es) to which the drug belongs. When appropriate, the chemical and/or pharmacological class designations are also given. You will find it helpful to recognize the class of the drug you are taking because many actions, reactions, and interactions with other drugs are often shared by drugs of the same class. Throughout this book (and in most literature on drug information) you will find reference to drugs by their class designation. (Section Three provides alphabetically arranged listings of the classes of drugs referred to in this guide.)

PRESCRIPTION REQUIRED

This indicates whether a drug is a prescription or a non-prescription (over-the-counter) purchase. Drugs subject to regulation under the Controlled Substances Act of 1970 (those with potential for abuse) are so designated in parentheses, and the particular schedule that governs their dispensing in the United States is cited. (A description of the Schedules of Controlled Drugs will be found inside the back cover of this guide.)

AVAILABLE FOR PURCHASE BY GENERIC NAME

Increasing interest in the availability of prescription drugs for purchase by their generic names has been prompted by two issues of major significance. The first is concerned with the cost of prescription drugs. The comparison shopper realizes that in general the cost of prescription medication is significantly less when a generic equivalent of a brand name product is purchased. The second issue relates to what is termed "bioavailability and bioequivalence"—the comparative composition, quality, and effectiveness of the generic versus the brand name drug product. Further discussion of bioavailability and bioequivalence of drug products will be found in the Glossary, Section Four.

AVAILABLE DOSAGE FORMS AND STRENGTHS

This represents a composite of available manufacturers' dosage forms (tablets, capsules, elixirs, etc.) and strengths, without company identification. Included are those dosage forms appropriate for use by outpatients and in extended care facilities and nursing homes. Dosage forms limited to hospital use are not included. Refer to Dosage Forms and Strengths in the Glossary (Section Four) for an explanation of those few abbreviations used to designate the strengths of each dosage form.

TABLET MAY BE CRUSHED OR CAPSULE OPENED FOR ADMINISTRATION

There are occasions when an individual finds it difficult or impossible to swallow a tablet or a capsule, and the drug to be taken is not available in a liquid dosage form. This problem occurs frequently in medical institutions caring for the elderly. On those occasions when the patient's condition urgently requires the medication, the attending nurse (or family member) may wish to crush the tablet or open the capsule and mix the contents with a palatable food or beverage for administration. Many of today's drugs are available in a bewildering array of solid dosage forms, some of which should *not* be altered to accommodate administration. This information category identifies those dosage forms of each drug which may be and those which should not be altered for administration. In addition, your pharmacist can provide appropriate guidance if you should need it.

HOW THIS DRUG WORKS

This simplified explanation is limited to consideration of where and how the drug acts to produce its principal (intended) therapeutic effect(s). A drug may be available as a single drug product or in combination with other drugs. In this section of the profile under the designation As a Single Drug Product, you will find the primary use(s) of the drug when used alone. Under the designation As a Combination Drug Product [CD], you will find the primary use(s) when combined with other active drugs within the same tablet, capsule, etc. The uses stated are those determined by consensus within the medical community and substantiated by current scientific study. Combination drugs have been developed because some conditions that warrant drug therapy have more than one cause, are characterized by a variety of symptoms, or may be treated in more than one way. Where appropriate, in this guide, the logic for combining certain drugs to enhance their theraputic value is explained. When you find the designation for Combination Drugs [CD] in the Brand Name list at the beginning of the Drug Profile, read under the Principal Uses of This Drug section to learn more about the drug's use in combination products.

THIS DRUG SHOULD NOT BE TAKEN IF

This category consists of the *absolute* contraindications to the use of the drug (see Contraindications in Glossary). It is most important that you alert your physician or dentist if any information in this category applies to you.

INFORM YOUR PHYSICIAN BEFORE TAKING THIS DRUG IF

This category lists the *relative* contraindications to the use of the drug. Here again, it is important that you communicate all relevant information to your physician or dentist.

TIME REQUIRED FOR APPARENT BENEFIT

The time stated represents a range that covers the shortest to the longest estimates that are generally recognized. Many factors influence the period of time required for any drug to exert beneficial effects. Among them are the nature and severity of the symptoms being treated, the formulation and strength of the drug, the presence or absence of food in the stomach, the ability of the patient to respond, and the concurrent use of other drugs. The information in this category is helpful in preventing premature termination of medication in treatment situations where improvement may seem to you to be unreasonably delayed.

POSSIBLE SIDE-EFFECTS

This category describes the natural, expected, and usually unavoidable actions of the drug—the normal and anticipated consequences of taking it. It is important that you maintain a realistic perspective that balances properly the occurrence of side-effects and the goals of treatment. Consult your physician for guidance whenever side-effects are troublesome or distressing, so that appropriate adjustments of your treatment program can be made.

POSSIBLE ADVERSE EFFECTS

This category includes those unusual, unexpected, and infrequent drug effects which are commonly referred to as adverse drug reactions. For the sake of evaluation, adverse effects are classified as mild or serious in nature. It is always wise to inform your physician as soon as you have reason to suspect you may be experiencing an adverse drug effect. Serious adverse reactions usually announce their development initially in the form of mild, unthreatening symptoms. It is important that you remain alert to significant changes in your well-being when you are taking a drug that is known to be capable of producing a serious adverse effect. It is also possible to experience an adverse reaction that has not yet been reported. Do not discount the possibility of an adverse effect just because it is not listed in this category. Following standard practice, some adverse reactions (and interactions) of certain drugs are listed, as a precaution, because these reactions are associated with the use of a particular class of drugs. Although the literature may not document such reactions in connection with the use of an individual drug within that class, the possibility of their occurrence must be considered.

A word of caution is appropriate here. You have consulted your physician for medical evaluation and management. He or she has advised you to take a drug (or administer it to someone else). It is important that you recognize and understand that *in the vast majority of instances a properly selected drug has a comparatively small chance of producing serious harm.* Most of the drugs included in this book produce serious adverse effects rarely. Knowledge that a drug is capable of causing a serious adverse reaction should not deter you from using it when it has been properly selected and its use will be carefully supervised.

Occasionally a dagger (†) will precede a serious adverse effect. It serves as a warning flag of an especially hazardous or frequent reaction.

CAUTION

This category provides information on certain aspects of drug action and/or drug use that require special emphasis. Occasionally these warnings may relate to information provided in other categories. When included here, such entries are of sufficient importance to warrant repetition.

PRECAUTIONS FOR USE BY INFANTS AND CHILDREN

In addition to mandatory adjustments of drug dosage for infants and children under twelve years of age, some drugs and/or treatment situations call for special precautions. This category provides such information for selected drugs. When administering *any* drug (whether prescription or over-the-counter drug), it is advisable to ask the attending physician about precautions to observe or procedures to follow.

PRECAUTIONS FOR USE BY THOSE OVER 60 YEARS OF AGE

Changes in body composition and function occur naturally as part of normal aging. As would be expected, there is enormous individual variation in the speed with which such changes occur and the degree of these changes. With regard to medical management—and to drug therapy in particular—the assessment of one's "age" must be based upon the individual's mental and physical condition and never upon years alone. In general, however, it should be recognized that changes that accompany aging may affect the actions of the body on the drug, as well as the actions of the drug on the body. Appropriate precautions are outlined in this category.

ADVISABILITY OF USE DURING PREGNANCY: PREGNANCY CATEGORY

Information regarding the safe use of a particular drug during pregnancy was one of the most forceful concerns that led to the formal petitioning of the Food and Drug Administration in 1975 for the provision of such guidance to the public. This section of each Profile is the first publication in either lay or professional literature that attempts to utilize the newly defined FDA Pregnancy Categories for a large number of drugs in common use. All category designations are labeled "tentative" at this time in recognition of the fact that data not readily available now may be advanced by pharmaceutical manufacturers as they negotiate with the FDA to eventually determine final category assignments. The FDA definitions of the five pregnancy categories are listed inside the back cover of the book. It should be noted that the FDA does not make the initial category assignment; this is the responsibility of the manufacturer that markets the drug. The initial designation is then subject to review and modification by the FDA as deemed appropriate. The Pregnancy Category designations presented in each Profile were determined by the author after thorough review of pertinent literature and consultation with appropriate authorities. They are offered at this time for initial guidance only. They are in no sense "official" and do not have the endorsement of either the manufacturer or the FDA.

SUGGESTED PERIODIC EXAMINATIONS WHILE TAKING THIS DRUG

This category lists those examinations your physician may recommend you undergo while taking the drug(s) he or she has prescribed, in order to monitor your reaction to them and the course of your condition. You should remember that the advisability of performing such examinations varies greatly from one situation to another, and is best left to the judgment of your physician. The selection and timing of examinations are based on many variables, including your past and present medical history, the nature of the condition under treatment, the dosage and anticipated duration of drug use, and your physician's observations of your response to treatment. There may be many occasions when he or she will feel no examinations are necessary.

To assure optimal results from drug treatment, it is important that you keep your physician informed of all developments you think may be drug-related.

WHILE TAKING THIS DRUG, OBSERVE THE FOLLOWING: MARIJUANA SMOKING

The widespread "social" use of marijuana by virtually all age groups has led to inquiries regarding the possibility of interactions between the pharmacologically active chemicals in marijuana smoke and medicinal drugs in common use. Currently available literature on the health aspects of marijuana use contains very little practical information concerning the potential for drug interactions. The information presented in this category of each Drug Profile represents those *possible interactions* that are considered likely to occur in view of the known pharmacological effects of the principal components of marijuana and of the medicinal drug reviewed in the Profile. In most instances, the interaction statements are not based on documented evidence since none is available. However, the conclusions stated—derived by logical inductive reasoning—represent the concurrence of authorities with expertise in this field.

WHILE TAKING THIS DRUG, OBSERVE THE FOLLOWING: OTHER DRUGS

For clarification of this confusing and often controversial area of drug information, this category is divided into five subcategories of possible interactions between drugs. Observe carefully the wording of each subcategory heading (see also Interaction in Glossary). Some of the drugs listed as possible interactants do not have a representative Profile in Section Two. If you are using one of these drugs, consult your physician for guidance regarding potential interactions. A brand name or names that follows the generic name of an interacting drug is given for purposes of illustration only. It is not intended to mean that the particular brand(s) named have interactions which are different from other brands of the same generic drug. If you are taking the generic drug, *all* brand names under which it is marketed are to be considered as possible interactants.

DRIVING A VEHICLE, OPERATING MACHINERY, ENGAGING IN HAZARDOUS ACTIVITIES

In addition to these specific activities, the information in this category applies to any activity of a dangerous nature such as working on ladders, using power tools, and handling weapons.

AVIATION NOTE

Until the publication of Dr. Stanley Mohler's *Medication and Flying: A Pilot's Drug Guide* in 1982, there was no authoritative source of current drug information written specifically to serve the needs of civil aviation. The military airman enjoys the expert guidance and surveillance provided by the flight surgeon, but no tightly structured control system exists for his civilian counterpart. However, the need for practical information regarding the possible effects of medicinal drugs on flight performance is the same for pilots in all settings. This category is designed to inform the civilian pilot how a particular drug may affect his or her eligibility to fly and when it is advisable or necessary to consult a designated Aviation Medical Examiner or an FAA medical officer.

OCCURRENCE OF UNRELATED ILLNESS

This category relates to those drugs which require careful regulation of daily doses to maintain a constant drug effect within critical limits. Anticoagulants, anti-diabetic medication, and digitalis are examples of such drugs. Emphasis is given to those interim illnesses, separate from the condition for which the drug has been prescribed, that might affect the established schedule of drug use.

DISCONTINUATION

This aspect of drug use is often overlooked when a plan of drug therapy is first discussed. However, for some drugs it is mandatory that the patient be fully informed on *when* to discontinue, when *not* to discontinue, and precisely *how* to discontinue use of the drug.

Another consideration in discontinuation is the need to adjust the dosage schedules of other drugs being taken concurrently. The physician who is primarily responsible for your overall management must be kept informed of *all* the drugs you are taking at a given time.

Other information categories in the Drug Profile are self-explanatory.

Section Three is a presentation of Drug Classes arranged alphabetically according to their chemical or therapeutic class designation. The drugs within each class are listed alphabetically by their brand and generic names. Because of their chemical composition and biological activities, some drugs will appear in two or more classes. For example, the drug product with the brand name Diuril will be represented by its generic name, chlorothiazide, in three drug classes: the Thiazide

Diuretics (a chemical classification), the Diuretics (a drug action classification), and the Anti-hypertensives (a disease-oriented classification).

Frequently in the Drug Profiles in Section Two you are advised to "See (a particular) Drug Class." This alerts you to a possible contraindication for drug use, or to possible interactions with certain foods, alcohol, or other drugs. In each case, you can determine the more readily recognized brand names for each drug listed generically within a drug class by consulting the appropriate Drug Profile. Timely use of these references will enable you to avoid many possible hazards of medication.

Section Four is a glossary of drug-related terms used throughout the book. Each term is explained, and in most instances an example is provided to illustrate the preferred use of the term. Frequent references to the glossary are made in the Drug Profiles. Use of the glossary will increase your understanding of how to recognize and interpret significant drug effects.

Section Five consists of tables of drug information. The title and introductory material explain the content and purpose of each table. The information in the tables is drawn from certain information categories in the Profiles and is rearranged to emphasize pertinent aspects of drug behavior. The tables are intended to provide another source of ready reference.

Section Six offers a method of recording personal histories of drug use for each member of the family. Model forms are provided for keeping records of drug intake during pregnancy, drug administration to the infant and child, and drug use by adults. In addition, there is a Medical Alert form suitable for carrying in your wallet or purse which can serve as an immediate source of information regarding (1) your current use of certain critical drugs and (2) the names of drugs to which you are allergic. Table 19 in Section Five lists the names of those drugs which should be entered on your personal identification card and carried with you at all times. This information can be of vital importance in the event of accident or serious illness, especially if you are unable to communicate with those providing you with medical care.

The index of Brand and Generic names in the back of the book is a single alphabetical listing that provides page references to the appropriate Drug Profile(s) for all drugs found in this book. Its usefulness will be enhanced if you read first the introductory explanation of the special features of this combined index.

SECTION TWO

DRUG PROFILES

NOTE

A dagger (†) that occasionally precedes an adverse effect, or an effect of extended use, signifies an especially hazardous or frequent reaction.

The designation [CD] following the brand names of any drugs in these Profiles indicates a combination drug (a drug product with more than one active ingredient).

ACETAMINOPHEN
(Paracetamol)

Year Introduced: 1893

Brand Names

USA

Datril (Bristol-Myers)
Panadol (Glenbrook)
Phenaphen (Robins)
SK-APAP (Smith
  Kline & French)
Tapar (Parke-Davis)
Tempra (Mead
  Johnson)
Tylenol (McNeil)
Valadol (Squibb)
Arthralgen [CD]
  (Robins)
CoTylenol [CD]
  (McNeil)
Darvocet-N [CD]
  (Lilly)
Excedrin [CD]
  (Bristol-Myers)

Parafon Forte [CD]
  (McNeil)
Percocet-5 [CD]
  (Endo)
Sinarest [CD]
  (Pharmacraft)
Sine-Off Extra
  Strength [CD]
  (Menley & James)
Sinutab [CD]
  (Warner/Chilcott)
(Numerous other
  brand and
  combination brand
  names)

Canada

Apo-Acetaminophen
  (Apotex)
Atasol (Horner)
Atasol Forte (Horner)
Campain (Winthrop)
Exdol (Frosst)
Robigesic (Robins)
Rounox (Rougier)
Tempra (Mead
  Johnson)
Tylenol (McNeil)
Parafon Forte [CD]
  (McNeil)
Percocet [CD] (Endo)
Percocet-Demi [CD]
  (Endo)
Sine-Aid [CD]
  (Johnson &
  Johnson)
Sinutab [CD] (P.D.)

Common Synonyms ("Street Names"):   None

Drug Class: Analgesic, Mild; Fever Reducer (Antipyretic)

Prescription Required: No (some combinations require prescription)

Available for Purchase by Generic Name: Yes

Available Dosage Forms and Strengths

Tablets — 80 mg., 120 mg., 300 mg., 325 mg., 500 mg., 650 mg.
Chewable tablets — 80 mg., 120 mg.
Capsules — 325 mg., 500 mg.
Elixir — 120 mg., 160 mg., 325 mg. per teaspoonful (5 ml.)
Drops — 100 mg. per ml., 120 mg. per 2.5 ml.
Suppositories — 120 mg., 125 mg., 130 mg., 300 mg., 325 mg., 600
  mg., 650 mg.
Syrup — 120 mg. per teaspoonful (5 ml.)
Liquid — 165 mg. per teaspoonful (5 ml.)

Tablet May Be Crushed or Capsule Opened for Administration: Yes

How This Drug Works
Intended Therapeutic Effect(s)
Relief of mild to moderate pain.
Reduction of high fever.

Location of Drug Action(s):   Principal actions occur in
- areas of injury, muscle spasm, or inflammation in many body tissues.
- the heat-regulating center, located in the hypothalamus of the brain.

Method of Drug Action(s):   Not fully established. It is thought that this drug relieves both pain and fever by reducing the tissue concentration of prostaglandins, chemicals involved in the production of pain, fever, and inflammation.

Principal Uses of This Drug
As a Single Drug Product: To relieve mild to moderate pain from any cause, and to reduce high fever. It is often used instead of aspirin for these purposes.

As a Combination Drug Product [CD]:   Often combined with other analgesics to enhance pain relief. Also combined with antihistamines and decongestants to relieve the discomfort associated with respiratory tract infections; and with muscle relaxants to augment the relief of discomfort associated with muscle spasm.

THIS DRUG SHOULD NOT BE TAKEN IF
—you have had an allergic reaction to any dosage form of it previously.

INFORM YOUR PHYSICIAN BEFORE TAKING THIS DRUG IF
—you have impaired liver or kidney function.

Time Required for Apparent Benefit
Drug action begins in 15 to 30 minutes and persists for 3 to 4 hours.

Possible Side-Effects *(natural, expected, and unavoidable drug actions)*
Drowsiness (in sensitive individuals).

Possible Adverse Effects *(unusual, unexpected, and infrequent reactions)*

IF ANY OF THE FOLLOWING DEVELOP, DISCONTINUE DRUG AND NOTIFY YOUR PHYSICIAN AS SOON AS POSSIBLE

Mild Adverse Effects
Allergic Reactions: Skin rash, hives (rare).
Other Reactions: Impaired thinking and concentration.

Serious Adverse Effects
Allergic Reactions
Swelling of the vocal cords, resulting in difficult breathing, anaphylactic reaction (see Glossary).
Hemolytic anemia (see Glossary).
Other Reactions
Abnormally low white blood cells.
Abnormal bruising or bleeding due to reduced blood platelets (see Glossary).

CAUTION
1. If you have bronchial asthma and you are also allergic to aspirin, use this drug with caution until your sensitivity to it has been determined.
2. If you are taking an oral anticoagulant drug (see Anticoagulant Drug Class, Section Three), acetaminophen may alter your response to it and increase the risk of abnormal bleeding. Ask physician for guidance.

Precautions for Use by Those over 60 Years of Age
Do not exceed a total dose of 2600 mg. in 24 hours. This drug may be eliminated more slowly than by younger adults.
Prolonged use in excessive doses can cause anemia, liver damage with jaundice, and kidney damage.

Advisability of Use During Pregnancy
Pregnancy Category: B (tentative). See Pregnancy Code inside back cover. Animal reproduction studies in mice reveal no birth defects due to this drug. Information from adequate studies in pregnant women is not available. Ask physician for guidance.

Advisability of Use While Nursing Infant
This drug is known to be present in milk. Ask physician for guidance.

Habit-Forming Potential
None.

Effects of Overdosage
With Moderate Overdose: Nausea, vomiting, abdominal pain, chills, drowsiness.
With Large Overdose: Nervous irritability followed by stupor and convulsions. Coma may develop due to damage to liver and kidney tissues. Jaundice may occur in 2 to 5 days.

Possible Effects of Extended Use
Formation of abnormal hemoglobin (methemoglobin).
Development of anemia.

Suggested Periodic Examinations While Taking This Drug (at physician's discretion)
None required for short-term use.
During long-term use, examination for abnormal hemoglobin (methemoglobin), anemia, and reduced white blood cells or platelets is advisable.

While Taking This Drug, Observe the Following
Foods: No restrictions.
Beverages: No restrictions.
Alcohol: No interactions expected.
Tobacco Smoking: No interactions expected.
Marijuana Smoking
Occasional (once or twice weekly): No effect to mild increase in pain relief effect of this drug.
Daily: Moderate increase in pain relief effect of this drug.

Other Drugs

Acetaminophen may *increase* the effects of
- oral anticoagulants. Use with caution and monitor prothrombin times until combined effect has been determined.

The following drug may *decrease* the effects of acetaminophen:
- phenobarbital may hasten its elimination from the body.

Driving a Vehicle, Operating Machinery, Engaging in Hazardous Activities: Usually no restrictions. Be alert to the rare occurrence of drowsiness and/or impaired thinking, and restrict activities accordingly.

Aviation Note: Usually no restrictions. However, it is advisable to observe for the possible occurrence of drowsiness or impaired thinking and to restrict activities accordingly.

Exposure to Sun: No restrictions.

Special Storage Instructions

Keep in a tightly closed container. Protect from light.

ACETAZOLAMIDE

Year Introduced: 1953

Brand Names

USA	Canada
Diamox (Lederle)	Acetazolam (ICN)
	Apo-Acetazolamide (Apotex)
	Diamox (Lederle)

Common Synonyms ("Street Names"):   Glaucoma pills

Drug Class: Anti-glaucoma, Diuretic, Sulfonamides

Prescription Required: Yes

Available for Purchase by Generic Name: USA: Yes   Canada: No

Available Dosage Forms and Strengths

Tablets — 125 mg., 250 mg.
Prolonged-action capsules — 500 mg.
Injection — 500 mg. per vial

Tablet May Be Crushed or Capsule Opened for Administration

Tablets — Yes
Prolonged-action capsules — No
Diamox Sequels — Yes, but do not crush or chew contents

How This Drug Works
Intended Therapeutic Effect(s)
Reduction of elevated internal eye pressure, of benefit in the management of glaucoma.

Reduction of excessive fluid retention (edema) in the body.

Location of Drug Action(s)
The ciliary processes of the eye, the source of fluid in the anterior chamber.

The tubular systems of the kidney that determine the final composition of the urine.

Method of Drug Action(s):   By inhibiting the action of the enzyme carbonic anhydrase, this drug
- decreases the formation of fluid (the aqueous humor) in the eye, thus lowering the internal eye pressure.
- increases the sodium content of the urine, resulting in an associated increase in the excretion of water (increased urine volume).

Principal Uses of This Drug
As a Single Drug Product: Primarily to treat certain types of glaucoma. It is also used concurrently with other anticonvulsant drugs in the management of the common types of epilepsy. Less frequent uses include the treatment of familial periodic paralysis, and the prevention of altitude sickness.

THIS DRUG SHOULD NOT BE TAKEN IF
—you have had an allergic reaction to any dosage form of it previously.

—you have serious liver or kidney disease.

—you have Addison's disease.

INFORM YOUR PHYSICIAN BEFORE TAKING THIS DRUG IF
—you have had an allergic reaction to any "sulfa" drug in the past.

—you have lupus erythematosus.

—you have gout.

Time Required for Apparent Benefit
Drug action begins in approximately 2 hours and persists for 8 to 12 hours. The maximal fall in internal eye pressure occurs in 4 hours and may persist for 12 to 24 hours.

Possible Side-Effects *(natural, expected, and unavoidable drug actions)*
Drowsiness, temporary nearsightedness.

Possible Adverse Effects *(unusual, unexpected, and infrequent reactions)*

IF ANY OF THE FOLLOWING DEVELOP, DISCONTINUE DRUG AND NOTIFY YOUR PHYSICIAN AS SOON AS POSSIBLE

Mild Adverse Effects
Allergic Reactions: Skin rash, hives, drug fever.

Other Reactions
Reduced appetite, indigestion, nausea.

Fatigue, weakness, tingling of face, arms, or legs, dizziness.

Serious Adverse Effects
Allergic Reactions
Hemolytic anemia (see Glossary), spontaneous bruising (not due to injury).
Other Reactions
Bone marrow depression (see Glossary)—fatigue, weakness, fever, sore throat, abnormal bleeding or bruising.
Hepatitis with jaundice (see Glossary)—yellow eyes and skin, dark-colored urine, light-colored stools.

Precautions for Use by Those over 60 Years of Age
Do not exceed recommended doses. Increased dosage can cause excessive excretion of sodium and potassium with resultant loss of appetite, nausea, fatigue, weakness, confusion, and tingling in the extremities.
If you are also taking a digitalis preparation (digitoxin, digoxin), ensure an adequate intake of high-potassium foods to prevent potassium deficiency —a potential cause of digitalis toxicity.

Advisability of Use During Pregnancy
Pregnancy Category: C (tentative). See Pregnancy Code inside back cover. Animal reproduction studies reveal significant birth defects due to this drug. Information from adequate studies in pregnant women is not available. Avoid completely during first 3 months.
Ask physician for guidance.

Advisability of Use While Nursing Infant
Safety not established for infant. Avoid use or avoid nursing. Ask physician for guidance.

Habit-Forming Potential
None.

Effects of Overdosage
With Moderate Overdose: Drowsiness, numbness and tingling, thirst, nausea, vomiting.
With Large Overdose: Confusion, excitement, convulsions, coma.

Possible Effects of Extended Use
Formation of kidney stones.

Suggested Periodic Examinations While Taking This Drug (at physician's discretion)
Complete blood cell counts.
Measurements of blood sodium and potassium levels.
Liver function tests.

While Taking This Drug, Observe the Following
Foods: It is recommended that you include in your daily diet liberal servings of foods rich in potassium (unless directed otherwise by your physician). The following foods have a high potassium content:

All-bran cereals	Fish, fresh
Almonds	Lentils
Apricots (dried)	Liver, beef
Bananas, fresh	Lonalac
Beans (navy and lima)	Milk
Beef	Peaches (dried)
Carrots (raw)	Peanut butter
Chicken	Peas
Citrus fruits, juices	Pork
Coconut	Potato, sweet
Coffee	Prunes (dried), juice
Crackers (rye)	Raisins
Dates and figs (dried)	Tomato Juice

Beverages: No restrictions.

Alcohol: No interactions expected.

Tobacco Smoking: No interactions expected.

Marijuana Smoking

Occasional (once or twice weekly): No effect to mild and transient additional decrease in internal eye pressure.

Daily: Sustained additional decrease in internal eye pressure.

Other Drugs

Acetazolamide may *increase* the effects of

- amphetamines and related drugs, by delaying their elimination from the body.
- tricyclic antidepressants, by delaying their elimination from the body.

Acetazolamide may *decrease* the effects of

- aspirin, by hastening its elimination from the body.
- lithium, by hastening its elimination from the body. Consult physician regarding dosage adjustment.

Driving a Vehicle, Operating Machinery, Engaging in Hazardous Activities: Usually no restrictions. Be alert to the possible occurrence of drowsiness or dizziness.

Aviation Note: The use of this drug *may be a disqualification* for the piloting of aircraft. Consultation with a designated Aviation Medical Examiner is advised.

Exposure to Sun: No restrictions.

Special Storage Instructions

Keep in a dry, tightly closed container.

ACETOHEXAMIDE

Year Introduced: 1963

Brand Names

USA	Canada
Dymelor (Lilly)	Dimelor (Lilly)

Common Synonyms ("Street Names"):   Diabetes pills

Drug Class: Anti-diabetic, Oral (Hypoglycemic), Sulfonylureas

Prescription Required: Yes

Available for Purchase by Generic Name: No

Available Dosage Forms and Strengths
  Tablets — 250 mg., 500 mg.

Tablet May Be Crushed or Capsule Opened for Administration: Yes

How This Drug Works
  Intended Therapeutic Effect(s):   The correction of insulin deficiency in adult (maturity-onset) diabetes of moderate severity.
  Location of Drug Action(s):   The insulin-producing tissues of the pancreas.
  Method of Drug Action(s):   It is well established that sulfonylurea drugs stimulate the secretion of insulin (by a pancreas capable of responding to stimulation). Therapeutic doses may increase the amount of available insulin.

Principal Uses of This Drug
  As a Single Drug Product: To assist in the control of mild to moderately severe diabetes mellitus of the adult (maturity-onset) type that does not require insulin, but that cannot be adequately controlled by diet alone.

THIS DRUG SHOULD NOT BE TAKEN IF
—you have had an allergic reaction to any dosage form of it previously.
—you have a history of impaired liver function or kidney function.

INFORM YOUR PHYSICIAN BEFORE TAKING THIS DRUG IF
—your diabetes has been difficult to control in the past ("brittle type").
—you have a history of peptic ulcer of the stomach or duodenum.
—you have a history of porphyria.
—you do not know how to recognize or treat hypoglycemia (see Glossary).

Time Required for Apparent Benefit:
  A single dose may lower the blood sugar within 2 to 4 hours. Regular use for 1 to 2 weeks may be needed to determine this drug's effectiveness in controlling your diabetes.

Possible Side-Effects (*natural, expected, and unavoidable drug actions*)
  Usually none. If drug dosage is excessive or food intake is inadequate, abnormally low blood sugar (hypoglycemia) will occur as a predictable drug effect (see hypoglycemia in Glossary).

Possible Adverse Effects *(unusual, unexpected, and infrequent reactions)*

IF ANY OF THE FOLLOWING DEVELOP, DISCONTINUE DRUG AND NOTIFY YOUR PHYSICIAN AS SOON AS POSSIBLE

Mild Adverse Effects
Allergic Reactions: Skin rashes (various kinds), hives, itching, drug fever.
Other Reactions
Headache, ringing in ears.
Indigestion, heartburn, nausea, diarrhea.

Serious Adverse Effects
Allergic Reactions: Hepatitis with jaundice (see Glossary).
Idiosyncratic Reactions: Hemolytic anemia in susceptible individuals (see Glossary).
Other Reactions: Bone marrow depression (see Glossary)—fatigue, weakness, fever, sore throat, unusual bleeding or bruising.

CAUTION
1. This drug must be looked upon as only one part of the total program for the management of your diabetes. It is not a substitute for a properly prescribed diet.
2. Over a period of time (usually several months), this drug may lose its effectiveness in controlling blood sugar levels. Periodic follow-up examinations are necessary to monitor all aspects of response to drug treatment.
3. Individual response to this drug varies widely. The effects of overdosage—hypoglycemia—can occur in sensitive individuals taking doses well within the recommended range.
4. Do not begin treatment with a large or "loading" dose. This is unnecessary and can be dangerous.
5. The total daily dose should not exceed 1500 mg.

Precautions for Use by Those over 60 Years of Age
The natural decline in kidney function that occurs after 60 years of age, together with the duration of this drug's action, require that both initial and maintenance dosage be less than those normally used in the younger adult. Do not exceed a total dosage of 1500 mg. per 24 hours.
The aging brain adapts well to the higher blood sugar levels associated with diabetes. Attempts to achieve "normal" blood sugar levels can result in unrecognized hypoglycemia that is manifested by confusion and abnormal behavior. Repeated episodes of hypoglycemia in the elderly can cause brain damage.

Advisability of Use During Pregnancy
Pregnancy Category: B (tentative). See Pregnancy Code inside back cover.
Animal reproduction studies reveal no birth defects due to this drug.
Information from adequate studies in pregnant women is not available.
Use during pregnancy is not recommended by manufacturer.

Advisability of Use While Nursing Infant
Drug is known to be present in milk. Ask physician for guidance.

Habit-Forming Potential
None.

Effects of Overdosage

With Moderate Overdose: Symptoms of mild to moderate hypoglycemia: headache, lightheadedness, faintness, nervousness, confusion, tremor, sweating, heart palpitation, weakness, and hunger.

With Large Overdose: Hypoglycemic coma (see Glossary).

Possible Effects of Extended Use

Reduced function of the thyroid gland (hypothyroidism) resulting in lowered metabolism.

Reports of increased frequency and severity of heart and blood vessel diseases associated with long-term use of the members of this drug family are highly controversial and inconclusive. A direct cause-and-effect relationship (see Glossary) has not been established to date. Ask your physician for guidance regarding extended use.

Suggested Periodic Examinations While Taking This Drug (at physician's discretion)

Complete blood cell counts.
Liver function tests.
Thyroid function tests.
Periodic evaluation of heart and circulatory system.

While Taking This Drug, Observe the Following

Foods: Follow the diabetic diet prescribed by your physician.

Beverages: As directed in the diabetic diet prescribed by your physician.

Alcohol: Use with extreme caution until the combined effect has been determined. This drug can cause a marked intolerance to alcohol resulting in a disulfiram-like reaction (see Glossary).

Tobacco Smoking: No restrictions unless imposed as part of your overall treatment program. Ask physician for guidance.

Marijuana Smoking

Occasional (once or twice weekly): No significant interactions expected.
Daily: Possible increase in blood sugar.

Other Drugs

Acetohexamide may *increase* the effects of

- sedatives and sleep-inducing drugs, by slowing their elimination from the body.
- "sulfa" drugs, by slowing their elimination from the body.

Acetohexamide *taken concurrently* with

- oral anticoagulants, may cause unpredictable changes in anticoagulant drug actions. Ask physician for guidance regarding prothrombin blood tests and dosage adjustment.
- propranolol (Inderal), may allow hypoglycemia to develop without adequate warning. Follow diet and dosage schedules very carefully.

The following drugs may *increase* the effects of acetohexamide:

- bishydroxycoumarin (Dicumarol, Dufalone)
- chloramphenicol (Chlormomycetin, etc.)

- clofibrate (Atromid-S)
- mono-amine oxidase (MAO) inhibitors (see Drug Class, Section Three)
- oxyphenbutazone (Oxalid, Tandearil)
- phenformin (DBI)
- phenylbutazone (Azolid, Butazolidin, etc.)
- phenyramidol (Analexin)
- probenecid (Benemid)
- propranolol (Inderal)
- salicylates (aspirin, sodium salicylate)
- sulfaphenazole (Orisul, Sulfabid)
- sulfisoxazole (Gantrisin, Novosoxazole, etc.)

The following drugs may *decrease* the effects of acetohexamide:
- chlorpromazine (Thorazine, Largactil, etc.)
- cortisone and related drugs (see Drug Class, Section Three)
- estrogens (Premarin, Menotrol, Ogen, etc.)
- isoniazid (INH, Isozide, etc.)
- nicotinic acid (niacin, etc.)
- oral contraceptives (see Drug Profile)
- pyrazinamide (Aldinamide)
- thiazide diuretics (see Drug Class, Section Three)

Driving a Vehicle, Operating Machinery, Engaging in Hazardous Activities: Regulate your dosage schedule, eating schedule, and physical activities very carefully to prevent hypoglycemia. Be able to recognize the early symptoms of hypoglycemia and avoid hazardous activities if you suspect that hypoglycemia is developing.

Aviation Note: Diabetes *is a disqualification* for the piloting of aircraft. Consultation with a designated Aviation Medical Examiner is advised.

Exposure to Sun: Use caution until sensitivity has been determined. This drug can cause photosensitivity (see Glossary).

Heavy Exercise or Exertion: Use caution. Excessive exercise may result in hypoglycemia.

Occurrence of Unrelated Illness: Acute infections, illnesses causing vomiting or diarrhea, serious injuries, and the need for surgery can interfere with diabetic control and may require a change in medication. If any of these conditions occur, ask your physician for guidance regarding the continued use of this drug.

Discontinuation: If you find it necessary to discontinue this drug for any reason, notify your physician and ask for guidance regarding necessary changes in your treatment program for diabetic control.

Special Storage Instructions
Keep in a dry, tightly closed container.

ALLOPURINOL

Year Introduced: 1963

Brand Names

USA	Canada
Zyloprim (Burroughs Wellcome)	Alloprin (ICN)
	Apo-Allopurinol (Apotex)
	Novopurol (Novopharm)
	Purinol (Horner)
	Roucol (Rougier)
	Zyloprim (B.W. Ltd.)

Common Synonyms ("Street Names"):   Gout pills

Drug Class: Anti-gout

Prescription Required: Yes

Available for Purchase by Generic Name: USA: Yes   Canada: No

Available Dosage Forms and Strengths
Tablets — 100 mg., 300 mg.

Tablet May Be Crushed or Capsule Opened for Administration: Yes

How This Drug Works
Intended Therapeutic Effect(s): Prevention of acute episodes of gout through maintenance of normal uric acid blood levels.

Location of Drug Action(s): Tissues throughout the body in which sufficient concentration of the drug can be achieved to reduce the production of uric acid.

Method of Drug Action(s): By inhibiting the action of the tissue enzyme xanthine oxidase, this drug decreases the conversion of purines (protein nutrients) to uric acid.

Principal Uses of This Drug
As a Single Drug Product: Used primarily in the long-term management of gout to *prevent* episodes of acute gout. (It does not relieve the symptoms of acute gout attacks.) Also used to prevent abnormally high blood levels of uric acid in individuals who have recurrent uric acid kidney stones, and in those receiving chemotherapy or radiation therapy for cancer.

THIS DRUG SHOULD NOT BE TAKEN IF
—you have had an allergic reaction to any dosage form of it previously.
—you are experiencing an attack of acute gout at the present time.

INFORM YOUR PHYSICIAN BEFORE TAKING THIS DRUG IF
—you have a history of liver or kidney disease, or impaired function of the liver or kidneys.

Time Required for Apparent Benefit
Blood uric acid levels usually begin to decrease in 48 to 72 hours and reach a normal range in 1 to 3 weeks. However, regular use for several months may be necessary to prevent attacks of acute gout.

Possible Side-Effects *(natural, expected, and unavoidable drug actions)*
An increase in the frequency and severity of episodes of acute gout may occur during the first several weeks of drug use. Consult physician regarding use of colchicine during this period.

Possible Adverse Effects *(unusual, unexpected, and infrequent reactions)*

IF ANY OF THE FOLLOWING DEVELOP, DISCONTINUE DRUG AND NOTIFY YOUR PHYSICIAN AS SOON AS POSSIBLE

Mild Adverse Effects
Allergic Reactions: Skin rash (various kinds), hives, itching, drug fever.
Other Reactions
Nausea, vomiting, diarrhea, abdominal cramping.
Drowsiness, headache, dizziness.
Loss of scalp hair.

Serious Adverse Effects
Allergic Reactions: Severe skin reactions, high fever, chills, joint pains, swollen glands, kidney damage.
Other Reactions
Hepatitis with or without jaundice (see Glossary)—yellow coloration of eyes and skin, dark-colored urine, light-colored stools.
Bone marrow depression (see Glossary).

Precautions for Use by Those over 60 Years of Age
The natural decline in kidney function that occurs after 60 may make it necessary to use smaller initial and maintenance doses. Do not exceed a total dose of 800 mg. per 24 hours.

Advisability of Use During Pregnancy
Pregnancy Category: C (tentative). See Pregnancy Code inside back cover.
Animal reproduction studies reveal significant birth defects due to this drug.
Information from adequate studies in pregnant women is not available.
Avoid completely during first 3 months.
Ask physician for guidance.

Advisability of Use While Nursing Infant
Safety for infant not established. Avoid use.

Habit-Forming Potential
None.

Effects of Overdosage
With Moderate Overdose: No significant symptoms reported in non-sensitive individuals. Nausea, vomiting, or diarrhea may occur as a result of individual sensitivity.

With Large Overdose: No serious toxic effects known and none anticipated in the presence of normal kidney function.

Possible Effects of Extended Use
No serious effects reported.

Suggested Periodic Examinations While Taking This Drug (at physician's discretion)
Liver and kidney function tests.
Complete blood cell counts.
Complete examination of the eyes for the development of cataract. (A cause-and-effect relationship [see Glossary] between this drug and the development of cataracts has not been established.)

While Taking This Drug, Observe the Following
Foods: Follow physician's advice regarding the need for a low purine diet. Drug may be taken after eating to reduce stomach irritation or nausea.

Beverages: A large intake of coffee, tea, or cola beverages may reduce the effectiveness of treatment. It is advisable to drink no less than 5 to 6 pints of liquid every 24 hours.

Alcohol: No interactions expected with this drug, but alcohol may impair successful management of gout.

Tobacco Smoking: No interactions expected.

Marijuana Smoking
Occasional (once or twice weekly):   No significant interactions expected.
Daily: Possible increase in blood uric acid level.

Other Drugs
Allopurinol may *increase* the effects of
- azathioprine (Imuran) and mercaptopurine (Purinethol), making it necessary to reduce their dosages to one-third or one-quarter the usual amount.
- oral anticoagulants (see Drug Class, Section Three), in some individuals. Ask physician for guidance regarding prothrombin time testing and dosage adjustment to prevent abnormal bleeding.
- theophylline (aminophylline, Elixophyllin, etc.), and prolong its action.

Allopurinol *taken concurrently* with
- iron preparations, may cause excessive accumulation of iron in body tissues. Avoid iron while taking this drug unless advised otherwise by your physician.

The following drugs may *increase* the effects of allopurinol
- acetohexamide (Dymelor) may increase its effectiveness in eliminating uric acid.
- probenecid (Benemid) adds to the elimination of uric acid.

The following drugs may *decrease* the effects of allopurinol
- thiazide diuretics (see Drug Class, Section Three) may reduce its effectiveness in controlling gout.
- ethacrynic acid (Edecrin) may reduce its effectiveness in controlling gout.

Driving a Vehicle, Operating Machinery, Engaging in Hazardous Activities:
Drowsiness may occur in some individuals. Determine sensitivity before
engaging in hazardous activities.

Aviation Note: The use of this drug *may be a disqualification* for the
piloting of aircraft. Consultation with a designated Aviation Medical Examiner is advised.

Exposure to Sun: No restrictions.

Special Storage Instructions
Keep in a dry, tightly closed container.

AMITRIPTYLINE

Year Introduced: 1961

Brand Names

USA	Canada
Amitril (Warner/Chilcott)	Apo-Amitriptyline
Elavil (Merck Sharp &	(Apotex)
Dohme)	Elavil (MSD)
Endep (Roche)	Levate (ICN)
Etrafon [CD] (Schering)	Meravil (Medic)
Limbitrol [CD] (Roche)	Novotriptyn (Novopharm)
Triavil [CD] (Merck	Etrafon [CD] (Schering)
Sharp & Dohme)	Triavil [CD] (MSD)

Common Synonyms ("Street Names"):   None

Drug Class: Antidepressant, Tricyclic

Prescription Required: Yes

Available for Purchase by Generic Name: Yes

Available Dosage Forms and Strengths
Tablets — 10 mg., 25 mg., 50 mg., 75 mg., 100 mg., 150 mg.
Injection — 10 mg. per ml.

Tablet May Be Crushed or Capsule Opened for Administration: Yes

How This Drug Works
Intended Therapeutic Effect(s): Gradual improvement of mood and relief
of emotional depression.

Location of Drug Action(s): Those areas of the brain that determine mood
and emotional stability.

Method of Drug Action(s): Not established. Present thinking is that this
drug slowly restores to normal levels certain constituents of brain tissue
(such as norepinephrine) that transmit nerve impulses.

Principal Uses of This Drug

As a Single Drug Product: To relieve the symptoms associated with spontaneous (endogenous) depression, and to initiate the restoration of normal mood. This drug should be used only when a diagnosis of a true, primary depression of significant degree has been established. It should not be used to treat the symptoms of mild and transient (reactive) depression that may be associated with many life situations in the absence of a bona fide affective illness.

As a Combination Drug Product [CD]:   This drug is available in combination with chlordiazepoxide, a mild tranquilizer of the benzodiazepine class. This combination is designed to relieve anxiety that may accompany depression. This drug is also available in combination with perphenazine, a strong tranquilizer of the phenothiazine class. This combination is effective in relieving severe agitation that may accompany depression.

THIS DRUG SHOULD NOT BE TAKEN IF

—you are allergic to any of the drugs bearing the brand names listed above.

—you are taking or have taken within the past 14 days any mono-amine oxidase (MAO) inhibitor drug (see Drug Class, Section Three).

—you are recovering from a recent heart attack.

—you have glaucoma (narrow-angle type).

—it is prescribed for a child under 12 years of age.

INFORM YOUR PHYSICIAN BEFORE TAKING THIS DRUG IF

—you are allergic or sensitive to any other tricyclic antidepressant (see Drug Class, Section Three).

—you have a history of any of the following: diabetes, epilepsy, glaucoma, heart disease, prostate gland enlargement, or overactive thyroid function.

—you plan to have surgery under general anesthesia in the near future.

Time Required for Apparent Benefit

Some benefit may be apparent within 1 to 2 weeks. Adequate response may require continuous treatment for 4 to 6 weeks or longer.

Possible Side-Effects *(natural, expected, and unavoidable drug actions)*

Drowsiness, blurring of vision, dryness of mouth, constipation, impaired urination.

Possible Adverse Effects *(unusual, unexpected, and infrequent reactions)*

IF ANY OF THE FOLLOWING DEVELOP, DISCONTINUE DRUG AND NOTIFY YOUR PHYSICIAN AS SOON AS POSSIBLE

Mild Adverse Effects

Allergic Reactions: Skin rash, hives, swelling of face or tongue, drug fever (see Glossary).

Other Reactions

Nausea, indigestion, irritation of tongue or mouth, peculiar taste.

Headache, dizziness, weakness, fainting, unsteady gait, tremors.

Swelling of testicles, breast enlargement, milk formation.

Fluctuation of blood sugar levels.

Serious Adverse Effects
    Allergic Reactions: Hepatitis with jaundice (see Glossary).
    Other Reactions
        Confusion (especially in the elderly over 60 years of age), hallucinations,
            agitation, restlessness, nightmares.
        Heart palpitation and irregular rhythm.
        Bone marrow depression (see Glossary)—fatigue, weakness, fever, sore
            throat, unusual bleeding or bruising.
        Peripheral neuritis (see Glossary)—numbness, tingling, pain, loss of
            strength in arms and legs.
        Parkinson-like disorders (see Glossary)—usually mild and infrequent;
            more likely to occur in the elderly.

Precautions for Use by Those over 60 Years of Age
    During the first 2 weeks of treatment observe for the development of confu-
        sional reactions—restlessness, agitation, forgetfulness, disorientation, delu-
        sions and hallucinations. Reduction of dosage or discontinuation may be
        necessary.
    Observe for incoordination and instability in stance and gait which may
        predispose to falling and injury.
    This drug can increase the degree of impaired urination associated with
        prostate gland enlargement (prostatism).

Advisability of Use During Pregnancy
    Pregnancy Category: C (tentative). See Pregnancy Code inside back cover.
        Animal reproduction studies reveal significant birth defects due to this
        drug.
        Information from adequate studies in pregnant women is not available.
        Avoid completely during first 3 months.
        Ask physician for guidance.

Advisability of Use While Nursing Infant
    This drug may be present in milk in small quantities. Ask physician for
    guidance.

Habit-Forming Potential
    Psychological or physical dependence is rare and unexpected.

Effects of Overdosage
    With Moderate Overdose: Confusion, hallucinations, extreme drowsiness,
        drop in body temperature, heart palpitation, dilated pupils, tremors.
    With Large Overdose: Stupor, deep sleep, coma, convulsions.

Possible Effects of Extended Use
    None reported.

Suggested Periodic Examinations While Taking This Drug (at physician's discretion)
    Complete blood cell counts.
    Liver function tests.
    Serial blood pressure readings and electrocardiograms.

While Taking This Drug, Observe the Following

Foods: No restrictions.

Beverages: No restrictions.

Alcohol: Avoid completely. This drug can increase markedly the intoxicating effects of alcohol and accentuate its depressant action on brain function.

Tobacco Smoking: No interactions expected.

Marijuana Smoking

Occasional (once or twice weekly):   Transient increase in drowsiness and dryness of mouth.

Daily: Persistent drowsiness, increased dryness of mouth; possible reduced effectiveness of this drug.

Other Drugs

Amitriptyline may *increase* the effects of

- amphetamine-like drugs (see Drug Class, Section Three).
- atropine-like drugs (see Drug Class, Section Three).
- levodopa (Dopar, Larodopa, etc.), in its control of Parkinson's disease.
- oral anticoagulants of the coumarin family (see Drug Family, Section Three).
- sedatives, sleep-inducing drugs, tranquilizers, anthihistamines, and narcotic drugs, and cause oversedation. Dosage adjustments may be necessary.

Amitriptyline may *decrease* the effects of

- clonidine (Catapres).
- guanethidine (Ismelin).
- other commonly used anti-hypertensive drugs. Ask physician for guidance regarding the need to monitor blood pressure readings and to adjust dosage of anti-hypertensive medications. (The action of methyldopa [Aldomet] is not decreased by amitriptyline or other tricyclic antidepressants.)
- phenytoin (Dantoin, Dilantin, etc.).

Amitriptyline *taken concurrently* with

- ethchlorvynol (Placidyl), may cause delirium.
- mono-amine oxidase (MAO) inhibitor drugs, may cause high fever, delirium, and convulsions (see Drug Class, Section Three).
- quinidine, may impair heart rhythm and function. Avoid the concurrent use of these two drugs.
- thyroid preparations, may impair heart rhythm and function. Ask physician for guidance regarding thyroid dosage adjustment.

The following drugs may *increase* the effects of amitriptyline

- thiazide diuretics (see Drug Class, Section Three) may slow its elimination from the body. Overdosage may occur.

Driving a Vehicle, Operating Machinery, Engaging in Hazardous Activities: This drug may impair mental alertness, judgment, physical coordination, and reaction time. Avoid hazardous activities.

Aviation Note: The use of this drug *is a disqualification* for the piloting of aircraft. Consultation with a designated Aviation Medical Examiner is advised.

Exposure to Sun: Use caution until sensitivity to sun has been determined. This drug may cause photosensitivity (see Glossary).

Discontinuation: If it has been necessary to use this drug for an extended period of time, do not discontinue it abruptly. Ask physician for guidance regarding dosage reduction and withdrawal. It may be necessary to adjust the dosage of other drugs taken concurrently with amitriptyline.

Special Storage Instructions
Keep in a dry, tightly closed container.

AMOBARBITAL

Year Introduced: 1925

Brand Names

USA	Canada
Amytal (Lilly)	Amytal (Lilly)
Tuinal [CD] (Lilly)	Isobec (Pharbec)
(Numerous other	Novamobarb
combination brand	(Novopharm)
names)	Tuinal [CD] Lilly

Common Synonyms ("Street Names"):   Barbs, blue angels, bluebirds, blue devils, blue heaven, blues, candy, downers, goofballs, peanuts, sleepers, stoppers, stumblers; for Tuinal, a brand of amobarbital with secobarbital: Christmas trees, double trouble, jelly beans, rainbows, tooies, tuies; for Dexamyl, a brand of amobarbital with dextroamphetamine: purple hearts

Drug Class: Sedative, Mild, Sleep Inducer (Hypnotic), Barbiturates

Prescription Required: Yes (Controlled Drug, U.S. Schedule II)*

Available for Purchase by Generic Name: Yes

Available Dosage Forms and Strengths
Tablets — 15 mg., 30 mg., 50 mg., 60 mg., 100 mg.
Capsules — 65 mg., 200 mg.
Elixir — 44 mg. per teaspoonful (5 ml.) (Alcohol 34%)
Injection — 250 mg., 500 mg. per vial

Tablet May Be Crushed or Capsule Opened for Administration: Yes

*See Schedules of Controlled Drugs inside back cover.

How This Drug Works
Intended Therapeutic Effect(s)
With low dosage, relief of mild to moderate anxiety or tension (sedative effect).

With higher dosage taken at bedtime, sedation sufficient to induce sleep (hypnotic effect).

Location of Drug Action(s):   The connecting points (synapses) in the nerve pathways that transmit impulses between the wake-sleep centers of the brain.

Method of Drug Action(s):   Not completely established. Present thinking is that this drug selectively blocks the transmission of nerve impulses by reducing the amount of available norepinephrine, one of the chemicals responsible for impulse transmission.

Principal Uses of This Drug
As a Single Drug Product: Primarily to relieve anxiety and nervous tension (daytime sedative), and to prevent insomnia (bedtime hypnotic).

As a Combination Drug Product [CD]:   May be combined with another sedative of the same class to provide a more rapid onset of sleep and a longer duration of sleep.

THIS DRUG SHOULD NOT BE TAKEN IF
—you have had an allergic reaction to any dosage form of it previously.
—you have a history of porphyria.

INFORM YOUR PHYSICIAN BEFORE TAKING THIS DRUG IF
—you are allergic or sensitive to any barbiturate drug.
—you are taking sedatives, sleep-inducing drugs, tranquilizers, antihistamines, pain relievers, or narcotic drugs of any kind.
—you have epilepsy.
—you have a history of liver or kidney disease.
—you plan to have surgery under general anesthesia in the near future.

Time Required for Apparent Benefit
Approximately 1 hour.

Possible Side-Effects *(natural, expected, and unavoidable drug actions)*
Drowsiness, lethargy, and sense of mental and physical sluggishness as "hangover" effect.

Possible Adverse Effects *(unusual, unexpected, and infrequent reactions)*
IF ANY OF THE FOLLOWING DEVELOP, DISCONTINUE DRUG AND NOTIFY YOUR PHYSICIAN AS SOON AS POSSIBLE
Mild Adverse Effects
Allergic Reactions: Skin rash (various kinds), hives, localized swelling of eyelids, face, or lips, drug fever.

Other Reactions
"Hangover" effect, dizziness, unsteadiness.

Nausea, vomiting, diarrhea.

Joint and muscle pains, most often in the neck, shoulders, and arms.

Serious Adverse Effects
  Allergic Reactions
    Hepatitis with jaundice (see Glossary).
    Severe skin reactions.
  Idiosyncratic Reactions: Paradoxical excitement and delirium (rather than sedation).
  Other Reactions
    Anemia—weakness and fatigue.
    Abnormally low blood platelets (see Glossary)—unusual bleeding or bruising.

Precautions for Use by Those over 60 Years of Age
  Small doses are advisable until tolerance has been determined. The elderly or debilitated may experience agitation, excitement, confusion, and delirium with standard doses (paradoxical reaction).
  This drug may also cause excessive lowering of body temperature (hypothermia). Keep dosage to a minimum during winter, and dress warmly.
  The natural decline in liver function that may occur after 60 can slow the elimination of this drug. Longer intervals between doses may be necessary to avoid overdosage and toxicity.
  Note: A barbiturate is not the drug of choice as a sedative or sleep inducer in this age group.

Advisability of Use During Pregnancy
  Pregnancy Category: B (tentative). See Pregnancy Code inside back cover.
  Animal reproduction studies reveal no birth defects due to this drug.
  Information from adequate studies in pregnant women is not available.
  Avoid completely during first 3 months.
  Ask physician for guidance.

Advisability of Use While Nursing Infant
  Drug is known to be present in milk. Avoid use if possible. Ask physician for guidance.

Habit-Forming Potential
  This drug can cause both psychological and physical dependence (see Glossary).

Effects of Overdosage
  With Moderate Overdose: Behavior similar to alcoholic intoxication: confusion, slurred speech, physical incoordination, staggering gait, drowsiness.
  With Large Overdose: Deepening sleep, coma, slow and shallow breathing, weak and rapid pulse, cold and sweaty skin.

Possible Effects of Extended Use
  Psychological and/or physical dependence.
  Anemia.
  If dose is excessive, a form of chronic intoxication can occur—headache, impaired vision, slurred speech, and depression.

Suggested Periodic Examinations While Taking This Drug (at physician's discretion)
Complete blood cell counts.
Liver function tests.

While Taking This Drug, Observe the Following
Foods: No restrictions.

Beverages: No restrictions.

Alcohol: Avoid completely. Alcohol can increase greatly the sedative and depressant actions of this drug on brain function.

Tobacco Smoking: No interactions expected.

Marijuana Smoking
Occasional (once or twice weekly):   Mild increase in sedative effect of this drug.

Daily: Marked increase in sedative effect of this drug.

Other Drugs
Amobarbital may *increase* the effects of
- other sedatives, sleep-inducing drugs, tranquilizers, antihistamines, pain relievers, and narcotic drugs, and cause oversedation. Ask your physician for guidance regarding dosage adjustments.

Amobarbital may *decrease* the effects of
- oral anticoagulants of the coumarin family (see Drug Class, Section Three). Ask physician for guidance regarding prothrombin time testing and adjustment of the anticoagulant dosage.
- aspirin, and reduce its pain-relieving action.
- cortisone and related drugs, by hastening their elimination from the body.
- oral contraceptives, by hastening their elimination from the body.
- griseofulvin (Fulvicin, Grisactin, etc.), and reduce its effectiveness in treating fungus infections.
- phenylbutazone (Azolid, Butazolidin, etc.), and reduce its effectiveness in treating inflammation and pain.

Amobarbital *taken concurrently* with
- anti-convulsants, may cause a change in the pattern of epileptic seizures. Careful dosage adjustments are necessary to achieve a balance of actions that will give the best protection from seizures.

The following drugs may *increase* the effects of amobarbital:
- both mild and strong tranquilizers may increase the sedative and sleep-inducing actions and cause oversedation.
- isoniazid (INH, Isozide, etc.) may prolong the action of barbiturate drugs.
- antihistamines may increase the sedative effects of barbiturate drugs.
- oral anti-diabetic drugs of the sulfonylurea type may prolong the sedative effect of barbiturate drugs.

Driving a Vehicle, Operating Machinery, Engaging in Hazardous Activities:
This drug can produce drowsiness and can impair mental alertness, judgment, physical coordination, and reaction time. Avoid hazardous activities.

Aviation Note: The use of this drug *is a disqualification* for the piloting of aircraft. Consultation with a designated Aviation Medical Examiner is advised.

Exposure to Sun: Use caution until sensitivity has been determined. Some barbiturates can cause photosensitivity (see Glossary).

Exposure to Heat: No restrictions.

Exposure to Cold: The elderly (over 60 years of age) may experience excessive lowering of body temperature while taking this drug. Keep dosage to a minimum during winter and dress warmly.

Heavy Exercise or Exertion: No restrictions.

Discontinuation: If it has been necessary to use this drug for an extended period of time, do not discontinue it abruptly. Ask physician for guidance regarding dosage adjustment and withdrawal. It may also be necessary to adjust the doses of other drugs taken concurrently with it.

Special Storage Instructions

Keep tablets and capsules in a dry, tightly closed container. Keep the elixir in a tightly closed, amber glass bottle.

AMOXAPINE

Year Introduced: 1970

Brand Names

USA	Canada
Asendin (Lederle)	Asendin (Lederle)

Common Synonyms ("Street Names"):   Depression pills

Drug Class: Antidepressants, Tricyclic

Prescription Required: USA: Yes   Canada: Yes

Available for Purchase by Generic Name: USA: No   Canada: No

Available Dosage Forms and Strengths

Tablets — 25 mg., 50 mg., 100 mg., 150 mg.

Tablet May Be Crushed or Capsule Opened for Administration: Yes

How This Drug Works

Intended Therapeutic Effect(s):   The relief of emotional depression and the gradual improvement of mood in all types of depressive disorders.

Location of Drug Action(s):   Those areas of the brain that control mood and emotional stability.

Method of Drug Action(s):   Not established. It is thought that by increasing the availability of certain nerve impulse transmitters (norepinephrine and serotonin), this drug relieves the symptoms associated with depression.

Principal Uses of This Drug

As a Single Drug Product: To provide symptomatic relief in all types of depression, and to initiate the restoration of normal mood.

THIS DRUG SHOULD NOT BE TAKEN IF

—you have had an allergic reaction to it previously.
—you are taking or have taken within the past 14 days any mono-amine oxidase (MAO) inhibitor drug (see Drug Class, Section Three).
—you are recovering from a recent heart attack.
—it is prescribed for a child under 16 years of age.

INFORM YOUR PHYSICIAN BEFORE TAKING THIS DRUG IF

—you are allergic or abnormally sensitive to any other tricyclic antidepressant drug (see Drug Class, Section Three).
—you have a history of any of the following: diabetes, epilepsy, glaucoma, heart disease, paranoia, prostate gland enlargement, schizophrenia, or overactive thyroid function.
—you plan to have surgery under general anesthesia in the near future.

Time Required for Apparent Benefit

Drug action usually begins in 30 minutes and reaches its peak in 2 hours. Continuous use on a regular schedule for 14 to 21 days is usually necessary to determine this drug's effectiveness in relieving depression. However, benefit may be apparent within 4 to 7 days in some individuals.

Possible Side-Effects *(natural, expected, and unavoidable drug actions)*

Drowsiness, blurring of vision, dryness of mouth, constipation, impaired urination.

Possible Adverse Effects *(unusual, unexpected, and infrequent reactions)*

IF ANY OF THE FOLLOWING DEVELOP, DISCONTINUE DRUG AND NOTIFY YOUR PHYSICIAN AS SOON AS POSSIBLE

Mild Adverse Effects

Allergic Reactions: Skin rash, hives, swelling, drug fever (see Glossary).
Other Reactions: Insomnia, nervousness, palpitations, dizziness, unsteadiness, tremors, fainting.
Peculiar taste, nausea, indigestion, vomiting.
Altered libido, breast enlargement, milk formation.

Serious Adverse Effects

Behavioral effects: anxiety, confusion, excitement, disorientation, hallucinations, delusions.
Aggravation of paranoid psychosis and schizophrenia.
Aggravation of epilepsy (seizures).
Altered menstrual pattern, impotence.
Parkinson-like disorders (see Glossary).
Peripheral neuritis (see Glossary)—numbness, tingling, pain, loss of strength in arms and legs.
Reduced white blood cell count—fever, sore throat.

Natural Diseases or Disorders That May Be Activated By This Drug
Latent epilepsy, glaucoma, prostatism.

CAUTION
1. The dosage of this drug should be adjusted carefully for each person individually. This requires observation of symptom improvement and, in some instances, the measurement of drug levels in the blood.
2. Observe for early indications of toxicity: confusion, agitation, rapid heart beat.
3. It is advisable to withold this drug if electroconvulsive therapy (ECT) is to be used.

Precautions for Use by Infants and Children
Safety and effectiveness in children below the age of 16 years have not been established.

Precautions for Use by Those over 60 Years of Age
During the first 2 weeks of treatment observe for the development of confusional reactions—restlessness, agitation, forgetfulness, disorientation, delusions and hallucinations. Reduction of dosage or discontinuation may be necessary.

Observe for unsteadiness and incoordination which may predispose to falling and injury.

This drug can increase the degree of impaired urination associated with prostate gland enlargement (prostatism).

It is advisable to take the total daily dose at bedtime to reduce the risks of postural hypotension (see Glossary).

Advisability of Use During Pregnancy
Pregnancy Category: C (tentative). See Pregnancy Code inside back cover.
Animal reproduction studies reveal toxic effects on the embryo in rats and rabbits but no birth defects in the newborn.
Information from adequate studies in pregnant women is not available.
Avoid completely during the first 3 months if possible.
Ask physician for guidance.

Advisability of Use While Nursing Infant
This drug is present in milk in small amounts. Nursing is permitted with careful observation of the infant for drowsiness or failure to feed.

Habit-Forming Potential
None.

Effects of Overdosage
With Moderate Overdose: Confusion, hallucinations, marked drowsiness, tremors, dilated pupils, cold skin.
With Large Overdose: Stupor, coma, convulsions, rapid heart rate, low blood pressure.

Possible Effects of Extended Use
None reported.

Suggested Periodic Examinations While Taking This Drug (at physician's discretion)

Complete blood cell counts.

Serial blood pressure readings and electrocardiograms.

While Taking This Drug, Observe the Following

Foods: No restrictions. May be taken without regard to meals.

Beverages: No restrictions. May be taken with milk.

Alcohol: Avoid completely. This drug can increase markedly the intoxicating effects of alcohol and accentuate its depressant action on brain function.

Tobacco Smoking: The elimination of this drug from the body may be accelerated by smoking. Consult your physician regarding the need to adjust your dosage.

Marijuana Smoking

Occasional (once or twice weekly): Transient increase in drowsiness and dryness of the mouth.

Daily: Persistent drowsiness, increased dryness of mouth; possible reduced effectiveness of this drug.

Other Drugs

Amoxapine may *increase* the effects of

• atropine-like drugs (see Drug Class, Section Three).

• sedatives, sleep-inducing drugs, tranquilizers, antihistamines, and narcotic drugs, and cause oversedation. Dosage adjustments may be necessary.

Amoxapine may *decrease* the effects of

• clonidine

• guanethidine

Amoxapine *taken concurrently* with

• amphetamine-like drugs may cause severe high blood pressure and/or high fever (see Drug Class, Section Three).

• anti-seizure (anticonvulsant) drugs requires careful monitoring for changes in siezure patterns; dosage of the anticonvulsant may need adjustment.

• ethchlorvynol may cause delirium; avoid concurrent use.

• mono-amine oxidase (MAO) inhibitor drugs may cause high fever, delirium, and convulsions (see Drug Class, Section Three). Avoid the concurrent use of these drugs. Do not begin to take any tricyclic antidepressant drug within 14 days after the last dose of any MAO inhibitor drug.

• thyroid preparations may impair heart rhythm and function; ask physician for guidance regarding adjustment of thyroid dosage.

The following drugs may *increase* the effects of amoxapine

• methylphenidate (Ritalin).

• phenothiazines (see Drug Class, Section Three).

The following drugs may *decrease* the effects of amoxapine
- barbiturates (see Drug Class, Section Three).
- chloral hydrate.
- estrogen.
- lithium.
- oral contraceptives.
- reserpine.

Driving a Vehicle, Operating Machinery, Engaging in Hazardous Activities: This drug may impair mental alertness, judgment, physical coordination, and reaction time. Avoid hazardous activities.

Aviation Note: The use of this drug *is a disqualification* for the piloting of aircraft. Consultation with a designated Aviation Medical Examiner is advised.

Exposure to Sun: Use caution until sensitivity to sun has been determined. This drug may cause photosensitivity.

Exposure to Heat: Caution advised. This drug can inhibit sweating and impair the body's adaptation to hot environments, increasing the risk of heat stroke. Avoid saunas.

Exposure to Cold: The elderly should use caution to avoid conditions that could cause hypothermia.

Exposure to Environmental Chemicals: This drug can mask the early indications of poisoning due to organophosphorus insecticides; observe the label of any insecticides you use.

Heavy Exercise or Exertion: No restrictions in temperate environment.

Occurrence of Unrelated Illness: In any condition that tends to lower the blood pressure, this drug may exaggerate the response and cause additional reduction of pressure beyond the expected.

Discontinuation: It is advisable to discontinue this drug gradually. Sudden withdrawal after prolonged use may cause headache, malaise and nausea. When this drug is discontinued, it may be necessary to adjust the doses of other drugs taken concurrently.

Special Storage Instructions
Keep tablets in a dry, tightly closed container at room temperature. Protect from light.

AMOXICILLIN

Year Introduced: 1969

Brand Names

USA	Canada
Amoxil (Beecham)	Amoxil (Ayerst)
Larotid (Roche)	Moxilean (Organon)
Polymox (Bristol)	Novamoxin (Novopharm)
Sumox (Reid-Provident)	Penamox (Beecham)
Trimox (Squibb)	Polymox (Bristol)
Utimox (Parke-Davis)	
Wymox (Wyeth)	

Common Synonyms ("Street Names"):   None

Drug Class: Antibiotic (Anti-infective), Penicillins

Prescription Required: Yes

Available for Purchase by Generic Name: USA: Yes   Canada: No

Available Dosage Forms and Strengths
Capsules — 250 mg., 500 mg.
Chewable tablets — 125 mg., 250 mg.
Oral suspension — 125 mg., 250 mg. per teaspoonful (5 ml.)
Pediatric drops — 50 mg. per ml.

Tablet May Be Crushed or Capsule Opened for Administration: Yes

How This Drug Works
Intended Therapeutic Effect(s):   The elimination of infections responsive to the action of this drug.
Location of Drug Action(s):   Any body tissue or fluid in which sufficient concentration of the drug can be achieved.
Method of Drug Action(s):   This drug destroys susceptible infecting bacteria by interfering with their ability to produce new protective cell walls as they multiply and grow.

Principal Uses of This Drug
As a Single Drug Product: To treat certain infections of the skin and soft tissues, of the ear, nose and throat, and of the genito-urinary tract, including gonorrhea.

THIS DRUG SHOULD NOT BE TAKEN IF
—you have had an allergic reaction to any dosage form of it previously.
—you are certain you are allergic to *any* form of penicillin.

INFORM YOUR PHYSICIAN BEFORE TAKING THIS DRUG IF
—you suspect you may be allergic to penicillin or you have a history of a previous "reaction" to penicillin.

—you are allergic to cephalosporin antibiotics (Ancef, Ceporan, Ceporex, Kafocin, Keflex, Keflin, Kefzol, Loridine).
—you are allergic by nature (hayfever, asthma, hives, eczema).

Time Required for Apparent Benefit
Varies with the nature of the infection under treatment; usually from 2 to 5
days.

Possible Side-Effects *(natural, expected, and unavoidable drug actions)*
Superinfections (see Glossary).

Possible Adverse Effects *(unusual, unexpected, and infrequent reactions)*

**IF ANY OF THE FOLLOWING DEVELOP, DISCONTINUE DRUG AND NOTIFY
YOUR PHYSICIAN AS SOON AS POSSIBLE**

Mild Adverse Effects
Allergic Reactions: Skin rashes (various kinds).
Other Reactions: Irritations of mouth or tongue, "black tongue," nausea,
vomiting, diarrhea, dizziness (rare).
Serious Adverse Effects
Allergic Reactions: †Anaphylactic reaction (see Glossary), severe skin
reactions, high fever, swollen painful joints, sore throat, unusual bleeding
or bruising.

Precautions for Use by Those over 60 Years of Age
It is advisable to evaluate kidney function before and during use of this drug
to determine the need for dosage adjustment.
Natural changes in the skin after 60 may predispose to severe and prolonged
itching reactions in the genital and anal regions. This reaction should be
reported promptly.

Advisability of Use During Pregnancy
Pregnancy Category: B (tentative). See Pregnancy Code inside back cover.
Animal reproduction studies: No data available.
Information from adequate studies in pregnant women indicates no in-
creased risk of defects in 3546 pregnancies exposed to penicillin deriva-
tives.
Ask physician for guidance.

Advisability of Use While Nursing Infant
Drug may be present in milk and may sensitize infant to penicillin. Ask
physician for guidance.

Habit-Forming Potential
None.

Effects of Overdosage
Possible nausea, vomiting, and/or diarrhea.

†A rare but potentially dangerous reaction characteristic of penicillins.

Possible Effects of Extended Use
Superinfections (see Glossary).

Suggested Periodic Examinations While Taking This Drug (at physician's discretion)
Complete blood cell counts.
Liver and kidney function tests.

While Taking This Drug, Observe the Following
Foods: No restrictions of food selection. Drug is absorbed better if taken 1 hour before eating or 2 hours after eating.

Beverages: No restrictions.

Alcohol: No interactions expected.

Tobacco Smoking: No interactions expected.

Marijuana Smoking: No interactions expected.

Other Drugs

The following drugs may *decrease* the effects of amoxicillin

• antacids reduce absorption of amoxicillin.

• chloramphenicol (Chloromycetin)

• erythromycin (Erythrocin, E-Mycin, etc.)

• tetracyclines (Achromycin, Aureomycin, Declomycin, Minocin, etc.; see Drug Class, Section Three)

Driving a Vehicle, Operating Machinery, Engaging in Hazardous Activities: Usually no restrictions. Be alert to the rare occurrence of dizziness and/or nausea, and restrict activities accordingly.

Aviation Note: The use of this drug *may be a disqualification* for the piloting of aircraft. Consultation with a designated Aviation Medical Examiner is advised.

Exposure to Sun: No restrictions.

Discontinuation: When used to treat infections that predispose to rheumatic fever or kidney disease, take continuously in full dosage for no less than 10 days. Ask physician for guidance regarding recommended duration of therapy.

Special Storage Instructions
Capsules should be kept in a tightly closed container at room temperature. Oral suspension and pediatric drops should be refrigerated.

Observe the Following Expiration Times
Do not take the oral suspension or drops of this drug if it is older than 7 days —when kept at room temperature; 14 days—when kept refrigerated.

AMPICILLIN

Year Introduced: 1961

Brand Names

USA

Amcill (Parke-Davis)
Omnipen (Wyeth)
Polycillin (Bristol)
Principen (Squibb)
SK-Ampicillin (Smith
   Kline & French)

Supen
   (Reid-Provident)
Totacillin (Beecham)
Polycillin-PRB [CD]
   (Bristol)

Canada

Amcill (P.D.)
Ampicin (Bristol)
Ampilean (Harris)
Novo-Ampicillin
   (Novopharm)
Penbritin (Ayerst)

Common Synonyms ("Street Names"):   None

Drug Class: Antibiotic (Anti-infective), Penicillins

Prescription Required: Yes

Available for Purchase by Generic Name: Yes

Available Dosage Forms and Strengths
   Capsules — 250 mg., 500 mg.
   Oral suspension — 125 mg., 250 mg., 500 mg. per teaspoonful (5 ml.)
   Pediatric drops — 100 mg. per ml.
   Injection — 125 mg., 250 mg., 1 g., 2 g. vials

Tablet May Be Crushed or Capsule Opened for Administration: Yes

How This Drug Works
   Intended Therapeutic Effect(s):   The elimination of infections responsive to
   the action of this drug.
   Location of Drug Action(s):   Any body tissue or fluid in which sufficient
   concentration of the drug can be achieved.
   Method of Drug Action(s):   This drug destroys susceptible infecting bacteria
   by interfering with their ability to produce new protective cell walls as they
   multiply and grow.

Principal Uses of This Drug
   As a Single Drug Product: To treat certain infections of the skin and soft
   tissues, of the respiratory tract, of the gastrointestinal tract, and of the
   genito-urinary tract (including gonorrhea in females). Also used to treat
   certain types of septicemia and meningitis.
   As a Combination Drug Product [CD]:   May be combined with probenecid
   (Benemid) to delay the elimination of ampicillin by the kidney and thereby
   increase its level in the blood. This combination drug is designed primarily
   for the treatment of gonorrhea in males and females.

THIS DRUG SHOULD NOT BE TAKEN IF
—you are allergic to any of the drugs bearing the brand names listed above.
—you are certain you are allergic to any form of penicillin.
—you have infectious mononucleosis (glandular fever).

INFORM YOUR PHYSICIAN BEFORE TAKING THIS DRUG IF
—you suspect you may be allergic to penicillin or you have a history of a previous "reaction" to penicillin.
—you are allergic to cephalosporin antibiotics (Ancef, Ceporan, Ceporex, Kafocin, Keflex, Keflin, Kefzol, Loridine).
—you are allergic by nature (hayfever, asthma, hives, eczema).

Time Required for Apparent Benefit
Varies with the nature of the infection under treatment; usually 2 to 5 days.

Possible Side-Effects *(natural, expected, and unavoidable drug actions)*
Superinfections (see Glossary).

Possible Adverse Effects *(unusual, unexpected, and infrequent reactions)*

IF ANY OF THE FOLLOWING DEVELOP, DISCONTINUE DRUG AND NOTIFY YOUR PHYSICIAN AS SOON AS POSSIBLE

Mild Adverse Effects
Allergic Reactions: Skin rashes (various kinds).
Other Reactions: Irritations of mouth and tongue, "black tongue," nausea, vomiting, diarrhea, dizziness (rare).
Note: A generalized rash occurs commonly (approximately 90% of the time) when ampicillin is taken in the presence of infectious mononucleosis.
Serious Adverse Effects
Allergic Reactions: †Anaphylactic reaction (see Glossary), severe skin reactions, high fever, swollen painful joints, sore throat, unusual bleeding or bruising.

Precautions for Use by Those over 60 Years of Age
It is advisable to evaluate kidney function before and during use of this drug to determine the need for dosage adjustment.
Natural changes in the skin after 60 may predispose to severe and prolonged itching reactions in the genital and anal regions. This reaction should be reported promptly.

Advisability of Use During Pregnancy
Pregnancy Category: B (tentative). See Pregnancy Code inside back cover.
Animal reproduction studies in mice and rats reveal no birth defects due to this drug.
Information from adequate studies in pregnant women indicates no increased risk of defects in 3546 pregnancies exposed to penicillin derivatives.
Ask physician for guidance.

Advisability of Use While Nursing Infant
Drug may be present in milk and could sensitize infant to penicillin. Ask physician for guidance.

†A rare but potentially dangerous reaction characteristic of penicillins.

Habit-Forming Potential
None.

Effects of Overdosage
Possible nausea, vomiting, and/or diarrhea.

Possible Effects of Extended Use
Superinfections (see Glossary).

Suggested Periodic Examinations While Taking This Drug (at physician's discretion)
Complete blood cell counts
Liver and kidney function tests.

While Taking This Drug, Observe the Following
Foods: No restrictions of food selection. Drug is absorbed better if taken 1 hour before or 2 hours after eating.

Beverages: No restrictions.

Alcohol: No interactions expected.

Tobacco Smoking: No interactions expected.

Marijuana Smoking: No interactions expected.

Other Drugs

The following drugs may *decrease* the effects of ampicillin

- antacids may reduce its absorption.
- chloramphenicol (Chloromycetin)
- erythromycin (Erythrocin, E-Mycin, etc.)
- tetracyclines (Achromycin, Aureomycin, Declomycin, Minocin, etc.; see Drug Class, Section Three)

Driving a Vehicle, Operating Machinery, Engaging in Hazardous Activities: Usually no restrictions. Be alert to the rare occurrence of dizziness and/or nausea, and restrict activities accordingly.

Aviation Note: The use of this drug *may be a disqualification* for the piloting of aircraft. Consultation with a designated Aviation Medical Examiner is advised.

Exposure to Sun: No restrictions.

Discontinuation: When used to treat infections that predispose to rheumatic fever or kidney disease, take continuously in full dosage for no less than 10 days. Ask physician for guidance regarding recommended duration of therapy.

Special Storage Instructions
Tablets and capsules should be kept in tightly closed containers. Oral suspension and pediatric drops should be refrigerated. Keep bottles tightly closed.

Observe the Following Expiration Times
Do not take the oral suspension or drops of this drug if it is older than 7 days —when kept at room temperature: 70°F. (21°C.); 14 days—when kept refrigerated: 40°F. (4°C.).

ANDROGENS

Fluoxymesterone   **Testosterone cypionate**
Methyltestosterone   **Testosterone enanthate**
Testosterone   **Testosterone propionate**

Year Introduced: Fluoxymesterone, 1956
Methyltestosterone, 1941
Testosterone, 1936
Testosterone cypionate, 1958
Testosterone enanthate, 1954
Testosterone propionate, 1972

Brand Names

USA

Fluoxymesterone
Android-F (Brown)
Halodrin [CD]
(Upjohn)
Halotestin (Upjohn)
Ora-Testryl
(Squibb)
Methyltestosterone
Android-5 (Brown)
Android-10 (Brown)
Android-25 (Brown)
Estratest [CD]
(Reid-Provident)
Metandren (CIBA)
Oreton Methyl
(Schering)
Testred (ICN)
Premarin with
Methyltestoster-
one [CD] (Ayerst)
Tylosterone [CD]
(Lilly)

Testosterone
Oreton (Schering)
Testosterone
cypionate
Depo-Testosterone
(Upjohn)
Testosterone
enanthate
Android-T (Brown)
Delatestryl (Squibb)

Canada

Fluoxymesterone
Halotestin (Upjohn)
Methyltestosterone
Metandren (CIBA)
Oestrilin with
Methyltestoster-
one [CD]
(Desbergers)
Premarin with
Methyltestoster-
one [CD] (Ayerst)
Testosterone
Malogen (Stickley)
Testosterone
cypionate
Depo-Testosterone
(Upjohn)
Testosterone
enanthate
Delatestryl (Squibb)
Malogex (Stickley)
Testosterone
propionate
Malogen in Oil
(Stickley)

Common Synonyms ("Street Names"):   None

Drug Class: Male Sex Hormones, Androgens

Prescription Required: Yes

Available for Purchase by Generic Name: USA: Yes   Canada: No

Available Dosage Forms and Strengths
Tablets — 2 mg., 5 mg., 10 mg., 25 mg.
Buccal tablets — 5 mg., 10 mg.
Capsules — 10 mg.
Pellets for implantation — 75 mg.
Injection — 25 mg., 50 mg., 100 mg., 200 mg. per ml.

Tablet May Be Crushed or Capsule Opened for Administration: Yes

How This Drug Works
Intended Therapeutic Effect(s):   Principal uses include
- replacement therapy in known testosterone-deficient states (masculinizing effect).
- correction of delayed descent of the testicles into the scrotum—undescended testes.
- relief of symptoms associated with the male menopause—hot flushes, sweats, reduced sexual interest and potency.
- stimulation of growth, weight gain, muscular development, physical stamina, and red blood cell production in selected individuals (anabolic effect).
- prevention and treatment of osteoporosis—loss of calcium from bones with resultant weakening and predisposition to breaking.
- control of female breast cancer in selected individuals (anti-estrogen effect).

Location of Drug Action(s):   Principal actions occur in
- the male reproductive organs.
- the skin, hair follicles, and sebaceous glands.
- the larynx (voice box) and vocal cords.
- the bones.
- the muscles.

Method of Drug Action(s):   By stimulating the nucleus of responsive cells, this hormone activates appropriate tissues to (1) develop the sexual characteristics of the adult male, and (2) increase the production of certain tissue proteins. Androgens, taken to restore normal tissue levels of the male sex hormone, reduce the frequency and severity of menopausal symptoms in the male. By suppressing the production of female sex hormones (estrogens), androgens retard the growth and spread of female breast cancer in certain selected individuals.

Principal Uses of This Drug

As a Single Drug Product: Used primarily to treat disorders due to testosterone deficiency. These include eunuchism, undescended testes, delayed puberty, and selected cases of impotence. Also used in the management of cancer of the breast in postmenopausal women. Used less frequently to stimulate the production of red blood cells.

As a Combination Drug Product [CD]:   May be combined with estrogen for use in the prevention and treatment of postmenopausal osteoporosis.

THIS DRUG SHOULD NOT BE TAKEN IF

—you have had an allergic reaction to any dosage form of it previously.
—you have a history of male breast cancer.
—you have a history of prostate gland cancer.
—you have active liver disease.
—you are or think you may be pregnant.

INFORM YOUR PHYSICIAN BEFORE TAKING THIS DRUG IF

—you have any form of heart disease, with or without a history of heart failure.
—you have high blood pressure.
—you have impaired liver or kidney function.
—you have enlargement of the prostate gland with or without difficult urination.
—you have epilepsy.
—you have migraine headaches.
—you have an abnormally high level of blood calcium.

Time Required for Apparent Benefit

Methyltestosterone by mouth reaches peak blood levels in 1 to 2 hours.
Early effects may be seen in 2 to 3 days. With continuous administration, additional effects are apparent in 2 to 3 weeks.
In treatment of female breast cancer, beneficial effects usually occur within 3 months.

Possible Side-Effects *(natural, expected and unavoidable drug actions)*

Retention of salt and water (edema) causing gain in weight.
Enlargement and tenderness of male breast tissue.
Development of male characteristics in the female—facial acne, oily skin, loss of scalp hair, growth of facial and body hair, deepening of the voice, prominent muscles and veins.

Possible Adverse Effects *(unusual, unexpected and infrequent reactions)*

**IF ANY OF THE FOLLOWING DEVELOP, DISCONTINUE DRUG AND NOTIFY
YOUR PHYSICIAN AS SOON AS POSSIBLE**

Mild Adverse Effects
   Allergic Reactions: Hives, itching.
   Other Reactions
      Nausea, vomiting, indigestion.
      Sustained and painful penile erections (priapism).
      Menstrual irregularity; vaginal bleeding in the post-menopausal woman.
      Mouth irritation from buccal tablets.
      Local tissue irritation from implanted pellets.
Serious Adverse Effects
   Allergic Reactions: Anaphylactic reaction (see Glossary).
   Idiosyncratic Reactions: Acute porphyria (see Glossary).
   Other Reactions: Hepatitis with jaundice (see Glossary)—yellow dis-
   coloration of eyes and skin, dark-colored urine, light-colored stools.
   Note: This reaction is associated with fluoxymesterone and methyltestos-
   terone.

   Possible Delayed Adverse Effects
   Liver cancer has been reported following prolonged administration of
   some androgens.

CAUTION
1. To be fully effective, the androgen in buccal tablets must be absorbed
   through the lining of the mouth and not swallowed. Eating, drinking,
   chewing, and smoking should be avoided until the tablet is completely
   absorbed.
2. The female user of androgens should observe for deepening of the voice
   and enlargement of the clitoris. These are permanent changes.
3. Excessive use of androgens in post-menopausal women can cause vaginal
   bleeding resembling menstruation.

Precautions for Use by Those over 60 Years of Age
   Androgens can increase the degree of impaired urination in men with prostate gland enlargement (prostatism).
   By causing retention of salt and water, androgens can aggravate high blood
   pressure, heart disease, and impaired liver or kidney function.
   The excessive physical and sexual stimulation caused by androgens may create demands beyond individual capacity to respond.

Advisability of Use During Pregnancy
   Pregnancy Category: X (tentative). See Pregnancy Code inside back
   cover.
      Animal reproduction studies reveal significant birth defects due to this
      drug.

Information from studies in pregnant women indicates that androgens can masculinize the female fetus during development.
Avoid completely during entire pregnancy.

Advisability of Use While Nursing Infant
These drugs are known to be present in milk and can affect the infant adversely. Avoid drug or refrain from nursing.

Habit-Forming Potential
None.

Effects of Overdosage
With Moderate Overdose: Nausea, vomiting, indigestion. Priapism—inappropriate, prolonged, and painful erection of the penis. Fluid retention, weight gain.
With Large Overdose: No serious or dangerous effects reported.

Possible Effects of Extended Use
Reduced production of semen and sperm.
Increased levels of calcium in blood and urine with formation of kidney stones.

Suggested Periodic Examinations While Taking This Drug (at physician's discretion)
Liver function tests.
Measurement of calcium levels in blood and urine.

While Taking This Drug, Observe the Following
Foods: The diet should be high in total calories, proteins, vitamins, and minerals to obtain the maximal anabolic effect from androgens. Ask physician for guidance regarding salt intake if you experience fluid retention (edema).
Beverages: No restrictions.
Alcohol: No interactions expected.
Tobacco Smoking: No interactions expected. Refrain from smoking during absorption of buccal tablets.
Marijuana Smoking
Occasional (once or twice weekly):   No significant interactions expected.
Daily: Possible decrease in blood testosterone levels.
Other Drugs
Fluoxymesterone may *increase* the effects of
• oral anticoagulants (Coumadin, etc.), and make it necessary to reduce the dosage of the anticoagulant.

The following drugs may *decrease* the effects of androgens:
- chlorcyclizine (Fedrazil, Perazil).
- chlorzoxazone (Paraflex).
- phenobarbital (Luminal, etc.)
- phenylbutazone (Butazolidin, etc.)

Driving a Vehicle, Operating Machinery, Engaging in Hazardous Activities: No restrictions or precautions.

Aviation Note: The use of this drug *may be a disqualification* for the piloting of aircraft. Consultation with a designated Aviation Medical Examiner is advised.

Exposure to Sun: No restrictions.

Exposure to Heat: No restrictions.

Exposure to Cold: No restrictions.

Heavy Exercise or Exertion: No restrictions.

Discontinuation: The desired therapeutic response to androgens may require continuous use on a regular schedule for 2 to 5 months. Do not discontinue before an adequate trial has been completed and evaluated. On the other hand, do not continue androgens if an adequate trial shows them to be ineffective.

Special Storage Instructions

Keep tablets and capsules in dry, tightly closed container. Protect from light.

ANTACIDS

Aluminum hydroxide	Magnesium hydroxide
Calcium carbonate	Magnesium trisilicate
Magaldrate	Sodium bicarbonate
Magnesium carbonate	Sodium carbonate

Year Introduced: Aluminum hydroxide, 1936
Calcium carbonate, 1825
Magaldrate, 1960
Magnesium hydroxide, 1873
Magnesium trisilicate, 1936
Sodium bicarbonate, 1886

Brand Names

USA

Absorbable Antacids:
Sodium bicarbonate*:
   Alka-Seltzer Antacid
      (Miles)
   Bell-Ans (C. S. Dent)
   BiSoDol Powder
      (Whitehall)
   Bromo-Seltzer
      (Warner-Lambert)
   Eno (Beecham)
   Fizrin (Glenbrook)
   Soda Mint (Numerous
      mfrs.)

Less Absorbable Antacids:
Aluminum hydroxide:
   ALternaGEL (Stuart)
   Amphojel (Wyeth)
Calcium carbonate*:
   Alka-2 (Miles)
   Amitone
      (Mitchum-Thayer)
   Dicarbosil (Norcliff
      Thayer)
   Gustalac (Geriatric)
   Pepto-Bismol Tablets
      (Norwich)
   Ratio (Warren-Teed)
   Titralac (Riker)
   Tums (Lewis-Howe)

Canada

Absorbable Antacids:
Sodium bicarbonate*:
   Alka-Seltzer (Miles)
   BiSoDol Powder (Whitehall)
   Brioschi (Brioschi, Inc.)
   Bromo-Seltzer
      (Warner-Lambert)
   Chembicarb (Chemo)
   Eno (Beecham)
   Soda Mint (Numerous mfrs.)

Less Absorbable Antacids:
Aluminum hydroxide:
   A-H GEL (Dymond)
   Alu-Tab (Riker)
   Amphojel (Wyeth)
   Chemgel (Chemo)
   Pepsogel (C & C)
   Robalate (Robins)
Calcium carbonate*:
   Pepto-Bismol Tablets
      (Norwich)
   Titralac (Riker)
   Tums (Lewis-Howe)
Magnesium hydroxide:
   Milk of Magnesia (Numerous
      mfrs.)

*The principal antacid component.

USA

Magnesium carbonate:
Marblen (Fleming)
Magnesium hydroxide:
Milk of Magnesia
(Numerous mfrs.)

Antacid Combinations:
Aluminum hydroxide +
Magnesium carbonate:
Silain-Gel (Robins)
Aluminum hydroxide +
Magnesium hydroxide:
Aludrox (Wyeth)
Creamalin (Winthrop)
Delcid (Merrell-National)
Di-Gel Liquid (Plough)
Kolantyl (Merrell-National)
Maalox (Rorer)
Maxamag (Vitarine)
Mylanta (Stuart)
Win-Gel (Winthrop)
Aluminum hydroxide +
Magnesium trisilicate:
A-M-T (Wyeth)
Gaviscon (Marion)
Gelusil (Warner/Chilcott)
Aluminum hydroxide +
Sodium carbonate:
Rolaids (American Chicle)
Aluminum hydroxide +
Calcium carbonate +
Magnesium hydroxide:
Camalox (Rorer)
Aluminum hydroxide +
Magnesium carbonate +
Magnesium hydroxide:
Di-Gel Tablets (Plough)
Aluminum hydroxide +
Magnesium hydroxide +
Magnesium trisilicate:
Magnatril (Lannett)
Calcium carbonate +
Magnesium carbonate +
Magnesium oxide:
Alkets (Upjohn)

Canada

Antacid Combinations:
Aluminum hydroxide + Calcium
carbonate:
Duatrol (SK&F)
Aluminum hydroxide +
Magnesium carbonate:
Antamel (Elliott-Marion)
Magnesed (M & M)
Aluminum hydroxide +
Magnesium hydroxide:
Alsimox (ICI)
A.M.H. Suspension (M & M)
Di-Gel Liquid (Plough)
Diovol (Horner)
Kolantyl (Merrell)
Maalox (Rorer)
Mylanta (P.D. & Co.)
Neutralca-S (Desbergers)
Univol (Horner)
Aluminum hydroxide +
Magnesium trisilicate:
Gelusil (Warner/Chilcott)
Aluminum hydroxide + Sodium
carbonate:
Rolaids (Adams)
Aluminum hydroxide + Calcium
carbonate + Magnesium
hydroxide:
Camalox (Rorer)
Aluminum hydroxide +
Magnesium carbonate +
Magnesium hydroxide:
Amphojel 65 (Wyeth)
Di-Gel Tablets (Plough)
Calcium carbonate +
Magnesium hydroxide:
BiSoDol Tablets (Whitehall)
Magaldrate:
Riopan (Ayerst)

Common Synonyms ("Street Names"):   Stomach medicine

Drug Class: Antacids, Stomach

Prescription Required: No

Available for Purchase by Generic Name: Yes

Available Dosage Forms and Strengths
Tablets
Chewable tablets
Wafers
Granules
Powders
Liquid suspensions
Available in a large variety of formulations and strengths. See package label for product composition and individual component strengths.

Tablet May Be Crushed or Capsule Opened for Administration: Yes

How This Drug Works
Intended Therapeutic Effect(s)
Relief of heartburn, sour stomach, and acid indigestion.
Relief of discomfort associated with peptic ulcer, gastritis, esophagitis, and hiatal hernia.
Location of Drug Action(s):   Within the digestive juices of the stomach.
Method of Drug Action(s)
By neutralizing some of the hydrochloric acid in the stomach, these drugs reduce the degree of acidity and thus lessen the irritant effect of digestive juices on inflamed and ulcerated tissues.
By reducing the action of the digestive enzyme pepsin, these drugs are thought to create a more favorable environment for the healing of peptic ulcer.

Principal Uses of This Drug
As a Single Drug Product: Used primarily to provide symptomatic relief in the treatment of peptic ulcer disease, gastritis, esophagitis, hiatal hernia, and conditions associated with the production of excessive stomach acid.
As a Combination Drug Product [CD]:   Antacids of different chemical composition are often combined to reduce unwanted side effects of each other. For example, the constipating effect of aluminum antacids can correct the laxative effects of magnesium antacids—hence their frequent combination in popular antacid products. Antacids are sometimes combined with drugs that cause stomach irritation, such as aspirin and related compounds, to make such drugs less irritating.

THIS DRUG SHOULD NOT BE TAKEN IF
—you have a known allergy or sensitivity to any of its components. (Brand names listed above are arranged according to generic components.)
—it contains a calcium compound, and you are known to have a high blood calcium level.

INFORM YOUR PHYSICIAN BEFORE TAKING THIS DRUG IF
—you have a history of chronic kidney disease or reduced kidney function.
—you have a history of kidney stones.
—you have chronic constipation or chronic diarrhea.
—you have any disorder that causes fluid retention.
—you have high blood pressure.
—you have a history of congestive heart failure.

Time Required for Apparent Benefit
Depending upon the composition and dose of the antacid, relief can begin in 5 to 15 minutes and persist for 45 minutes to 3 hours. Liquid preparations give relief more rapidly than tablets.

Possible Side-Effects *(natural, expected, and unavoidable drug actions)*
Aluminum preparations may cause constipation. Calcium carbonate may cause belching and constipation. Magnesium carbonate may cause belching and diarrhea. Magnesium preparations may cause diarrhea. Sodium bicarbonate may cause belching and weight gain.

Possible Adverse Effects *(unusual, unexpected, and infrequent reactions)*

IF ANY OF THE FOLLOWING DEVELOP, DISCONTINUE DRUG AND NOTIFY YOUR PHYSICIAN AS SOON AS POSSIBLE

Mild Adverse Effects
Aluminum hydroxide may cause nausea and/or vomiting.
Calcium carbonate may cause nausea.

Serious Adverse Effects
Aluminum hydroxide taken in large doses and with inadequate fluids can cause intestinal obstruction.
Calcium carbonate taken in large doses can cause abnormally high calcium levels in the blood; chronic use can lead to kidney stones and impaired kidney function.
Sodium bicarbonate taken in large doses or on a regular basis can cause elevation of the blood pressure, fluid retention (edema), and serious disturbance of the acid-alkaline balance of body chemistry (alkalosis).

CAUTION
1. Do not use any antacid regularly for more than 2 weeks without your physician's guidance.
2. If symptoms requiring the use of antacids persist, consult your physician for definitive diagnosis and appropriate treatment.
3. If frequent and continuous use of antacids is necessary, it is advisable to use aluminum and/or magnesium preparations.
4. Calcium carbonate and sodium bicarbonate preparations should be limited to occasional use by healthy individuals. Their frequent or continuous use should be avoided.
5. The elderly and individuals with high blood pressure, fluid retention, or a history of congestive heart failure should avoid antacids with a high sodium content. These include:

Alka-Seltzer   Eno
Bell-Ans   Fizrin
BiSoDol Powder   Rolaids
Brioschi   Soda Mints
Bromo-Seltzer

6. Do not exceed the maximal daily dose stated on the product label.
7. Do not swallow chewable tablets and wafers whole. These preparations must be thoroughly sucked or chewed before swallowing, and preferably followed by a small amount of water or milk. (Antacid tablets designed for chewing can cause intestinal obstruction if swallowed whole.)
8. Shake all liquid suspensions of antacids well before measuring dose.
9. In the presence of reduced kidney function: (1) antacids may accumulate in the blood and cause an excessive shift in the acid-alkaline balance of body chemistry to the alkaline side (alkalosis); (2) antacids containing magnesium may lead to excessive retention of magnesium and resulting toxicity.
10. Individuals sensitive to aspirin should note that these antacids contain aspirin: Alka-Seltzer (original formulation; see label), Cama Inlay-Tabs, and Fizrin.
11. Bromo-Seltzer also contains acetaminophen.

Precautions for Use by Those over 60 Years of Age
If you have been advised to restrict your use of salt, refer to paragraph 5 under Caution for those antacids you should avoid.
If you develop either constipation or diarrhea with the use of any antacid, consult your physician or pharmacist for guidance. Do not allow either condition to go uncorrected.

Advisability of Use During Pregnancy
Pregnancy Category: C (tentative). See Pregnancy Code inside back cover.
Animal reproduction studies: No data available.
Information from studies in pregnant women indicates the possibility of fetal damage from antacids containing magnesium.
Ask physician for guidance.
Select antacid preparations with contents limited to aluminum and magnesium compounds. Avoid antacid preparations containing sodium compounds and aspirin. If you have impaired kidney function, ask your physician for guidance in selecting an antacid.

Advisability of Use While Nursing Infant
As for pregnancy.

Habit-Forming Potential
None. However, frequent use of sodium bicarbonate, and large doses of calcium carbonate or magnesium hydroxide, may cause "acid rebound," which requires repeated use of the antacid to sustain relief from recurring hyperacidity.

Effects of Overdosage

With Moderate Overdose: Aluminum hydroxide may cause nausea, vomiting, and/or severe constipation. Magnesium compounds may cause severe diarrhea.

With Large Overdose: Moderate alkalosis, manifested by loss of appetite, weakness, fatigue, and dizziness. Severe alkalosis, manifested by nervous irritability, restlessness, and muscle spasms. Magnesium overdose may cause dryness of the mouth, stupor, and slow, shallow breathing.

Possible Effects of Extended Use

Aluminum hydroxide may cause decreased levels of blood phosphates, resulting in loss of calcium and phosphate from bone with weakening of bone structure (osteomalacia).

Calcium carbonate may cause an abnormally high blood level of calcium, disturbance of the acid-alkaline balance of body chemistry (alkalosis), impaired kidney function, and the formation of kidney stones.

Magnesium hydroxide may cause toxic effects on the nervous system (if used in the presence of reduced kidney function).

Magnesium trisilicate may cause the formation of kidney stones.

Sodium bicarbonate may predispose to recurrent urinary tract infections, kidney stones, excessive retention of sodium leading to elevated blood pressure, and fluid retention.

Suggested Periodic Examinations While Taking This Drug (at physician's discretion)

Measurements of blood calcium and phosphorus levels.

Measurements of blood acid-alkaline status.

Kidney function tests and urine analyses.

While Taking This Drug, Observe the Following

Foods: Follow the diet prescribed by your physician. Maintain regular intake of high phosphate foods such as meats, poultry, fish, eggs, dairy products, and cereals. When used on a regular basis for continuous effect, antacids are most effective when taken 1 hour after eating.

Beverages: As directed by your physician.

Alcohol: No interactions with antacids. However, alcoholic beverages may increase stomach acidity and thus increase antacid requirements.

Tobacco Smoking: No interactions with antacids. However, nicotine may increase stomach acidity and thus increase antacid requirements.

Marijuana Smoking: No interactions expected.

Other Drugs

Aluminum hydroxide may *increase* the effects of

• meperidine (pethidine, Demerol).

• pseudoephedrine (Sudafed).

Magnesium hydroxide may *increase* the effects of

• dicumarol.

Sodium bicarbonate may *increase* the effects of
• quinidine.

Antacids may *decrease* the effects of
• chlorpromazine.
• digitalis preparations.
• iron preparations.
• isoniazid.
• nalidixic acid.
• para-aminosalicylic acid.
• penicillins.
• pentobarbital.
• phenylbutazone.
• sulfonamides ("sulfa" drugs).
• tetracyclines.
• Vitamins A and C.

Antacids *taken concurrently* with
• anticoagulants, may cause impaired absorption and reduced effectiveness of the anticoagulant. Consult physician regarding need for prothrombin time determinations.

Driving a Vehicle, Operating Machinery, Engaging in Hazardous Activities: No precautions or restrictions.

Aviation Note: Usually no restrictions. However, it is advisable to observe for the possible occurrence of diarrhea and to restrict activities accordingly.

Exposure to Sun: No restrictions.

Special Storage Instructions
Keep all antacids in tightly closed containers. Store liquid suspensions in a cool place; avoid freezing.

ASPIRIN*
(Acetylsalicylic Acid)

Year Introduced: 1899

Brand Names

USA

A.S.A. Preparations (Lilly)
Aspergum (Plough)
Aspirjen Jr. (Jenkins)
Bayer Aspirin (Glenbrook)
Bayer Children's Aspirin
   (Glenbrook)
Bayer Timed-Release Aspirin
   (Glenbrook)
Easprin (Parke-Davis)
Ecotrin (Smith Kline &
   French)
Empirin (Burroughs
   Wellcome)
Measurin (Breon)
St. Joseph Children's Aspirin
   (Plough)
Synalgos-DC (Ives)

Canada

Acetophen (Frosst)
Ancasal (Anca)
Astrin (Medic)
Bayer Aspirin* (Sterling)
Ecotrin (SK&F)
Entrophen (Frosst)
Novasen (Novopharm)
Sal-Adult (Beecham)
Sal-Infant (Beecham)
Supasa (Nordic)
Triaphen-10 (Trianon)

OTC Preparations containing Aspirin

Alka-Seltzer [CD] (Miles)
Anacin [CD] (Whitehall)
A.P.C. Tablets [CD]
   (Various
   manufacturers)
Ascriptin [CD] (Rorer)
Bufferin [CD] (Bristol
   Labs)
Cama-Inlay-Tabs [CD]
   (Dorsey)
Cope [CD] (Glenbrook)

Excedrin [CD]
   (Bristol-Myers)
4-Way Tablets [CD]
   (Bristol-Myers)
Midol [CD] (Glenbrook)
Stanback (Stanback)
Synalgos (Ives)
Vanquish [CD]
   (Glenbrook)
(Numerous others)

Common Synonyms ("Street Names"):   None

Drug Class: Analgesic, Mild; Anti-inflammatory; Fever Reducer (Antipyretic); Salicylates

Prescription Required: No

Available for Purchase by Generic Name: Yes

*In the United States *aspirin* is an official generic designation. In Canada *Aspirin* is the Registered Trade Mark of the Bayer Company Division of Sterling Drug Ltd.

Available Dosage Forms and Strengths

Tablets — 65 mg. (1 gr.), 81 mg. (1.3 gr.), 210 mg. (3.2 gr.), 325 mg. (5 gr.), 500 mg. (7.7 gr.), 650 mg. (10 gr.)

Tablets (Prolonged-action) — 650 mg.

Enteric-coated tablets — 325 mg. (5 gr.), 500 mg. (7.7 gr.), 650 mg. (10 gr.), 975 mg. (15 gr.)

Capsules — 325 mg. (5 gr.)

Suppositories — 65 mg. (1 gr.), 130 mg. (2 gr.), 195 mg. (3.3 gr.), 325 mg. (5 gr.), 650 mg. (10 gr.), 1200 mg. (18.4 gr.)

Tablet May Be Crushed or Capsule Opened for Administration

Regular tablets and capsules — Yes

Enteric-coated tablets — No

A.S.A. Enseals — No

Cama — No

Ecotrin — No

How This Drug Works

Intended Therapeutic Effect(s)

Reduction of high fever.

Relief of mild to moderate pain and inflammation.

Prevention of blood clots (as in phlebitis, heart attack, and stroke).

Location of Drug Action(s):   Principal actions occur in:

• a major control center of the brain known as the hypothalamus.

• areas of injury, inflammation, or spasm, in many body tissues.

• blood platelets (see Glossary).

Method of Drug Action(s)

Aspirin, by indirect action on the hypothalamus, reduces fever by dilating blood vessels in the skin. This hastens the loss of body heat.

Aspirin reduces the tissue concentration of prostaglandins, chemicals involved in the production of inflammation and pain.

Aspirin interferes with the blood clotting mechanism by its action on blood platelets.

Principal Uses of This Drug

As a Single Drug Product: To relieve mild to moderate pain from any cause, to reduce high fever, and to provide symptomatic relief in conditions characterized by inflammation. A major use is to treat musculoskeletal disorders, especially acute and chronic arthritis. Because aspirin inhibits the aggregation of blood platelets (blood clots), it is used selectively in low dosage to prevent platelet embolism to the brain (in men) and to reduce the risk of thromboembolism in patients with artificial heart valves and those undergoing hip surgery. (See Blood Platelets in the Glossary.)

As a Combination Drug Product [CD]:   Frequently combined with other mild or strong analgesic drugs to enhance pain relief.

THIS DRUG SHOULD NOT BE TAKEN IF
—you have had an allergic reaction or an unfavorable response to it previously.
—you have any type of bleeding disorder (such as hemophilia).
—you are taking anticoagulant drugs.
—you have an active peptic ulcer (stomach or duodenum).

INFORM YOUR PHYSICIAN BEFORE TAKING THIS DRUG IF
—you have a history of peptic ulcer disease.
—you have a history of gout.
—you are taking oral anti-diabetic drugs.
—you are pregnant or planning pregnancy.
—you plan to have surgery of any kind in the near future.

Time Required for Apparent Benefit
Drug action begins in 15 to 20 minutes, reaches a maximum in approximately 1 to 2 hours, and persists for 3 to 4 hours.

Possible Side-Effects (*natural, expected, and unavoidable drug actions*)
Mild drowsiness in sensitive individuals.

Possible Adverse Effects (*unusual, unexpected, and infrequent reactions*)

IF ANY OF THE FOLLOWING DEVELOP, DISCONTINUE DRUG AND NOTIFY YOUR PHYSICIAN AS SOON AS POSSIBLE

Mild Adverse Effects
Allergic Reactions: Skin rash, hives, nasal discharge (resembling hay fever), nasal polyps.
Other Reactions: Stomach irritation, heartburn, nausea, vomiting.

Serious Adverse Effects
Allergic Reactions: Acute anaphylactic reaction (see Glossary), asthma, unusual bruising due to allergic destruction of blood platelets (see Glossary).
Idiosyncratic Reactions: Hemolytic anemia (see Glossary).
Other Reactions
Erosion of stomach lining, with silent bleeding.
Activation of peptic ulcer, with and without hemorrhage.
Bone marrow depression (see Glossary)—fatigue, weakness, fever, sore throat, abnormal bruising or bleeding.
Hepatitis with jaundice (see Glossary)—yellow skin and eyes, dark-colored urine, light-colored stools.
Kidney damage, if used in large doses or for a prolonged time.

CAUTION
1. It is most important to understand that aspirin is a drug. While it is one of our most useful drugs, we have an unrealistic sense of safety and unconcern regarding its actions within the body and its potential for adverse effects. This is due to its unlimited availability in over 400 products and its extremely wide use (100 million aspirin tablets taken daily in the United States).
2. In order to know if you are taking aspirin, make it a point to learn the

contents of all drugs you take—those prescribed by your physician and those you purchase over-the-counter (OTC) without prescription.

3. Limit the dosage of aspirin to no more than 3 tablets (15 grs.) at one time, allow at least 4 hours between doses, and take no more than 10 tablets (50 grs.) in 24 hours.

4. Remember that aspirin can
   • cause new illnesses.
   • complicate existing illnesses.
   • complicate pregnancy.
   • complicate surgery.
   • interact unfavorably with many other drugs.

5. When your physician asks "Are you taking any drugs?," the answer is yes if you are taking aspirin. This also applies to any non-prescription drug you are taking (see OTC drugs in Glossary).

Precautions for Use by Those over 60 Years of Age

The natural decline in kidney function that may occur can reduce your tolerance to aspirin. Observe for indications of excessive dosage: nervous irritability, confusion, ringing in the ears, deafness, loss of appetite, nausea, and stomach irritation.

Aspirin can cause excessive bleeding from the stomach in sensitive individuals. This can occur as "silent" bleeding of small amounts over an extended period of time, resulting in anemia. It may also occur as sudden hemorrhage, even without a history of stomach ulcer. Observe stools for gray to black discoloration—an indication of stomach bleeding.

Advisability of Use During Pregnancy

Pregnancy Category: B (tentative). See Pregnancy Code inside back cover.

Animal reproduction studies reveal significant birth defects due to this drug.

Information from studies in pregnant women indicates no increased risk of defects in 32,164 pregnancies exposed to this drug.

Studies indicate that the regular use of salicylates during pregnancy is often detrimental to the health of the mother and to the welfare of the infant. Excessive use of salicylate drugs can cause anemia, hemorrhage before and after delivery, and an increased incidence of still births. It is advisable to limit the use of aspirin during pregnancy to small doses and to brief periods of time, and to avoid aspirin altogether during the last month of pregnancy.

Advisability of Use While Nursing Infant

This drug is present in milk and may cause adverse effects in the nursing infant. It is advisable to avoid use if nursing.

Habit-Forming Potential

Use of this drug in large doses for a prolonged period of time may cause a form of psychological dependence (see Glossary).

Effects of Overdosage

With Moderate Overdose: Stomach distress, nausea, vomiting, ringing in the ears, dizziness, impaired hearing, drowsiness, sweating.

With Large Overdose: Stupor, warm and dry skin, fever, deep and rapid breathing, fast pulse, muscular twitching, delirium, hallucinations, convulsions.

Possible Effects of Extended Use

A form of psychological dependence (see Glossary).

Anemia due to chronic blood loss from erosion of stomach lining.

The development of stomach ulcer.

The development of "aspirin allergy"—nasal discharge, nasal polyps, asthma.

Kidney damage.

Excessive prolongation of bleeding time, of major importance in the event of injury or surgical procedure.

Suggested Periodic Examinations While Taking This Drug (at physician's discretion)

Complete blood cell counts.

Kidney function tests and urine analysis.

Liver function tests.

While Taking This Drug, Observe the Following

Foods: No restrictions. Stomach irritation can be reduced by taking aspirin with milk or after food. Supplement diet, if necessary, with no more than the recommended daily allowance of Vitamin C. Do not take large doses of Vitamin C while taking aspirin on a regular basis.

Beverages: No restrictions. It is advisable to drink a full glass of water with each dose of aspirin to reduce its irritant effect on the stomach lining.

Alcohol: No interactions expected. However, the concurrent use of alcohol and aspirin may significantly increase the possibility of erosion and ulceration of the stomach lining and result in bleeding.

Tobacco Smoking: No interactions expected.

Marijuana Smoking

Occasional (once or twice weekly): No effect to mild increase in pain relief effect of this drug.

Daily: Moderate increase in pain relief effect of this drug.

Other Drugs

Aspirin may *increase* the effects of

- oral anticoagulants, and cause abnormal bleeding. Dosage adjustment is often necessary.
- oral anti-diabetic drugs and insulin, and cause hypoglycemia (see Glossary). Dosage adjustment is often necessary.
- cortisone-like drugs, by raising their blood levels. Monitor cortisone effects to determine the need for dosage adjustment. Withdrawal of corti-

sone drugs may cause aspirin toxicity and require a reduction of aspirin dosage.
- methotrexate, and increase its toxicity on the bone marrow.
- penicillin drugs, by raising their blood levels.
- phenytoin (Dantoin, Dilantin, etc.), by raising its blood level.
- "sulfa" drugs, by raising their blood levels.

Aspirin may *decrease* the effects of
- allopurinol (Zyloprim), and reduce its effectiveness in the treatment of gout—with aspirin doses of less than 2 grams per 24 hours.
- probenecid (Benemid), and reduce its effectiveness in the treatment of gout—with aspirin doses of less than 2 grams per 24 hours.
- spironolactone (Aldactone), and impair its ability to lower the blood pressure.
- sulfinpyrazone (Anturane), and reduce its effectiveness in the treatment of gout—with aspirin doses of less than 2 grams per 24 hours.

Aspirin *taken concurrently* with
- para-aminosalicylic acid (PAS), may cause salicylate toxicity. Dosage reduction may be necessary.
- cortisone-like drugs, may increase the risk of stomach ulceration and bleeding. Monitor stomach reaction carefully.
- furosemide (Lasix), may cause aspirin toxicity.
- indomethacin (Indocin), may increase the risk of stomach ulceration and bleeding.
- phenylbutazone (Azolid, Butazolidin, etc.), may increase the risk of stomach ulceration and bleeding.

The following drug may *increase* the effects of aspirin
- Vitamin C, taken as ascorbic acid and in large doses, may acidify the urine in some individuals and cause aspirin accumulation and toxicity.

The following drugs may *decrease* the effects of aspirin
- antacid preparations may reduce the absorption of aspirin.
- phenobarbital may hasten the elimination of aspirin.
- propranolol (Inderal) may abolish aspirin's ability to reduce inflammation.
- reserpine and related drugs may reduce aspirin's ability to relieve pain.

Driving a Vehicle, Operating Machinery, Engaging in Hazardous Activities: No restrictions or precautions.

Aviation Note: Usually no restrictions. However, it is advisable to observe for the possible occurrence of mild drowsiness and to restrict activities accordingly.

Exposure to Sun: No restrictions.

Discontinuation: The use of aspirin should be discontinued completely at least 1 week before surgery of any kind.

Special Storage Instructions
Keep in a dry, tightly closed container. Keep suppositories in a cool place.

Do Not Take This Drug If
it has an odor resembling vinegar. This is due to the presence of acetic acid, and indicates the decomposition of aspirin.

ATENOLOL

Year Introduced: 1973

Brand Names

USA	Canada
Tenormin (Stuart)	None

Common Synonyms ("Street Names"):   Blood pressure pills

Drug Class: Anti-hypertensive, Beta-Adrenergic Blocker

Prescription Required: USA: Yes

Available for Purchase by Generic Name: USA: No

Available Dosage Forms and Strengths
Tablets — 50 mg., 100 mg.

Tablet May Be Crushed or Capsule Opened for Administration: Yes

How This Drug Works
Intended Therapeutic Effect(s)
Reduction of high blood pressure.
Location of Drug Action(s)
Principal sites of therapeutic actions include
- the heart pacemaker and tissues that comprise the electrical conduction system.
- the heart muscle.
- the vasomotor center in the brain that influences the control of the sympathetic nervous system over blood vessels (principally arterioles) throughout the body.
- sympathetic nerve terminals in blood vessel walls.
- the site of renin production in the kidneys.
Method of Drug Action(s)
Not completely established. By blocking certain actions of the sympathetic nervous system, this drug
- reduces the rate and the contraction force of the heart, thus lowering the ejection pressure of the blood leaving the heart.
- reduces the degree of contraction of blood vessel walls, resulting in their relaxation and expansion and consequent lowering of the blood pressure.
- inhibits the release of renin by the kidney and thus contributes further to reduction of the blood pressure.

Principal Uses of This Drug

As a Single Drug Product: The treatment of mild to moderately severe high blood pressure. This drug may be used alone or concurrently with other anti-hypertensive drugs, such as diuretics.

THIS DRUG SHOULD NOT BE TAKEN IF

—you have had an allergic reaction to it previously.

—you have Prinzmetal's type of angina (coronary artery spasm).

—you have congestive heart failure.

—you have an abnormally slow heart rate, or a serious form of heart block.

—you are taking, or have taken within the past 2 weeks, any mono-amine oxidase (MAO) inhibitor drug (see Drug Class, Section Three).

INFORM YOUR PHYSICIAN BEFORE TAKING THIS DRUG IF

—you have had an adverse reaction to any "beta-blocker" drug in the past (see Drug Class, Section Three).

—you have a history of serious heart disease, with or without episodes of heart failure.

—you have a history of hay fever (allergic rhinitis), asthma, chronic bronchitis, or emphysema.

—you have a history of overactive thyroid function (hyperthyroidism).

—you have a history of low blood sugar (hypoglycemia).

—you have a history of impaired liver or kidney function.

—you have diabetes or myasthenia gravis.

—you are currently taking any form of digitalis, quinidine or reserpine, or any "calcium-blocker" drug (see Drug Class, Section Three).

—you plan to have surgery under general anesthesia in the near future.

Time Required for Apparent Benefit

Drug action usually begins in 1 hour and reaches its peak in 2 to 4 hours. Continuous use on a regular schedule for 10 to 14 days is usually necessary to determine this drug's effectiveness in lowering the blood pressure. During this period the dosage must be carefully adjusted according to individual response. This can vary widely from person to person.

Possible Side-Effects *(natural, expected, and unavoidable drug actions)*

Lethargy and fatigability, cold hands and feet, slow heart rate, lightheadedness in upright position (see orthostatic hypotension in Glossary).

Possible Adverse Effects *(unusual, unexpected, and infrequent reactions)*

IF ANY OF THE FOLLOWING DEVELOP, DISCONTINUE DRUG AND NOTIFY YOUR PHYSICIAN AS SOON AS POSSIBLE

Mild Adverse Effects

Allergic Reactions: Skin rash

Other Reactions: Headache, dizziness, vertigo, drowsiness, increased dreaming.

Indigestion, nausea, diarrhea.

Leg pain, fluid retention (edema).

Serious Adverse Effects
Idiosyncratic Reactions: Acute behavioral disturbances: confusion, disorientation, hallucinations, amnesia, (reported for other "beta-blocker" drugs, not for atenolol to date).
Other Reactions: Reduced heart strength and reserve, precipitation of congestive heart failure.
Mental depression.
Shortness of breath, induction of bronchial asthma.
Reduction of white blood cells and blood platelets (reported for other "beta-blocker" drugs, not for atenolol to date).

Adverse Effects That May Mimic Natural Diseases or Disorders
Impaired circulation in the extremities (cold hands and feet) may resemble Raynaud's disorder.

Natural Diseases or Disorders That May Be Activated By This Drug
Prinzmetal's type of angina (coronary artery spasm), Raynaud's disease, peripheral arterial circulatory disease, possibly myasthenia gravis.

CAUTION
1. *Do not discontinue this drug suddenly* without the knowledge and guidance of your physician. Include a notation on your card of personal identification that you are taking this drug (see Table 19 and Section Six).
2. Hot weather and the fever associated with infection can reduce the blood pressure significantly, requiring adjustment of dosage.
3. Report the development of any tendency to emotional depression.

Precautions for Use by Infants and Children
Safety and effectiveness in children under 12 years of age have not been established. However, if this drug is used, observe for the development of low blood sugar (hypoglycemia) during periods of reduced food intake.

Precautions for Use by Those over 60 Years of Age
The basic rule in treating high blood pressure after 60 is to proceed *cautiously.* The elevated systolic blood pressure often present after 60 is not necessarily a threat to health, and can serve as an adaptive and compensatory change with age that should not be altered drastically. The goals of treatment must be adjusted to the natural changes in body function that occur with aging. Unacceptably high blood pressure should be reduced without creating the risks associated with excessively low blood pressure.
It is advisable to start treatment with small doses and to monitor the blood pressure response frequently. Sudden, rapid, and excessive reduction of blood pressure can predispose to stroke or heart attack.
You may be more susceptible to the development of orthostatic hypotension with resultant lightheadedness, dizziness, unsteadiness, fainting, and falling. Report such symptoms to your physician promptly.
The incidence of adverse effects from drugs of this class in those over 60 is twice that in individuals under 50 years of age. Observe for the develop-

ment of lethargy, confusion, illusions, hallucinations, unusual dreams, nightmares, urinary frequency, and loss of bladder control.

The long-term use of high doses can cause depression and worsening of circulation.

Advisability of Use During Pregnancy

Pregnancy Category: C (tentative). See Pregnancy Code inside back cover.

Animal reproduction studies reveal an increased incidence of embryo and fetal resorptions in rats, but no birth defects.

Information from adequate studies in pregnant women is not available.

Avoid use of drug during the first 3 months if possible. Avoid use during labor and delivery because of the possible effects on the newborn infant.

Advisability of Use While Nursing Infant

This drug is present in milk. Avoid drug if possible. If drug is necessary, observe nursing infant for slow heart rate and indications of low blood sugar.

Habit-Forming Potential

None.

Effects of Overdosage

With Moderate Overdose: General weakness, slow pulse, low blood pressure.

With Large Overdose: Marked drop in blood pressure, fainting, slow and weak pulse, cold and sweaty skin, congestive heart failure, possible coma and convulsions.

Possible Effects of Extended Use

Reduced reserve of heart muscle strength may result from prolonged use of high doses.

Suggested Periodic Examinations While Taking This Drug (at physician's discretion)

Complete blood cell counts, evaluations of heart function.

While Taking This Drug, Observe the Following

Foods: No restrictions. Avoid excessive salt intake. May be taken without regard to eating.

Beverages: No restrictions. May be taken with milk.

Alcohol: Use with caution until the combined effect has been determined. Alcohol may exaggerate this drug's ability to lower the blood pressure and may increase its mild sedative effect.

Tobacco Smoking: Nicotine may reduce this drug's effectiveness in treating high blood pressure. In addition, this drug may potentiate the constriction of the bronchial tubes caused by regular smoking.

Marijuana Smoking

Occasional (once or twice weekly): No effect to mild and transient increase in lethargy.

Daily: More marked and persistent drowsiness and lethargy. Possible accentuation of cold hands and feet.

Other Drugs

Atenolol may *increase* the effects of
- other anti-hypertensive drugs and cause excessive lowering of the blood pressure. Dosage adjustments may be necessary.
- other drugs with sedative effects: tranquilizers, sleep-inducers, analgesics, narcotics, etc; observe for excessive sedation.
- digitalis preparations and cause additional slowing of the heart rate.
- ergot preparations (Cafergot, etc.) and cause excessive constriction of blood vessels.
- phenothiazines and cause excessive lowering of the blood pressure.
- reserpine and cause sedation, emotional depression, and excessive lowering of the blood pressure.

Atenolol may *decrease* the effects of
- aminophylline and reduce its effectiveness in relieving asthma.
- isoproterenol (Isuprel, etc.) and reduce its effectiveness in relieving asthma.

Atenolol *taken concurrently* with
- anti-diabetic drugs (insulin, oral hypoglycemia agents) requires close monitoring to avoid undetected hypoglycemia (see Glossary).
- clonidine (Catapres) requires close monitoring for rebound high blood pressure if clonidine is withdrawn while atenolol is still being taken.
- disopyramide (Norpace) can cause serious impairment of heart function.

The following drugs may *decrease* the effects of atenolol
- aluminum hydroxide gel (ALternaGEL, Amphojel, etc.) may inhibit its absorption.
- indomethacin (Indocin) and other "aspirin substitutes" (prostaglandin inhibitors) may impair atenolol's anti-hypertensive effect.

Driving a Vehicle, Operating Machinery, Engaging in Hazardous Activities: Caution advised until the full extent of drowsiness, lethargy, and blood pressure change has been determined.

Aviation Note: The use of this drug and the disorder for which this drug is prescribed *are disqualifications* for the piloting of aircraft. Consultation with a designated Aviation Medical Examiner is advised.

Exposure to Sun: No restrictions.

Exposure to Heat: Caution advised. Hot environments can induce lowering of the blood pressure and exaggerate the effects of this drug.

Exposure to Cold: Caution advised. Cold environments can enhance the circulatory deficiency in the extremities caused by this drug. The elderly should take precautions to prevent hypothermia.

Heavy Exercise or Exertion: It is advisable to avoid exertion that produces lightheadedness, excessive fatigue, or muscle cramping. The use of this drug may intensify the hypertensive response to isometric exercise.

Occurrence of Unrelated Illness: The fever that accompanies systemic infections can lower the blood pressure and require adjustment of dosage. Illnesses that cause nausea or vomiting may interrupt the regular dosage schedule. Ask your physician for guidance.

Discontinuation: It is advisable to avoid sudden discontinuation of this drug in all situations. If possible, gradual reduction of dose over a period of 2 or more weeks is recommended. Ask your physician for specific guidance.

Special Storage Instructions
Keep in a dry, tightly closed container at room temperature. Protect from light, excessive heat and moisture.

ATROPINE
(Belladonna, Hyoscyamine, Scopolamine)

Year Introduced: 1831 (Belladonna preparations have been in use for many centuries)

Brand Names

USA	Canada
Barbidonna [CD] (Mallinckrodt)	Isopto Atropine (Alcon)
Belladenal [CD] (Sandoz)	SMP Atropine (Cooper Vision)
Bellergal [CD] (Dorsey)	Belladenal [CD] (Sandoz)
Bellergal-S [CD] (Dorsey)	Bellergal [CD] (Sandoz)
Butibel [CD] (McNeil)	Donnagel [CD] (Robins)
Chardonna-2 [CD] (Rorer)	Donnagel-PG [CD] (Robins)
Donnagel [CD] (Robins)	Donnagel w/Neomycin [CD] (Robins)
Donnagel-PG [CD] (Robins)	Donnatal [CD] (Robins)
Donnatal [CD] (Robins)	Donnazyme [CD] (Robins)
Kinesed [CD] (Stuart)	(Numerous other combination brand names)
Urised [CD] (Webcon)	
(Numerous other combination brand names)	

Common Synonyms ("Street Names"):   Stomach relaxer

Drug Class: Antispasmodic; Atropine-like Drug [Anticholinergics]

Prescription Required: USA: For low-strength formulations—No
For high-strength formulations—Yes
Canada: No

Available for Purchase by Generic Name: Yes

Available Dosage Forms and Strengths
Numerous combination drugs are available in a wide variety of dosage forms and strengths including tablets, capsules, prolonged-action forms, elixirs, suspensions, eye drops, etc.

Tablet May Be Crushed or Capsule Opened for Administration
Regular tablets and capsules — Yes
Prolonged-action forms — No
Belladenal-S and Bellergal-S — No
Contac — Yes, but do not crush or chew contents

How This Drug Works
Intended Therapeutic Effect(s):   Relief of discomfort associated with
- excessive activity and spasm of the digestive tract (esophagus, stomach, intestine, colon and gall bladder).
- irritation and spasm of the lower urinary tract (bladder and urethra).
- painful menstruation (cramping of the uterus).

Location of Drug Action(s):   The terminal nerve fibers of the parasympathetic nervous system that control the activity of the gastrointestinal tract and the genitourinary tract.

Method of Drug Action(s):   By blocking the action of the chemical (acetylcholine) that transmits impulses at parasympathetic nerve endings, this drug prevents stimulation of muscular contraction and glandular secretion within the organs involved. This results in reduced overall activity, including the prevention or relief of muscle spasm.

Principal Uses of This Drug
As a Single Drug Product: Used primarily for its antispasmodic effect in the treatment of spastic disorders of the digestive tract and lower urinary tract.

As a Combination Drug Product [CD]:   Frequently combined with mild sedatives (especially barbiturates) to utilize their calming effect in the management of functional disorders associated with anxiety and nervous tension. The combination of a mild tranquilizer and an antispasmodic medication is more effective than either drug used alone.

THIS DRUG SHOULD NOT BE TAKEN IF
—you have had an allergic reaction or unfavorable response to any atropine or belladonna preparation in the past.
—your stomach cannot empty properly into the intestine (pyloric obstruction).
—you are unable to empty the urinary bladder completely.
—you have glaucoma (narrow-angle type).
—you have severe ulcerative colitis.

INFORM YOUR PHYSICIAN BEFORE TAKING THIS DRUG IF
—you have glaucoma (open-angle type).
—you have angina or coronary heart disease.
—you have chronic bronchitis.
—you have a hiatal hernia.
—you have enlargement of the prostate gland.
—you have myasthenia gravis.
—you have a history of peptic ulcer disease.
—you plan to have surgery under general anesthesia in the near future.

Time Required for Apparent Benefit
Drug action begins in 1 to 2 hours and persists for approximately 4 hours.

Possible Side-Effects *(natural, expected, and unavoidable drug actions)*
Blurring of vision (impairment of focus), dryness of the mouth and throat, constipation, hesitancy in urination. (Nature and degree of side-effects depend upon individual susceptibility and drug dosage.)

Possible Adverse Effects *(unusual, unexpected, and infrequent reactions)*
IF ANY OF THE FOLLOWING DEVELOP, DISCONTINUE DRUG AND NOTIFY YOUR PHYSICIAN AS SOON AS POSSIBLE

Mild Adverse Effects
Allergic Reactions: Skin rash, hives.
Other Reactions
Dilation of pupils, causing sensitivity to light.
Flushing and dryness of the skin (reduced sweating).
Rapid heart action.
Lightheadedness, dizziness, unsteady gait.

Serious Adverse Effects
Idiosyncratic Reactions: Acute confusion, delirium, and behavioral abnormalities.
Other Reactions: Development of acute glaucoma (in susceptible individuals).

CAUTION
Many over-the-counter medications (see OTC drugs in Glossary) for allergies, colds, and coughs contain drugs that can interact unfavorably with this drug. Ask your physician or pharmacist for guidance before using any such medication.

Precautions for Use by Those over 60 Years of Age
You may be more sensitive to all of the actions of this drug. Small doses are advisable until your individual response has been determined.
This drug can increase the degree of impaired urination associated with prostate gland enlargement (prostatism).

Advisability of Use During Pregnancy
Pregnancy Category: B (tentative). See Pregnancy Code inside back cover.
Animal reproduction studies reveal significant birth defects due to this drug.
Information from studies in pregnant women indicates no association between defects and 1198 exposures to this drug.
Avoid completely during first 3 months.
Ask physician for guidance.

Advisability of Use While Nursing Infant
This drug may impair the formation of milk and make nursing difficult.
Sufficient quantities of drug may be present in the milk to affect the infant.
Avoid drug or avoid nursing as directed by your physician.

Habit-Forming Potential
None.

Effects of Overdosage
With Moderate Overdose: Marked dryness of the mouth, dilated pupils, blurring of near vision, rapid pulse, heart palpitation, headache, difficulty in urination.
With Large Overdose: Extremely dilated pupils, rapid pulse and breathing, hot skin, high fever, excitement, confusion, hallucinations, delirium, eventual loss of consciousness, convulsions, and coma.

Possible Effects of Extended Use
Chronic constipation, severe enough to result in fecal impaction. (Constipation should be treated promptly with effective laxatives.)

Suggested Periodic Examinations While Taking This Drug (at physician's discretion)
Measurement of internal eye pressure to detect any significant increase that could indicate developing glaucoma.

While Taking This Drug, Observe the Following
Foods: No interaction with drug. Effectiveness is greater if drug is taken one-half to 1 hour before eating. Follow diet prescribed for condition under treatment.
Beverages: No interactions. Follow prescribed diet.
Alcohol: No interactions expected with this drug. Follow physician's advice regarding use of alcohol (based upon its effect on the condition under treatment).
Tobacco Smoking: No interactions expected. Follow physician's advice regarding smoking.
Marijuana Smoking
Occasional (once or twice weekly):   Mild increase in drowsiness and dryness of mouth.
Daily: Moderate to marked increase in drowsiness and dryness of mouth.
Other Drugs
Atropine may *increase* the effects of
• all other drugs having atropine-like actions (see Drug Class, Section Three).

Atropine may *decrease* the effects of
• pilocarpine eye drops, and reduce their effectiveness in lowering internal eye pressure in the treatment of glaucoma.

Atropine *taken concurrently* with
• mono-amine oxidase (MAO) inhibitor drugs, may cause an exaggerated response to normal doses of atropine-like drugs. It is best to avoid atropine-like drugs for 2 weeks after the last dose of any MAO inhibitor drug (see Drug Class, Section Three).
• haloperidol (Haldol), may significantly increase internal eye pressure (dangerous in glaucoma).

The following drugs may *increase* the effects of atropine
- tricyclic antidepressants
- those antihistamines that have an atropine-like action
- meperidine (Demerol, pethidine)
- methylphenidate (Ritalin)
- orphenadrine (Disipal, Norflex)
- those phenothiazines that have an atropine-like action (see Drug Class, Section Three).

The following drug may *decrease* the effects of atropine
- Vitamin C reduces its effectiveness by hastening its elimination from the body. Avoid large doses of Vitamin C during treatment with this drug.

Driving a Vehicle, Operating Machinery, Engaging in Hazardous Activities: This drug may produce blurred vision, drowsiness, or dizziness. Avoid hazardous activities if these drug effects occur.

Aviation Note: The use of this drug *is a disqualification* for the piloting of aircraft. Consultation with a designated Aviation Medical Examiner is advised.

Exposure to Sun: No restrictions.

Exposure to Heat: Use extreme caution. The use of this drug in hot environments may significantly increase the risk of heat stroke.

Heavy Exercise or Exertion: Use caution in warm or hot environments. This drug may impair normal perspiration (heat loss) and interfere with the regulation of body temperature.

Special Storage Instructions
Keep in a tightly closed container. Protect from light.

BACAMPICILLIN

Note: This is an Abbreviated Drug Profile of a modified member of the penicillin class of drugs, namely ampicillin. During its absorption from the gastrointestinal tract, bacampicillin is converted to ampicillin. However, the unique chemical modification that characterizes bacampicillin permits its more rapid and complete absorption than ampicillin. When given in equivalent doses, bacampicillin provides peak blood levels that are 3 times the levels provided by unmodified ampicillin. Thus bacampicillin can be effective when given every 12 hours; ampicillin requires a dosage schedule of every 6 hours.

The information categories provided in this abbreviated Profile are appropriate for bacampicillin. For specific information that is normally found in those categories that have been omitted from this Profile, the reader is referred to the Drug Profile of ampicillin.

Year Introduced: 1979

Brand Names

USA	Canada
Spectrobid (Roerig)	None

Common Synonyms ("Street Names"):   Penicillin pills

Drug Class: Anti-infectives, Penicillins

Prescription Required: USA: Yes

Available for Purchase by Generic Name: USA: No

Available Dosage Forms and Strengths
Tablets — 400 mg.
Oral Suspension — 125 mg. per teaspoonful (5 ml.)

Tablet May Be Crushed or Capsule Opened for Administration: Yes

Principal Uses of This Drug
As a Single Drug Product: To treat certain infections of the skin and soft tissues, of the upper and lower respiratory tract, and of the genito-urinary tract, including gonorrhea.

While Taking This Drug, Observe the Following
Foods: No restrictions. The tablets may be taken without regard to eating. The oral suspension should be taken on an empty stomach.
Other Drugs
Bacampicillin *taken concurrently* with
• allopurinol (Zyloprim) substantially increases the incidence of skin rash.
• disulfiram (Antabuse) can cause a disulfiram-like reaction (see Glossary). Avoid the concurrent use of these two drugs.

The following drugs may *decrease* the effects of bacampicillin
• chloramphenicol (Chloromycetin).
• erythromycins (Erythrocin, E-Mycin, etc.).

• sulfonamides ("Sulfa" drugs, see Drug Class, Section Three).
• tetracyclines (see Drug Class, Section Three).

Special Storage Instructions
Keep the tablets in a dry, tightly closed container.
Keep the oral suspension in the refrigerator; do not freeze.

Observe the Following Expiration Times
The oral suspension must be stored under refrigeration and discarded after 10 days.

BECLOMETHASONE

Year Introduced: 1976

Brand Names

USA	Canada
Beclovent Inhaler (Glaxo)	Beclovent Inhaler (A&H)
Beconase Nasal Inhaler (Glaxo)	Beconase Nasal Spray (A&H)
Vancenase Nasal Inhaler (Schering)	Vancenase Nasal Inhaler (Schering)
Vanceril Inhaler (Schering)	Vanceril Oral Inhaler (Schering)

Common Synonyms ("Street Names"):   Asthma inhaler

Drug Class: Anti-allergic, Anti-asthmatic, Cortisone-like Drug, Adrenocortical Steroids

Prescription Required: Yes

Available for Purchase by Generic Name: No

Available Dosage Forms and Strengths
Nasal Inhaler — 10 mg. (200 doses of 50 mcg. each)
Oral Inhaler — 8.4 mg. (200 doses of 42 mcg. each)

How This Drug Works
Intended Therapeutic Effect(s): The control of allergic rhinitis, and of bronchial asthma in those individuals who require the continuous use of cortisone-like drugs to reduce the frequency and severity of asthmatic attacks.

Location of Drug Action(s): Those tissues that line the nasal passages, mouth, trachea, and bronchial tubes.

Method of Drug Action(s):   Not established. One possibility is that by increasing the amount of cyclic AMP in appropriate tissues, this drug may thereby increase the concentration of epinephrine, which is an effective bronchodilator and anti-asthmatic. Additional benefit may be due to the drug's ability to reduce local inflammation in the bronchial tubes.

Principal Uses of This Drug

As a Single Drug Product: Used primarily to treat bronchial asthma in those individuals who do not respond to bronchodilators and who require cortisone-like drugs for asthma control. This inhalation dosage form is significantly more advantageous than cortisone taken by mouth (swallowed) or by injection in that it works locally on the tissues of the respiratory tract and does not require absorption and systemic distribution. This prevents the more serious adverse effects that usually result from the long-term use of cortisone taken for systemic use.

THIS DRUG SHOULD NOT BE TAKEN IF

—you have had an allergic reaction to any of the drugs bearing the brand names listed above.

—you are experiencing severe acute asthma or status asthmaticus that requires more intensive treatment for prompt relief.

—your asthma can be controlled by bronchodilators and other anti-asthmatic drugs that are not related to cortisone.

—your asthma requires cortisone-like drugs infrequently for control.

—you have a form of non-allergic bronchitis with asthmatic features.

INFORM YOUR PHYSICIAN BEFORE TAKING THIS DRUG IF

—you are now taking or have recently taken any cortisone-related drugs (including ACTH by injection) for any reason (see Drug Class, Section Three).

—you have a history of tuberculosis of the lungs.

—you have bronchiectasis.

—you think you may have an active infection of any kind, especially a respiratory infection.

Time Required for Apparent Benefit

Continuous use on a regular schedule for 1 to 4 weeks is usually necessary to determine this drug's effectiveness in relieving allergic rhinitis or chronic asthma and improving breathing.

Possible Side-Effects *(natural, expected, and unavoidable drug actions)*

Fungus infections (thrush) of the mouth and throat.

Note: The risk of this development can be reduced by thoroughly rinsing the mouth and gargling with water after each inhalation of the drug.

Possible Adverse Effects *(unusual, unexpected, and infrequent reactions)*

IF ANY OF THE FOLLOWING DEVELOP, DISCONTINUE DRUG AND NOTIFY YOUR PHYSICIAN AS SOON AS POSSIBLE

Mild Adverse Effects

Allergic Reactions: Skin rash (rare).

Other Reactions: Dryness of the mouth, hoarseness, sore throat.

Serious Adverse Effects
 Allergic Reactions: Localized areas of "allergic" pneumonitis (lung inflammation).
 Idiosyncratic Reactions: None reported.
 Other Reactions: Bronchospasm, asthmatic wheezing (rare).

Natural Diseases or Disorders That May Be Activated by This Drug

Cortisone-related drugs that have systemic effects can impair immunity and lead to the reactivation of "healed" or quiescent tuberculosis of the lungs. Individuals with a history of tuberculosis must be observed closely during use of this drug by inhalation.

CAUTION

1. This drug does not act primarily as a bronchodilator and should not be relied upon for the immediate relief of acute asthma.
2. If you were using any cortisone-related drugs for treatment of your asthma *before* transferring to this inhaler-drug, it may be necessary to resume the former cortisone-related drug if you experience injury or infection of any kind, or if you require surgery. Be sure to notify your attending physician of your prior use of cortisone-related drugs taken either by mouth or by injection.
3. If you experience a return of severe asthma while using this drug, notify your physician immediately so that additional supportive treatment with cortisone-related drugs by mouth or injection can be provided as needed.
4. It is advisable to carry a card of personal identification with a notation (if applicable) that you have used cortisone-related drugs within the past year. During periods of stress it may be necessary to resume cortisone treatment in adequate dosage.
5. The adult daily dose of this drug should not exceed 20 inhalations.
6. An interval of approximately 5 to 10 minutes should separate the inhalation of bronchodilators such as epinephrine, isoetharine, or isoproterenol (which should be used first) and the inhalation of this drug. This sequence will permit greater penetration of beclomethasone into the bronchial tubes. The delay between inhalations will also reduce the possibility of adverse effects from the propellants used in the two inhalers.

Precautions for Use by Infants and Children

The maximal daily dose in children 6 to 12 years of age should not exceed 10 inhalations.
Use of this drug in children under 6 years of age is not recommended.

Precautions for Use by Those over 60 Years of Age

Individuals with bronchiectasis should be observed closely for the development of lung infections.

Advisability of Use During Pregnancy

Pregnancy Category: C (tentative). See Pregnancy Code inside back cover.
 Animal reproduction studies in mice, rats, and rabbits reveal significant birth defects due to this drug.

Information from adequate studies in pregnant women is not available.

Ask physician for guidance.

Advisability of Use While Nursing Infant
This drug is probably present in the mother's milk. It is advisable to avoid use of this drug or to refrain from breast-feeding.

Habit-Forming Potential
With recommended dosage a state of functional dependence (see Glossary) is not likely to develop.

Effects of Overdosage
With Moderate Overdose: Increased risk of fungus infections of the mouth, throat, and air passages.

With Large Overdose: Indications of cortisone excess—fluid retention, flushing of the face, nervousness, stomach irritation.

Possible Effects of Extended Use
Unknown at this time.

Suggested Periodic Examinations While Taking This Drug (at physician's discretion)
Inspection of nose, mouth, and throat for evidence of fungus infection (thrush).

Assessment of status of adrenal function in individuals who have used cortisone-related drugs over an extended period prior to using this drug.

X-ray examination of the lungs of individuals with a prior history of tuberculosis.

While Taking This Drug, Observe the Following
Foods: No specific restrictions beyond those advised by your physician. Timing of Drug and Food: May be used without regard to time of eating.

Nutritional Support: No specific requirements.

Beverages: No specific restrictions beyond those advised by your physician.

Alcohol: No interactions expected.

Tobacco Smoking: No interactions expected. However, smoking can affect the condition under treatment and reduce the effectiveness of this drug. Follow your physician's advice.

Marijuana Smoking

Occasional (once or twice weekly): No effect to mild and transient improvement in breathing.

Daily: Unpredictable. Irritant effects of continued smoking may reduce beneficial effects of drug.

Other Drugs

Beclomethasone may *increase* the effects of

• other antiasthmatic drugs (see Drug Class, Section Three).

The following drugs may *increase* the effects of beclomethasone:
- inhalant bronchodilators—epinephrine, isoetharine, and isoproterenol.
- oral bronchodilators—aminophylline, ephedrine, terbutaline, theophylline, etc.

Driving a Vehicle, Operating Machinery, Engaging in Hazardous Activities: Usually no restrictions. However, it is advisable to observe for the rare occurrence of paradoxical asthma and to restrict activities accordingly.

Aviation Note: The use of this drug and the disorder for which this drug is prescribed *may be disqualifications* for the piloting of aircraft. Consultation with a designated Aviation Medical Examiner is advised.

Exposure to Sun: No restrictions.

Exposure to Heat: No restrictions.

Exposure to Cold: No restrictions.

Heavy Exercise or Exertion: No interactions with drug. However, excessive exertion can induce asthma in sensitive individuals.

Occurrence of Unrelated Illness: Acute infections, serious injuries, and surgical procedures can create an urgent need for the administration of additional supportive cortisone-related drugs given by mouth and/or injection. Notify your physician immediately in the event of new illness or injury of any kind.

Discontinuation: If the regular use of this drug has made it possible to reduce or discontinue maintenance doses of cortisone-like drugs by mouth, do not discontinue this drug abruptly. If you find it necessary to discontinue this drug for any reason, consult your physician promptly. It may be necessary to resume cortisone preparations and to institute other measures for satisfactory management.

Special Storage Instructions

Store at room temperature. Avoid exposure to temperatures above 120°F. (49°C.). Do not store or use this inhaler near heat or open flame. Protect from light.

BENZTROPINE

Year Introduced: 1954

Brand Names

USA	Canada
Cogentin (Merck Sharp & Dohme)	Apo-Benztropine (Apotex)
	Bensylate (ICN)
	Cogentin (MSD)

Common Synonyms ("Street Names"):   None

Drug Class: Anti-parkinsonism; Atropine-like Drug (Anticholinergics)

Prescription Required: USA: Yes   Canada: No

Available for Purchase by Generic Name: No

Available Dosage Forms and Strengths
　　Tablets — 0.5 mg., 1 mg., 2 mg.
　　Injection — 1 mg. per ml.

Tablet May Be Crushed or Capsule Opened for Administration: Yes

How This Drug Works
　　Intended Therapeutic Effect(s):   Relief of the rigidity, tremor, sluggish movement, and impaired gait associated with Parkinson's disease.
　　Location of Drug Action(s):   The principal site of the desired therapeutic action is the regulating center in the brain (the basal ganglia) which governs the coordination and efficiency of bodily movements.
　　Method of Drug Action(s):   The improvement in Parkinson's disease results from the restoration of a more normal balance of the chemical activities responsible for the transmission of nerve impulses within the basal ganglia.

Principal Uses of This Drug
　　As a Single Drug Product: Used adjunctively in the management of all types of parkinsonism to relieve the characteristic rigidity, tremor, and sluggish movement. Should it fail to provide adequate relief, it may be supplemented with more potent drugs such as levodopa or bromocriptine. This drug is also used to control the parkinsonian reactions that can result from the use of certain antipsychotic drugs, such as the phenothiazines and related compounds.

THIS DRUG SHOULD NOT BE TAKEN IF
—you have had an allergic reaction to any dosage form of it previously.
—it is prescribed for a child under 3 years of age.

INFORM YOUR PHYSICIAN BEFORE TAKING THIS DRUG IF
—you have experienced an unfavorable response to atropine or atropine-like drugs in the past.
—you have glaucoma.
—you have high blood pressure or heart disease.
—you have a history of liver or kidney disease.
—you have difficulty emptying the urinary bladder.

Time Required for Apparent Benefit
　　Drug action begins in 1 to 2 hours and persists for approximately 24 hours. Daily dosage may be cumulative in some individuals. Regular use for 2 to 4 weeks may be needed to determine optimal dosage schedule.

Possible Side-Effects (*natural, expected, and unavoidable drug actions*)
　　Nervousness, blurring of vision, dryness of the mouth, constipation. (These often subside as drug use continues.)

Possible Adverse Effects *(unusual, unexpected, and infrequent reactions)*

IF ANY OF THE FOLLOWING DEVELOP, DISCONTINUE DRUG AND NOTIFY YOUR PHYSICIAN AS SOON AS POSSIBLE

Mild Adverse Effects
  Allergic Reactions: Skin rashes.
  Other Reactions
    Drowsiness, dizziness, headache.
    Nausea, vomiting.
    Urinary hesitancy, difficulty emptying bladder.
Serious Adverse Effects
  Idiosyncratic Reactions: Confusion, delusions, hallucinations, agitation, abnormal behavior.

CAUTION
Many over-the-counter (OTC) medications for allergies, colds, and coughs contain drugs that can interact unfavorably with this drug. Ask your physician or pharmacist for guidance before using any such medications.

Precautions for Use by Those over 60 Years of Age
You may be more sensitive to all of the actions of this drug. Small doses are advisable until your individual response has been determined.
This drug can increase the degree of impaired urination associated with prostate gland enlargement (prostatism).
You may be more susceptible to the development of impaired thinking, confusion, nightmares, and hallucinations. Careful dosage adjustments are mandatory.

Advisability of Use During Pregnancy
Pregnancy Category: C (tentative). See Pregnancy Code inside back cover.
  Animal reproduction studies: No data available.
  Information from adequate studies in pregnant women is not available. Ask physician for guidance.

Advisability of Use While Nursing Infant
Presence of drug in milk is not known. Safety for infant not established. Ask physician for guidance.

Habit-Forming Potential
None.

Effects of Overdosage
With Moderate Overdose: Drowsiness, stupor, weakness, impaired vision, rapid pulse.
With Large Overdose: Excitement, confusion, agitation, hallucinations, dry and hot skin, generalized skin rash, markedly dilated pupils.

Possible Effects of Extended Use
Increased internal eye pressure—possibly glaucoma.

Suggested Periodic Examinations While Taking This Drug (at physician's discretion)
Measurement of internal eye pressure at regular intervals.

While Taking This Drug, Observe the Following
Foods: No restrictions. Drug may be taken after food if it causes indigestion.
Beverages: No restrictions.
Alcohol: No interactions expected.
Tobacco Smoking: No interactions expected.
Marijuana Smoking
Occasional (once or twice weekly): Mild increase in drowsiness and dryness of mouth.
Daily: Moderate to marked increase in drowsiness and dryness of mouth.
Other Drugs
Benztropine may *increase* the effects of
- levodopa (Dopar, Larodopa, etc.), and improve its effectiveness in the treatment of parkinsonism.
- the mild and strong tranquilizers, and cause excessive sedation.

Benztropine *taken concurrently* with
- cortisone (and related drugs), on an extended basis, may cause an increase in internal eye pressure—possibly glaucoma.
- primidone (Mysoline), may cause excessive sedation.
- a phenothiazine drug, may cause (in sensitive individuals) severe behavioral disturbances (toxic psychosis).

The following drugs may *increase* the effects of benztropine:
- antihistamines may add to the dryness of mouth and throat.
- tricyclic antidepressants may add to the effects on the eye and further increase internal eye pressure (dangerous in glaucoma).
- mono-amine oxidase (MAO) inhibitor drugs may intensify all effects of this drug (see Drug Family, Section Three).
- meperidine (Demerol)
- methylphenidate (Ritalin)
- orphenadrine (Disipal, Norflex)
- quinidine

Driving a Vehicle, Operating Machinery, Engaging in Hazardous Activities: Drowsiness and dizziness may occur in sensitive individuals. Avoid hazardous activities until full effects and tolerance have been determined.
Aviation Note: The use of this drug *is a disqualification* for the piloting of aircraft. Consultation with a designated Aviation Medical Examiner is advised.
Exposure to Sun: No restrictions.
Exposure to Heat: Use caution. This drug may reduce sweating, cause an increase in body temperature, and contribute to the development of heat stroke.
Heavy Exercise or Exertion: Avoid in hot environments.

Discontinuation: Do not discontinue this drug suddenly. Ask physician for guidance in reducing dose gradually.

Special Storage Instructions
Keep in a dry, tightly closed container. Protect from light.

BROMOCRIPTINE

Year Introduced: 1975

Brand Names

USA	Canada
Parlodel (Sandoz)	Parlodel (Sandoz)

Common Synonyms ("Street Names"):   None

Drug Class: Anti-Parkinsonism, Dopamine Agonist, Ergot Derivative

Prescription Required: USA: Yes   Canada: Yes

Available for Purchase by Generic Name: USA: No   Canada: No

Available Dosage Forms and Strengths
Tablets — 2.5 mg.
Capsules — 5 mg.

Tablet May Be Crushed or Capsule Opened for Administration: Yes

How This Drug Works
Intended Therapeutic Effect(s)
Reduction of the rigidity, tremor, sluggish movement, and gait disturbances characteristic of Parkinson's disease.
Prevention of milk production following childbirth.
Restoration of normal menstrual cycles and fertility in women with abnormally high production of the pituitary hormone prolactin.
Location of Drug Action(s)
Principal sites include
- a regulating center in the brain (the corpus striatum) that governs the coordination and efficiency of bodily movements.
- the cells of the anterior pituitary gland in the brain that produce the hormone prolactin.
Method of Drug Action(s)
By directly stimulating the dopamine receptor sites in the corpus striatum, this drug helps to offset the deficiency of dopamine that is responsible for the symptoms of Parkinson's disease.
By inhibiting the production of the hormone prolactin by the anterior pituitary gland, this drug

- reduces the amount of prolactin in the blood to below the level required to stimulate the breast glands to produce milk.
- reduces the abnormally high levels of prolactin in the blood, restoring it to normal levels that permit menstrual regularity and fertility.

Principal Uses of This Drug

As a Single Drug Product: This drug is used primarily to

1. Treat the manifestations of Parkinson's disease. It may be used as the initial drug in treating those with early-stage symptoms. More often it is used in conjunction with levodopa when it is found that levodopa is losing its effectiveness, or the patient cannot tolerate the adverse effects of levodopa and dosage reduction or withdrawal is necessary.
2. Suppress the production of milk and thereby prevent the breast congestion and engorgement that normally follow childbirth.
3. Treat those disorders that are due to excessive production of prolactin by the pituitary gland, mainly absence of menstruation, infertility, and inappropriate production of milk.

THIS DRUG SHOULD NOT BE TAKEN IF

—you have had an allergic reaction to it previously.
—you have had an adverse effect from any ergot preparation in the past.
—you have severe coronary artery disease or peripheral vascular disease.
—you are pregnant.

INFORM YOUR PHYSICIAN BEFORE TAKING THIS DRUG IF

—you have constitutionally low blood pressure.
—you are taking any anti-hypertensive drugs or phenothiazines (see Drug Class, Section Three).
—you have any degree of coronary artery disease, especially with a history of a "heart attack" (myocardial infarction).
—you have a history of heart rhythm abnormalities.
—you have impaired liver function.
—you have a seizure disorder.

Time Required for Apparent Benefit

Improvement may occur within the first 2 to 4 weeks. However, regular use for 3 to 4 months, with careful dosage adjustments, may be necessary to determine this drug's maximal effectiveness.

Possible Side-Effects *(natural, expected, and unavoidable drug actions)*

Fatigue, lethargy, lightheadedness in upright position (see orthostatic hypotension in Glossary).

Possible Adverse Effects *(unusual, unexpected, and infrequent reactions)*

IF ANY OF THE FOLLOWING DEVELOP, DISCONTINUE DRUG AND NOTIFY YOUR PHYSICIAN AS SOON AS POSSIBLE

Mild Adverse Effects

Allergic Reactions: Skin rash.
Other Reactions: Headache, dizziness, fainting, nervousness, nightmares.

Loss of appetite, nausea, vomiting, abdominal cramps, constipation, diarrhea, nasal congestion, dry mouth.

Serious Adverse Effects
Abnormal, involuntary movements, confusion, hallucinations, incoordination, visual disturbances, depression, epileptic-like seizures.
Swelling of the feet and ankles (edema).
Loss of urinary bladder control, inability to empty bladder.
Indications of "ergotism": numbness and tingling of fingers, cold hands and feet, muscle cramps of legs and feet.

Natural Diseases or Disorders That May Be Activated By This Drug
Coronary artery disease with anginal syndrome. Raynaud's syndrome.

CAUTION
1. During treatment to reduce the blood level of prolactin and restore normal menstruation and fertility, it is mandatory that you use a barrier method of contraception to prevent pregnancy. Oral contraceptives should not be used while taking bromocriptine.
2. If pregnancy occurs, discontinue this drug immediately and notify your physician.
3. During treatment of parkinsonism, avoid excessive and hurried activity as improvement occurs; this will reduce the risk of falls and injuries.

Precautions for Use by Infants and Children
Safety and effectiveness in children under 15 years of age have not been established.

Precautions for Use by Those over 60 Years of Age
You may be more sensitive to the actions of this drug.
Small doses are advisable until your individual response has been determined.
You may be more susceptible to the development of impaired thinking, confusion, agitation, nightmares, and hallucinations. Close monitoring and careful dosage adjustments are mandatory.

Advisability of Use During Pregnancy
Pregnancy Category: X (tentative). See Pregnancy Code inside back cover.
Serious birth defects have been reported in infants whose mothers took this drug during early pregnancy. Because the incidence of these defects (3.3%) does not exceed that reported for the general population, a cause-and-effect relationship is uncertain.
Until further studies clarify this issue, it is recommended that this drug not be taken during the entire pregnancy.

Advisability of Use While Nursing Infant
This drug prevents the production of milk and makes nursing impossible.

Habit-Forming Potential
None.

Effects of Overdosage
With Moderate Overdose: Weakness, low blood pressure, nausea, vomiting, diarrhea.

With Large Overdose: Confusion, agitation, hallucinations, loss of consciousness.

Possible Effects of Extended Use
Drug-induced changes in the lung tissue, thickening of the pleura, and pleural effusion (fluid formation). These effects appear to be reversible after discontinuation of the drug.

Suggested Periodic Examinations While Taking This Drug (at physician's discretion)
Complete blood cell counts.
Evaluations of heart, liver and kidney functions.

While Taking This Drug, Observe the Following
Foods: No restrictions. Take this drug with meals or food.

Beverages: No restrictions. May be taken with milk.

Alcohol: Use caution until the combined effects have been determined. Alcohol can exaggerate the blood pressure-lowering effect of this drug.

Tobacco Smoking: No interactions expected.

Marijuana Smoking
Occasional (once or twice weekly): No effect to mild increase in fatigue and lethargy.

Daily: Moderate to marked increase in lethargy; possible accentuation of orthostatic hypotension.

Other Drugs
Bromocriptine *taken concurrently* with
- anti-hypertensive drugs (and other drugs that can lower the blood pressure) requires careful monitoring for excessive drops in pressure. Dosage adjustments may be necessary.

The following drugs may *decrease* the effects of bromocriptine:
- phenothiazines may reduce the effectiveness of bromocriptine (see Drug Class, Section Three). Avoid the concurrent use of these drugs.

Driving a Vehicle, Operating Machinery, Engaging in Hazardous Activities: Be alert to the possible occurrence of orthostatic hypotension, dizziness, or impaired coordination. Be prepared to stop and lie down to prevent fainting.

Aviation Note: Parkinsonism *is a disqualification* for the piloting of aircraft. Consultation with a designated Aviation Medical Examiner is advised.

Exposure to Sun: No restrictions.

Exposure to Heat: Caution advised. Hot environments can lower the blood pressure and exaggerate this drug's effect.

Discontinuation: When used to treat Parkinson's disease, safety has not been established for continuous use beyond 2 years. When used to prevent milk production following childbirth, limit treatment to 21 days or less. When used to restore normal menstruation and fertility, the duration of treatment should not exceed 6 months.

Special Storage Instructions

Keep tablets and capsules in a dry, tightly closed container at room temperature. Protect from light.

BROMPHENIRAMINE

Year Introduced: 1957

Brand Names

USA	Canada
Dimetane (Robins)	Dimetane (Robins)
Veltane (Lannett)	Dimetapp [CD] (Robins)
Dimetapp [CD] (Robins)	
Disophrol [CD]* (Schering)	
Drixoral [CD]* (Schering)	
(Numerous other brand and combination brand names)	

Common Synonyms ("Street Names"):   Allergy pills

Drug Class: Antihistamines

Prescription Required: for 4 mg. tablet and elixir—No
for prolonged-action tablets—Yes

Available for Purchase by Generic Name: USA: Yes   Canada: No

Available Dosage Forms and Strengths

Tablets — 4 mg.
Prolonged-action tablets — 8 mg., 12 mg.
Elixir — 2 mg. per teaspoonful (5 ml.)
Injection — 10 mg. per ml.

Tablet May Be Crushed or Capsule Opened for Administration

Regular tablets — Yes
Prolonged-action tablets — No
Dimetapp and Disophrol Chronotab — No
Drixoral — No

*Contains dexbrompheniramine, which has the same actions as brompheniramine.

How This Drug Works

Intended Therapeutic Effect(s): Relief of symptoms associated with hayfever (allergic rhinitis) and with allergic reactions in the skin, such as itching, swelling, hives, and rash.

Location of Drug Action(s): Those hypersensitive tissues that release excessive histamine as part of an allergic reaction. The principal tissue sites are the eyes, the nose, and the skin.

Method of Drug Action(s): This drug reduces the intensity of the allergic response by blocking the action of histamine after it has been released from sensitized tissue cells.

Principal Uses of This Drug

As a Single Drug Product: Used primarily to provide symptomatic relief in allergic and related disorders: seasonal and perennial allergic rhinitis (hay fever), allergic conjunctivitis, and vasomotor rhinitis; also in hives and localized swellings (angioedema) of allergic origin. This drug is not effective in the treatment of allergically-induced bronchial asthma.

As a Combination Drug Product [CD]: Often combined with decongestant drugs to enhance their ability to reduce tissue swelling and secretions in allergic and infectious disorders of the upper respiratory tract. Also combined with decongestants, expectorants, and codeine to increase their effectiveness in the symptomatic treatment of allergic and infectious disorders of the lower respiratory tract, often with associated coughing.

THIS DRUG SHOULD NOT BE TAKEN IF

—you have had an allergic reaction to any dosage form of it previously.
—it is prescribed for a newborn infant.

INFORM YOUR PHYSICIAN BEFORE TAKING THIS DRUG IF

—you have had any unfavorable reaction to previous use of antihistamines.
—you have glaucoma (narrow-angle type).
—you have difficulty in emptying the urinary bladder.
—you plan to have surgery under general anesthesia in the near future.

Time Required for Apparent Benefit

Drug action usually begins in 15 to 30 minutes, reaches maximal effect in 1 to 2 hours, and subsides in 3 to 6 hours.

Possible Side-Effects *(natural, expected, and unavoidable drug actions)*

Drowsiness, sense of weakness, dryness of the nose, mouth, and throat.

Possible Adverse Effects *(unusual, unexpected, and infrequent reactions)*

IF ANY OF THE FOLLOWING DEVELOP, DISCONTINUE DRUG AND NOTIFY YOUR PHYSICIAN AS SOON AS POSSIBLE

Mild Adverse Effects
  Allergic Reactions: Skin rash (rare).
  Other Reactions
    Headache, nervous agitation, dizziness, double vision, blurred vision, ringing in the ears, tremors.

Reduced appetite, heartburn, nausea, vomiting, diarrhea.
Reduced tolerance for contact lenses.

Serious Adverse Effects

Reduced production of white blood cells possibly resulting in fever and/or sore throat.

Precautions for Use by Those over 60 Years of Age

You may be more susceptible to the development of drowsiness, dizziness, and lethargy and to impairment of thinking, judgment, and memory.

This drug can increase the degree of impaired urination associated with prostate gland enlargement (prostatism).

Advisability of Use During Pregnancy

Pregnancy Category: C (tentative). See Pregnancy Code inside back cover.

Animal reproduction studies: No data available.

Information from adequate studies in pregnant women is not available. Ask physician for guidance.

Advisability of Use While Nursing Infant

Drug is present in milk in small quantities. Avoid use or discontinue nursing. Ask physician for guidance.

Habit-Forming Potential

None.

Effects of Overdosage

With Moderate Overdose: Excitement, incoordination, staggering gait, hallucinations, muscular tremors and spasms.

With Large Overdose: Stupor progressing to coma, convulsions, dilated pupils, flushed face, fever, shallow respiration, weak and rapid pulse.

Possible Effects of Extended Use

Tardive dyskinesia (see Glossary).

Bone marrow depression (see Glossary).

Note: Prolonged, continuous use of antihistamines should be avoided.

Suggested Periodic Examinations While Taking This Drug (at physician's discretion)

Complete blood cell counts.

While Taking This Drug, Observe the Following

Foods: No restrictions.

Beverages: Coffee and tea can help to offset the drowsiness produced by most antihistamines.

Alcohol: Use with extreme caution until combined effects have been determined. The combination of alcohol and antihistamine can produce rapid and marked sedation.

Tobacco Smoking: No interactions expected.

Marijuana Smoking
  Occasional (once or twice weekly):   Mild increase in drowsiness and dryness of mouth.
  Daily: Moderate to marked increase in drowsiness and dryness of mouth; possible accentuation of impaired thinking.

Other Drugs
  Brompheniramine may *increase* the effects of
  • all sedatives, sleep-inducing drugs, tranquilizers, analgesics, and narcotic drugs, and produce oversedation.

  Brompheniramine may *decrease* the effects of
  • oral anticoagulants, by hastening their elimination from the body. Consult physician regarding prothrombin time testing and dosage adjustment.

  The following drugs may *increase* the effects of brompheniramine
  • all sedatives, sleep-inducing drugs, tranquilizers, analgesics, and narcotic drugs exaggerate its sedative action.
  • mono-amine oxidase (MAO) inhibitor drugs (see Drug Class, Section Three) may prolong the action of antihistamines.

Driving a Vehicle, Operating Machinery, Engaging in Hazardous Activities: This drug can impair mental alertness, judgment, coordination, and reaction time. Avoid hazardous activities until full sedative effects have been determined.

Aviation Note: The use of this drug *may be a disqualification* for the piloting of aircraft. Consultation with a designated Aviation Medical Examiner is advised.

Exposure to Sun: No photosensitivity reactions reported.

Special Storage Instructions
Keep tablets and capsules in a dry, tightly closed container. Protect liquid drug preparations from light to prevent discoloration.

BUMETANIDE

Year Introduced: 1983

Brand Names

USA	Canada
Bumex (Roche)	None

Common Synonyms ("Street Names"):   Water pills

Drug Class: Diuretic

Prescription Required: USA: Yes

Available for Purchase by Generic Name: USA: No

Available Dosage Forms and Strengths
Tablets — 0.5 mg., 1 mg.
Injection — 2 ml. ampule (0.25 mg/ml)

Tablet May Be Crushed or Capsule Opened for Administration: Yes

How This Drug Works
Intended Therapeutic Effect(s):   Elimination of excessive fluid retention (edema).
Location of Drug Action(s):   The tubular systems of the kidney that determine the final composition of the urine.
Method of Drug Action(s):   By increasing the elimination of salt and water from the body (through increased urine production), this drug reduces the volume of fluid in the blood and body tissues and lowers the sodium content throughout the body.

Principal Uses of This Drug
As a Single Drug Product: To relieve edema associated with congestive heart failure, liver disease, or kidney disease.

THIS DRUG SHOULD NOT BE TAKEN IF
—you have had an allergic reaction to either dosage form previously.
—your kidneys are unable to produce urine.

INFORM YOUR PHYSICIAN BEFORE TAKING THIS DRUG IF
—you are allergic to any form of "sulfa" drug.
—you are pregnant or planning pregnancy.
—you have a history of liver or kidney disease, or impaired liver or kidney function.
—you have diabetes or a tendency to diabetes.
—you have a history of gout.
—you have impaired hearing.
—you are taking any form of cortisone, digitalis, oral anti-diabetic drugs, insulin, probenecid, indomethacin, lithium, or drugs for high blood pressure.
—you plan to have surgery under general anesthesia in the near future.

Time Required for Apparent Benefit
Increased urine volume begins within 30 to 60 minutes, reaches a maximum within 1 to 2 hours, and subsides within 4 hours.

Possible Side-Effects (*natural, expected, and unavoidable drug actions*)
Lightheadedness on arising from sitting or lying position (see orthostatic hypotension in Glossary).
Increase in level of blood sugar, affecting control of diabetes.
Increase in level of blood uric acid, affecting control of gout.
Decrease in levels of blood potassium and sodium, resulting in muscle weakness and cramping.

Possible Adverse Effects *(unusual, unexpected, and infrequent reactions)*

IF ANY OF THE FOLLOWING DEVELOP, DISCONTINUE DRUG AND NOTIFY
YOUR PHYSICIAN AS SOON AS POSSIBLE

Mild Adverse Effects
Allergic Reactions: Skin rashes, hives, itching.
Other Reactions
Headache, dizziness, vertigo, fatigue, weakness, sweating, earache.
Nausea, vomiting, abdominal pain, diarrhea.
Nipple tenderness, joint and muscle pains.

Serious Adverse Effects
Impaired hearing, precipitation of liver coma (in preexisting liver disease),
reduced sexual potency, premature ejaculation.

Natural Diseases or Disorders That May Be Activated By This Drug
Diabetes mellitus, gout.

CAUTION
1. Do not exceed recommended doses. Increased dosage can cause excessive
excretion of water, sodium, and potassium with resultant loss of appetite,
nausea, weakness, confusion, and profound drop in blood pressure (circulatory collapse).
2. If you are also taking a digitalis preparation (digitoxin, digoxin), ensure an
adequate intake of high-potassium foods to prevent potassium deficiency
—a potential cause of digitalis toxicity.
3. If you are being treated for cirrhosis of the liver, do not increase your dose
without consulting your physician. Excessive dosage can alter blood chemistry significantly and induce liver coma.

Precautions for Use by Infants and Children
Safety and effectiveness for use under 18 years of age have not been established.

Precautions for Use by Those over 60 Years of Age
You may be more sensitive to the actions of this drug.
Small doses are advisable until your individual response has been determined.
You may be more susceptible to the development of impaired thinking,
orthostatic hypotension, potassium loss, and elevation of blood sugar.
Overdosage and extended use of this drug can cause excessive loss of body
water, thickening of the blood, and an increased tendency of the blood to
clot, predisposing to stroke, heart attack, or thrombophlebitis.

Advisability of Use During Pregnancy
Pregnancy Category: C (tentative). See Pregnancy Code inside back cover.
Animal reproduction studies do not reveal significant birth defects due to
this drug. However, high-dose studies in rats and rabbits revealed some
lethal effect on developing embryos.
Information from adequate studies in pregnant women is not available.

This drug should not be used during pregnancy unless a very serious complication of pregnancy occurs for which this drug is significantly beneficial.

Advisability of Use While Nursing Infant

This drug may be present in milk. Avoid drug or refrain from nursing. Ask physician for guidance.

Habit-Forming Potential None.

Effects of Overdosage

With Moderate Overdose: Weakness, lethargy, dizziness, confusion, nausea, vomiting, muscle cramps, thirst.

With Large Overdose: Drowsiness progressing to stupor or deep sleep, weak and rapid pulse.

Possible Effects of Extended Use

Impaired balance of water, salt, and potassium in blood and body tissues.
Dehydration with resultant increase in blood viscosity and the potential for abnormal clotting.
Development of diabetes (in predisposed individuals).

Suggested Periodic Examinations While Taking This Drug (at physician's discretion)

Complete blood cell counts.
Measurements of blood levels of sodium, potassium, chloride, sugar, uric acid.
Liver and kidney function tests.

While Taking This Drug, Observe the Following

Foods: It is recommended that you include in your daily diet liberal servings of foods rich in potassium (unless directed otherwise by your physician).

The following foods have a high potassium content:

All-bran cereals	Fish, fresh
Almonds	Lentils
Apricots (dried)	Liver, beef
Bananas, fresh	Lonalac
Beans (navy and lima)	Milk
Carrots (raw)	Peanut butter
Chicken	Peas
Citrus fruits, juices	Pork
Coconut	Potato, sweet
Coffee	Prunes (dried)
Crackers (rye)	Raisins
Dates and figs (dried)	Tomato juice

Note: Avoid licorice in large amounts while taking this drug.
Follow your physician's instructions regarding the use of salt.

Nutritional Support: Ask your physician for guidance regarding the need for potassium and/or magnesium supplements.

Beverages: No restrictions unless directed by your physician. This drug may be taken with milk.

Alcohol: Use with caution until the combined effect has been determined. Alcohol can exaggerate the blood pressure-lowering effect of this drug and cause orthostatic hypotension (see Glossary).

Tobacco Smoking: No interactions expected with this drug. Follow your physician's advice regarding smoking.

Marijuana Smoking

Occasional (once or twice weekly): No effect to mild increase in thirst and/or urinary frequency.

Daily: Moderate increase in thirst and/or urinary frequency; possible accentuation of orthostatic hypotension (see Glossary).

Other Drugs

Bumetanide may *increase* the effects of

- anti-hypertensive drugs. Careful adjustment of dosages is necessary to prevent excessive lowering of the blood pressure.

Bumetanide may *decrease* the effects of

- oral antidiabetic drugs and insulin, by raising the level of blood sugar. Careful dosage adjustment is necessary to maintain proper control of diabetes.
- allopurinol (Zyloprim), by raising the level of blood uric acid. Careful dosage adjustments are necessary to maintain control of gout.

Bumetanide *taken concurrently* with

- aminoglycoside antibiotics (amikacin, gentamicin, kanamycin, neomycin, streptomycin, tobramycin, viomycin) may increase the risk of hearing loss.
- cortisone and cortisone-related drugs may cause excessive loss of potassium from the body.
- digitalis and related drugs require very careful monitoring and dosage adjustments to prevent serious disturbances of heart rhythm.
- lithium may increase the risk of lithium toxicity. Avoid the concurrent use of these drugs.

The following drugs may *increase* the effects of bumetanide:

- barbiturates may increase its blood pressure-lowering effect.
- narcotic drugs may increase its blood pressure-lowering effect.

The following drugs may *decrease* the effects of bumetanide:

- probenecid (Benemid), reduced diuretic effect.
- indomethacin (Indocin), reduced diuretic effect.

Driving a Vehicle, Operating Machinery, Engaging in Hazardous Activities: Use caution until the possible occurrence of dizziness, weakness, or orthostatic hypotension has been determined.

Aviation Note: The use of this drug *may be a disqualification* for the piloting of aircraft. Consultation with a designated Aviation Medical Examiner is advised.

Exposure to Sun: No restrictions.

Exposure to Heat: Avoid excessive perspiring which could cause additional loss of water and salt from the body.

Exposure to Cold: The elderly should use caution and dress warmly. The hypotensive effect of this drug could predispose to hypothermia.

Heavy Exercise or Exertion: Avoid exertion that produces lightheadedness, excessive fatigue, or muscle cramping.

Occurrence of Unrelated Illness: Illnesses which cause vomiting or diarrhea can produce a serious imbalance of important body chemistry. Discontinue this drug and ask your physician for guidance.

Discontinuation: It may be advisable to discontinue this drug 5 to 7 days before major surgery. Ask your physician, surgeon, and/or anesthesiologist for guidance regarding dosage reduction or withdrawal.

Special Storage Instructions

Keep tablets in a dry, tightly closed, light-resistant container. Protect ampules from light.

BUTABARBITAL

Year Introduced: 1939

Brand Names

USA		Canada
BBS (Reid-Provident)	Intasedol (Elder)	Buta-Barb (Dymond)
Bubartal TT (Philips Roxane)	Medarsed (Medar)	Butisol (McNeil)
	Quiebar (Nevin)	Day-Barb (Anca)
Buticaps (McNeil)	Renbu (Wren)	Neo-Barb (Neo)
Butisol (McNeil)	(Numerous	
Butte (Scrip)	combination brand	
Da-Sed (Sheryl)	names)	
Expansatol (Merit)		

Common Synonyms ("Street Names"):   Barbs, candy, goofballs, nerve pills, peanuts, stoppers, stumblers

Drug Class: Sedative, Mild; Sleep Inducer (Hypnotic); Barbiturates

Prescription Required: Yes (Controlled Drug, U.S. Schedule III)*

Available for Purchase by Generic Name: USA: Yes   Canada: No

Available Dosage Forms and Strengths

Tablets — 15 mg., 30 mg., 50 mg., 100 mg.
Prolonged-action tablets — 130 mg.
Capsules — 15 mg., 30 mg., 65 mg.
Elixir — 30 mg. per teaspoonful (5 ml.)

*See Schedules of Controlled Drugs inside back cover.

Tablet May Be Crushed or Capsule Opened for Administration
Regular tablets and capsules — Yes
    Prolonged-action tablets — No

How This Drug Works

Intended Therapeutic Effect(s)
With low dosage, relief of mild to moderate anxiety or tension (sedative effect).
With higher dosage taken at bedtime, sedation sufficient to induce sleep (hypnotic effect).

Location of Drug Action(s): The connecting points (synapses) in the nerve pathways that transmit impulses between the wake-sleep centers of the brain.

Method of Drug Action(s): Not completely established. Present thinking is that this drug selectively blocks the transmission of nerve impulses by reducing the amount of available norepinephrine, one of the chemicals responsible for impulse transmission.

Principal Uses of This Drug

As a Single Drug Product: This barbiturate, with intermediate duration of action, is used primarily as a mild sedative to relieve anxiety and nervous tension. Used infrequently at bedtime to induce sleep.

As a Combination Drug Product [CD]: Frequently combined with atropine and its derivatives to utilize their antispasmodic effect in the management of functional disorders associated with anxiety and nervous tension, such as "nervous stomach" and "spastic colon." Also combined with ephedrine and theophylline in the treatment of bronchial asthma. The addition of a mild sedative renders such combinations more effective by relieving the emotional component that contributes to the disorder.

THIS DRUG SHOULD NOT BE TAKEN IF

—you have had an allergic reaction to any dosage form of it previously.
—you have a history of porphyria.

INFORM YOUR PHYSICIAN BEFORE TAKING THIS DRUG IF

—you are sensitive or allergic to any barbiturate drug.
—you are taking any sedative, sleep-inducing drugs, tranquilizers, antihistamines, pain relievers, or narcotic drugs of any kind.
—you have epilepsy.
—you have a history of liver or kidney disease.
—you plan to have surgery under general anesthesia in the near future.

Time Required for Apparent Benefit
Approximately 30 minutes.

Possible Side-Effects *(natural, expected, and unavoidable drug actions)*
Drowsiness, lethargy, and sense of mental or physical sluggishness as "hangover" effect.

Possible Adverse Effects *(unusual, unexpected, and infrequent reactions)*

IF ANY OF THE FOLLOWING DEVELOP, DISCONTINUE DRUG AND NOTIFY YOUR PHYSICIAN AS SOON AS POSSIBLE

Mild Adverse Effects
　　Allergic Reactions: Skin rash (various kinds), hives, localized swelling of eyelids, face, or lips, drug fever.
　　Other Reactions
　　"Hangover" effect, dizziness, unsteadiness.
　　Nausea, vomiting, diarrhea.
　　Joint and muscle pains, most often in the neck, shoulders, and arms.
Serious Adverse Effects
　　Allergic Reactions
　　Hepatitis with jaundice (see Glossary).
　　Severe skin reactions.
　　Idiosyncratic Reactions: Paradoxical excitement and delirium (rather than sedation).
　　Other Reactions
　　Anemia—weakness and fatigue.
　　Abnormally low blood platelets (see Glossary)—unusual bleeding or bruising.

Precautions for Use by Infants and Children
This drug should not be given to the hyperkinetic child.
Observe for possible paradoxical hyperactivity.

Precautions for Use by Those over 60 Years of Age
Small doses are advisable until tolerance has been determined. The elderly or debilitated may experience agitation, excitement, confusion, and delirium with standard doses (paradoxical reaction).
This drug may also cause excessive lowering of body temperature (hypothermia). Keep dosage to a minimum during winter, and dress warmly.
The natural decline in liver function that may occur after 60 can slow the elimination of this drug. Longer intervals between doses may be necessary to avoid overdosage and toxicity.
Note: A barbiturate is not the drug of choice as a sedative or sleep inducer in this age group.

Advisability of Use During Pregnancy
Pregnancy Category: C (tentative). See Pregnancy Code inside back cover.
　　Animal reproduction studies: No data available.
　　Information from adequate studies in pregnant women is not available.
　　Ask physician for guidance.

Advisability of Use While Nursing Infant
Drug is known to be present in milk. Ask physician for guidance.

Habit-Forming Potential
This drug can cause both psychological and physical dependence (see Glossary).

Effects of Overdosage

With Moderate Overdose: Behavior similar to alcoholic intoxication: confusion, slurred speech, physical incoordination, staggering gait, drowsiness.

With Large Overdose: Deepening sleep, coma, slow and shallow breathing, weak and rapid pulse, cold and sweaty skin.

Possible Effects of Extended Use

Psychological and/or physical dependence.

Anemia.

If dose is excessive, a form of chronic drug intoxication can occur: headache, impaired vision, slurred speech, and depression.

Suggested Periodic Examinations While Taking This Drug (at physician's discretion)

Complete blood cell counts. Liver function tests.

While Taking This Drug, Observe the Following

Foods: No restrictions.

Beverages: No restrictions.

Alcohol: Avoid completely. Alcohol can increase greatly the sedative and depressant actions of this drug on brain function.

Tobacco Smoking: No interactions expected.

Marijuana Smoking

Occasional (once or twice weekly): Mild increase in sedative effect of this drug.

Daily: Marked increase in sedative effect of this drug.

Other Drugs

Butabarbital may *increase* the effects of

- other sedatives, sleep-inducing drugs, tranquilizers, antihistamines, pain relievers, and narcotic drugs, and cause oversedation. Ask your physician for guidance regarding dosage adjustments.

Butabarbital may *decrease* the effects of

- oral anticoagulants of the coumarin drug family. Ask physician for guidance regarding prothrombin time testing and adjustment of the anticoagulant dosage.
- aspirin, and reduce its pain-relieving action.
- cortisone and related drugs, by hastening their elimination from the body.
- oral contraceptives, by hastening their elimination from the body.
- griseofulvin (Fulvicin, Grisactin, etc.), and reduce its effectiveness in treating fungus infections.
- phenylbutazone (Azolid, Butazolidin, etc.), and reduce its effectiveness in treating inflammation and pain.

Butabarbital *taken concurrently* with

- anti-convulsants, may cause a change in the pattern of epileptic seizures. Careful dosage adjustments are necessary to achieve a balance of actions that will give the best protection from seizures.

The following drugs may *increase* the effects of butabarbital
- both mild and strong tranquilizers may increase the sedative and sleep-inducing actions and cause oversedation.
- isoniazid (INH, Isozide, etc.) may prolong the action of barbiturate drugs.
- antihistamines may increase the sedative effects of barbiturate drugs.
- oral anti-diabetic drugs of the sulfonylurea type may prolong the sedative effect of barbiturate drugs.

Driving a Vehicle, Operating Machinery, Engaging in Hazardous Activities: This drug can produce drowsiness and can impair mental alertness, judgment, physical coordination, and reaction time. Avoid hazardous activities.

Aviation Note: The use of this drug *is a disqualification* for the piloting of aircraft. Consultation with a designated Aviation Medical Examiner is advised.

Exposure to Sun: Use caution until sensitivity has been determined. Some barbiturates can cause photosensitivity (see Glossary).

Exposure to Heat: No restrictions.

Exposure to Cold: The elderly may experience excessive lowering of body temperature while taking this drug. Keep dosage to a minimum during winter and dress warmly.

Heavy Exercise or Exertion: No restrictions.

Discontinuation: If it has been necessary to use this drug for an extended period of time, do not discontinue it abruptly. Ask physician for guidance regarding dosage adjustment and withdrawal. It may also be necessary to adjust the doses of other drugs taken concurrently with it.

Special Storage Instructions

Keep tablets and capsules in a dry, tightly closed container. Keep the elixir in a tightly closed, amber glass bottle.

BUTALBITAL
(Talbutal)

Year Introduced: 1954

Brand Names

USA	Canada
Lotusate (Winthrop)	Fiorinal [CD] (Sandoz)
Fiorinal [CD] (Sandoz)	Fiorinal-C ¼ [CD] (Sandoz)
Fiorinal with Codeine [CD] (Sandoz)	Fiorinal-C ½ [CD] (Sandoz)

Common Synonyms ("Street Names"):   Barbs, candy, downers, goofballs, peanuts, sleepers, stoppers, stumblers

Drug Class: Sedative, Mild; Sleep Inducer (Hypnotic), Barbiturates

Prescription Required: Yes (Controlled Drug, U.S. Schedule III)*

Available for Purchase by Generic Name: No

Available Dosage Forms and Strengths
Tablets — 50 mg. (in combination), 120 mg.
Capsules — 120 mg.; 50 mg. (in combination)

Tablet May Be Crushed or Capsule Opened for Administration: Yes

How This Drug Works
Intended Therapeutic Effect(s)
With low dosage, relief of mild to moderate anxiety or tension (sedative effect).
With higher dosage taken at bedtime, sedation sufficient to induce sleep (hypnotic effect).
Location of Drug Action(s):   The connecting points (synapses) in the nerve pathways that transmit impulses between the wake-sleep centers of the brain.
Method of Drug Action(s):   Not completely established. Present thinking is that this drug selectively blocks the transmission of nerve impulses by reducing the amount of available norepinephrine, one of the chemicals responsible for impulse transmission.

Principal Uses of This Drug
As a Single Drug Product: This barbiturate, with short to intermediate duration of action, is a mild sedative that is infrequently used alone to relieve anxiety and nervous tension.
As a Combination Drug Product [CD]:   This drug is used primarily in combination with aspirin, caffeine, and codeine to treat headaches associated with nervous tension. Because of the significant emotional component in the perception of pain, the addition of a mild sedative to a mixture of analgesics renders the combination more effective in relieving pain.

THIS DRUG SHOULD NOT BE TAKEN IF
—you have had an allergic reaction to any dosage form of it previously.
—you have a history of porphyria.

INFORM YOUR PHYSICIAN BEFORE TAKING THIS DRUG IF
—you are allergic or sensitive to any barbiturate drug.
—you are taking any sedative, sleep-inducing drugs, tranquilizers, antihistamines, pain relievers, or narcotic drugs of any kind.
—you have epilepsy.
—you have a history of liver or kidney disease.
—you plan to have surgery under general anesthesia in the near future.

*See Schedules of Controlled Drugs inside back cover.

Time Required for Apparent Benefit
Drug action begins in 15 to 30 minutes, reaches a maximum in approximately 1 hour, and subsides in 2 to 6 hours.

Possible Side-Effects *(natural, expected, and unavoidable drug actions)*
Drowsiness, lethargy, and sense of mental and physical sluggishness as "hangover" effect.

Possible Adverse Effects *(unusual, unexpected, and infrequent reactions)*

IF ANY OF THE FOLLOWING DEVELOP, DISCONTINUE DRUG AND NOTIFY YOUR PHYSICIAN AS SOON AS POSSIBLE

Mild Adverse Effects
Allergic Reactions: Skin rash, hives, localized swellings of eyelids, face, or lips, drug fever.
Other Reactions
Nausea, vomiting, diarrhea.
Headache, dizziness, mild "hangover" effect.

Serious Adverse Effects
Idiosyncratic Reactions: Paradoxical excitement and delirium (rather than sedation). This is more likely to occur in the presence of pain and in the elderly.

Precautions for Use by Those over 60 Years of Age
Small doses are advisable until tolerance has been determined. The elderly or debilitated may experience agitation, excitement, confusion, and delirium with standard doses (paradoxical reaction).
This drug may also cause excessive lowering of body temperature (hypothermia). Keep dosage to a minimum during winter, and dress warmly.
The natural decline in liver function that may occur after 60 can slow the elimination of this drug. Longer intervals between doses may be necessary to avoid overdosage and toxicity.
Note: A barbiturate is not the drug of choice as a sedative or sleep inducer in this age group.

Advisability of Use During Pregnancy
Pregnancy Category: C (tentative). See Pregnancy Code inside back cover.
Animal reproduction studies: No data available.
Information from adequate studies in pregnant women is not available.
Ask physician for guidance.

Advisability of Use While Nursing Infant
Drug is probably present in milk. Ask physician for guidance.

Habit-Forming Potential
If used for an extended period of time, this drug can cause both psychological and physical dependence (see Glossary).

Effects of Overdosage
With Moderate Overdose: Behavior similar to alcoholic intoxication: confusion, slurred speech, physical incoordination, staggering gait, drowsiness.

With Large Overdose: Deepening sleep, coma, slow and shallow breathing, weak and rapid pulse, cold and sweaty skin.

Possible Effects of Extended Use

Psychological and/or physical dependence. If dose is excessive, a form of chronic intoxication can occur: headache, impaired vision, slurred speech, and depression.

Suggested Periodic Examinations While Taking This Drug (at physician's discretion)

With frequent or continual use, complete blood cell counts and liver function tests are desirable.

While Taking This Drug, Observe the Following

Foods: No restrictions.

Beverages: No restrictions.

Alcohol: Avoid completely. Alcohol can increase greatly the sedative and depressant actions of this drug on brain function.

Tobacco Smoking: No interactions expected.

Marijuana Smoking

Occasional (once or twice weekly):   Mild increase in sedative effect of this drug.

Daily: Marked increase in sedative effect of this drug.

Other Drugs

Butalbital may *increase* the effects of

• other sedatives, sleep-inducing drugs, tranquilizers, antihistamines, pain relievers, and narcotic drugs, and cause oversedation. Ask your physician for guidance regarding dosage adjustments.

Butalbital may *decrease* the effects of

• oral anticoagulants of the coumarin drug family. Ask physician for guidance regarding prothrombin time testing and adjustment of the anticoagulant dose.
• aspirin, and reduce its pain-relieving action.
• cortisone and related drugs, by hastening their elimination from the body.
• oral contraceptives, by hastening their elimination from the body.
• griseofulvin (Fulvicin, Grisactin, etc.), and reduce its effectiveness in treating fungus infections.
• phenylbutazone (Azolid, Butazolidin, etc.), and reduce its effectiveness in treating inflammation and pain.

Butalbital *taken concurrently* with

• anti-convulsants, may cause a change in the pattern of epileptic seizures. Careful dosage adjustments are necessary to achieve a balance of actions that will give the best protection from seizures.

The following drugs may *increase* the effects of butalbital:

• both mild and strong tranquilizers may increase its sedative and sleep-inducing actions and cause oversedation.

• isoniazid (INH, Isozide, etc.) may prolong the action of barbiturate drugs.
• antihistamines may increase the sedative effects of barbiturate drugs.
• oral anti-diabetic drugs of the sufonylurea type may prolong the sedative effect of barbiturate drugs.

Driving a Vehicle, Operating Machinery, Engaging in Hazardous Activities: This drug can produce drowsiness and can impair mental alertness, judgment, physical coordination, and reaction time. Avoid hazardous activities.

Aviation Note: The use of this drug *is a disqualification* for the piloting of aircraft. Consultation with a designated Aviation Medical Examiner is advised.

Exposure to Sun: Use caution until sensitivity has been determined. Some barbiturates can cause photosensitivity (see Glossary).

Exposure to Heat: No restrictions.

Exposure to Cold: The elderly (over 60 years of age) may experience excessive lowering of body temperature while taking this drug. Keep dosage to a minimum during winter and dress warmly.

Heavy Exercise or Exertion: No restrictions.

Discontinuation: If it has been necessary to use this drug for an extended period of time, do not discontinue it abruptly. Ask physician for guidance regarding dosage adjustment and withdrawal. It may also be necessary to adjust the doses of other drugs taken concurrently with it.

Special Storage Instructions
Keep tablets and capsules in a dry, tightly closed container.

CAFFEINE

Year Introduced: In use for many centuries in the form of coffee, tea, and cocoa.

Brand Names

USA	Canada
Cafecon (Consol. Midland)	Cafergot [CD] (Sandoz)
Nodoz (Bristol-Myers)	
Cafergot [CD] (Sandoz)	
(Numerous other combination brand names)	

Common Synonyms ("Street Names"):   None

Drug Class: Stimulant, Xanthines

Prescription Required: Preparations without ergot—No
                              Preparations with ergot—Yes

Available for Purchase by Generic Name: Yes

Available Dosage Forms and Strengths
                    Tablets — 65 mg., 100 mg., 200 mg., 250 mg.
                    Capsules — 100 mg.
        Prolonged-action capsules — 200 mg., 250 mg.

Tablet May Be Crushed or Capsule Opened for Administration
    Regular tablets and capsules — Yes
        Prolonged-action capsules — No

How This Drug Works
  Intended Therapeutic Effect(s)
    Prevention and early relief of blood vessel (vascular) headaches, such as
      migraine and variations of migraine.
    Relief of drowsiness and mental fatigue (stimulant effect).
  Location of Drug Action(s)
    The walls of blood vessels in the head.
    The wake-sleep centers and the thought-association areas of the brain.
  Method of Drug Action(s)
    By constricting the walls of blood vessels, this drug corrects the excessive
      expansion (dilation) responsible for the pain of vascular headache.
    By increasing the energy level of the chemical systems responsible for
      nerve tissue activity, this drug induces wakefulness and improves alert-
      ness and mental acuity.

Principal Uses of This Drug
  As a Single Drug Product: This stimulant of brain activity is used primarily
    to prolong wakefulness and delay the onset of sleep.
  As a Combination Drug Product [CD]:   This drug is used most commonly
    in combination with ergotamine to treat vascular headaches, such as mi-
    graine and cluster headaches. Caffeine increases the absorption of ergota-
    mine by the gastrointestinal tract and renders it more effective.

THIS DRUG SHOULD NOT BE TAKEN IF
—you have had an allergic reaction to any dosage form of it previously.
—you have severe heart disease.
—you have an active stomach ulcer.

INFORM YOUR PHYSICIAN BEFORE TAKING THIS DRUG IF
—you experience severe disturbances of heart rhythm.
—you have a history of peptic ulcer disease.
—you are subject to hypoglycemia.
—you have epilepsy.

Time Required for Apparent Benefit
  Drug action begins in approximately 30 minutes and reaches a maximum in
  50 to 75 minutes.

Possible Side-Effects *(natural, expected, and unavoidable drug actions)*
Sense of nervousness, insomnia, increased urine output.
(Nature and degree of side-effects depend upon the dose of the drug and the susceptibility of the individual.)

Possible Adverse Effects *(unusual, unexpected, and infrequent reactions)*

IF ANY OF THE FOLLOWING DEVELOP, DISCONTINUE DRUG AND NOTIFY YOUR PHYSICIAN AS SOON AS POSSIBLE

Mild Adverse Effects
Headache, irritability, lightheadedness, feeling of drunkenness, impaired thinking.
Nausea, heartburn, indigestion, stomach irritation.
Serious Adverse Effects
Development of stomach ulcer.

CAUTION
Do not exceed 250 mg. per dose or 500 mg. per 24 hours.

Precautions for Use by Those over 60 Years of Age
Tolerance for caffeine often decreases after 60. You may be more susceptible to the development of nervousness, irritability, impaired thinking, tremor, insomnia, disturbed heart rhythm, and acid indigestion.

Advisability of Use During Pregnancy
Pregnancy Category: C (tentative). See Pregnancy Code inside back cover.
Animal reproduction studies reveal significant birth defects due to this drug.
Information from studies in pregnant women indicates no increased defects in 12,696 exposures to this drug.
Avoid completely during first 3 months.
Ask physician for guidance.
One study suggests that heavy coffee consumption (in excess of 3 cups daily) during pregnancy may increase the frequency of complications. Do not exceed recommended doses, including the use of caffeine beverages.

Advisability of Use While Nursing Infant
This drug is present in milk in very small amounts. The blood level in the nursing infant is too small to be significant, if the mother adheres to recommended dosage.

Habit-Forming Potential
Varying degrees of tolerance and psychological dependence (see Glossary) may occur with prolonged use.

Effects of Overdosage
With Moderate Overdose: Nervousness, restlessness, insomnia (followed by depression in some individuals), tremor, sweating, ringing in the ears, spots before the eyes, heart palpitation, diarrhea.

With Large Overdose: Excitement, rapid and irregular pulse, rapid breathing, fever, delirium, hallucinations, convulsions.

Possible Effects of Extended Use
Development of tolerance and psychological dependence (see Glossary).
Development of stomach irritation (gastritis) and peptic ulcer in stomach or duodenum.
Aggravation and perpetuation of fibrocystic breast disease.

Suggested Periodic Examinations While Taking This Drug (at physician's discretion)
None.

While Taking This Drug, Observe the Following
Foods: No restrictions. Chocolate contains 5 to 10 mg. of caffeine per ounce.

Beverages: Keep in mind that caffeine beverages (coffee, tea, and cola) will add to the total intake of caffeine used in medicinal form. Avoid possible overdosage. The approximate caffeine content of popular beverages is as follows:

Regular coffee	(average cup)	100–150 mg.
Instant coffee	(average cup)	80–100 mg.
Coffee-grain blends	(average cup)	14–37 mg.
Decaffeinated coffee	(average cup)	3–5 mg.
Tea	(average cup)	60–75 mg.
Regular cola	(6 ounces)	36 mg.
Diet cola	(6 ounces)	18 mg.
Cocoa	(6 ounces)	10 mg.

Alcohol: No harmful interactions expected. Caffeine can counteract the depressant action of alcohol on the brain.

Tobacco Smoking: Consult physician regarding possible adverse effects of combined nicotine and caffeine.

Marijuana Smoking
Occasional (once or twice weekly):   No effect to mild increase in heart rate.
Daily: Persistent rapid heart rate; possible heart rhythm disturbance (in sensitive individuals).

Other Drugs
Caffeine may *increase* the effects of
- thyroid preparations, by raising the body metabolism approximately 10%.
- amphetamines (and related drugs), and cause excessive nervousness. Dosage adjustment may be necessary.

Caffeine may *decrease* the effects of
- sedatives, tranquilizers, sleep-inducing drugs, pain relievers, and narcotic drugs.

Caffeine *taken concurrently* in large doses with
- mono-amine oxidase (MAO) inhibitor drugs (see Drug Family, Section Three), may cause an excessive rise in blood pressure. Use caffeine in small doses or discontinue the MAO inhibitor drug.

The following drugs may *increase* the effects of caffeine:
- isoniazid (INH, Isozide, etc.) may delay its elimination from the body.
- meprobamate (Equanil, Miltown) may increase the concentration of caffeine in the brain.

Driving a Vehicle, Operating Machinery, Engaging in Hazardous Activities: No restrictions.

Aviation Note: Usually no restrictions. However, it is advisable to observe for the possible occurrence of nervousness and to restrict activities accordingly.

Exposure to Sun: No restrictions.

Discontinuation: Sudden discontinuation of this drug following extended use can produce a "caffeine-withdrawal" headache. This is readily relieved by coffee or caffeine in medicinal form.

Special Storage Instructions
Keep in a dry, tightly closed container.

CALCIUM

Note: This is an Abbreviated Drug Profile of a mineral that is sometimes used as a drug. Calcium is one of the most common and most important elements in the human body. It is essential for numerous functions: the development and maintenance of healthy bone, the transmission of nerve impulses, the contraction of all types of muscles, lung function (respiration), kidney function, and blood coagulation. Most of the body calcium (96%–97%) is found in the bones. In those conditions that are characterized by inadequate bone development or excessive bone loss (such as rickets, osteoporosis, and osteomalacia), calcium is given to correct the deficiency and to promote bone replacement. It is also used preventively as a dietary supplement during pregnancy, while breast-feeding, and following menopause. Calcium carbonate is used most frequently because it is the most effective form of calcium taken by mouth. It is also one of the three most commonly used antacids. (See the Drug Profile of Antacids if you are taking it for this purpose.)

Year Introduced: 1951

Brand Names

USA	Canada
Os-Cal 500 Tablets (Marion)	Os-Cal (Ayerst)
Os-Cal Forte Tablets [CD] (Marion)	
Os-Cal-Gesic Tablets [CD] (Marion)	
Os-Cal Plus Tablets [CD] (Marion)	
Os-Cal Tablets [CD] (Marion)	

Common Synonyms ("Street Names"):   Calcium pills

Drug Class: Calcium Preparations

Prescription Required: No

Available for Purchase by Generic Name: Yes

Available Dosage Forms and Strengths
Tablets — 650 mg., 1250 mg.
Chewable Tablets — 330 mg., 350 mg., 420 mg., 500 mg.
Chewing Gum — 500 mg.
Oral Suspension — 1 gram per teaspoonful (5 ml.)

Tablet May Be Crushed or Capsule Opened for Administration: Yes

How This Drug Works
Intended Therapeutic Effect(s): Sufficient supplementation of dietary calcium to prevent or treat calcium-deficient bone disorders.

Location of Drug Action(s):   The bone cells and matrix that constitute the framework for the development of skeletal bone.

Method of Drug Action(s):   By preventing or correcting calcium deficiency throughout the body, this drug provides the level of calcium needed to ensure the development and continuous maintenance of normal bone texture.

Principal Uses of This Drug

As a Single Drug Product: Within the limited scope of this Drug Profile, this drug is used as a dietary supplement to meet the body's requirements for calcium in the formation and maintenance of normal bone. It is used in children primarily to prevent or treat rickets, and in adults to prevent or treat osteoporosis or osteomalacia.

As a Combination Drug Product [CD]:   Vitamin D increases the intestinal absorption of calcium. For this reason, they are often combined in one dosage form. Calcium is also available in combination with the entire spectrum of essential vitamins and minerals.

THIS DRUG SHOULD NOT BE TAKEN IF
—your calcium blood level is abnormally high.
—you have severe kidney disease.
—you have calcified kidney stones.
—you are immobilized for an extended period of time.

INFORM YOUR PHYSICIAN BEFORE TAKING THIS DRUG IF
—you have a history of kidney stones.
—you have impaired kidney function.
—you have any form of heart disease.
—you have sarcoidosis.
—you are prone to constipation.
—you are taking any other oral medications at this time, especially thiazide diuretics, quinidine, or tetracycline.
—you have deficient or absent stomach acid.

Possible Side-Effects *(natural, expected, and unavoidable drug actions)*
Constipation (may be severe with large doses).

Possible Adverse Effects *(unusual, unexpected, and infrequent reactions)*

IF ANY OF THE FOLLOWING DEVELOP, DISCONTINUE DRUG AND NOTIFY YOUR PHYSICIAN AS SOON AS POSSIBLE

Mild Adverse Effects
Chalky taste in mouth, belching, intestinal gas.

Serious Adverse Effects
With normal dosage—none.

CAUTION
1. The need for supplemental calcium and its correct dosage must be determined for each person individually. Ask your physician for guidance. The recommended daily dietary allowances are as follows:

Infants up to 6 months of age: 360 mg.
Infants 6 months to 1 year of age: 540 mg.
Children 1 to 10 years of age: 800 mg.
Males 11 to 18 years of age: 1200 mg.
Males 19 years of age and older: 800 mg.
Females 11 to 18 years of age: 1200 mg.
Females 19 to 50 years of age: 800 mg.
Females after 50 years of age (post-menopausal): 1500 mg.
During pregnancy: 1200 mg.
While breast-feeding: 1200 mg.

2. Calcium can interfere with the absorption of many drugs. Do not take any other oral medication within 2 hours of a dose of calcium carbonate.
3. Avoid large doses of Vitamin D while taking any form of calcium. Ask your physician for guidance regarding Vitamin D dosage.

Advisability of Use During Pregnancy

Pregnancy Category: C (tentative). See Pregnancy Code inside back cover.
Animal reproduction studies: No data available.
Information from adequate studies in pregnant women is not available.
This drug is considered safe for use during the last 6 months of pregnancy in dosages not to exceed 1200 mg. daily. The calcium content of the diet must be considered. Ask your physician for guidance.

Advisability of Use While Nursing Infant

Calcium is a normal constituent of breast milk. This drug does not increase the calcium content of milk to any significant degree.

Effects of Overdosage

With Moderate Overdose: Unusual fatigue and weakness, nervousness, muscle twitching, abdominal discomfort, constipation.

With Large Overdose: Headache, nausea, vomiting, weakness, mental disturbances, rapid heart rate, low blood pressure, reduced urine formation, delirium, coma.

Possible Effects of Extended Use

The development of calcium-containing kidney stones.

While Taking This Drug, Observe the Following

Foods: Avoid frequent and excessive intake of spinach, rhubarb, bran, and whole-grain cereals; these can interfere with the absorption of calcium. This drug should be taken 1 to 2 hours after meals.

Beverages: Avoid large quantities of milk while taking calcium.

Other Drugs

Calcium may *increase* the effects of
- levodopa (Larodopa, Sinemet) by increasing its absorption.
- quinidine by delaying its elimination.

Calcium may *decrease* the effects of
- cimetidine (Tagamet) by reducing its absorption.
- iron preparations by interfering with their absorption.

• phenothiazines by reducing their absorption (see Drug Class, Section Three).
• salicylates (aspirin, etc.) by hastening their elimination.
• tetracyclines by reducing their absorption.

Calcium *taken concurrently* with
• thiazide diuretics can cause abnormally high blood levels of calcium (see Drug Class, Section Three).

The following drugs may *decrease* the effects of calcium:
• cortisone-like drugs, by interfering with its absorption (see Drug Class, Section Three).
• furosemide (Lasix), by increasing its elimination.

CARBAMAZEPINE

Year Introduced: 1968

Brand Names

USA	Canada
Tegretol (Geigy)	Apo-Carbamazepine (Apotex)
	Mazepine (ICN)
	Tegretol (Geigy)

Common Synonyms ("Street Names"):   None

Drug Class: Analgesic, Anti-convulsant

Prescription Required: Yes

Available for Purchase by Generic Name: No

Available Dosage Forms and Strengths
Tablets — 200 mg.
Tablets, Chewable — 100 mg.

Tablet May Be Crushed or Capsule Opened for Administration: Yes

How This Drug Works
Intended Therapeutic Effect(s)
Reduction in the frequency, severity, and duration of facial pain associated with trigeminal neuralgia (tic douloureux)—an analgesic effect.
Prevention of certain complex types of epileptic seizures—an anti-convulsant effect.
Location of Drug Action(s):   The principal sites of therapeutic action include
• the trigeminal nerve terminals in the spinal cord.
• those areas of the brain that initiate and sustain episodes of excessive electrical discharges responsible for epileptic seizures.

Method of Drug Action(s)

The mechanism of its analgesic effect is not established. It is thought that by reducing the transmission of impulses at certain nerve terminals, this drug relieves the pain of trigeminal neuralgia.

The mechanism of its anti-convulsant effect is not established. It is thought that this drug lowers and stabilizes the excitability of nerve fibers in the brain and inhibits the repetitious spread of electrical impulses along nerve pathways. This action may prevent seizures altogether, or it may reduce their frequency and severity.

Principal Uses of This Drug

As a Single Drug Product: This drug is used primarily in the management of two uncommon but serious disorders: (1) for relief of pain in true trigeminal neuralgia (tic douloureux) and glossopharyngeal neuralgia; (2) for control of several types of epilepsy, namely grand mal, psychomotor or temporal lobe, and mixed seizure patterns. Because of its potential for toxic effects, precise diagnosis and careful management are mandatory for its proper use.

THIS DRUG SHOULD NOT BE TAKEN IF

—you have had an allergic reaction to it previously.

—you have active liver disease.

—you have a history of previous bone marrow depression (see Glossary) or serious blood disorder due to any cause, but especially due to a drug.

—you are taking now, or have taken during the past 14 days, any monoamine oxidase (MAO) inhibiting drug (see Drug Class, Section Three).

INFORM YOUR PHYSICIAN BEFORE TAKING THIS DRUG IF

—you have had an allergic reaction to any tricyclic antidepressant drug: Aventyl, Elavil, Endep, Norpramin, Pertofrane, Presamine, Tofranil, Vivactil.

—you have high blood pressure.

—you have any type of heart disease.

—you have glaucoma.

—you have a history of serious emotional or mental disorder.

—you have impaired liver or kidney function.

—you have a history of thrombophlebitis.

—you take more than 2 alcoholic drinks a day.

Time Required for Apparent Benefit

In treating trigeminal neuralgia, relief of pain begins in 24 to 72 hours and usually continues for as long as the drug is taken.

In treating epilepsy, continuous use on a regular schedule may be necessary for 1 to 2 weeks to determine this drug's effectiveness in preventing and/or reducing the occurrence of seizures.

Possible Side-Effects *(natural, expected, and unavoidable drug actions)*

Dryness of the mouth and throat, constipation, impairment of urination.

Possible Adverse Effects *(unusual, unexpected, and infrequent reactions)*

IF ANY OF THE FOLLOWING DEVELOP, DISCONTINUE DRUG AND NOTIFY YOUR PHYSICIAN AS SOON AS POSSIBLE

Mild Adverse Effects
Allergic Reactions: Skin rash, hives, itching, drug fever.
Other Reactions
  Headache, dizziness, drowsiness, unsteadiness, fatigue, blurred vision, confusion.
  Exaggerated hearing, ringing in ears.
  Loss of appetite, nausea, vomiting, indigestion, diarrhea.
  Water retention (edema), frequent urination, impaired sexual function.
  Changes in skin pigmentation, hair loss.
  Aching of muscles and joints, leg cramps.
Serious Adverse Effects
Allergic Reactions: Severe dermatitis with peeling of skin, irritation of mouth and tongue, swelling of lymph glands.
Other Reactions
  Bone marrow depression (see Glossary)—fatigue, weakness, fever, sore throat, unusual bleeding or bruising.
  Hepatitis with jaundice (see Glossary)—yellow eyes and skin, dark-colored urine, light-colored stools.
  Kidney damage—reduced urine volume, uremic poisoning.
  Mental depression and agitation.
  Double vision, visual hallucinations.
  Speech disturbances, peripheral neuritis (see Glossary).
  Thrombophlebitis.

CAUTION
1. Because this drug can cause serious adverse effects, it should be used only after a trial of less hazardous drugs has been ineffective.
2. Before the first dose is taken, pre-treatment blood cell counts, liver function tests, and kidney function tests should be performed.
3. Do not exceed a total dose of 1200 mg. per 24 hours unless you are under very close medical supervision.
4. During periods of spontaneous remission from trigeminal neuralgia, this drug should **not** be used preventively.

Precautions for Use by Infants and Children
Do not exceed a total dose of 1000 mg. per 24 hours.
Because of the high frequency of adverse effects (up to 25%), frequent and careful monitoring of blood cell production, liver function, and kidney function must be performed regularly. Complete blood cell counts, and liver and kidney function studies should be obtained weekly during the first 3 months and monthly thereafter until the drug is discontinued.

Precautions for Use by Those over 60 Years of Age

Confusion and agitation may occur more frequently.

The anginal pain associated with coronary heart disease may occur with greater frequency and severity, requiring reduced activity and increased dosage of anti-anginal medication.

The impairment of urination associated with enlargement of the prostate gland (prostatism) may be increased and lead to an inability to void.

Advisability of Use During Pregnancy

Pregnancy Category: C (tentative). See Pregnancy Code inside back cover.

Animal reproduction studies in rats reveal significant birth defects due to this drug.

Information from adequate studies in pregnant women is not available.

Avoid completely during first 3 months.

Ask physician for guidance.

Advisability of Use While Nursing Infant

This drug is known to be present in milk. It is advisable to avoid this drug or to refrain from nursing.

Habit-Forming Potential

None.

Effects of Overdosage

With Moderate Overdose: Increased dizziness, unstable stance and gait, excessive drowsiness, nausea, vomiting.

With Large Overdose: Disorientation, tremor, involuntary movements, dilated pupils, flushing of skin, stupor progressing to coma.

Possible Effects of Extended Use

Impairment of liver function, possible liver damage with jaundice (see Glossary).

Suggested Periodic Examinations While Taking This Drug (at physician's discretion)

Complete blood cell counts weekly during the first 3 months of treatment, and monthly thereafter until the drug is discontinued.

Liver function tests.

Kidney function tests.

Complete eye examinations.

Measurement of internal eye pressure in presence of glaucoma.

While Taking This Drug, Observe The Following

Foods: This drug may be taken with or immediately following food to minimize stomach irritation.

Beverages: No restrictions as to kind of beverage. May be taken with milk.

Note: This drug can cause retention of water in body tissues. Do not exceed a total liquid intake of 2 quarts per 24 hours unless advised otherwise by your physician.

Alcohol: Use caution until the combined effect has been determined. This drug may increase the sedative effect of alcohol.

Tobacco Smoking: No interactions expected.

Marijuana Smoking

Occasional (once or twice weekly):   No effect to mild increase in drowsiness and unsteadiness; little influence on anti-convulsant effect of drug; intensified anti-convulsant effect on temporal lobe epilepsy (dependent upon composition of marijuana).

Daily: Moderate increase in drowsiness, unsteadiness, and impaired thinking; possible decrease of anti-convulsant effect of drug; marked intensification of anti-convulsant effect in temporal lobe epilepsy (dependent upon composition of marijuana).

Other Drugs

Carbamazepine may *decrease* the effects of

- doxycycline (Doxy-II, Vibramycin, etc.).
- phenytoin (Dantoin, Dilantin, etc.).
- warfarin (Coumadin, Panwarfin, etc.).

Carbamazepine *taken concurrently* with

- a digitalis preparation (digitoxin, digoxin), may cause excessive slowing of the heart rate.
- mono-amine oxidase (MAO) inhibiting drugs (see Drug Class, Section Three), may cause severe toxic reactions. An interval of at least 2 weeks should elapse between the last dose of any MAO inhibitor and the first dose of carbamazepine.
- tricyclic antidepressant drugs (see Drug Class, Section Three), may cause confusion or activate a latent mental disorder. An interval of at least 1 week should elapse between the use of any tricyclic antidepressant and carbamazepine.

The following drug may *increase* the effects of carbamazepine:

- propoxyphene (Darvocet, Darvon, etc.).

The following drug may *decrease* the effects of carbamazepine:

- phenytoin (Dantoin, Dilantin, etc.).

Driving a Vehicle, Operating Machinery, Engaging in Hazardous Activities: This drug can cause dizziness and drowsiness. Avoid hazardous activities if these drug effects occur.

Aviation Note: The use of this drug *is a disqualification* for the piloting of aircraft. Consultation with a designated Aviation Medical Examiner is advised.

Exposure to Sun: This drug can cause photosensitivity (see Glossary). Use caution until sensitivity to sun has been determined.

Exposure to Heat: No restrictions.

Exposure to Cold: No restrictions.

Heavy Exercise or Exertion: Use caution if you have coronary artery disease. This drug can intensify angina and reduce tolerance for physical activity.

Occurrence of Unrelated Illness: Because of this drug's potential for serious adverse effects, it is mandatory that you inform each physician and dentist you consult that you are taking carbamazepine (Tegretol).

Discontinuation   While taking this drug for trigeminal neuralgia, attempts should be made every 3 months to reduce the maintenance dose or to discontinue it altogether.

While taking this drug for epilepsy or seizure disorders, do *not* discontinue it abruptly. Sudden withdrawal of any anti-convulsant drug can cause severe and repeated seizures.

Special Storage Instructions
Keep in a dry, tightly closed container.

CARBENICILLIN

Year Introduced: 1964

Brand Names

USA	Canada
Geocillin (Roerig)	Geopen (Pfizer)
Geopen (Roerig)	Pyopen (Ayerst)
Pyopen (Beecham)	

Common Synonyms ("Street Names"):   None

Drug Class: Antibiotic (Anti-infective), Penicillins

Prescription Required: Yes

Available for Purchase by Generic Name: No

Available Dosage Forms and Strengths
Tablets — 382 mg.

Tablet May Be Crushed or Capsule Opened for Administration: Yes

How This Drug Works
Intended Therapeutic Effect(s):   The elimination of infections responsive to the action of this drug.

Location of Drug Action(s):   Any body tissue or fluid in which sufficient concentration of the drug can be achieved.

Method of Drug Action(s):   This drug destroys susceptible infecting bacteria by interfering with their ability to produce new protective cell walls as they multiply and grow.

Principal Uses of This Drug
As a Single Drug Product: To treat certain acute and chronic infections of the upper and lower urinary tract, including prostatitis. Effective use of this drug depends upon the precise identification of the infecting organism and determination of its sensitivity to this form of penicillin.

THIS DRUG SHOULD NOT BE TAKEN IF
—you are certain you are allergic to any form of penicillin.

INFORM YOUR PHYSICIAN BEFORE TAKING THIS DRUG IF
—you suspect you may be allergic to penicillin, or you have a history of a previous "reaction" to penicillin.
—you are allergic to cephalosporin antibiotics (Ancef, Ceporan, Ceporex, Kafocin, Keflex, Keflin, Kefzol, Loridine).
—you are allergic by nature (hayfever, asthma, hives, eczema).

Time Required for Apparent Benefit
Varies with the nature of the infection under treatment; usually from 2 to 5 days.

Possible Side-Effects *(natural, expected, and unavoidable drug actions)*
Superinfections (see Glossary).

Possible Adverse Effects *(unusual, unexpected, and infrequent reactions)*

IF ANY OF THE FOLLOWING DEVELOP, DISCONTINUE DRUG AND NOTIFY YOUR PHYSICIAN AS SOON AS POSSIBLE

Mild Adverse Effects
  Allergic Reactions: Skin rashes (various kinds).
  Other Reactions: Irritations of mouth or tongue, "black tongue," nausea, vomiting, diarrhea, dizziness (rare).
Serious Adverse Effects
  Allergic Reactions: †Anaphylactic reaction (see Glossary), severe skin reactions, high fever, swollen painful joints, sore throat, unusual bleeding or bruising.

Precautions for Use by Those over 60 Years of Age
It is advisable to evaluate kidney function before and during use of this drug to determine the need for dosage adjustment.
Natural changes in the skin after 60 may predispose to severe and prolonged itching reactions in the genital and anal regions. This reaction should be reported promptly.

Advisability of Use During Pregnancy
Pregnancy Category: B (tentative). See Pregnancy Code inside back cover.
Animal reproduction studies: No data available.
Information from studies in pregnant women indicates no increased risk of defects in 3546 exposures to penicillin derivatives.
Ask physician for guidance.

Advisability of Use While Nursing Infant
Drug may be present in milk and may sensitize infant to penicillin. Ask physician for guidance.

---

†A rare but potentially dangerous reaction characteristic of penicillins.

Habit-Forming Potential
None.

Effects of Overdosage
Possible nausea, vomiting, and/or diarrhea.

Possible Effects of Extended Use
Superinfections (see Glossary).

Suggested Periodic Examinations While Taking This Drug (at physician's discretion)
Complete blood cell counts.
Liver and kidney function tests.

While Taking This Drug, Observe the Following
Foods: No restrictions of food selection. Drug is absorbed better if taken 1 hour before or 2 hours after eating.

Beverages: No restrictions.

Alcohol: No interactions expected.

Tobacco Smoking: No interactions expected.

Marijuana Smoking: No interactions expected.

Other Drugs

The following drugs may *decrease* the effects of carbenicillin
- antacids reduce absorption of carbenicillin.
- chloramphenicol (Chloromycetin)
- erythromycin (Erythrocin, E-Mycin, etc.)
- tetracyclines (Achromycin, Aureomycin, Declomycin, Minocin, etc.; see Drug Class, Section Three)

Driving a Vehicle, Operating Machinery, Engaging in Hazardous Activities: Usually no restrictions. Be alert to the rare occurrence of dizziness and/or nausea, and restrict activities accordingly.

Aviation Note: The use of this drug *may be a disqualification* for the piloting of aircraft. Consultation with a designated Aviation Medical Examiner is advised.

Exposure to Sun: No restrictions.

Special Storage Instructions
Keep in a tightly closed container at room temperature.

CARISOPRODOL

Year Introduced: 1959

Brand Names

USA	Canada
Rela (Schering)	Soma (Horner)
Soma (Wallace)	Soma Compound [CD]
Soma Compound [CD] (Wallace)	(Horner)
Soma Compound with/Codeine [CD] (Wallace)	

Common Synonyms ("Street Names"):   None

Drug Class: Muscle Relaxant

Prescription Required: Yes

Available for Purchase by Generic Name: Yes

Available Dosage Forms and Strengths
    Tablets — 350 mg.

Tablet May Be Crushed or Capsule Opened for Administration: Yes

How This Drug Works
Intended Therapeutic Effect(s):   Relief of discomfort resulting from spasm of voluntary muscles.

Location of Drug Action(s):   Not completely established. This drug is thought to act on those nerve pathways in the brain and spinal cord that are involved in the reflex activity of voluntary muscles.

Method of Drug Action(s):   Not completely established. It is thought that this drug may relieve muscle spasm and pain by blocking the transmission of nerve impulses over reflex pathways and/or by producing a sedative effect that decreases the perception of pain.

Principal Uses of This Drug
As a Single Drug Product: Used primarily to relieve the pain and stiffness associated with spasm of voluntary muscles, such as that resulting from accidental injury of musculoskeletal structures. It is often necessary to supplement the use of this drug with other treatment measures, such as rest, support, and physiotherapy.

As a Combination Drug Product [CD]:   May be combined with caffeine and codeine to enhance its effectiveness in relieving discomfort. Codeine is an effective analgesic and may be required to control the pain that is not relieved by carisoprodol alone. Caffeine is added to offset the sedative effects of the analgesic drugs.

THIS DRUG SHOULD NOT BE TAKEN IF
—you have had an allergic reaction to any dosage form of it previously.
—you have a history of acute intermittent porphyria.
—it is prescribed for a child under 5 years of age.

INFORM YOUR PHYSICIAN BEFORE TAKING THIS DRUG IF
—you are allergic or sensitive to any chemically related drugs: meprobamate, tybamate.
—you have cerebral palsy.
—you are taking sedatives, sleep-inducing drugs, tranquilizers, antidepressants, or anti-convulsants.

Time Required for Apparent Benefit
Approximately 30 to 60 minutes.

Possible Side-Effects *(natural, expected, and unavoidable drug actions)*
Drowsiness, lethargy, sense of weakness.

Possible Adverse Effects *(unusual, unexpected, and infrequent reactions)*

IF ANY OF THE FOLLOWING DEVELOP, DISCONTINUE DRUG AND NOTIFY YOUR PHYSICIAN AS SOON AS POSSIBLE

Mild Adverse Effects
Allergic Reactions: Skin rashes (various kinds), fever, burning of eyes.
Other Reactions
Dizziness, unsteadiness in stance and gait, tremor, headache, fainting. Heart palpitation, nausea, indigestion.

Serious Adverse Effects
Allergic Reactions: Anaphylactic reaction (see Glossary), high fever, asthmatic breathing.
Idiosyncratic Reactions (may occur with first dose):   Extreme weakness, temporary paralysis of arms and legs, dizziness, temporary loss of vision, slurred speech, confusion.

Precautions for Use by Those over 60 Years of Age
You may be more sensitive to the sedative effects of this drug. Small doses are advisable until your individual response has been determined.
You may be more susceptible to the development of drowsiness, dizziness, muscular weakness, unsteadiness, and falling.

Advisability of Use During Pregnancy
Pregnancy Category: C (tentative). See Pregnancy Code inside back cover.
Animal reproduction studies: No data available.
Information from adequate studies in pregnant women is not available.
Ask physician for guidance.

Advisability of Use While Nursing Infant
Drug is known to be present in milk. Ask physician for guidance.

Habit-Forming Potential

This drug can produce psychological and (possibly) physical dependence if used in large doses for an extended period of time.

Effects of Overdosage

With Moderate Overdose: Dizziness, impaired stance, staggering gait, slurred speech, marked drowsiness.

With Large Overdose: Stupor progressing to deep sleep and coma, depression of breathing and heart function.

Possible Effects of Extended Use

Psychological and (possibly) physical dependence (see Glossary).

Suggested Periodic Examinations While Taking This Drug (at physician's discretion)

None.

While Taking This Drug, Observe the Following

Foods: No restrictions.

Beverages: No restrictions.

Alcohol: Use with extreme caution until combined effect is determined. Alcohol combined with carisoprodol can cause severe impairment of mental and physical functions.

Tobacco Smoking: No interactions expected.

Marijuana Smoking

Occasional (once or twice weekly): No effect to mild and transient increase in drowsiness, muscle weakness, and orthostatic hypotension (see Glossary).

Daily: Moderate to marked drowsiness, muscle weakness and incoordination, and significant accentuation of orthostatic hypotension.

Other Drugs

Carisoprodol may *increase* the effects of

- sedatives, sleep-inducing drugs, tranquilizers, antidepressants, and narcotic drugs. Use such drugs with caution until combined effect has been determined. Ask physician for guidance regarding dosage adjustment.

The following drugs may *increase* the effects of carisoprodol:

- tricyclic antidepressants (see Drug Class, Section Three) may increase the sedative action of carisoprodol.
- mono-amine oxidase (MAO) inhibitor drugs (see Drug Class, Section Three) may increase the muscle relaxant and sedative actions of carisoprodol.

The following drugs may *decrease* the effects of carisoprodol

- barbiturate drugs, especially phenobarbital, may hasten its destruction and elimination.
- some antihistamines, such as Benadryl and Fedrazil, may hasten its destruction and elimination.

Driving a Vehicle, Operating Machinery, Engaging in Hazardous Activities: This drug may impair mental alertness, judgment, and physical coordination. Avoid hazardous activities.

Aviation Note: The use of this drug *may be a disqualification* for the piloting of aircraft. Consultation with a designated Aviation Medical Examiner is advised.

Exposure to Sun: No restrictions.

Exposure to Heat: No restrictions.

Heavy Exercise or Exertion: No restrictions, but muscular strength and endurance may appear reduced.

Special Storage Instructions
Keep in a dry, tightly closed container.

CEFACLOR

Year Introduced: 1979

Brand Names

USA	Canada
Ceclor (Lilly)	Ceclor (Lilly)

Common Synonyms ("Street Names"):   None

Drug Class: Antibiotic (Anti-infective), Cephalosporin

Prescription Required: Yes

Available for Purchase by Generic Name: No

Available Dosage Forms and Strengths
Capsules — 250 mg., 500 mg.
Oral suspension — 125 mg., 250 mg. per teaspoonful (5 ml.)

Tablet May Be Crushed or Capsule Opened for Administration: Yes

How This Drug Works
Intended Therapeutic Effect(s):   The elimination of infections responsive to the action of this drug.

Location of Drug Action(s):   Any body tissue or fluid in which sufficient concentration of the drug can be achieved.

Method of Drug Action(s):   This drug destroys susceptible infecting bacteria by interfering with their ability to produce new protective cell walls as they multiply and grow.

Principal Uses of This Drug
As a Single Drug Product: To treat certain infections of the skin and soft tissues, the upper and lower respiratory tract (including middle ear infections and "strep" throat), and certain infections of the urinary tract.

THIS DRUG SHOULD NOT BE TAKEN IF
—you are allergic to any cephalosporin antibiotics (Ancef, Anspor, Ceclor, Cefadyl, Ceporan, Ceporex, Duricef, Kafocin, Keflex, Keflin, Kefzol, Loridine,
Mandol, Mefoxin, Velosef).

INFORM YOUR PHYSICIAN BEFORE TAKING THIS DRUG IF
—you have a history of allergy to any form of penicillin (see Drug Class, Section
Three).
—you have impaired kidney function.

Time Required for Apparent Benefit
Drug action usually begins in 30 minutes and reaches its peak in 1 to 2 hours.
Continuous use on a regular schedule for 2 to 5 days is usually necessary to
determine this drug's effectiveness in controlling the infection under treatment. Response varies with the nature of the infection.

Possible Side-Effects *(natural, expected, and unavoidable drug actions)*
Superinfections (see Glossary).

Possible Adverse Effects *(unusual, unexpected, and infrequent reactions)*

**IF ANY OF THE FOLLOWING DEVELOP, DISCONTINUE DRUG AND NOTIFY
YOUR PHYSICIAN AS SOON AS POSSIBLE**

Mild Adverse Effects
  Allergic Reactions: Skin rash (various kinds), itching, hives.
  Other Reactions: Nausea and vomiting (1 in 90), mild diarrhea (1 in 70),
  sore mouth or tongue.
Serious Adverse Effects
  Allergic Reactions: Drug fever (see Glossary), joint aches and pains, ana-
  phylactic reaction (see Glossary).
  Idiosyncratic Reactions: Minor and temporary changes in white blood
  cell counts and liver function tests (infrequent).
  Other Reactions: Genital itching (may represent a superinfection). Se-
  vere diarrhea indicating a drug-induced form of colitis (rare).

Adverse Effects That May Mimic Natural Diseases or Disorders
Skin rash and fever may resemble measles.

CAUTION
1. In the management of diabetes it should be noted that this drug can cause
a false positive test result for urine sugar when testing with Clinitest tablets,
Benedict's solution or Fehling's solution, but not with Tes-Tape.
2. The maximal dosage in adults should not exceed 4 grams per 24 hours.

Precautions for Use by Infants and Children
Not recommended for use in infants less than one month old.
The maximal dose in children should not exceed 1 gram per 24 hours.

Precautions for Use by Those over 60 Years of Age

The natural decline in kidney function that occurs after 60 may require some reduction in dosage and lengthening of dosage intervals. Dosage must be carefully individualized and based upon measurements of kidney function.

Natural changes in the skin after 60 may predispose to severe and prolonged itching reactions in the genital and anal regions. This reaction should be reported promptly.

Advisability of Use During Pregnancy

Pregnancy Category: B (tentative). See Pregnancy Code inside back cover.

Animal reproduction studies reveal no birth defects due to this drug. Information from adequate studies in pregnant women is not available. Ask physician for guidance.

Advisability of Use While Nursing Infant

This drug is probably present in the mother's milk. It is advisable to proceed with breast-feeding under physician's supervision.

Habit-Forming Potential

None.

Effects of Overdosage

Nausea, vomiting, abdominal cramping, and/or diarrhea.

Possible Effects of Extended Use

Superinfections (see Glossary).

Suggested Periodic Examinations While Taking This Drug (at physician's discretion)

Complete blood cell counts.

While Taking This Drug, Observe the Following

Foods: No restrictions of food selection. Drug is most effective when taken 1 hour before or 2 hours after eating, but may be taken at any time.

Beverages: No restrictions. This drug may be taken with milk.

Alcohol: No interactions expected.

Tobacco Smoking: No interactions expected.

Marijuana Smoking: No interactions expected.

Other Drugs

Cefaclor *taken concurrently* with

- probenecid (Benemid) will slow the elimination of cefaclor, resulting in higher blood levels and prolonged effect.

Driving a Vehicle, Operating Machinery, Engaging in Hazardous Activities: Usually no restrictions. However, it is advisable to observe for the possible occurrence of nausea, vomiting, or diarrhea and to restrict activities accordingly.

Aviation Note: The use of this drug *may be a disqualification* for the piloting of aircraft. Consultation with a designated Aviation Medical Examiner is advised.

Exposure to Sun: No restrictions.

Occurrence of Unrelated Illness: If you experience another illness or injury of any kind, notify *all* your attending physicians that you have been taking this drug.

Discontinuation: Certain infections require that this drug be taken for 10 days to prevent the development of rheumatic fever. Ask your physician for guidance regarding the recommended duration of treatment.

Special Storage Instructions

Capsules should be kept in a dry, tightly closed container. Oral suspension should be refrigerated.

Observe the Following Expiration Times

Do not take the oral suspension of this drug if it is older than 14 days.

CEFADROXIL

Year Introduced: 1977

Brand Names

USA	Canada
Duricef (Mead Johnson)	Duricef (Bristol)
Ultracef (Bristol)	

Common Synonyms ("Street Names"):   Antibiotic

Drug Class: Anti-infectives, Cephalosporins

Prescription Required: USA: Yes
Canada: Yes

Available for Purchase by Generic Name: USA: No   Canada: No

Available Dosage Forms and Strengths
Tablets — 1000 mg. (1 gram)
Capsules — 500 mg.
Oral suspension — 125 mg., 250 mg., 500 mg. per teaspoonful (5 ml.)

Tablet May Be Crushed or Capsule Opened for Administration: Yes

How This Drug Works

Intended Therapeutic Effect(s):   The elimination of infections responsive to the action of this drug.

Location of Drug Action(s):   Any body tissue or fluid in which sufficient concentration of the drug can be achieved.

Method of Drug Action(s):   This drug destroys susceptible infecting bacteria by interfering with their ability to produce new protective cell walls as they multiply and grow.

Principal Uses of This Drug

As a Single Drug Product: To treat certain infections of the skin and soft tissues, "strep" throat and tonsillitis, and certain infections of the urinary tract.

THIS DRUG SHOULD NOT BE TAKEN IF
—you are allergic to *any* cephalosporin or related drug (see Drug Class, Section Three).

INFORM YOUR PHYSICIAN BEFORE TAKING THIS DRUG IF
—you have a history of allergy to any form of penicillin (see Drug Class, Section Three).
—you have impaired kidney function.
—you have a history of any form of colitis.

Time Required for Apparent Benefit
Varies with the nature of the infection under treatment; usually from 2 to 5 days.

Possible Side-Effects *(natural, expected, and unavoidable drug actions)*
Superinfections (see Glossary).

Possible Adverse Effects *(unusual, unexpected, and infrequent reactions)*

IF ANY OF THE FOLLOWING DEVELOP, DISCONTINUE DRUG AND NOTIFY YOUR PHYSICIAN AS SOON AS POSSIBLE

Mild Adverse Effects
Allergic Reactions: Skin rashes, hives, localized swellings.

Other Reactions: Headache, drowsiness, dizziness.
Irritation of mouth or tongue, indigestion, abdominal cramping, nausea, vomiting, diarrhea.

Serious Adverse Effects
Allergic Reactions: Anaphylactic reaction (see Glossary), fever, sore throat.
Other Reactions: Genital itching, vaginitis (may be yeast infection), abdominal pain and cramping accompanied by severe diarrhea—possible pseudomembranous colitis (rare).

Precautions for Use by Those over 60 Years of Age
The natural decline in kidney function that occurs after 60 may require significant reduction in dosage and lengthening of dosage intervals. Dosage must be carefully individualized and based upon measurements of kidney function.
Natural changes in the skin after 60 may predispose to severe and prolonged itching reactions in the genital and anal regions. Such reactions should be reported promptly.

Advisability of Use During Pregnancy
Pregnancy Category: B (tentative). See Pregnancy Code inside back cover. Animal reproduction studies in mice and rats reveal no birth defects due to this drug.

Information from adequate studies in pregnant women is not available. This drug is considered safe for use during entire pregnancy. Ask physician for guidance.

Advisability of Use While Nursing Infant

This drug is present in human milk and can sensitize the infant to cephalosporin antibiotics (and possibly to penicillin). Ask physician for guidance.

Habit-Forming Potential

None.

Effects of Overdosage

Nausea, vomiting, abdominal cramping, and/or diarrhea.

Possible Effects of Extended Use

Superinfections (see Glossary).

Suggested Periodic Examinations While Taking This Drug (at physician's discretion)

Complete blood cell counts.
Liver and kidney function tests.

While Taking This Drug, Observe the Following

Foods: No restrictions. May be taken without regard to eating.
Beverages: No restrictions. May be taken with milk.
Alcohol: No interactions expected.
Tobacco Smoking: No interactions expected.
Marijuana Smoking: No interactions expected.
Other Drugs
The following drugs may *increase* the effects of cefadroxil:
  • probenecid (Benemid) may increase its blood level and prolong its action.

Driving a Vehicle, Operating Machinery, Engaging in Hazardous Activities: No restrictions unless drug causes drowsiness or dizziness.

Aviation Note: The use of this drug *may be a disqualification* for the piloting of aircraft. Consultation with a designated Aviation Medical Examiner is advised.

Exposure to Sun: No restrictions.

Discontinuation: Certain infections require that this drug be taken for 10 days to prevent the development of rheumatic fever. Ask your physician for guidance regarding the recommended duration of treatment.

Special Storage Instructions

Keep tablets and capsules in dry, tightly closed containers at room temperature.
Keep the oral suspension in the refrigerator; do not freeze.

Observe the Following Expiration Times

The oral suspension should be stored under refrigeration and discarded after 14 days.

CEPHALEXIN

Year Introduced: 1971

Brand Names

USA	Canada
Keflex (Lilly)	Ceporex (Glaxo)
	Keflex (Lilly)
	Novolexin (Novopharm)

Common Synonyms ("Street Names"): None

Drug Class: Antibiotic (Anti-infective), Cephalosporins

Prescription Required: Yes

Available for Purchase by Generic Name: No

Available Dosage Forms and Strengths

Tablets — 1000 mg. (1 gram)
Capsules — 250 mg., 500 mg.
Oral suspension — 125 mg., 250 mg. per teaspoonful (5 ml.)
Pediatric drops — 100 mg. per ml.

Tablet May Be Crushed or Capsule Opened for Administration: Yes

How This Drug Works

Intended Therapeutic Effect(s): The elimination of infections responsive to the action of this drug.

Location of Drug Action(s): Any body tissue or fluid in which sufficient concentration of the drug can be achieved.

Method of Drug Action(s): This drug destroys susceptible infecting bacteria by interfering with their ability to produce new protective cell walls as they multiply and grow.

Principal Uses of This Drug

As a Single Drug Product: To treat certain infections of the skin and soft tissues, of the upper respiratory tract (including middle ear infections and "strep" throat), of the genito-urinary tract, and certain infections involving bones and joints.

THIS DRUG SHOULD NOT BE TAKEN IF

—you are allergic to any cephalosporin antibiotics (Ancef, Anspor, Ceclor, Cefadyl, Ceporan, Ceporex, Duricef, Kafocin, Keflex, Keflin, Kefzol, Loridine, Mandol, Mefoxin, Velosef).

INFORM YOUR PHYSICIAN BEFORE TAKING THIS DRUG IF

—you have a history of allergy to any form of penicillin (see Drug Class, Section Three).
—you have impaired kidney function.

Time Required for Apparent Benefit
Varies with nature of infection under treatment; usually from 2 to 5 days.

Possible Side-Effects *(natural, expected, and unavoidable drug actions)*
Superinfections (see Glossary).

Possible Adverse Effects *(unusual, unexpected, and infrequent reactions)*

IF ANY OF THE FOLLOWING DEVELOP, DISCONTINUE DRUG AND NOTIFY YOUR PHYSICIAN AS SOON AS POSSIBLE

Mild Adverse Effects
Allergic Reactions: Skin rashes (various kinds).
Other Reactions: Headache, drowsiness, dizziness, nausea, vomiting, diarrhea, indigestion, abdominal cramping, irritation of mouth or tongue.
Serious Adverse Effects
Allergic Reactions: Anaphylactic reaction (see Glossary), fever, sore throat.

Precautions for Use by Those over 60 Years of Age
The natural decline in kidney function that occurs after 60 may require significant reduction in dosage and lengthening of dosage intervals. Dosage must be carefully individualized and based upon measurements of kidney function.
Natural changes in the skin after 60 may predispose to severe and prolonged itching reactions in the genital and anal regions. This reaction should be reported promptly.

Advisability of Use During Pregnancy
Pregnancy Category: B (tentative). See Pregnancy Code inside back cover.
Animal reproduction studies in mice and rats reveal no birth defects due to this drug.
Information from adequate studies in pregnant women is not available.
Ask physician for guidance.

Advisability of Use While Nursing Infant
Drug may be present in milk and may sensitize infant to cephalosporins (and possibly to penicillin). Ask physician for guidance.

Habit-Forming Potential
None.

Effects of Overdosage
Nausea, vomiting, abdominal cramping, and/or diarrhea.

Possible Effects of Extended Use
Superinfections (see Glossary).

Suggested Periodic Examinations While Taking This Drug (at physician's discretion)
Complete blood cell counts.
Liver and kidney function tests.

While Taking This Drug, Observe the Following

Foods: No restrictions of food selection. Drug is most effective when taken 1 hour before or 2 hours after eating, but may be taken at any time.

Beverages: No restrictions.

Alcohol: No interactions expected.

Tobacco Smoking: No interactions expected.

Marijuana Smoking: No interactions expected.

Other Drugs

Cephalexin may *increase* the effects of oral anticoagulants, and make it necessary to reduce their dosage.

The following drug may *increase* the effects of cephalexin:
- probenecid (Benemid) may increase its blood level and prolong its action.

Driving a Vehicle, Operating Machinery, Engaging in Hazardous Activities: No restrictions unless drug causes dizziness or drowsiness.

Aviation Note: The use of this drug *may be a disqualification* for the piloting of aircraft. Consultation with a designated Aviation Medical Examiner is advised.

Exposure to Sun: No restrictions.

Discontinuation: Certain infections require that this drug be taken for 10 days to prevent the development of rheumatic fever. Ask your physician for guidance regarding the recommended duration of treatment.

Special Storage Instructions

Tablets and capsules should be kept in a tightly closed container. Oral suspension and drops should be refrigerated.

Observe the Following Expiration Times

Do not take the oral suspension or drops of this drug if it is older than 14 days —when kept at room temperature or refrigerated.

CEPHRADINE

Year Introduced: 1974

Brand Names

USA	Canada
Anspor (Smith Kline & French)	Velosef (Squibb)
Velosef (Squibb)	

Common Synonyms ("Street Names"): None

Drug Class: Antibiotic (Anti-infective), Cephalosporins

Prescription Required: Yes

Available for Purchase by Generic Name: No

Available Dosage Forms and Strengths
Tablets — 1 gram
Capsules — 250 mg., 500 mg.
Oral suspension — 125 mg., 250 mg. per teaspoonful (5 ml.)

Tablet May Be Crushed or Capsule Opened for Administration: Yes

How This Drug Works
Intended Therapeutic Effect(s):   The elimination of infections responsive to the action of this drug.
Location of Drug Action(s):   Any body tissue or fluid in which sufficient concentration of the drug can be achieved.
Method of Drug Action(s):   This drug destroys susceptible infecting bacteria by interfering with their ability to produce new protective cell walls as they multiply and grow.

Principal Uses of This Drug
As a Single Drug Product: To treat certain infections of the skin and soft tissues, of the upper and lower respiratory tracts (including middle ear infections and "strep" throat), of the urinary tract, and certain infections involving the blood stream (septicemia), the bones, and the joints.

THIS DRUG SHOULD NOT BE TAKEN IF
—you are allergic to any cephalosporin antibiotic (Ancef, Anspor, Ceclor, Cefadyl, Ceporan, Ceporex, Duricef, Kafocin, Keflex, Keflin, Kefzol, Loridine, Mandol, Mefoxin, Velosef).

INFORM YOUR PHYSICIAN BEFORE TAKING THIS DRUG IF
—you have a history of allergy to any form of penicillin (see Drug Class, Section Three).
—you have impaired kidney function.

Time Required for Apparent Benefit
Varies with nature of infection under treatment; usually from 2 to 5 days.

Possible Side-Effects *(natural, expected, and unavoidable drug actions)*
Superinfections (see Glossary).

Possible Adverse Effects *(unusual, unexpected, and infrequent reactions)*
IF ANY OF THE FOLLOWING DEVELOP, DISCONTINUE DRUG AND NOTIFY YOUR PHYSICIAN AS SOON AS POSSIBLE
Mild Adverse Effects
Allergic Reactions: Skin rashes (various kinds).
Other Reactions: Headache, drowsiness, dizziness, nausea, vomiting, diarrhea, indigestion, abdominal cramping, irritation of mouth or tongue.
Serious Adverse Effects
Allergic Reactions: Anaphylactic reaction (see Glossary), fever, sore throat.

Precautions for Use by Those over 60 Years of Age

The natural decline in kidney function that occurs after 60 may require significant reduction in dosage and lengthening of dosage intervals. Dosage must be carefully individualized and based upon measurements of kidney function.

Natural changes in the skin after 60 may predispose to severe and prolonged itching reactions in the genital and anal regions. This reaction should be reported promptly.

Advisability of Use During Pregnancy

Pregnancy Category: B (tentative). See Pregnancy Code inside back cover. Animal reproduction studies in mice and rats reveal no birth defects due to this drug.

Information from adequate studies in pregnant women is not available. Ask physician for guidance.

Advisability of Use While Nursing Infant

Drug may be present in milk and can sensitize infant to cephalosporins (and possibly to penicillin). Ask physician for guidance.

Habit-Forming Potential

None.

Effects of Overdosage

Nausea, vomiting, abdominal cramping, and/or diarrhea.

Possible Effects of Extended Use

Superinfections (see Glossary).

Suggested Periodic Examinations While Taking This Drug (at physician's discretion)

Complete blood cell counts.

Liver and kidney function tests.

While Taking This Drug, Observe the Following

Foods: No restrictions of food selection. Drug is most effective when taken 1 hour before or 2 hours after eating, but may be taken at any time.

Beverages: No restrictions.

Alcohol: No interactions expected.

Tobacco Smoking: No interactions expected.

Marijuana Smoking: No interactions expected.

Other Drugs

Cephradine may *increase* the effects of
- oral anticoagulants, and make it necessary to reduce their dosage.

The following drug may *increase* the effects of cephradine:
- probenecid (Benemid) may increase its blood level and prolong its action.

Driving a Vehicle, Operating Machinery, Engaging in Hazardous Activities:
No restrictions unless drug causes dizziness or drowsiness.

Aviation Note: The use of this drug *may be a disqualification* for the piloting of aircraft. Consultation with a designated Aviation Medical Examiner is advised.

Exposure to Sun: No restrictions.

Discontinuation: Certain infections require that this drug be taken continuously for 10 days to prevent the development of rheumatic fever or nephritis. Ask your physician for guidance regarding the recommended duration of treatment.

Special Storage Instructions

Capsules should be kept in a tightly closed container. Oral suspension should be refrigerated.

Observe the Following Expiration Times

Do not take the oral suspension of this drug if it is older than 14 days—when kept at room temperature or refrigerated.

CHLORAL HYDRATE

Year Introduced: 1860

Brand Names

USA	Canada
Aquachloral (Webcon)	Noctec (Squibb)
Noctec (Squibb)	Novochlorhydrate
Oradrate (Coast)	(Novopharm)
SK-Chloral Hydrate	
(Smith Kline & French)	

Common Synonyms ("Street Names"):   Chloral, Mickey, Peter; combined with alcohol: knockout drops, Mickey Finn

Drug Class: Sleep Inducer (Hypnotic)

Prescription Required: Yes (Controlled Drug, U.S. Schedule IV)*

Available for Purchase by Generic Name: Yes

Available Dosage Forms and Strengths

Capsules — 250 mg., 500 mg.
     Syrup — 250 mg., 500 mg. per teaspoonful (5 ml.)
     Elixir — 500 mg. per teaspoonful (5 ml.)
Suppositories — 325 mg., 500 mg., 650 mg., 975 mg., 1.3 Gms.

Tablet May Be Crushed or Capsule Opened for Administration: No

*See Schedules of Controlled Drugs inside back cover.

How This Drug Works
Intended Therapeutic Effect(s)
With low dosage, relief of mild to moderate anxiety or tension (sedative effect).

With higher dosage taken at bedtime, relief of insomnia (hypnotic effect).

Location of Drug Action(s):   Not completely established. Thought to be the wake-sleep centers of the brain, possibly the reticular activating system.

Method of Drug Action(s):   Not established.

Principal Uses of This Drug
As a Single Drug Product: Used most commonly as a bedtime sedative in sufficient dosage to induce sleep. It is the drug of choice for use in the elderly because it produces less "hangover" effect and does not cause the confusion so commonly seen with use of the barbiturates.

THIS DRUG SHOULD NOT BE TAKEN IF
—you have had an allergic reaction to any dosage form of it previously.
—you have a history of severe impairment of liver or kidney function.
—you have active inflammation of the stomach (gastritis).

INFORM YOUR PHYSICIAN BEFORE TAKING THIS DRUG IF
—you are taking sedatives, other sleep-inducing drugs, tranquilizers, pain relievers, antihistamines, or narcotic drugs of any kind.
—you plan to have surgery under general anesthesia in the near future.

Time Required for Apparent Benefit
Approximately 30 to 60 minutes.

Possible Side-Effects (natural, expected, and unavoidable drug actions)
Lightheadedness in upright position, unsteadiness in stance and gait, weakness.

Possible Adverse Effects (unusual, unexpected, and infrequent reactions)

IF ANY OF THE FOLLOWING DEVELOP, DISCONTINUE DRUG AND NOTIFY YOUR PHYSICIAN AS SOON AS POSSIBLE

Mild Adverse Effects
Allergic Reactions: Skin rashes (various kinds), hives.
Other Reactions
Indigestion, nausea, heartburn, vomiting.
Nightmares, "hangover" effects.
Serious Adverse Effects
Allergic Reactions: Severe skin reactions.
Idiosyncratic Reactions: Paradoxical excitement and delirium, sleepwalking.

Precautions for Use by Those over 60 Years of Age
You may be more sensitive to the actions of this drug. Small doses are advisable until your individual response has been determined.

You may be more susceptible to the "hangover" effect caused by most sleep-inducing (hypnotic) drugs.

Natural changes in body functions may make you more susceptible to the development of dizziness, confused thinking, impaired memory, incoordination, unsteady gait and balance, falling, loss of bladder control, and constipation.

Advisability of Use During Pregnancy
Pregnancy Category: C (tentative). See Pregnancy Code inside back cover.
Animal reproduction studies: No data available.
Information from adequate studies in pregnant women is not available.
Ask physician for guidance.

Advisability of Use While Nursing Infant
This drug is known to be present in milk. Observe nursing infant for indications of sedation. Ask physician for guidance.

Habit-Forming Potential
This drug can cause psychological and/or physical dependence (see Glossary). Avoid large doses and continuous use.

Effects of Overdosage
With Moderate Overdose: Marked drowsiness, confusion, incoordination, slurred speech, staggering gait, weakness, vomiting.
With Large Overdose: Stupor, deep sleep, flushing of the skin, weak pulse, slow and shallow breathing, dilated pupils.

Possible Effects of Extended Use
Psychological and/or physical dependence.
Kidney damage.

Suggested Periodic Examinations While Taking This Drug (at physician's discretion)
Kidney function studies.

While Taking This Drug, Observe the Following
Foods: No restrictions.
Beverages: Capsules should be taken with a full glass of liquid (water, milk, or fruit juice) to reduce stomach irritation that might occur in some individuals. The syrup and elixir should be taken in one-half glass of water, milk, or fruit juice.
Alcohol: Avoid completely for 6 hours before taking this drug. Alcohol can increase greatly the sedative and depressant actions of this drug on brain function.
Tobacco Smoking: No interactions expected.
Marijuana Smoking
Occasional (once or twice weekly): Mild, transient increase in drowsiness, unsteadiness, and impairment of mental and physical performance.
Daily: Marked, prolonged drowsiness, unsteadiness, and significantly impaired mental and physical performance.

Other Drugs

Chloral hydrate may *increase* the effects of

- oral anticoagulants, and cause abnormal bleeding or hemorrhage. Ask physician for guidance regarding prothrombin time testing and adjustment (reduction) of anticoagulant dosage.
- other sedatives, sleep-inducing drugs, tranquilizers, antihistamines, pain relievers, and narcotic drugs. Dosage adjustments may be necessary.

Chloral hydrate may *decrease* the effects of

- cortisone and related drugs, by hastening their elimination from the body. Dosage adjustments may be necessary.

The following drugs may *increase* the effects of chloral hydrate:

- mono-amine oxidase (MAO) inhibitor drugs (see Drug Class, Section Three) may increase the sedative action of chloral hydrate and cause oversedation.
- some phenothiazine and antihistamine drugs may increase the sedative action of chloral hydrate. It is advisable to use this combination with caution.

Driving a Vehicle, Operating Machinery, Engaging in Hazardous Activities: This drug can impair mental alertness, judgment, physical coordination, and reaction time. Avoid hazardous activities until all sensation of drowsiness has disappeared.

Aviation Note: The use of this drug *is a disqualification* for the piloting of aircraft. Consultation with a designated Aviation Medical Examiner is advised.

Exposure to Sun: No restrictions.

Discontinuation: If it has been necessary to use this drug for an extended period of time, do not discontinue abruptly. Ask physician for guidance regarding dosage reduction and withdrawal. Ask physician for guidance regarding dosage adjustment of certain other drugs taken concurrently with chloral hydrate, such as oral anticoagulants and cortisone.

Special Storage Instructions

Keep in a tightly closed container.

Keep suppositories refrigerated.

CHLORAMPHENICOL

Year Introduced: 1947

Brand Names

USA	Canada
Amphicol (McKesson)	Chloromycetin (P.D. &
Antibiopto (Softcon)	Co.)
Chloromycetin	Chloroptic (Allergan)
(Parke-Davis)	Fenicol (Alcon)
Chloroptic (Allergan)	Isopto Fenicol (Alcon)
Econochlor (Alcon)	Minims (S & N)
Mychel (Rachelle)	Nova-Phenicol (Nova)
Ophthochlor	Novochlorocap
(Parke-Davis)	(Novopharm)
	Pentamycetin
	(Pentagone)
	Sopamycetin (Nordic)

Common Synonyms ("Street Names"):   None

Drug Class: Antibiotic (Anti-infective)

Prescription Required: Yes

Available for Purchase by Generic Name: USA: Yes   Canada: No

Available Dosage Forms and Strengths

Capsules — 250 mg., 500 mg.
Oral suspension — 150 mg. per teaspoonful (5 ml.)
Eye solution — 0.5%
Eye ointment — 1%
Ear solution — 0.5%
Cream — 1%

Tablet May Be Crushed or Capsule Opened for Administration: Yes

How This Drug Works

Intended Therapeutic Effect(s):   The elimination of infections responsive to the action of this drug.

Location of Drug Action(s):   Any body tissue or fluid in which sufficient concentration of the drug can be achieved.

Method of Drug Action(s):   This drug prevents the growth and multiplication of susceptible bacteria by interfering with their formation of essential proteins.

Principal Uses of This Drug

As a Single Drug Product: This drug is quite effective in a very broad spectrum of infections. However, because of its potential for serious toxicity (fatal aplastic anemia), its use is now reserved for life-threatening infections caused by organisms that are resistant to safer antibiotics, and for infections in individuals who, for one reason or another, cannot take other appropriate anti-infective drugs.

THIS DRUG SHOULD NOT BE TAKEN IF
—you have had an allergic reaction to any dosage form of it previously.
—it is prescribed for a mild or trivial infection such as a cold, sore throat, or "flu"-like illness.
—it is prescribed for a premature or newborn infant (under 2 weeks of age).

INFORM YOUR PHYSICIAN BEFORE TAKING THIS DRUG IF
—you have a history of liver or kidney disease.
—you have a history of a blood or bone marrow disease.
—you are taking anticoagulants.

Time Required for Apparent Benefit
Varies with nature of infection under treatment; usually 2 to 5 days.

Possible Side-Effects *(natural, expected, and unavoidable drug actions)*
Superinfections (see Glossary).

Possible Adverse Effects *(unusual, unexpected, and infrequent reactions)*

IF ANY OF THE FOLLOWING DEVELOP, DISCONTINUE DRUG AND NOTIFY YOUR PHYSICIAN AS SOON AS POSSIBLE

Mild Adverse Effects
Allergic Reactions: Skin rash (various kinds), hives, swelling of face or extremities, fever.
Other Reactions
Nausea, vomiting, diarrhea, irritation of mouth or tongue, "black tongue."
Headache, confusion.
Peripheral neuritis (see Glossary), numbness, tingling, pain (often burning), weakness in hands and/or feet.

Serious Adverse Effects
Allergic Reactions: Anaphylactic reaction (see Glossary), jaundice (rare).
Other Reactions: Bone marrow depression (see Glossary)—weakness, fever, sore throat, unusual bleeding or bruising.

CAUTION
1. This drug can cause serious bone marrow depression and aplastic anemia (see Glossary). It must not be used to treat trivial infections or as a preventive medication under any circumstances. Its use must be restricted to the treatment of serious or life-threatening infections which fail to respond to other anti-infective drugs.
2. Troublesome and persistent diarrhea can develop in sensitive individuals. If diarrhea persists more than 24 hours, discontinue this drug and consult your physician for guidance.

Precautions for Use by Those over 60 Years of Age
The natural decline in liver and kidney function that occurs after 60 may require reduction in dosage and adjustment of dosage interval.
Natural changes in the skin after 60 may predispose to severe and prolonged itching reactions in the genital and anal regions. This reaction should be reported promptly.

Advisability of Use During Pregnancy

Pregnancy Category: C (tentative). See Pregnancy Code inside back cover.

Animal reproduction studies are inconclusive.

Information from adequate studies in pregnant women is not available.

It is advisable to avoid this drug during first 3 months.

Ask physician for guidance.

Advisability of Use While Nursing Infant

Drug can be present in milk and can have adverse effects on infant. Ask physician for guidance.

Habit-Forming Potential

None.

Effects of Overdosage

Possible nausea, vomiting, and/or diarrhea.

Possible Effects of Extended Use

Impaired vision, bone marrow depression, superinfections.

Suggested Periodic Examinations While Taking This Drug (at physician's discretion)

Complete blood cell counts, which should be performed before treatment is started and repeated every 2 days during administration of drug.

Periodic liver and kidney function tests.

While Taking This Drug, Observe the Following

Foods: No restrictions.

Beverages: No restrictions.

Alcohol: Avoid while taking chloramphenicol if

• you have a history of liver disease.

• you do not know your sensitivity to this combination. In some people, the concurrent use of chloramphenicol and alcohol can produce a "disulfiram-like" reaction (see Glossary). Use alcohol cautiously until combined effect is determined.

Tobacco Smoking: No interactions expected.

Marijuana Smoking: No interactions expected.

Other Drugs

Chloramphenicol may *increase* the effects of

• oral anti-diabetic (hypoglycemic) drugs; these are: chlorpropamide (Diabinese), acetohexamide (Dymelor), tolbutamide (Orinase), tolazamide (Tolinase).

• dicumarol.

• phenytoin (Dantoin, Dilantin, etc.).

Chloramphenicol may *decrease* the effects of

• cyclophosphamide (Cytoxan).

• penicillin drugs.

Driving a Vehicle, Operating Machinery, Engaging in Hazardous Activities: Usually no restrictions. Be alert to the rare occurrence of nausea and/or confusion, and restrict activities accordingly.

Aviation Note: The use of this drug *may be a disqualification* for the piloting of aircraft. Consultation with a designated Aviation Medical Examiner is advised.

Exposure to Sun: No restrictions.

Special Storage Instructions

Keep in a tightly closed, light-resistant container.

CHLORDIAZEPOXIDE

Year Introduced: 1960

Brand Names

USA		Canada
A-poxide (Abbott)	SK-Lygen (Smith	Apo-Chlordiazepoxide
Librax [CD] (Roche)	Kline & French)	(Apotex)
Libritabs (Roche)	Tenax	Librium (Roche)
Librium (Roche)	(Reid-Provident)	Medilium (Medic)
Limbitrol [CD]		Novopoxide
(Roche)		(Novopharm)
		Relium (Riva)
		Solium (Horner)

Common Synonyms ("Street Names"):   Downs, nerve pills, tranks

Drug Class: Tranquilizer, Mild (Anti-anxiety), Benzodiazepines

Prescription Required: Yes (Controlled Drug, U.S. Schedule IV)*

Available for Purchase by Generic Name: Yes

Available Dosage Forms and Strengths

Tablets — 5 mg., 10 mg., 25 mg.

Capsules — 5 mg., 10 mg., 25 mg.

Injection — 100 mg. per ampule

Tablet May Be Crushed or Capsule Opened for Administration: Yes

How This Drug Works

Intended Therapeutic Effect(s): Relief of mild to moderate anxiety and nervous tension, without significant sedation.

Location of Drug Action(s): Thought to be the limbic system of the brain, one of the centers that influence emotional stability.

*See Schedules of Controlled Drugs inside back cover.

Method of Drug Action(s):   Not established. Present thinking is that this drug may reduce the activity of certain parts of the limbic system.

Principal Uses of This Drug
As a Single Drug Product: This mild tranquilizer is used primarily to (1) provide short-term relief of mild to moderate anxiety, and (2) relieve the symptoms of acute alcohol withdrawal: agitation, tremors, hallucinations, incipient delirium tremens.

As a Combination Drug Product [CD]:   Used in combination with amitriptyline (an antidepressant) to allay the anxiety that is often a troublesome feature in the agitated and depressed patient. Also used in combination with clidinium (a synthetic atropine-like antispasmodic) to treat peptic ulcer disease and the irritable bowel syndrome.

THIS DRUG SHOULD NOT BE TAKEN IF
—you have had an allergic reaction to any dosage form of it previously.
—you are subject to acute intermittent porphyria.
—you have myasthenia gravis.
—it is prescribed for a child under 6 years of age.

INFORM YOUR PHYSICIAN BEFORE TAKING THIS DRUG IF
—you are allergic to any drugs chemically related to chlordiazepoxide: clorazepate, diazepam, flurazepam, oxazepam (see Drug Profiles for brand names).
—you have diabetes.
—you have epilepsy.
—you are taking sedative, sleep-inducing, tranquilizer, or anti-convulsant drugs of any kind.
—you are taking anticoagulant drugs.
—you plan to have surgery under general or spinal anesthesia in the near future.

Time Required for Apparent Benefit
Approximately 2 to 4 hours. For severe symptoms of some duration, benefit may require regular medication for several days.

Possible Side-Effects *(natural, expected, and unavoidable drug actions)*
Drowsiness, lethargy, unsteadiness in stance and gait.
Increase in the level of blood sugar in some cases of diabetes.

Possible Adverse Effects *(unusual, unexpected, and infrequent reactions)*

IF ANY OF THE FOLLOWING DEVELOP, DISCONTINUE DRUG AND NOTIFY YOUR PHYSICIAN AS SOON AS POSSIBLE
Mild Adverse Effects
Allergic Reactions: Skin rashes (various kinds).
Other Reactions: Dizziness, fainting, blurred vision, double vision, slurred speech, nausea, menstrual irregularity, vivid dreaming.
Serious Adverse Effects
Allergic Reactions: Jaundice (see Glossary), impaired resistance to infection manifested by fever and/or sore throat, unusual bleeding or bruising.

Paradoxical Reactions: Acute excitement, hallucinations, rage.
Other Reactions: Parkinson-like disorders (see Glossary), depression.

Precautions for Use by Infants and Children
Safety and effectiveness in children below the age of 6 years has not been established.
This drug is contraindicated in the hyperactive or psychotic child of any age.
If this drug is used concurrently with a narcotic analgesic, the initial dose of the narcotic should be reduced by one-third.

Precautions for Use by Those over 60 Years of Age
Natural changes in body functions increase the duration of this drug's action. It is necessary to use smaller doses with longer intervals between doses to avoid excessive accumulation of the drug in body tissues. Dosage must be carefully individualized and limited to the smallest effective amount.
You may be more susceptible to the development of lightheadedness, impaired thinking and memory, confusion, lethargy, drowsiness, incoordination, unsteady gait and balance, impaired bladder control, and constipation.
Be alert to the possibility of paradoxical responses consisting of excitement, agitation, anger, hostility, and rage.

Advisability of Use During Pregnancy
Pregnancy Category: C (tentative). See Pregnancy Code inside back cover.
Animal reproduction studies in mice reveal significant birth defects due to this drug.
Information from adequate studies in pregnant women is not available.
Ask physician for guidance.
The findings of some recent studies suggest a possible association between the use of this drug during early pregnancy and the occurrence of birth defects, such as cleft lip. It is advisable to avoid this drug completely during the first 3 months of pregnancy.

Advisability of Use While Nursing Infant
With recommended dosage, drug is present in milk and can affect infant. Avoid use if possible. Ask physician for guidance.

Habit-Forming Potential
This drug can produce psychological and/or physical dependence (see Glossary) if used in large doses for an extended period of time.

Effects of Overdosage
With Moderate Overdose: Marked drowsiness, weakness, feeling of drunkenness, staggering gait, tremor.
With Large Overdose: Stupor progressing to deep sleep and coma.

Possible Effects of Extended Use
Psychological and/or physical dependence.
Impairment of blood cell production.
Impairment of liver function.

Suggested Periodic Examinations While Taking This Drug (at physician's discretion)

Blood cell counts and liver function tests during long-term use.

Blood sugar measurements (in presence of diabetes).

While Taking This Drug, Observe the Following

Food: No restrictions.

Beverages: Large intake of coffee, tea, or cola drinks (because of their caffeine content) may reduce the calming action of this drug.

Alcohol: Use with extreme caution until the combined effect is determined. Alcohol may increase the sedative effects of chlordiazepoxide. Chlordiazepoxide may increase the intoxicating effects of alcohol.

Tobacco Smoking: Heavy smoking may reduce the calming action of chlordiazepoxide.

Marijuana Smoking

Occasional (once or twice weekly):   Mild increase in sedative effect of this drug.

Daily: Marked increase in sedative effect of this drug.

Other Drugs

Chlordiazepoxide may *increase* the effects of

- other sedatives, sleep-inducing drugs, tranquilizers, anti-convulsants, and narcotic drugs. Use these only under supervision of a physician. Careful dosage adjustment is necessary.
- oral anticoagulants of the coumarin class; ask physician for guidance regarding need for dosage adjustment to prevent bleeding.
- anti-hypertensives, producing excessive lowering of the blood pressure.

Chlordiazepoxide *taken concurrently* with

- anti-convulsants, may cause an increase in the frequency or severity of seizures; an increase in the dose of the anti-convulsant may be necessary.
- mono-amine oxidase (MAO) inhibitor drugs (see Drug Class, Section Three), may cause extreme sedation, convulsions, or paradoxical excitement or rage.

The following drugs may *increase* the effects of chlordiazepoxide

- disulfiram (Antabuse) may delay the elimination of chlordiazepoxide.
- tricyclic antidepressants (see Drug Class, Section Three) may increase the sedative effects of chlordiazepoxide.

Driving a Vehicle, Operating Machinery, Engaging in Hazardous Activities: This drug can impair mental alertness, judgment, physical coordination, and reaction time. Avoid hazardous activities.

Aviation Note: The use of this drug *is a disqualification* for the piloting of aircraft. Consultation with a designated Aviation Medical Examiner is advised.

Exposure to Sun: Use caution until sensitivity is determined. Chlordiazepoxide may cause photosensitivity (see Glossary).

Exposure to Heat: Use caution until effect of excessive perspiration is determined. Because of reduced urine volume, chlordiazepoxide may accumulate in the body and produce effects of overdosage.

Heavy Exercise or Exertion: No restrictions in cool or temperate weather.

Discontinuation: If it has been necessary to use this drug for an extended period of time, do not discontinue it abruptly. Ask physician for guidance regarding dosage reduction and withdrawal. The dosage of other drugs taken concurrently with chlordiazepoxide may also require adjustment.

Special Storage Instructions
Keep in a dry, tightly closed, light-resistant container.

CHLOROTHIAZIDE

Year Introduced: 1958

Brand Names

USA	Canada
Diuril (Merck Sharp & Dohme)	Diuril (Frosst)
Aldoclor [CD] (Merck Sharp & Dohme)	
Diupres [CD] (Merck Sharp & Dohme)	
SK-chlorothiazide (SKF)	

Common Synonyms ("Street Names"):   Water pills

Drug Class: Anti-hypertensive (Hypotensive), Diuretic, Thiazides

Prescription Required: Yes

Available for Purchase by Generic Name: USA: Yes   Canada: No

Available Dosage Forms and Strengths
Tablets — 250 mg., 500 mg.
Oral suspension — 250 mg. per teaspoonful (5 ml.)

Tablet May Be Crushed or Capsule Opened for Administration: Yes

How This Drug Works
Intended Therapeutic Effect(s)
Elimination of excessive fluid retention (edema).
Reduction of high blood pressure.
Location of Drug Action(s):   Principal actions occur in
- the tubular systems of the kidney that determine the final composition of the urine
- the walls of the smaller arteries.

Method of Drug Action(s)

By increasing the elimination of salt and water from the body (through increased urine production), this drug reduces the volume of fluid in the blood and body tissues and lowers the sodium content throughout the body.

By relaxing the walls of the smaller arteries and allowing them to expand, this drug significantly increases the total capacity of the arterial system.

The combined effect of these two actions (reduced blood volume in expanded space) results in lowering of the blood pressure.

Principal Uses of This Drug

As a Single Drug Product: The thiazide diuretics are used primarily to (1) increase the volume of urine (diuresis) to correct the excessive fluid retention associated with congestive heart failure and certain types of liver and kidney disease; and (2) initiate treatment for high blood pressure (hypertension). They are usually the first drugs to be tried in treating mild to moderate hypertension. Less frequent uses include the treatment of diabetes insipidus and the prevention of kidney stones that contain calcium.

As a Combination Drug Product [CD]:   When this drug is used alone to treat hypertension, it is referred to as a "step 1" anti-hypertensive. Should it fail to reduce the blood pressure adequately, a "step 2" anti-hypertensive drug is added to be taken concurrently with the "step 1" drug. These drugs may be combined in one drug product. Chlorothiazide is available in combination with methyldopa and with reserpine to increase its effectiveness as an anti-hypertensive.

THIS DRUG SHOULD NOT BE TAKEN IF

—you have had an allergic reaction to any dosage form of it previously.

INFORM YOUR PHYSICIAN BEFORE TAKING THIS DRUG IF

—you are allergic to any form of "sulfa" drug.

—you are pregnant and your physician does not know it.

—you have a history of kidney disease or liver disease, or impaired kidney or liver function.

—you have diabetes (or a tendency to diabetes).

—you have a history of gout.

—you have a history of lupus erythematosus.

—you are taking any form of cortisone, digitalis, oral anti-diabetic drugs, or insulin.

—you plan to have surgery under general anesthesia in the near future.

Time Required for Apparent Benefit

Increased urine volume begins in 2 hours, reaches a maximum in 4 to 6 hours, and subsides in 8 to 12 hours. Continuous use on a regular schedule will be necessary for 2 to 3 weeks to determine this drug's effectiveness in lowering your blood pressure.

Possible Side-Effects *(natural, expected, and unavoidable drug actions)*

Lightheadedness on arising from sitting or lying position (see orthostatic hypotension in Glossary).

Increase in level of blood sugar, affecting control of diabetes.

Increase in level of blood uric acid, affecting control of gout.

Decrease in the level of blood potassium, resulting in muscle weakness and cramping.

Possible Adverse Effects (unusual, unexpected, and infrequent reactions)

IF ANY OF THE FOLLOWING DEVELOP, DISCONTINUE DRUG AND NOTIFY YOUR PHYSICIAN AS SOON AS POSSIBLE

Mild Adverse Effects

Allergic Reactions: Skin rashes (various kinds), hives, drug fever.

Other Reactions

Reduced appetite, indigestion, nausea, vomiting, diarrhea.

Headache, dizziness, yellow vision, blurred vision.

Serious Adverse Effects

Allergic Reactions: Hepatitis with jaundice (see Glossary), anaphylactic reaction (see Glossary), severe skin reactions.

Other Reactions

Inflammation of the pancreas—severe abdominal pain.

Bone marrow depression (see Glossary)—fatigue, weakness, fever, sore throat, unusual bleeding or bruising.

CAUTION

1. Do not exceed recommended doses. Increased dosage can cause excessive excretion of sodium and potassium with resultant loss of appetite, nausea, fatigue, weakness, confusion, and tingling in the extremities.
2. If you are also taking a digitalis preparation (digitoxin, digoxin), ensure an adequate intake of high potassium foods to prevent potassium deficiency —a potential cause of digitalis toxicity.

Precautions for Use by Those over 60 Years of Age

You may be more sensitive to the actions of this drug. Small doses are advisable until your individual response has been determined.

You may be more susceptible to the development of impaired thinking, orthostatic hypotension, potassium loss, and elevation of blood sugar, complicating the management of diabetes.

If you are taking this drug to treat high blood pressure, remember that warm weather and fever can reduce your blood pressure and make it necessary to adjust your dosage.

Overdosage and extended use of this drug can cause excessive loss of body water, thickening (increased viscosity) of the blood, and an increased tendency of the blood to clot, predisposing to stroke, heart attack, or thrombophlebitis.

Advisability of Use During Pregnancy

Pregnancy Category: B (tentative). See Pregnancy Code inside back cover.

Animal reproduction studies in rats reveal no birth defects due to this drug. Information from studies in pregnant women indicates no increased defects in 5283 exposures to this drug.

Ask physician for guidance.

This drug should not be used during pregnancy unless a very serious complication of pregnancy occurs for which this drug is significantly beneficial. This type of diuretic can have adverse effects on the fetus.

Advisability of Use While Nursing Infant

This drug is known to be present in milk. Prudent use is best determined by the physician's evaluation.

Habit-Forming Potential

None.

Effects of Overdosage

With Moderate Overdose: Dryness of mouth, thirst, lethargy, weakness, muscle pain and cramping, nausea, vomiting.

With Large Overdose: Drowsiness progressing to stupor and coma, weak and rapid pulse.

Possible Effects of Extended Use

Impaired balance of water, salt, and potassium in blood and body tissues. Development of diabetes (in predisposed individuals).

Suggested Periodic Examinations While Taking This Drug (at physician's discretion)

Complete blood cell counts.
Measurements of blood levels of sodium, potassium, chloride, sugar, and uric acid.
Liver function tests.
Kidney function tests.

While Taking This Drug, Observe the Following

Foods: It is recommended that you include in your daily diet liberal servings of foods rich in potassium (unless directed otherwise by your physician). The following foods have a high potassium content:

All-bran cereals	Fish, fresh
Almonds	Lentils
Apricots (dried)	Liver, beef
Bananas, fresh	Lonalac
Beans (navy and lima)	Milk
Beef	Peaches (dried)
Carrots (raw)	Peanut butter
Chicken	Peas
Citrus fruits, juices	Pork
Coconut	Potato, sweet
Coffee	Prunes (dried), juice
Crackers (rye)	Raisins
Dates and figs (dried)	Tomato juice

Note: Avoid licorice in large amounts while taking this drug. Follow your physician's instructions regarding the use of salt.

Beverages: No restrictions unless directed by your physician.

Alcohol: Use with caution until the combined effect has been determined. Alcohol can exaggerate the blood pressure-lowering effect of this drug and cause orthostatic hypotension.

Tobacco Smoking: No interactions expected with this drug. Follow your physician's advice regarding smoking.

Marijuana Smoking

Occasional (once or twice weekly): No effect to mild increase in thirst and/or urinary frequency.

Daily: Moderate increase in thirst and/or urinary frequency; possible accentuation of orthostatic hypotension (see Glossary).

Other Drugs

Chlorothiazide may *increase* the effects of

- other anti-hypertensive drugs. Careful adjustment of dosages is necessary to prevent excessive lowering of the blood pressure.
- drugs of the phenothiazine class, and cause excessive lowering of the blood pressure. (The thiazides and related drugs and the phenothiazines may both cause orthostatic hypotension.)

Chlorothiazide may *decrease* the effects of

- oral anti-diabetic drugs and insulin, by raising the level of blood sugar. Careful dosage adjustment is necessary to maintain proper control of diabetes.
- allopurinol (Zyloprim), by raising the level of blood uric acid. Careful dosage adjustment is required to maintain proper control of gout.
- probenecid (Benemid), by raising the level of blood uric acid. Careful dosage adjustments are necessary to maintain control of gout.

Chlorothiazide *taken concurrently* with

- cortisone and cortisone-related drugs, may cause excessive loss of potassium from the body.
- digitalis and related drugs, requires very careful monitoring and dosage adjustments to prevent serious disturbances of heart rhythm.
- tricyclic antidepressants (Elavil, Sinequan, etc.), may cause excessive lowering of the blood pressure.

The following drugs may *increase* the effects of chlorothiazide:

- barbiturates may exaggerate its blood pressure-lowering action.
- mono-amine oxidase (MAO) inhibitor drugs (see Drug Class, Section Three) may increase urine volume by delaying this drug's elimination from the body.
- pain relievers (analgesics), both narcotic and non-narcotic, may exaggerate its blood pressure-lowering action.

The following drug may *decrease* the effects of chlorothiazide:

- cholestyramine (Cuemid, Questran) may interfere with its absorption. Take cholestyramine 30 to 60 minutes before any oral diuretic.

Driving a Vehicle, Operating Machinery, Engaging in Hazardous Activities: Use caution until the possibility of orthostatic hypotension (lightheadedness, dizziness, incoordination) or impaired vision has been determined.

Aviation Note: The use of this drug *may be a disqualification* for the piloting of aircraft. Consultation with a designated Aviation Medical Examiner is advised.

Exposure to Sun: Use caution until sensitivity has been determined. This drug can cause photosensitivity (see Glossary).

Exposure to Heat: Avoid excessive perspiring which could cause additional loss of water and salt from the body.

Heavy Exercise or Exertion: Avoid exertion that produces lightheadedness, excessive fatigue, or muscle cramping. Isometric exercises—the "overload" technique for strengthening individual muscles—can raise the blood pressure significantly. Ask your physician for guidance regarding participation in this form of exercise.

Occurrence of Unrelated Illness: Illnesses which cause vomiting or diarrhea can produce a serious imbalance of important body chemistry. Discontinue this drug and ask your physician for guidance.

Discontinuation: It may be advisable to discontinue this drug approximately 5 to 7 days before major surgery. Ask your physician, surgeon, and/or anesthesiologist for guidance regarding dosage reduction or withdrawal.

Special Storage Instructions

Keep in a dry, tightly closed container.

CHLORPHENIRAMINE

Year Introduced: 1950

Brand Names

USA

Chlor-Trimeton
(Schering)
Histaspan (USV)
Polaramine* (Schering)
Teldrin (Smith Kline
& French)
Allerest [CD]
(Pennwalt)
Contac [CD] (Menley
& James)
Deconamine [CD]
(Cooper)
Demazin [CD]
(Schering)
Isoclor [CD]
(Arnar-Stone)
Naldecon [CD]
(Bristol)

Novafed A [CD]
(Dow)
Ornade [CD] (Smith
Kline & French)
Rynatan [CD]
(Mallinckrodt)
Sine-Off [CD]
(Menley & James)
Sine-Off Extra
Strength [CD]
(Menley & James)
Singlet [CD] (Dow)
(Numerous other
brand and
combination brand
names)

Canada

Chlorphen (Pro Doc)
Chlor-Tripolon
(Schering)
Novopheniram
(Novopharm)
Ornade [CD] (SKF)
Ornade-A.F. [CD]
(SKF)
Ornade-DM [CD]
(SKF)
Ornade Expectorant
[CD] (SKF)

Common Synonyms ("Street Names"):   Allergy pills

Drug Class: Antihistamines

Prescription Required: For tablets of 2 mg. and 4 mg. and for syrup—No
For all other dosage forms—Yes

Available for Purchase by Generic Name: USA: Yes   Canada: No

Available Dosage Forms and Strengths

Tablets — 2 mg., 4 mg.
Tablets, chewable — 2 mg.
Prolonged-action tablets — 4 mg., 6 mg., 8 mg., 12 mg.
Prolonged-action capsules — 8 mg., 12 mg.
Syrup — 2 mg. per teaspoonful (5 ml.)
Injection — 10 mg. per ml., 20 mg. per ml., 100 mg. per ml.

Tablet May Be Crushed or Capsule Opened for Administration

Regular tablets — Yes
Prolonged-action tablets and capsules — No
Demazin — No
Naldecon — No
Allerest, Contac, Isoclor Timesules,
Ornade and Teldrin Spansules — Yes, but do not crush or chew
contents

*A brand of the closely related generic drug dexchlorpheniramine.

How This Drug Works

Intended Therapeutic Effect(s):   Relief of symptoms associated with hayfever (allergic rhinitis) and with allergic reactions in the skin, such as itching, swelling, hives, and rash.

Location of Drug Action(s):   Those hypersensitive tissues that release excessive histamine as part of an allergic reaction. The principal tissue sites are the eyes, the nose, and the skin.

Method of Drug Action(s):   This drug reduces the intensity of the allergic response by blocking the action of histamine after it has been released from sensitized tissue cells.

Principal Uses of This Drug

As a Single Drug Product: Used primarily to provide symptomatic relief in allergic and related disorders: seasonal and perennial allergic rhinitis (hayfever), allergic conjunctivitis, and vasomotor rhinitis; also in hives and localized swellings (angioedema) of allergic origin. This drug is not effective in the treatment of allergically-induced bronchial asthma.

As a Combination Drug Product [CD]:   Often combined with decongestant drugs to enhance their ability to reduce tissue swelling and secretions in allergic and infectious disorders of the upper respiratory tract. Also combined with decongestants, expectorants, and codeine to increase their effectiveness in the symptomatic relief of allergic and infectious disorders of the lower respiratory tract, often with associated coughing.

THIS DRUG SHOULD NOT BE TAKEN IF

—you have had an allergic reaction to any dosage form of it previously.

INFORM YOUR PHYSICIAN BEFORE TAKING THIS DRUG IF

—you have had any unfavorable reaction to previous use of antihistamines.
—you have glaucoma (narrow-angle type).
—you have difficulty in emptying the urinary bladder.
—you plan to have surgery under general anesthesia in the near future.

Time Required for Apparent Benefit

Drug action usually begins in 15 to 30 minutes, reaches maximal effect in 1 to 2 hours, and subsides in 3 to 6 hours.

Possible Side-Effects *(natural, expected, and unavoidable drug actions)*

Drowsiness, sense of weakness, dryness of the nose, mouth, and throat.

Possible Adverse Effects *(unusual, unexpected, and infrequent reactions)*

IF ANY OF THE FOLLOWING DEVELOP, DISCONTINUE DRUG AND NOTIFY YOUR PHYSICIAN AS SOON AS POSSIBLE

Mild Adverse Effects
  Allergic Reactions: Skin rashes (rare).
  Other Reactions
    Headache, nervous agitation, dizziness, double vision, blurred vision, ringing in the ears, tremors.
    Reduced appetite, heartburn, nausea, vomiting, diarrhea.
    Reduced tolerance for contact lenses.

Serious Adverse Effects
Reduced production of white blood cells possibly resulting in fever and/or sore throat.

Precautions for Use by Those over 60 Years of Age
You may be more susceptible to the development of drowsiness, dizziness, and lethargy and to impairment of thinking, judgment, and memory.
This drug can increase the degree of impaired urination associated with prostate gland enlargement (prostatism).

Advisability of Use During Pregnancy
Pregnancy Category: B (tentative). See Pregnancy Code inside back cover. Animal reproduction studies in mice reveal no birth defects due to this drug. Information from studies in pregnant women indicates no significant increase in defects in 3931 exposures to this drug.
Ask physician for guidance.

Advisability of Use While Nursing Infant
Drug is present in milk in small quantities. Ask physician for guidance.

Habit-Forming Potential
None.

Effects of Overdosage
With Moderate Overdose: Excitement, incoordination, staggering gait, hallucinations, muscular tremors and spasms.
With Large Overdose: Stupor progressing to coma, convulsions, dilated pupils, flushed face, fever, shallow respiration, weak and rapid pulse.

Possible Effects of Extended Use
Tardive dyskinesia (see Glossary).
Bone marrow depression (see Glossary).
Note: Prolonged, continuous use of antihistamines should be avoided.

Suggested Periodic Examinations While Taking This Drug (at physician's discretion)
Complete blood cell counts.

While Taking This Drug, Observe the Following
Foods: No restrictions.
Beverages: Coffee and tea can help to offset the drowsiness produced by most antihistamines.
Alcohol: Use with extreme caution until combined effects have been determined. The combination of alcohol and antihistamines can produce rapid and marked sedation.
Tobacco Smoking: No interactions expected.
Marijuana Smoking
Occasional (once or twice weekly):   Mild increase in drowsiness and dryness of mouth.
Daily: Moderate to marked increase in drowsiness and dryness of mouth; possible accentuation of impaired thinking.

Other Drugs

Chlorpheniramine may *increase* the effects of

- all sedatives, sleep-inducing drugs, tranquilizers, analgesics, and narcotic drugs, and produce oversedation.

Chlorpheniramine may *decrease* the effects of

- oral anticoagulants, by hastening their elimination from the body. Consult physician regarding prothrombin time testing and dosage adjustment.

The following drugs may *increase* the effects of chlorpheniramine

- all sedatives, sleep-inducing drugs, tranquilizers, analgesics, and narcotic drugs may exaggerate its sedative action.
- mono-amine oxidase (MAO) inhibitor drugs (see Drug Class, Section Three) may prolong the action of antihistamines.

Driving a Vehicle, Operating Machinery, Engaging in Hazardous Activities: This drug can impair mental alertness, judgment, coordination, and reaction time. Avoid hazardous activities until full sedative effects have been determined.

Aviation Note: The use of this drug *may be a disqualification* for the piloting of aircraft. Consultation with a designated Aviation Medical Examiner is advised.

Exposure to Sun: No restrictions.

Special Storage Instructions

Keep tablets and capsules in a dry, tightly closed container.
Protect liquid drug preparations from light to prevent discoloration.

CHLORPROMAZINE

Year Introduced: 1951

Brand Names

USA	Canada
Promachlor (Geneva)	Apo-Chlorpromazine
Promapar (Parke-Davis)	(Apotex)
Sonazine (Tutag)	Chlor-Promanyl (Maney)
Thorazine (Smith Kline	Largactil (Poulenc)
& French)	Novochlorpromazine
	(Novopharm)

Common Synonyms ("Street Names"):   None

Drug Class: Tranquilizer, Strong (Anti-psychotic); Antinausea (Antiemetic), Phenothiazines

Prescription Required: Yes

Available for Purchase by Generic Name: Yes

Available Dosage Forms and Strengths
Tablets — 10 mg., 25 mg., 50 mg., 100 mg., 200 mg.
Prolonged-action capsules — 30 mg., 75 mg., 150 mg., 200 mg., 300 mg.
Suppositories — 25 mg., 100 mg.
Syrup — 10 mg. per teaspoonful (5 ml.)
Concentrated solution — 30 mg. per ml., 100 mg. per ml.
Injection — 25 mg. per ml.

Tablet May Be Crushed or Capsule Opened for Administration
Tablets — Yes
Prolonged-action capsules — No
Thorazine Spansules — Yes, but do not crush or chew contents

How This Drug Works
Intended Therapeutic Effect(s):   Restoration of emotional calm. Relief of severe anxiety, agitation, and psychotic behavior.
Location of Drug Action(s):   Those nerve pathways in the brain that utilize the tissue chemical dopamine for the transmission of nerve impulses.
Method of Drug Action(s):   Not completely established. Present theory is that by inhibiting the action of dopamine, this drug acts to correct an imbalance of nerve impulse transmissions that is thought to be responsible for certain mental disorders.

Principal Uses of This Drug
As a Single Drug Product: This anti-psychotic drug, the first of the phenothiazines, is used primarily to treat acute and chronic psychotic disorders such as agitated depression, schizophrenia, and similar states of mental dysfunction. It may be used as a tranquilizer in the management of agitated and disruptive behavior in the absence of true psychosis. Less frequently it may be used to relieve severe nausea or vomiting.

THIS DRUG SHOULD NOT BE TAKEN IF
—you are allergic to any of the drugs bearing the brand names listed above.
—you have a disorder of the blood or bone marrow.
—it is prescribed for a child under 6 months of age.

INFORM YOUR PHYSICIAN BEFORE TAKING THIS DRUG IF
—you are allergic or sensitive to any phenothiazine drug (see Drug Class, Section Three).
—you are taking sedatives, sleep-inducing drugs, tranquilizers, antidepressants, antihistamines, or narcotic drugs of any kind.
—you have glaucoma.
—you have epilepsy.
—you have a liver, heart, or lung disorder, especially asthma or emphysema.
—you have a history of peptic ulcer.
—you plan to have surgery under general or spinal anesthesia in the near future.

Time Required for Apparent Benefit

Approximately 1 to 2 hours. Maximal benefit may require regular use for several weeks.

Possible Side-Effects *(natural, expected, and unavoidable drug actions)*

Drowsiness (usually during the first 2 weeks), dryness of the mouth, nasal congestion, constipation, impaired urination.

Pink or purple coloration of the urine, of no significance.

Possible Adverse Effects *(unusual, unexpected, and infrequent reactions)*

IF ANY OF THE FOLLOWING DEVELOP, DISCONTINUE DRUG AND NOTIFY YOUR PHYSICIAN AS SOON AS POSSIBLE

Mild Adverse Effects

Allergic Reactions: Skin rashes (various kinds), hives, low-grade fever.

Other Reactions

Lowering of body temperature, especially in the elderly.

Increased appetite and weight gain.

Breast fullness, tenderness, and milk production.

Menstrual irregularity.

False positive pregnancy tests.

Serious Adverse Effects

Allergic Reactions: Hepatitis with jaundice (see Glossary)—usually occurs between second and fourth week, high fever, asthma, anaphylactic reaction (see Glossary).

Other Reactions

Bone marrow depression (see Glossary)—fatigue, weakness, fever, sore throat, unusual bleeding or bruising.

Parkinson-like disorders (see Glossary).

Muscle spasms affecting the jaw, neck, back, hands, or feet.

Eye-rolling, muscle twitching, convulsions.

Prolonged drop in blood pressure with weakness, perspiration, and fainting.

CAUTION

1. Many over-the-counter medications (see OTC drugs in Glossary) for allergies, colds, and coughs contain drugs that can interact unfavorably with this drug. Ask your physician for guidance before using any such medications.
2. Antacids that contain aluminum and/or magnesium can prevent the absorption of this drug and reduce its effectiveness.
3. Obtain prompt evaluation of any disturbance or change in vision.

Precautions for Use by Those over 60 Years of Age

You may be more sensitive to all of the actions of this drug. Small doses are advisable until your individual response has been determined.

You may be more susceptible to the development of drowsiness, lethargy, constipation, lowering of body temperature (hypothermia), and excessive drop in blood pressure on arising from a lying or sitting position (see orthostatic hypotension in Glossary).

This drug can increase the degree of impaired urination associated with prostate gland enlargement (prostatism).

You may also be more susceptible to the development of parkinson-like disorders and/or tardive dyskinesia (see discussion of these terms in Glossary). These conditions must be recognized early since they may become unresponsive to treatment and irreversible. Consult your physician promptly if suggestive symptoms develop.

Advisability of Use During Pregnancy
Pregnancy Category: C (tentative). See Pregnancy Code inside back cover. Animal reproduction studies reveal no birth defects due to this drug. Information from adequate studies in pregnant women is not available. Ask physician for guidance.

Advisability of Use While Nursing Infant
Drug is known to be present in milk. Ask physician for guidance.

Habit-Forming Potential
None.

Effects of Overdosage
With Moderate Overdose: Marked drowsiness, weakness, tremor, impairment of stance and gait, agitation.

With Large Overdose: Stupor, deep sleep, coma, convulsions.

Possible Effects of Extended Use
Tardive dyskinesia (see Glossary).

Pigmentation of skin, gray to violet in color, usually in exposed areas, more common in women.

Eye changes—cataracts and pigmentation of retina, with impairment of vision.

Severe ulcerative colitis.

Suggested Periodic Examinations While Taking This Drug (at physician's discretion)
Complete blood cell counts, especially between the fourth and tenth weeks of treatment.

Liver function tests.

Complete eye examinations, including eye structures and vision.

Careful inspection of the tongue for early evidence of fine, involuntary, wave-like movements that could indicate the beginning of tardive dyskinesia.

Periodic electrocardiograms.

While Taking This Drug, Observe the Following
Foods: No restrictions.

Beverages: No restrictions.

Alcohol: Avoid completely. Alcohol can increase the sedative action of chlorpromazine and accentuate its depressant effects on brain function and blood pressure. Chlorpromazine can increase the intoxicating effects of alcohol.

Tobacco Smoking: No interactions expected.

Marijuana Smoking

Occasional (once or twice weekly):   No effect to mild and transient increase in drowsiness and accentuation of orthostatic hypotension (see Glossary); some risk of precipitating latent psychoses (in predisposed individuals).

Daily: Moderate increase in drowsiness, significant accentuation of orthostatic hypotension; increased risk of precipitating latent psychoses, confusing interpretation of mental status and of drug responses.

Other Drugs

Chlorpromazine may *increase* the effects of

- all drugs containing atropine or having an atropine-like action (see Drug Class, Section Three).
- all sedatives, sleep-inducing drugs, other tranquilizers, antidepressants, antihistamines, and narcotic drugs, and produce oversedation.
- methyldopa (Aldomet), and cause excessive lowering of the blood pressure.
- pargyline (Eutonyl), and cause excessive lowering of the blood pressure.
- phenytoin (Dantoin, Dilantin, etc.).
- reserpine (and related drugs), and cause excessive lowering of the blood pressure.

Chlorpromazine may *decrease* the effects of

- oral anticoagulants, by hastening their destruction and elimination. Dosage adjustments of the anticoagulant may be necessary.
- oral anti-diabetic drugs and insulin, and reduce their effectiveness in regulating blood sugar.
- chlorphentermine (Pre-Sate), and reduce its effectiveness in controlling appetite.
- guanethidine (Ismelin), and reduce its effectiveness in lowering blood pressure.
- levodopa (Dopar, Larodopa, Parda), and reduce its effectiveness in the treatment of Parkinson's disease (shaking palsy).
- phenmetrazine (Preludin), and reduce its effectiveness in controlling appetite.

Chlorpromazine *taken concurrently* with

- quinidine, may impair heart function. Avoid the concurrent use of these two drugs.
- orphenadrine (Norflex, Norgesic, Disipal), may cause severe lowering of the blood sugar and unconsciousness (see hypoglycemia in Glossary).

Driving a Vehicle, Operating Machinery, Engaging in Hazardous Activities: This drug can impair mental alertness, judgment, and physical coordination. Avoid hazardous activities.

Aviation Note: The use of this drug *is a disqualification* for the piloting of aircraft. Consultation with a designated Aviation Medical Examiner is advised.

Exposure to Sun: Use caution until sensitivity has been determined. This drug can produce photosensitivity (see Glossary).

Exposure to Heat: Use caution and avoid excessive heat as much as possible. This drug may impair the regulation of body temperature and increase the risk of heat stroke.

Heavy Exercise or Exertion: Use caution. Ask physician for guidance.

Discontinuation: If it has been necessary to use this drug for an extended period of time, do not discontinue it suddenly. Ask physician for guidance regarding dosage reduction and withdrawal. Upon discontinuation of this drug, it may also be necessary to adjust the dosages of other drugs taken concurrently with it.

Special Storage Instructions
Keep in a tightly closed, light-resistant container.

CHLORPROPAMIDE

Year Introduced: 1958

Brand Names

USA	Canada
Diabinese (Pfizer)	Apo-Chlorpropamide (Apotex)
	Chloronase (Hoechst)
	Diabinese (Pfizer)
	Novopropamide (Novopharm)
	Stabinol (Horner)

Common Synonyms ("Street Names"):   Diabetes pills

Drug Class: Anti-diabetic, Oral (Hypoglycemic), Sulfonylureas

Prescription Required: Yes

Available for Purchase by Generic Name: Yes

Available Dosage Forms and Strengths
Tablets — 100 mg., 250 mg.

Tablet May Be Crushed or Capsule Opened for Administration: Yes

How This Drug Works
Intended Therapeutic Effect(s):   The correction of insulin deficiency in adult (maturity-onset) diabetes of moderate severity.

Location of Drug Action(s):   The insulin-producing tissues of the pancreas.

Method of Drug Action(s):   It is well established that sulfonylurea drugs stimulate the secretion of insulin (by a pancreas capable of responding to stimulation). Therapeutic doses may increase the amount of available insulin.

Principal Uses of This Drug

As a Single Drug Product: To assist in the control of mild to moderately severe diabetes mellitus of the adult (maturity-onset) type that does not require insulin, but that cannot be adequately controlled by diet alone.

THIS DRUG SHOULD NOT BE TAKEN IF

—you have had an allergic reaction to any dosage form of it previously.

—you have severe impairment of liver function or kidney function.

INFORM YOUR PHYSICIAN BEFORE TAKING THIS DRUG IF

—your diabetes has been difficult to control in the past ("brittle type").

—you have a history of peptic ulcer of the stomach or duodenum.

—you have a history of porphyria.

—you do not know how to recognize or treat hypoglycemia (see Glossary).

Time Required for Apparent Benefit

A single dose may lower the blood sugar within 2 to 4 hours. Regular use for 1 to 2 weeks may be needed to determine this drug's effectiveness in controlling your diabetes.

Possible Side-Effects *(natural, expected, and unavoidable drug actions)*

Usually none. If drug dosage is excessive or food intake is inadequate, abnormally low blood sugar (hypoglycemia) will occur as a predictable drug effect.

Possible Adverse Effects *(unusual, unexpected, and infrequent reactions)*

IF ANY OF THE FOLLOWING DEVELOP, DISCONTINUE DRUG AND NOTIFY YOUR PHYSICIAN AS SOON AS POSSIBLE

Mild Adverse Effects

Allergic Reactions: Skin rashes (various kinds), hives, itching, drug fever.
Other Reactions
   Headache, ringing in ears.
   Indigestion, heartburn, nausea, diarrhea.

Serious Adverse Effects

Allergic Reactions: Hepatitis with jaundice (see Glossary).
Idiosyncratic Reactions: Hemolytic anemia in susceptible individuals (see Glossary).
Other Reactions: Bone marrow depression (see Glossary)—fatigue, weakness, fever, sore throat, unusual bleeding or bruising.

CAUTION

1. This drug must be looked upon as only one part of the total program for the management of your diabetes. It is not a substitute for a properly prescribed diet.
2. Over a period of time (usually several months), this drug may lose its effectiveness in controlling blood sugar levels. Periodic follow-up examina-

tions are necessary to monitor all aspects of response to drug treatment.
3. Individual response to this drug varies widely. The effects of overdosage—hypoglycemia—can occur in sensitive individuals taking doses well within the recommended range.
4. Do not begin treatment with a large or "loading" dose. This is unnecessary and can be dangerous.
5. The total daily dose should not exceed 750 mgs.

Precautions for Use by Those over 60 Years of Age
The natural decline in kidney function that occurs after 60, together with the duration of this drug's action, require that both initial and maintenance dosage be less than those normally used in the younger adult.
Do not exceed a total dosage of 750 mg. in 24 hours.
The aging brain adapts well to the higher blood sugar levels associated with diabetes. Attempts to achieve "normal" blood sugar level can result in unrecognized hypoglycemia that is manifested by confusion and abnormal behavior. Repeated episodes of hypoglycemia in the elderly can cause brain damage.

Advisability of Use During Pregnancy
Pregnancy Category: X (tentative). See Pregnancy Code inside back cover.
Animal reproduction studies are inconclusive.
Information from adequate studies in pregnant women is not available.
The manufacturers state that this drug is contraindicated during entire pregnancy.
Ask physician for guidance.

Advisability of Use While Nursing Infant
Drug is known to be present in milk. Ask physician for guidance.

Habit-Forming Potential
None.

Effects of Overdosage
With Moderate Overdose: Symptoms of mild to moderate hypoglycemia: headache, lightheadedness, faintness, nervousness, confusion, tremor, sweating, heart palpitation, weakness, and hunger.
With Large Overdose: Hypoglycemic coma (see Glossary).

Possible Effects of Extended Use
Reduced function of the thyroid gland (hypothyroidism), resulting in lowered metabolism.
Reports of increased frequency and severity of heart and blood vessel diseases associated with long-term use of the members of this drug family are highly controversial and inconclusive. A direct cause-and-effect relationship (see Glossary) has not been established to date. Ask your physician for guidance regarding extended use.

Suggested Periodic Examinations While Taking This Drug (at physician's discretion)
Complete blood cell counts.
Liver function tests.

Thyroid function tests.
Periodic evaluation of heart and circulatory system.

While Taking This Drug, Observe the Following
Foods: Follow the diabetic diet prescribed by your physician.

Beverages: As directed in the diabetic diet prescribed by your physician.

Alcohol: Use with extreme caution until the combined effect has been determined. This drug can cause a marked intolerance to alcohol resulting in a disulfiram-like reaction (see Glossary).

Tobacco Smoking: No restrictions unless imposed as part of your overall treatment program. Ask physician for guidance.

Marijuana Smoking
Occasional (once or twice weekly):   No significant interactions expected.
Daily: Possible increase in blood sugar.

Other Drugs
Chlorpropamide may *increase* the effects of
• sedatives and sleep-inducing drugs, by slowing their elimination from the body.
• "sulfa" drugs, by slowing their elimination from the body.

Chlorpropamide *taken concurrently* with
• oral anticoagulants, may cause unpredictable changes in anticoagulant drug actions. Ask physician for guidance regarding prothrombin blood tests and dosage adjustment.
• propranolol (Inderal), may allow hypoglycemia to develop without adequate warning. Follow diet and dosage schedules very carefully.

The following drugs may *increase* the effects of chlorpropamide
• bishydroxycoumarin (Dicumarol, Dufalone)
• chloramphenicol (Chloromycetin, etc.)
• clofibrate (Atromid-S)
• mono-amine oxidase (MAO) inhibitors (see Drug Class, Section Three)
• oxyphenbutazone (Oxalid, Tandearil)
• phenformin (DBI)
• phenylbutazone (Azolid, Butazolidin, etc.)
• phenyramidol (Analexin)
• probenecid (Benemid)
• propranolol (Inderal)
• salicylates (aspirin, sodium salicylate)
• sulfaphenazole (Orisul, Sulfabid)
• sulfisoxazole (Gantrisin, Novosoxazole, etc.)

The following drugs may *decrease* the effects of chlorpropamide
• chlorpromazine (Thorazine, Largactil, etc.)
• cortisone and related drugs (see Drug Class, Section Three)
• estrogens (Premarin, Menotrol, Ogen, etc.)
• isoniazid (INH, Isozide, etc.)
• nicotinic acid (Niacin, etc.)
• oral contraceptives

- pyrazinamide (Aldinamide)
- thiazide diuretics (see Drug Class, Section Three)
- thyroid preparations

Driving a Vehicle, Operating Machinery, Engaging in Hazardous Activities: Regulate your dosage schedule, eating schedule, and physical activities very carefully to prevent hypoglycemia. Be able to recognize the early symptoms of hypoglycemia and avoid hazardous activities if you suspect that hypoglycemia is developing.

Aviation Note: Diabetes *is a disqualification* for the piloting of aircraft. Consultation with a designated Aviation Medical Examiner is advised.

Exposure to Sun: Use caution until sensitivity has been determined. This drug can cause photosensitivity (see Glossary).

Exposure to Heat: No restrictions.

Exposure to Cold: No restrictions.

Heavy Exercise or Exertion: Use caution. Excessive exercise may result in hypoglycemia.

Occurrence of Unrelated Illness: Acute infections, illnesses causing vomiting or diarrhea, serious injuries, and the need for surgery can interfere with diabetic control and may require a change in medication. If any of these conditions occur, ask your physician for guidance regarding the continued use of this drug.

Discontinuation: If you find it necessary to discontinue this drug for any reason, notify your physician and ask for guidance regarding necessary changes in your treatment program for diabetic control. If periodic examinations disclose that this drug is no longer effective, it should be discontinued.

Special Storage Instructions
Keep in a dry, tightly closed container.

CHLORTHALIDONE

Year Introduced: 1960

Brand Names

USA	Canada
Hygroton (USV)	Hygroton (Geigy)
Thalitone (Boehringer Ingelheim)	Novothalidone (Novopharm)
Demi-Regroton [CD] (USV)	Uridon (ICN)
Regroton [CD] (USV)	

Common Synonyms ("Street Names"):   Water pills

Drug Class: Anti-hypertensive (Hypotensive); Diuretic

Prescription Required: Yes

Available for Purchase by Generic Name: Yes

Available Dosage Forms and Strengths
  Tablets — 25 mg., 50 mg., 100 mg.

Tablet May Be Crushed or Capsule Opened for Administration: Yes

How This Drug Works

  Intended Therapeutic Effect(s)
    Elimination of excessive fluid retention (edema).
    Reduction of high blood pressure.
  Location of Drug Action(s):   Principal actions occur in
    • the tubular systems of the kidney that determine the final composition of
      the urine.
    • the walls of the smaller arteries.
  Method of Drug Action(s)
    By increasing the elimination of salt and water from the body (through
      increased urine production), this drug reduces the volume of fluid in the
      blood and body tissues and lowers the sodium content throughout the
      body.
    By relaxing the walls of the smaller arteries and allowing them to expand,
      this drug significantly increases the total capacity of the arterial system.
      The combined effect of these two actions (reduced blood volume in
      expanded space) results in lowering of the blood pressure.

Principal Uses of This Drug

  As a Single Drug Product: This drug is used primarily to (1) increase the
    volume of urine (diuresis) to correct the excessive fluid retention associated
    with congestive heart failure and certain types of liver and kidney disease;
    and (2) initiate treatment for high blood pressure (hypertension). It may be
    the first drug to be tried in treating mild to moderate hypertension. Less
    frequent uses include the treatment of diabetes insipidus and the preven-
    tion of kidney stones that contain calcium.
  As a Combination Drug Product [CD]:   When this drug is used alone to treat
    hypertension, it is referred to as a "step 1" anti-hypertensive. Should it fail
    to reduce the blood pressure adequately, a "step 2" anti-hypertensive drug
    is added to be taken concurrently with the "step 1" drug. These drugs may
    be combined in one drug product. Chlorthalidone is available in combina-
    tion with clonidine and with reserpine to increase its effectiveness as an
    anti-hypertensive.

THIS DRUG SHOULD NOT BE TAKEN IF
—you have had an allergic reaction to any dosage form of it previously.

INFORM YOUR PHYSICIAN BEFORE TAKING THIS DRUG IF
—you are allergic to any form of "sulfa" drug.
—you are pregnant and your physician does not know it.

—you have a history of kidney disease or liver disease, or impaired kidney or liver function.

—you have diabetes (or a tendency to diabetes).

—you have a history of gout.

—you have a history of lupus erythematosus.

—you are taking any form of cortisone, digitalis, oral anti-diabetic drugs, or insulin.

—you plan to have surgery under general anesthesia in the near future.

Time Required for Apparent Benefit

Increased urine volume begins in 2 hours, reaches a maximum in 6 to 18 hours, and gradually subsides within 48 to 72 hours. Continuous use on a regular schedule will be necessary for 2 to 3 weeks to determine this drug's effectiveness in lowering your blood pressure.

Possible Side-Effects *(natural, expected, and unavoidable drug actions)*

Lightheadedness on arising from sitting or lying position (see orthostatic hypotension in Glossary).

Increase in the level of blood sugar, affecting control of diabetes.

Increase in the level of blood uric acid, affecting control of gout.

Decrease in the level of blood potassium, resulting in muscle weakness and cramping.

Possible Adverse Effects *(unusual, unexpected, and infrequent reactions)*

IF ANY OF THE FOLLOWING DEVELOP, DISCONTINUE DRUG AND NOTIFY YOUR PHYSICIAN AS SOON AS POSSIBLE

Mild Adverse Effects

Allergic Reactions: Skin rash (various kinds), hives, drug fever.

Other Reactions

Reduced appetite, indigestion, nausea, vomiting, diarrhea.

Headache, dizziness, yellow vision, blurred vision.

Serious Adverse Effects

Allergic Reactions: Hepatitis with jaundice (see Glossary), anaphylactic reaction (see Glossary), severe skin reactions.

Other Reactions

Inflammation of the pancreas—severe abdominal pain.

Bone marrow depression (see Glossary)—fatigue, weakness, fever, sore throat, unusual bleeding or bruising.

CAUTION

1. Do not exceed recommended doses. Increased dosage can cause excessive excretion of sodium and potassium with resultant loss of appetite, nausea, fatigue, weakness, confusion, and tingling in the extremities.

2. If you are also taking a digitalis preparation (digitoxin, digoxin), ensure an adequate intake of high potassium foods to prevent potassium deficiency —a potential cause of digitalis toxicity.

Precautions for Use by Those over 60 Years of Age
You may be more sensitive to the actions of this drug. Small doses are advisable until your individual response has been determined.

You may be more susceptible to the development of impaired thinking, orthostatic hypotension, potassium loss, and elevation of blood sugar, complicating the management of diabetes.

If you are taking this drug to treat high blood pressure, remember that warm weather and fever can reduce your blood pressure and make it necessary to adjust your dosage.

Overdosage and extended use of this drug can cause excessive loss of body water, thickening (increased viscosity) of the blood, and an increased tendency of the blood to clot, predisposing to stroke, heart attack, or thrombophlebitis.

Advisability of Use During Pregnancy
Pregnancy Category: C (tentative). See Pregnancy Code inside back cover.

Animal reproduction studies reveal no birth defects due to this drug.

Information from adequate studies in pregnant women is not available.

This drug should not be used during pregnancy unless a very serious complication of pregnancy occurs for which this drug is significantly beneficial. This type of diuretic can have adverse effects on the fetus.

Ask physician for guidance.

Advisability of Use While Nursing Infant
This drug is known to be present in milk. Ask physician for guidance.

Habit-Forming Potential
None.

Effects of Overdosage
With Moderate Overdose: Dryness of mouth, thirst, lethargy, weakness, muscle pain and cramping, nausea, vomiting.

With Large Overdose: Drowsiness progressing to stupor and coma, weak and rapid pulse.

Possible Effects of Extended Use
Impaired balance of water, salt, and potassium in blood and body tissues.

Development of diabetes (in predisposed individuals).

Suggested Periodic Examinations While Taking This Drug (at physician's discretion)
Complete blood cell counts.

Measurements of blood levels of sodium, potassium, chloride, sugar, and uric acid.

Liver function tests.

Kidney function tests.

While Taking This Drug, Observe the Following

Foods: It is recommended that you include in your daily diet liberal servings of foods rich in potassium (unless directed otherwise by your physician). The following foods have a high potassium content

All-bran cereals	Fish, fresh
Almonds	Lentils
Apricots (dried)	Liver, beef
Bananas, fresh	Lonalac
Beans (navy and lima)	Milk
Beef	Peaches (dried)
Carrots (raw)	Peanut butter
Chicken	Peas
Citrus fruits, juices	Pork
Coconut	Potato, sweet
Coffee	Prunes (dried), juice
Crackers (rye)	Raisins
Dates and figs (dried)	Tomato Juice

Note: Avoid licorice in large amounts while taking this drug. Follow your physician's instructions regarding the use of salt.

Beverages: No restrictions unless directed by your physician.

Alcohol: Use with caution until the combined effect has been determined. Alcohol can exaggerate the blood pressure-lowering effect of this drug and cause orthostatic hypotension.

Tobacco Smoking: No interactions expected with this drug. Follow your physician's advice regarding smoking.

Marijuana Smoking

Occasional (once or twice weekly): No effect to mild increase in thirst and/or urinary frequency.

Daily: Moderate increase in thirst and/or urinary frequency; possible accentuation of orthostatic hypotension (see Glossary).

Other Drugs

Chlorthalidone may *increase* the effects of

- other anti-hypertensive drugs. Careful adjustment of dosages is necessary to prevent excessive lowering of the blood pressure.
- drugs of the phenothiazine class, and cause excessive lowering of the blood pressure. (The thiazides and related drugs and the phenothiazines may both cause orthostatic hypotension).

Chlorthalidone may *decrease* the effects of

- oral anti-diabetic drugs and insulin, by raising the level of blood sugar. Careful dosage adjustment is necessary to maintain proper control of diabetes.
- allopurinol (Zyloprim), by raising the level of blood uric acid. Careful dosage adjustment is required to maintain proper control of gout.
- probenecid (Benemid), by raising the level of blood uric acid. Careful dosage adjustments are necessary to maintain control of gout.

Chlorthalidone *taken concurrently* with
- cortisone and cortisone-related drugs, may cause excessive loss of potassium from the body.
- digitalis and related drugs, requires very careful monitoring and dosage adjustments to prevent serious disturbances of heart rhythm.
- tricyclic antidepressants (Elavil, Sinequan, etc.), may cause excessive lowering of the blood pressure.

The following drugs may *increase* the effects of chlorthalidone
- barbiturates may exaggerate its blood pressure-lowering action.
- mono-amine oxidase (MAO) inhibitor drugs (see Drug Class, Section Three) may increase urine volume by delaying this drug's elimination from the body.
- pain relievers (analgesics), both narcotic and non-narcotic, may exaggerate its blood pressure-lowering action.

The following drug may *decrease* the effects of chlorthalidone
- cholestyramine (Cuemid, Questran) may interfere with its absorption. Take cholestyramine 30 to 60 minutes before any oral diuretic.

Driving a Vehicle, Operating Machinery, Engaging in Hazardous Activities: Use caution until the possibility of orthostatic hypotension (lightheadedness, dizziness, incoordination) or impaired vision has been determined.

Aviation Note: The use of this drug *may be a disqualification* for the piloting of aircraft. Consultation with a designated Aviation Medical Examiner is advised.

Exposure to Sun: Use caution until sensitivity has been determined. This drug can cause photosensitivity (see Glossary).

Exposure to Heat: Avoid excessive perspiring which could cause additional loss of water and salt from the body.

Heavy Exercise or Exertion: Avoid exertion that produces lightheadedness, excessive fatigue, or muscle cramping. Isometric exercises—the "overload" technique for strengthening individual muscles—can raise the blood pressure significantly. Ask your physician for guidance regarding participation in this form of exercise.

Occurrence of Unrelated Illness: Illnesses which cause vomiting or diarrhea can produce a serious imbalance of important body chemistry. Discontinue this drug and ask your physician for guidance.

Discontinuation: It may be advisable to discontinue this drug approximately 5 to 7 days before major surgery. Ask your physician, surgeon, and/or anesthesiologist for guidance regarding dosage reduction or withdrawal.

Special Storage Instructions
Keep in a dry, tightly closed container.

CHLORZOXAZONE

Year Introduced: 1958

Brand Names

USA	Canada
Paraflex (McNeil)	Parafon Forte [CD]
Parafon Forte [CD]	(McNeil)
(McNeil)	

Common Synonyms ("Street Names"):   None

Drug Class: Muscle Relaxant

Prescription Required: USA: Yes   Canada: No

Available for Purchase by Generic Name: USA: Yes   Canada: No

Available Dosage Forms and Strengths
   Tablets — 250 mg.

Tablet May Be Crushed or Capsule Opened for Administration: Yes

How This Drug Works
   Intended Therapeutic Effect(s):   Relief of discomfort resulting from spasm
   of voluntary muscles.
   Location of Drug Action(s):   Not completely established. This drug is
   thought to act on those nerve pathways in the brain and spinal cord that
   are involved in the reflex activity of voluntary muscles.
   Method of Drug Action(s):   Not completely established. It is thought that
   this drug may relieve muscle spasm and pain by blocking the transmission
   of nerve impulses over reflex pathways and/or by producing a sedative
   effect that decreases the perception of pain.

Principal Uses of This Drug
   As a Single Drug Product: Used primarily to relieve the pain and stiffness
   associated with spasm of voluntary muscles, such as that resulting from
   accidental injury of musculoskeletal structures. It is often necessary to
   supplement the use of this drug with other treatment measures, such as
   rest, support, and physiotherapy.
   As a Combination Drug Product [CD]:   May be combined with acetaminophen to enhance its effectiveness in relieving discomfort. Acetaminophen
   is an effective analgesic and may be necessary to control the pain that is
   not relieved by chlorzoxazone alone.

THIS DRUG SHOULD NOT BE TAKEN IF
—you have had an allergic reaction to any dosage form of it previously.

INFORM YOUR PHYSICIAN BEFORE TAKING THIS DRUG IF
—you have experienced any unfavorable reactions to muscle relaxant drugs in
   the past.
—you have a history of liver disease or impaired liver function.

Time Required for Apparent Benefit
Drug action begins in 1 hour, reaches a maximal effect in 3 to 4 hours, and subsides in 5 to 6 hours.

Possible Side-Effects *(natural, expected, and unavoidable drug actions)*
Drowsiness, orange or red-purple discoloration of the urine (of no significance).

Possible Adverse Effects *(unusual, unexpected, and infrequent reactions)*

IF ANY OF THE FOLLOWING DEVELOP, DISCONTINUE DRUG AND NOTIFY YOUR PHYSICIAN AS SOON AS POSSIBLE

Mild Adverse Effects
Allergic Reactions: Skin rash, hives, itching.
Other Reactions
Lightheadedness, dizziness, lethargy.
Nausea, indigestion, heartburn.

Serious Adverse Effects
Allergic Reactions: Spontaneous bruising of skin (not due to injury).
Idiosyncratic Reactions: Overstimulation, disorientation, amnesia.
Other Reactions
Bleeding from the stomach or intestine—black or dark colored stools.
Hepatitis with or without jaundice (see Glossary)—yellow eyes and skin, dark colored urine, light colored stools.

Precautions for Use by Those over 60 Years of Age
You may be more sensitive to the sedative effects of this drug. Small doses are advisable until your individual response has been determined.
You may be more susceptible to the development of drowsiness, dizziness, muscular weakness, unsteadiness, and falling.

Advisability of Use During Pregnancy
Pregnancy Category: C (tentative). See Pregnancy Code inside back cover.
Animal reproduction studies: No data available.
Information from adequate studies in pregnant women is not available.
Ask physician for guidance.

Advisability of Use While Nursing Infant
This drug is known to be present in milk. Safety for infant not established. Ask physician for guidance.

Habit-Forming Potential
None.

Effects of Overdosage
With Moderate Overdose: Nausea, vomiting, diarrhea, drowsiness, dizziness, headache, sluggishness.
With Large Overdose: Marked weakness, sense of paralysis of arms and legs, rapid and irregular breathing.

Possible Effects of Extended Use
None reported.

Suggested Periodic Examinations While Taking This Drug (at physician's discretion)
Liver function tests.

While Taking This Drug, Observe the Following
Foods: No restrictions.

Beverages: No restrictions.

Alcohol: Use with caution until the combined effect has been determined. This drug may add to the depressant action of alcohol on the brain.

Tobacco Smoking: No interactions expected.

Marijuana Smoking
> Occasional (once or twice weekly): No effect to mild and transient increase in drowsiness, muscle weakness, and orthostatic hypotension (see Glossary).
>
> Daily: Moderate to marked drowsiness, muscle weakness, and incoordination, and significant accentuation of orthostatic hypotension.

Other Drugs
> The following drug may *decrease* the effects of chlorzoxazone:
> • testosterone is reported to reduce its ability to relax muscles in spasm.

Driving a Vehicle, Operating Machinery, Engaging in Hazardous Activities: This drug may cause drowsiness, lightheadedness, or dizziness in susceptible individuals. Avoid hazardous activities if these drug effects occur.

Aviation Note: The use of this drug *is a disqualification* for the piloting of aircraft. Consultation with a designated Aviation Medical Examiner is advised.

Exposure to Sun: No restrictions.

Special Storage Instructions
Keep in a dry, tightly closed container. Protect from light.

CIMETIDINE

Year Introduced: 1976

Brand Names

USA	Canada
Tagamet (Smith Kline & French)	Apo-Cimetidine (Apotex)
	Novocimetine (Novopharm)
	Peptol (Horner)
	Tagamet (SK&F)

Common Synonyms ("Street Names"):   Ulcer pill

Drug Class: Anti-peptic ulcer, Histamine Blocker (H-2 Receptor Antagonist)

Prescription Required: Yes

Available for Purchase by Generic Name: No

Available Dosage Forms and Strengths
Tablets — 200 mg., 300 mg., 400 mg.
Liquid — 300 mg. per 5 ml. teaspoonful
Injection — 300 mg. per 2 ml.

Tablet May Be Crushed or Capsule Opened for Administration: Yes

How This Drug Works
Intended Therapeutic Effect(s):   The relief of pain associated with active duodenal ulcer, the acceleration of ulcer healing, and the prevention of ulcer recurrence.
Note: The value of this drug in the treatment of stomach (gastric) ulcer has not been fully determined.
Location of Drug Action(s):   The acid-producing cells of the stomach lining that secrete acid when stimulated by histamines.
Method of Drug Action(s):   By blocking the action of histamine, this drug effectively inhibits the secretion of stomach acid and thus creates a more favorable environment for healing of duodenal ulcer.

Principal Uses of This Drug
As a Single Drug Product: Used primarily in the treatment of peptic ulcer disease, specifically to hasten the healing of duodenal ulcer and to prevent its recurrence. Also used to control the excessive production of stomach acid in the Zollinger-Ellison syndrome. Though its effectiveness has not been fully established, this drug is also widely used in the management of stomach (gastric) ulcer, esophagitis (as with hiatal hernia), and upper gastrointestinal bleeding.

THIS DRUG SHOULD NOT BE TAKEN IF
—you have had an allergic reaction to any dosage form of it previously.

INFORM YOUR PHYSICIAN BEFORE TAKING THIS DRUG IF
—you have impaired kidney function.
—you have a low sperm count.
—you are taking any digitalis preparation (digitoxin, digoxin) or propranolol (Inderal).
—you are taking any oral anticoagulant drug (see Anticoagulant Drug Class, Section Three).

Time Required for Apparent Benefit
Drug action begins within 1 hour and reaches a peak in 1 and one-half to 2 hours. Continuous use on a regular schedule for at least 6 weeks is recommended to allow for adequate healing of active duodenal ulcer.

Duration of Drug Effects After Last Dose

The daytime secretion of stomach acid following dosage with meals is inhibited for approximately 3 hours. The nighttime secretion is inhibited for 5 to 8 hours following bedtime dosage.

Possible Side-Effects *(natural, expected, and unavoidable drug actions)*

None reported.

Possible Adverse Effects *(unusual, unexpected, and infrequent reactions)*

IF ANY OF THE FOLLOWING DEVELOP, DISCONTINUE DRUG AND NOTIFY YOUR PHYSICIAN AS SOON AS POSSIBLE

Mild Adverse Effects

Allergic Reactions: Skin rash, hives, drug fever (see Glossary).
Other Reactions
Headache, dizziness, double vision, fatigue, muscular pains, diarrhea.
Breast secretion in women.
Breast swelling and soreness in men.

Serious Adverse Effects

Slowed heart rate.
Nervous agitation, confusion, delirium, hallucinations, coma.
Abnormally low white blood cell counts (leukopenia).
Abnormally low blood platelets (see Glossary).
Impaired absorption of Vitamin B-12, possibly leading to development of anemia.
Reduced sexual interest (libido) and potency.
Reduced formation of sperm—reduced fertility (temporary).

CAUTION

1. Do not exceed a total daily dose of 2400 mgs.
2. Do not discontinue this drug abruptly. Perforation of ulcer following abrupt cessation has been reported.
3. Hemodialysis (used in the management of chronic kidney disease) reduces the blood level of cimetidine. Drug is best taken at the end of a dialysis treatment.

Precautions for Use by Those over 60 Years of Age

The natural decline in kidney function that occurs after 60 makes it advisable to begin treatment with one-half the dose recommended for younger adults.
Observe closely for the occurrence of nervous agitation, depression, mental confusion, slurred speech, or excessive drowsiness. Report such developments promptly to the physician.

Advisability of Use During Pregnancy

Pregnancy Category: B (tentative). See Pregnancy Code inside back cover.
Animal reproduction studies reveal no birth defects due to this drug.
Information from adequate studies in pregnant women is not available.
Ask physician for guidance.

Advisability of Use While Nursing Infant
This drug is present in milk. Ask physician for guidance.

Habit-Forming Potential
None.

Effects of Overdosage
With Moderate Overdose: Mental confusion, delirium, slurred speech in sensitive individuals.
With Large Overdose: No serious or life-threatening effects reported.

Possible Effects of Extended Use
Liver damage (reversible).
Swelling and soreness of breast tissue in men.

Suggested Periodic Examinations While Taking This Drug (at physician's discretion)
Complete blood cell counts.
Liver function tests.
Sperm counts.
Prothrombin times, if taking an oral anticoagulant drug concurrently.

While Taking This Drug, Observe the Following
Foods: Protein-rich foods produce maximal stomach acid secretion. Follow the diet prescribed to derive optimal benefit from this drug and to promote ulcer healing. To obtain the longest period of stomach acid reduction, this drug should be taken with meals.

Beverages: Caffeine-containing beverages (coffee, tea, cola drinks) may increase stomach acidity, reduce the effectiveness of this drug, and delay ulcer healing. This drug may be taken with milk.

Alcohol: No interactions expected. However, alcoholic beverages may increase stomach acidity, reduce the effectiveness of this drug, and delay ulcer healing.

Tobacco Smoking: No interactions expected. However, nicotine may increase stomach acidity, reduce the effectiveness of this drug, and perpetuate peptic ulcer disease.

Marijuana Smoking
Occasional (once or twice weekly): No interactions expected.
Daily: Possible accentuation of reduced sperm production due to this drug.

Other Drugs
Cimetidine may *increase* the effects of
- diazepam (Valium, etc.), by delaying its elimination from the body with resultant accumulation and increased sedation.
- digitoxin (Crystodigin, etc.), by slowing its elimination.
- penicillin G, by increasing its absorption from the stomach.
- quinidine (Cardioquin, Quinidex, etc.), by slowing its elimination.
- warfarin (Coumadin, etc.), and increase the risk of bleeding. Ask physician for guidance.

Cimetidine may *decrease* the effects of
- bethanechol (Urecholine), by inhibiting its stimulation of stomach acid secretion.

Cimetidine *taken concurrently with*
- carmustine (BCNU) may cause severe bone marrow depression (see Glossary) with selective impairment of white blood cell production.

The following drugs may *increase* the effects of cimetidine:
- propantheline (Pro-Banthine), and other anticholinergic drugs, by augmenting cimetidine's inhibitory effect on stomach acid secretion.

Driving a Vehicle, Operating Machinery, Engaging in Hazardous Activities: This drug can cause erratic driving behavior. Use caution until it has been determined that dizziness, double vision, or confusion does not occur.

Aviation Note: The use of this drug *may be a disqualification* for the piloting of aircraft. Consultation with a designated Aviation Medical Examiner is advised.

Exposure to Sun: No restrictions.

Exposure to Heat: No restrictions.

Exposure to Cold: No restrictions.

Heavy Exercise or Exertion: No restrictions.

Occurrence of Unrelated Illness: Report the development of any illness that causes nausea, vomiting, or diarrhea.

Discontinuation: Do not discontinue this drug abruptly; ulcer perforation has been reported following abrupt cessation. This drug does not provide an extended protective effect. Be alert to the possibility of ulcer recurrence anytime after discontinuation.

Special Storage Instructions
Keep in a dry, tightly closed container.

CLIDINIUM

Year Introduced: 1961

Brand Names

USA	Canada
Quarzan (Roche)	Librax [CD] (Roche)
Librax [CD] (Roche)	

Common Synonyms ("Street Names"):   Stomach relaxer

Drug Class: Antispasmodic, Atropine-like Drug (Anticholinergics)

Prescription Required: Yes

Available for Purchase by Generic Name: No

Available Dosage Forms and Strengths
    Capsules — 2.5 mg., 5 mg.
  Capsules [CD] — 2.5 mg. (+ 5 mg. chlordiazepoxide)
Note: In Canada this drug is available only in combination with chlordiazepoxide. To be fully informed on the use of Librax, read Drug Profiles of both components.

Tablet May Be Crushed or Capsule Opened for Administration: Yes

How This Drug Works
  Intended Therapeutic Effect(s):   Relief of discomfort resulting from excessive activity and spasm of the digestive tract (esophagus, stomach, intestine, and colon).
  Location of Drug Action(s):   The terminal nerve fibers of the parasympathetic nervous system that control the activity of the gastrointestinal tract.
  Method of Drug Action(s):   By blocking the action of the chemical (acetylcholine) that transmits impulses at parasympathetic nerve endings, this drug prevents stimulation of muscular contraction and glandular secretion within the organs involved. This results in reduced overall activity, including the prevention or relief of muscle spasms.

Principal Uses of This Drug
  As a Single Drug Product: This atropine-like antispasmodic drug is used primarily in the management of peptic ulcer disease and the irritable bowel syndrome. Because it has been replaced by more effective drugs, it is seldom used alone.
  As a Combination Drug Product [CD]:   The major use of this drug is in combination with chlordiazepoxide. When combined, the tranquilizing effect of chlordiazepoxide and the atropine-like effects of clidinium are more effective than either drug used alone. Their actions complement each other in the treatment of peptic ulcer and functional disorders of the gastrointestinal tract.

THIS DRUG SHOULD NOT BE TAKEN IF
—you have had an allergic reaction to any dosage form of it previously.
—your stomach cannot empty properly into the intestine (pyloric obstruction).
—you are unable to empty the urinary bladder completely.
—you have glaucoma (narrow-angle type).
—you have severe ulcerative colitis.

INFORM YOUR PHYSICIAN BEFORE TAKING THIS DRUG IF
—you have glaucoma (open-angle type).
—you have angina or coronary heart disease.
—you have chronic bronchitis.
—you have a hiatal hernia.
—you have enlargement of the prostate gland.
—you have myasthenia gravis.
—you have a history of peptic ulcer disease.
—you plan to have surgery under general anesthesia in the near future.

Time Required for Apparent Benefit
Drug action begins in 1 to 2 hours and persists for approximately 4 hours.

Possible Side-Effects *(natural, expected, and unavoidable drug actions)*
Blurring of vision (impairment of focus), dryness of the mouth and throat, constipation, hesitancy in urination. (Nature and degree of side effects depend upon individual susceptibility and drug dosage.)

Possible Adverse Effects *(unusual, unexpected, and infrequent reactions)*

IF ANY OF THE FOLLOWING DEVELOP, DISCONTINUE DRUG AND NOTIFY YOUR PHYSICIAN AS SOON AS POSSIBLE

Mild Adverse Effects
Allergic Reactions: Skin rash, hives.
Other Reactions
Dilation of pupils, causing sensitivity to light.
Flushing and dryness of the skin (reduced sweating).
Rapid heart action.
Lightheadedness, dizziness, unsteady gait.
Serious Adverse Effects
Idiosyncratic Reactions: Acute confusion, delirium, and behavioral abnormalities.
Other Reactions: Development of acute glaucoma (in susceptible individuals).

CAUTION
Many over-the-counter medications (see OTC drugs in Glossary) for allergies, colds, and coughs contain drugs that can interact unfavorably with this drug. Ask your physician or pharmacist for guidance before using this medication.

Precautions for Use by Those over 60 Years of Age
You may be more sensitive to all of the actions of this drug. Small doses are advisable until your individual response has been determined.
This drug can increase the degree of impaired urination associated with prostate gland enlargement (prostatism).

Advisability of Use During Pregnancy
Pregnancy Category: B (tentative). See Pregnancy Code inside back cover.
Animal reproduction studies reveal no birth defects due to this drug.
Information from adequate studies in pregnant women is not available.
Ask physician for guidance.

Advisability of Use While Nursing Infant
Drug is known to be present in milk. Ask physician for guidance.

Habit-Forming Potential
For clidinium, none (see CHLORDIAZEPOXIDE Drug Profile).

Effects of Overdosage

With Moderate Overdose: Marked dryness of the mouth, dilated pupils, blurring of near vision, rapid pulse, heart palpitation, headache, difficulty in urination.

With Large Overdose: Extremely dilated pupils, rapid pulse and breathing, hot skin, high fever, excitement, confusion, hallucinations, delirium, eventual loss of consciousness, convulsions, and coma.

Possible Effects of Extended Use

Chronic constipation, severe enough to result in fecal impaction. (Constipation should be treated promptly with effective laxatives.)

Suggested Periodic Examinations While Taking This Drug (at physician's discretion)

Measurement of internal eye pressure to detect any significant increase that might indicate developing glaucoma.

While Taking This Drug, Observe the Following

Foods: No interaction with drug. Effectiveness is greater if drug is taken one-half to 1 hour before eating. Follow diet prescribed for condition under treatment.

Beverages: No interactions expected. As allowed by prescribed diet.

Alcohol: No interactions expected with this drug (see CHLORDIAZEPOXIDE Drug Profile).

Tobacco Smoking: No interactions expected with clidinium (see CHLORDIAZEPOXIDE Drug Profile).

Marijuana Smoking

Occasional (once or twice weekly):   Mild increase in drowsiness and dryness of mouth.

Daily: Moderate to marked increase in drowsiness and dryness of mouth.

Other Drugs

Clidinium may *increase* the effects of

• all other drugs having atropine-like actions (see Drug Class, Section Three).

Clidinium may *decrease* the effects of

• pilocarpine eye drops, and reduce their effectiveness in lowering internal eye pressure (in the treatment of glaucoma).

Clidinium *taken concurrently* with

• mono-amine oxidase (MAO) inhibitor drugs, may cause an exaggerated response to normal doses of atropine-like drugs. It is best to avoid atropine-like drugs for 2 weeks after the last dose of any MAO inhibitor drug (see Drug Class, Section Three).

• haloperidol (Haldol), may significantly increase internal eye pressure (dangerous in glaucoma).

The following drugs may *increase* the effects of clidinium:

• tricyclic antidepressants (see Drug Class, Section Three)

• those antihistamines that have an atropine-like action

- meperidine (Demerol, pethidine)
- methylphenidate (Ritalin)
- orphenadrine (Disipal, Norflex)
- those phenothiazines that have an atropine-like action (see Drug Class, Section Three)

The following drug may *decrease* the effects of clidinium:
- Vitamin C reduces its effectiveness by hastening its elimination from the body. Avoid large doses of Vitamin C during treatment with this drug.

Driving a Vehicle, Operating Machinery, Engaging in Hazardous Activities: This drug may produce blurred vision, drowsiness, or dizziness. Avoid hazardous activities if these drug effects occur.

Aviation Note: The use of this drug and the disorder for which this drug is prescribed *may be disqualifications* for the piloting of aircraft. Consultation with a designated Aviation Medical Examiner is advised.

Exposure to Sun: No restrictions.

Exposure to Heat: Use extreme caution. The use of this drug in hot environments may significantly increase the risk of heat stroke.

Heavy Exercise or Exertion: Use caution in warm or hot environments. This drug may impair normal perspiration (heat loss) and interfere with the regulation of body temperature.

Special Storage Instructions
Keep in a tightly closed container. Protect from light.

CLINDAMYCIN

Year Introduced: 1973

Brand Names

USA	Canada
Cleocin (Upjohn)	Dalacin C (Upjohn)
Cleocin T (Upjohn)	

Common Synonyms ("Street Names"):   None

Drug Class: Antibiotic (Anti-infective)

Prescription Required: Yes

Available for Purchase by Generic Name: No

Available Dosage Forms and Strengths
Capsules — 75 mg., 150 mg.
Oral solution — 75 mg. per teaspoonful (5 ml.)
Topical Solution — 10 mg. per ml.

Tablet May Be Crushed or Capsule Opened for Administration: Yes

How This Drug Works

Intended Therapeutic Effect(s):   The elimination of infections responsive to the action of this drug.

Location of Drug Action(s):   Any body tissue or fluid in which sufficient concentration of the drug can be achieved.

Method of Drug Action(s):   This drug prevents the growth and multiplication of susceptible bacteria by interfering with their formation of essential proteins.

Principal Uses of This Drug

As a Single Drug Product: To treat serious infections of the skin and soft tissues, of the lower respiratory tract, of the abdominal cavity, of the genital tract in women, and blood stream infections (septicemia). It is quite valuable in treating infections caused by unusual bacteria. Precise identification of the causative organism and determination of its sensitivity are mandatory to the safe and effective use of this drug.

THIS DRUG SHOULD NOT BE TAKEN IF
—you are allergic to lincomycin or clindamycin.
—it is prescribed for a mild or trivial infection such as a cold, sore throat, or "flu"-like illness.
—you have a history of ulcerative colitis.
—it is prescribed for an infant under 1 month of age.

INFORM YOUR PHYSICIAN BEFORE TAKING THIS DRUG IF
—you have a history of allergy to any drug.
—you are allergic by nature (hayfever, asthma, hives, eczema).
—you have a history of previous yeast infections.
—you have liver or kidney disease or impaired liver or kidney function.
—you plan to have surgery under general anesthesia in the near future.

Time Required for Apparent Benefit
Varies with nature of infection under treatment; usually 2 to 5 days.

Possible Side-Effects *(natural, expected, and unavoidable drug actions)*
Superinfections (see Glossary).

Possible Adverse Effects *(unusual, unexpected, and infrequent reactions)*

IF ANY OF THE FOLLOWING DEVELOP, DISCONTINUE DRUG AND NOTIFY YOUR PHYSICIAN AS SOON AS POSSIBLE

Mild Adverse Effects
   Allergic Reactions: Skin rashes (various kinds), hives.
   Other Reactions: Nausea, vomiting, diarrhea, abdominal pain.
Serious Adverse Effects
   Allergic Reactions: Painful, swollen joints, jaundice (see Glossary).
   Other Reactions: †*Severe colitis with persistent diarrhea;* stools may contain blood and/or mucus.

†An infrequent but potentially dangerous reaction characteristic of this drug.

CAUTION
1. Troublesome and persistent diarrhea can develop in sensitive individuals. If diarrhea persists more than 24 hours, discontinue this drug and consult your physician for guidance.
2. If surgery under general anesthesia is planned while taking this drug, the choice of anesthetic must be considered carefully to prevent excessive muscle relaxation and associated impairment of breathing.

Precautions for Use by Those over 60 Years of Age
The natural decline in liver function that occurs after 60 may require significant reduction in dosage and lengthening of dosage intervals. Dosage must be carefully individualized.

Natural changes in the skin after 60 may predispose to severe and prolonged itching reactions in the genital and anal regions. This reaction should be reported promptly.

Advisability of Use During Pregnancy
Pregnancy Category: B (tentative). See Pregnancy Code inside back cover. Animal reproduction studies in mice and rats reveal no birth defects due to this drug.

Information from adequate studies in pregnant women is not available. Ask physician for guidance.

Advisability of Use While Nursing Infant
Drug can be present in milk. Safety for infant not established. Ask physician for guidance.

Habit-Forming Potential
None.

Effects of Overdosage
Nausea, vomiting, cramping, diarrhea.

Possible Effects of Extended Use
†*Severe colitis with persistent diarrhea.*
Superinfections (see Glossary), especially from yeast organisms.

Suggested Periodic Examinations While Taking This Drug (at physician's discretion)
Complete blood cell counts.
Liver function tests.

While Taking This Drug, Observe the Following
Foods: No restrictions of food selection. Drug may be taken at any time with relationship to eating.
Beverages: No restrictions.
Alcohol: No interactions expected.
Tobacco Smoking: No interactions expected.
Marijuana Smoking: No interactions expected.

†An infrequent but potentially dangerous reaction characteristic of this drug.

Other Drugs
The following drugs may *decrease* the effects of clindamycin:
- anti-diarrheal preparations
- erythromycin

Driving a Vehicle, Operating Machinery, Engaging in Hazardous Activities: Usually no restrictions. Be alert to the possible occurrence of nausea and/or diarrhea.

Aviation Note: The use of this drug *may be a disqualification* for the piloting of aircraft. Consultation with a designated Aviation Medical Examiner is advised.

Exposure to Sun: Use caution until sensitivity is determined.

Discontinuation: When used to treat infections that predispose to rheumatic fever or kidney disease (nephritis), take continuously in full dosage for no less than 10 days. Ask physician for guidance regarding the recommended duration of therapy.

Special Storage Instructions
Capsules should be kept in a dry, tightly closed container.
Oral solution should be kept at room temperature; do *not* refrigerate.

Observe the Following Expiration Times
Do not take the oral solution of this drug if it is older than 14 days.

CLOFIBRATE

Year Introduced: 1967

Brand Names

USA	Canada
Atromid-S (Ayerst)	Atromid-S (Ayerst)
	Claripex (ICN)
	Novafibrate (Novopharm)

Common Synonyms ("Street Names"):   Cholesterol medicine

Drug Class: Cholesterol Reducer (Antihyperlipemic)

Prescription Required: Yes

Available for Purchase by Generic Name: No

Available Dosage Forms and Strengths
Capsules — 500 mg.

Tablet May Be Crushed or Capsule Opened for Administration: Yes

How This Drug Works

Intended Therapeutic Effect(s): Reduction of high blood levels of cholesterol and/or triglycerides.

Location of Drug Action(s): Not completely established. Thought to be those liver cells responsible for the production of cholesterol.

Method of Drug Action(s): Not completely established. It is thought that this drug may reduce blood levels of cholesterol and triglycerides by inhibiting their production and hastening their removal from the blood.

Principal Uses of This Drug

As a Single Drug Product: Used primarily in carefully selected individuals to reduce the blood levels of cholesterol and triglycerides. Its use should be restricted to those who have type III or IV hyperlipoproteinemia, have a significant risk of coronary artery disease, and have failed to respond to safer measures such as diet, weight control, and exercise. This drug is most effective in lowering triglyceride levels and should not be used when cholesterol alone is elevated.

THIS DRUG SHOULD NOT BE TAKEN IF

—you have had an allergic reaction to any dosage form of it previously.
—you have impaired function of the liver or kidneys.

INFORM YOUR PHYSICIAN BEFORE TAKING THIS DRUG IF

—you are taking any anticoagulant drug.
—you have a history of liver disease or jaundice.
—you have a history of peptic ulcer.
—you have diabetes.

Time Required for Apparent Benefit

Continuous use for 2 to 3 months may be needed to determine the extent of this drug's ability to lower blood levels of either cholesterol or triglycerides.

Possible Side-Effects *(natural, expected, and unavoidable drug actions)*

Gain in weight occurs frequently.

Possible Adverse Effects *(unusual, unexpected, and infrequent reactions)*

IF ANY OF THE FOLLOWING DEVELOP, DISCONTINUE DRUG AND NOTIFY YOUR PHYSICIAN AS SOON AS POSSIBLE

Mild Adverse Effects
  Allergic Reactions: Skin rash, hives, itching, loss of scalp hair.
  Other Reactions
    Nausea, vomiting, indigestion, diarrhea.
    Headache, dizziness, fatigue, drowsiness.
    "Flu"-like muscle and joint aching and cramping.
    Impairment of sexual function.

Serious Adverse Effects
Allergic Reactions: Kidney tissue injury (rare).
Other Reactions
Liver damage (without jaundice).
Abnormally low red blood cells (anemia) and white blood cells.

CAUTION
1. Recent reports indicate that an increase in serious diseases and disorders may be associated with the long-term use of this drug. Consult your physician regarding the consideration of benefit versus risk before using this drug.
2. It is advisable to prevent pregnancy while using this drug and for an additional 3 to 6 months after its discontinuation.

Precautions for Use by Those over 60 Years of Age
Before using this drug, discuss with your physician the exact nature of your "cholesterol disorder" and the justification for drug therapy. This drug can cause serious adverse effects and should be taken only if the anticipated benefits clearly outweigh the possible risks.

You may be more susceptible to the development of "flu"-like symptoms. These should not be mistaken for indications of actual infection. Consult your physician.

Advisability of Use During Pregnancy
Pregnancy Category: X (tentative). See Pregnancy Code inside back cover.
Animal reproduction studies reveal no birth defects due to this drug.
Information from adequate studies in pregnant women is not available.
The manufacturers state that this drug is contraindicated during entire pregnancy.
Ask physician for guidance.

Advisability of Use While Nursing Infant
Safety for infant not established. Ask physician for guidance.

Habit-Forming Potential
None.

Effects of Overdosage
With Moderate Overdose: Nausea, vomiting, abdominal distress, diarrhea.
With Large Overdose: Headache, muscular pain, weakness.

Possible Effects of Extended Use
None reported.

Suggested Periodic Examinations While Taking This Drug (at physician's discretion)
Complete blood cell counts.
Liver function tests.

While Taking This Drug, Observe the Following
Foods: Follow the low animal fat and/or low carbohydrate diet prescribed by your physician.

Beverages: No restrictions.

Alcohol: No interactions expected; follow diet prescribed.

Tobacco Smoking: No interactions expected; follow physician's advice regarding smoking.

Marijuana Smoking: No interactions expected.

Other Drugs

Clofibrate may *increase* the effects of

- oral anticoagulants of the coumarin family (see Drug Class, Section Three). The usual dose of the anticoagulant must be reduced by one-third or one-half to prevent abnormal bleeding or hemorrhage. Consult physician regarding prothrombin time testing and dosage adjustment.
- oral anti-diabetics of the sulfonylurea family (see Drug Class, Section Three). Dosage adjustments may be necessary to prevent hypoglycemia (see Glossary) and to establish correct control of diabetes.
- insulin preparations, which may also require dosage adjustments to prevent hypoglycemia.

The following drugs may *increase* the effects of clofibrate

- thyroid preparations may enhance the lowering of blood cholesterol.

The following drugs may *decrease* the effects of clofibrate

- oral contraceptives may prevent the lowering of blood cholesterol or triglycerides.
- estrogens (Premarin, etc.) may prevent the lowering of cholesterol.

Driving a Vehicle, Operating Machinery, Engaging in Hazardous Activities: Usually no restrictions, but be alert to the possible occurrence of drowsiness or dizziness. Avoid hazardous activities if these occur.

Aviation Note: The use of this drug *may be a disqualification* for the piloting of aircraft. Consultation with a designated Aviation Medical Examiner is advised.

Exposure to Sun: No restrictions.

Discontinuation: This drug should be discontinued after 3 months if significant lowering of the blood cholesterol and/or triglycerides has not occurred. Withdrawal should be gradual, not sudden. Ask physician for guidance.

Special Storage Instructions

Keep in a dry, tightly closed container. Protect from light.

CLONIDINE

Year Introduced: 1966 (Europe)
1974 (USA)

Brand Names

USA	Canada
Catapres (Boehringer Ingelheim)	Catapres (Boehringer)
Combipres [CD] (Boehringer Ingelheim)	Combipres [CD] (Boehringer)
	Dixarit (Boehringer)

Common Synonyms ("Street Names"):   Blood pressure pills

Drug Class: Anti-hypertensive (Hypotensive)

Prescription Required: Yes

Available for Purchase by Generic Name: No

Available Dosage Forms and Strengths
Tablets — 0.1 mg., 0.2 mg., 0.3 mg.

Tablet May Be Crushed or Capsule Opened for Administration: Yes

How This Drug Works
Intended Therapeutic Effect(s):   Reduction of high blood pressure.
Location of Drug Action(s):   The vasomotor center in the brain that influences the control of the sympathetic nervous system over blood vessels (principally arterioles) throughout the body.
Method of Drug Action(s):   By decreasing the activity of the vasomotor center, this drug reduces the ability of the sympathetic nervous system to maintain the degree of blood vessel constriction responsible for elevation of the blood pressure. This change results in relaxation of blood vessel walls and lowering of the blood pressure.

Principal Uses of This Drug
As a Single Drug Product: This anti-hypertensive drug is considered to be a "step 2" drug in the management of high blood pressure. It is generally not used to initiate treatment, but is added when a "step 1" drug proves to be inadequate. It may be used as a "step 3" or "step 4" drug in place of drugs that are more likely to cause marked orthostatic hypotension (see Glossary). This drug is sometimes used to prevent migraine headache, to prevent hot flushes of the menopause, and to treat menstrual cramps.
As a Combination Drug Product [CD]:   This "step 2" anti-hypertensive drug is available in combination with the "step 1" anti-hypertensive drug chlorthalidone. The differing methods of action complement each other to make the combination a more effective anti-hypertensive medication.

THIS DRUG SHOULD NOT BE TAKEN IF
—you have had an allergic reaction to any dosage form of it previously.
—it is prescribed for a child under 12 years of age.

INFORM YOUR PHYSICIAN BEFORE TAKING THIS DRUG IF
—you have a history of heart or circulatory disease (angina, heart attack, stroke).
—you plan to have surgery under general anesthesia in the near future.

Time Required for Apparent Benefit
Blood pressure is lowered within 1 to 4 hours. Drug action subsides in 6 to 8 hours.

Possible Side-Effects *(natural, expected, and unavoidable drug actions)*
Drowsiness, dryness of the nose and mouth, constipation, lightheadedness on arising from a sitting or lying position (see orthostatic hypotension in Glossary).

Possible Adverse Effects *(unusual, unexpected, and infrequent reactions)*

IF ANY OF THE FOLLOWING DEVELOP, NOTIFY YOUR PHYSICIAN AS SOON AS POSSIBLE

Mild Adverse Effects
  Allergic Reactions: Skin rash, hives, localized swellings, itching.
  Other Reactions
    Dizziness, depression, insomnia, nightmares.
    Nausea, vomiting.
    Dryness and burning of the eyes. Breast enlargement.
Serious Adverse Effects
  None reported.

CAUTION
1. *Do not discontinue this drug suddenly.* Be sure to keep an adequate supply on hand. Sudden withdrawal can produce a severe and possibly fatal reaction. Include notation of the use of this drug on your card of personal identification (see Table 19 and Section Six).
2. Hot weather and the fever associated with infection can reduce the blood pressure significantly, requiring adjustment of dosage.
3. Report the development of any tendency to emotional depression.

Precautions for Use by Those over 60 Years of Age
The basic rule in treating high blood pressure after 60 is to proceed *cautiously*. The elevated systolic blood pressure often present after 60 is not necessarily a threat to health, and can serve as an adaptive and compensatory change with age that should not be altered drastically. The goals of treatment must be adjusted to the natural changes in body function that occur with aging. Unacceptably high blood pressure should be reduced without creating the risks associated with excessively low blood pressure.
It is advisable to start treatment with small doses and to monitor the blood pressure response frequently. Sudden, rapid, and excessive reduction of blood pressure can predispose to stroke or heart attack.
You may be more susceptible to the development of orthostatic hypotension with resultant lightheadedness, dizziness, unsteadiness, fainting, and falling. Report such symptoms to your physician promptly.

Advisability of Use During Pregnancy
Pregnancy Category: C (tentative). See Pregnancy Code inside back cover.
Animal reproduction studies reveal possible injury to embryo.
Information from adequate studies in pregnant women is not available.
It is advisable to avoid this drug during first 3 months.
Ask physician for guidance.

Advisability of Use While Nursing Infant
Presence of drug in milk is not known. Ask physician for guidance.

Habit-Forming Potential
None.

Effects of Overdosage
With Moderate Overdose: Marked drowsiness, weakness, slow and weak
pulse.
With Large Overdose: Deep sleep, lowered body temperature.

Possible Effects of Extended Use
Weight gain due to salt and water retention.
Temporary sexual impotence.

Suggested Periodic Examinations While Taking This Drug (at physician's discretion)
Monitoring of weight to detect possible water retention.
Eye examinations for changes in retina or impairment of vision.

While Taking This Drug, Observe the Following
Foods: Follow prescribed diet. Ask physician for guidance regarding use of
salt.
Beverages: No restrictions.
Alcohol: Use with extreme caution until combined effect has been deter-
mined. This combination can cause marked drowsiness and exaggerated
reduction of blood pressure.
Tobacco Smoking: No interactions expected with this drug. Follow your
physician's advice regarding smoking.
Marijuana Smoking
Occasional (once or twice weekly):   No effect to mild and transient accentuation of orthostatic hypotension (see Glossary).
Daily: Significant accentuation of orthostatic hypotension, requiring dosage adjustment in sensitive individuals.
Other Drugs
Clonidine may *increase* the effects of
- sedatives, sleep-inducing drugs, tranquilizers, antihistamines, pain relievers, and narcotic drugs, and cause oversedation.
- thiazide diuretics and other anti-hypertensive drugs, and cause exaggerated lowering of the blood pressure. Careful dosage adjustments are
necessary.

The following drugs may *decrease* the effects of clonidine
- tricyclic antidepressants (Elavil, Tofranil, Sinequan, etc.) may interfere with its blood pressure-lowering action. Dosage adjustments may be necessary.

Driving a Vehicle, Operating Machinery, Engaging in Hazardous Activities: This drug can cause drowsiness and orthostatic hypotension (see Glossary). Avoid hazardous activities until its effect on mental alertness, judgment, and coordination have been determined.

Aviation Note: Hypertension (high blood pressure) *is a disqualification* for the piloting of aircraft. Consultation with a designated Aviation Medical Examiner is advised.

Exposure to Sun: No restrictions.

Exposure to Heat: No restrictions.

Exposure to Cold: Use caution until combined effect has been determined. This drug may cause painful blanching and numbness of the hands and feet on exposure to cold air or water.

Heavy Exercise or Exertion: Use caution. Isometric exercises—the "overload" technique for strengthening individual muscles—can raise the blood pressure significantly. The use of this drug may intensify the hypertensive response to isometric exercises. Ask your physician for guidance.

Occurrence of Unrelated Illness: If an illness causes vomiting and prevents the intake of this drug on a regular basis, notify your physician as soon as possible.

Discontinuation: Do not discontinue this drug suddenly. A severe withdrawal reaction can occur within 12 to 48 hours. If drug is to be discontinued for any reason, ask your physician for guidance regarding dosage reduction and gradual withdrawal.

Special Storage Instructions
Keep in a dry, tightly closed container.

CLORAZEPATE

Year Introduced: 1972

Brand Names

USA	Canada
Azene (Endo)	Tranxene (Abbott)
Tranxene (Abbott)	
Tranxene-SD (Abbott)	

Common Synonyms ("Street Names"):   Downs, nerve pills, tranks

Drug Class: Tranquilizer, Mild (Anti-anxiety), Benzodiazepines

Prescription Required: Yes (Controlled Drug, U.S. Schedule IV)*

Available for Purchase by Generic Name: No

Available Dosage Forms and Strengths
   Tablets — 3.75 mg., 7.5 mg., 11.25 mg., 15 mg., 22.5 mg.
   Capsules — 3.75 mg., 7.5 mg., 15 mg.

Tablet May Be Crushed or Capsule Opened for Administration: Yes

How This Drug Works
   Intended Therapeutic Effect(s):   Relief of mild to moderate anxiety and nervous tension, without significant sedation.
   Location of Drug Action(s):   Thought to be the limbic system of the brain, one of the centers that influence emotional stability.
   Method of Drug Action(s):   Not established. Present thinking is that this drug may reduce the activity of certain parts of the limbic system.

Principal Uses of This Drug
   As a Single Drug Product: This mild tranquilizer is used primarily to (1) provide short-term relief of mild to moderate anxiety, and (2) provide adjunctive treatment in controlling "partial" seizures, a type of epilepsy.

THIS DRUG SHOULD NOT BE TAKEN IF
—you have had an allergic reaction to any dosage form of it previously.
—you have glaucoma (narrow-angle type).
—you have myasthenia gravis.
—it is prescribed for an infant under 6 months of age.

INFORM YOUR PHYSICIAN BEFORE TAKING THIS DRUG IF
—you are allergic to any drugs chemically related to clorazepate: chlordiazepoxide, diazepam, flurazepam, oxazepam (see Drug Profiles for brand names).
—you have epilepsy.
—you have glaucoma (open-angle type).
—you are taking sedative, sleep-inducing, tranquilizer, antidepressant, or anticonvulsant drugs of any kind.
—you plan to have surgery under general anesthesia in the near future.

Time Required For Apparent Benefit
   Approximately 1 to 2 hours. For severe symptoms of some duration, relief may require regular medication for several days.

Possible Side-Effects (*natural, expected, and unavoidable drug actions*)
   Drowsiness, lethargy, unsteadiness in stance and gait.

*See Schedules of Controlled Drugs inside back cover.

Possible Adverse Effects *(unusual, unexpected, and infrequent reactions)*

IF ANY OF THE FOLLOWING DEVELOP, DISCONTINUE DRUG AND NOTIFY YOUR PHYSICIAN AS SOON AS POSSIBLE

Mild Adverse Effects
Allergic Reactions: Skin rashes (various kinds).
Other Reactions: Dizziness, fainting, blurred vision, double vision, slurred speech, nausea, menstrual irregularity.

Serious Adverse Effects
Allergic Reactions: Jaundice (see Glossary), fever, sore throat.
Paradoxical Reactions: Acute excitement, hallucinations, rage.
Other Reactions: Eye pain (possibly glaucoma), depression.

Precautions for Use by Those over 60 Years of Age
Natural changes in body functions increase the duration of this drug's action. It is necessary to use smaller doses with longer intervals between doses to avoid excessive accumulation of the drug in body tissues. Dosage must be carefully individualized and limited to the smallest effective amount.
You may be more susceptible to the development of lightheadedness, impaired thinking and memory, confusion, lethargy, drowsiness, incoordination, unsteady gait and balance, impaired bladder control, and constipation. Be alert to the possibility of paradoxical responses consisting of excitement, agitation, anger, hostility, and rage.

Advisability of Use During Pregnancy
Pregnancy Category: B (tentative). See Pregnancy Code inside back cover.
Animal reproduction studies in mice, rats, and rabbits reveal no birth defects due to this drug.
Information from adequate studies in pregnant women is not available.
The findings of some recent studies suggest a possible association between the use of a drug closely related to clorazepate during early pregnancy and the occurrence of birth defects, such as cleft lip. It is advisable to avoid this drug completely during the first 3 months of pregnancy.
Ask physician for guidance.

Advisability of Use While Nursing Infant
With recommended dosage, drug is present in milk. Avoid use if possible. Ask physician for guidance.

Habit-Forming Potential
This drug can cause psychological and/or physical dependence (see Glossary) if used in large doses for an extended period of time.

Effects of Overdosage
With Moderate Overdose: Marked drowsiness, weakness, drunkenness, impairment of stance and gait.
With Large Overdose: Stupor progressing to deep sleep and coma.

Possible Effects of Extended Use
Psychological and/or physical dependence.
Impairment of blood cell production.
Impairment of liver function.

Suggested Periodic Examinations While Taking This Drug (at physician's discretion)
Blood cell counts and liver function tests during long-term use.

While Taking This Drug, Observe the Following
Foods: No restrictions.

Beverages: Large intake of coffee, tea, or cola drinks (because of their caffeine content) may reduce the calming action of this drug.

Alcohol: Use with extreme caution until the combined effect is determined. Alcohol may increase the sedative effects of clorazepate. Clorazepate may increase the intoxicating effects of alcohol.

Tobacco Smoking: Heavy smoking may reduce the calming action of clorazepate.

Marijuana Smoking
Occasional (once or twice weekly):   Mild increase in sedative effect of this drug.
Daily: Marked increase in sedative effect of this drug.

Other Drugs
Clorazepate may *increase* the effects of
- other sedatives, sleep-inducing drugs, tranquilizers, anti-convulsants, and narcotic drugs. Use these only under supervision of a physician. Careful dosage adjustments are necessary.
- oral anticoagulants of the coumarin family (see Drug Class, Section Three). Ask physician for guidance regarding need for dosage adjustments to prevent bleeding.
- anti-hypertensives, producing excessive lowering of the blood pressure.

Clorazepate *taken concurrently* with
- anti-convulsants, may cause an increase in the frequency or severity of seizures; an increase in the dose of the anti-convulsant may be necessary.
- mono-amine oxidase (MAO) inhibitor drugs (see Drug Class, Section Three), may cause extreme sedation, convulsions, or paradoxical excitement or rage.

The following drugs may *increase* the effects of clorazepate
- tricyclic antidepressants (see Drug Class, Section Three) may increase the sedative effects of clorazepate.

The following drugs may *decrease* the effects of clorazepate
- antacids, by interfering with its absorption.

Driving a Vehicle, Operating Machinery, Engaging in Hazardous Activities: This drug can impair mental alertness, judgment, physical coordination, and reaction time. Avoid hazardous activities.

Aviation Note: The use of this drug *is a disqualification* for the piloting of aircraft. Consultation with a designated Aviation Medical Examiner is advised.

Exposure to Sun: No restrictions.

Exposure to Heat: Use caution until effect of excessive perspiration is determined. Because of reduced urine volume, clorazepate may accumulate in the body and produce effects of overdosage.

Heavy Exercise or Exertion: No restrictions in cool or temperate weather.

Discontinuation: If it has been necessary to use this drug for an extended period of time, ask physician for guidance regarding dosage reduction and withdrawal. The dosage of other drugs taken concurrently with clorazepate may also require adjustment.

Special Storage Instructions

Keep in a dry, tightly closed, light-resistant container.

CLOXACILLIN

Year Introduced: 1962

Brand Names

USA	Canada
Cloxapen (Beecham)	Bactopen (Beecham)
Tegopen (Bristol)	Cloxilean (Organon)
	Novocloxin (Novopharm)
	Orbenin (Ayerst)
	Tegopen (Bristol)

Common Synonyms ("Street Names"): None

Drug Class: Antibiotic (Anti-infective), Penicillins

Prescription Required: Yes

Available for Purchase by Generic Name: USA: Yes   Canada: No

Available Dosage Forms and Strengths
Capsules — 250 mg., 500 mg.
Oral solution — 125 mg. per teaspoonful (5 ml.)

Tablet May Be Crushed or Capsule Opened for Administration: Yes

How This Drug Works

Intended Therapeutic Effect(s): The elimination of infections responsive to the action of this drug.

Location of Drug Action(s): Any body tissue or fluid in which sufficient concentration of the drug can be achieved.

Method of Drug Action(s):   This drug destroys susceptible infecting bacteria by interfering with their ability to produce new protective cell walls as they multiply and grow.

Principal Uses of This Drug

As a Single Drug Product: This drug is used primarily to treat infections that are caused by bacteria (principally staphylococcus) that have developed resistance to the original types of penicillin. It is of value in treating infections of the skin and soft tissues, the upper and lower respiratory tracts (including "strep" throat), and infections that are widely scattered throughout the body.

THIS DRUG SHOULD NOT BE TAKEN IF
—you have had an allergic reaction to any dosage form of it previously.
—you are certain you are allergic to any form of penicillin.

INFORM YOUR PHYSICIAN BEFORE TAKING THIS DRUG IF
—you suspect you may be allergic to penicillin or you have a history of a previous "reaction" to penicillin.
—you are allergic to cephalosporin antibiotics (Ancef, Ceporan, Ceporex, Kafocin, Keflex, Keflin, Kefzol, Loridine).
—you are allergic by nature (hayfever, asthma, hives, eczema).

Time Required for Apparent Benefit
Varies with the nature of the infection under treatment; usually from 2 to 5 days.

Possible Side-Effects *(natural, expected, and unavoidable drug actions)*
Superinfections (see Glossary).

Possible Adverse Effects *(unusual, unexpected, and infrequent reactions)*

IF ANY OF THE FOLLOWING DEVELOP, DISCONTINUE DRUG AND NOTIFY YOUR PHYSICIAN AS SOON AS POSSIBLE

Mild Adverse Effects
Allergic Reactions: Skin rashes (various kinds).
Other Reactions: Irritation of mouth or tongue, "black tongue," nausea, vomiting, diarrhea, gaseous indigestion.
Serious Adverse Effects
Allergic Reactions: †Anaphylactic reaction (see Glossary), severe skin reactions, high fever, swollen painful joints, sore throat, unusual bleeding or bruising.

Precautions for Use by Those over 60 Years of Age
It is advisable to evaluate kidney function before and during use of this drug to determine the need for dosage adjustment.
Natural changes in the skin after 60 may predispose to severe and prolonged itching reactions in the genital and anal regions. This reaction should be reported promptly.

†A rare but potentially dangerous reaction characteristic of penicillins.

Advisability of Use During Pregnancy
Pregnancy Category: B (tentative). See Pregnancy Code inside back cover.
Animal reproduction studies in rabbits reveal no birth defects due to this drug.
Information from studies in pregnant women indicates no increased risk of defects in 3546 exposures to penicillin derivatives.
Ask physician for guidance.

Advisability of Use While Nursing Infant
Drug may be present in milk and may sensitize infant to penicillin. Ask physician for guidance.

Habit-Forming Potential
None.

Effects of Overdosage
Possible nausea, vomiting, and/or diarrhea.

Possible Effects of Extended Use
Superinfections (see Glossary).

Suggested Periodic Examinations While Taking This Drug (at physician's discretion)
Complete blood cell counts.
Liver and kidney function tests.

While Taking This Drug, Observe the Following
Foods: No restrictions of food selection. Drug is most effective when taken on empty stomach, 1 hour before or 2 hours after eating.
Beverages: No restrictions.
Alcohol: No interactions expected.
Tobacco Smoking: No interactions expected.
Marijuana Smoking: No interactions expected.
Other Drugs
The following drugs may *decrease* the effects of cloxacillin
- antacids can reduce absorption of cloxacillin.
- chloramphenicol (Chloromycetin)
- erythromycin (Erythrocin, E-Mycin, etc.)
- paromomycin (Humatin)
- tetracyclines (Achromycin, Declomycin, Minocin, etc.; see Drug Class, Section Three)
- troleandomycin (Cyclamycin, TAO)

Driving a Vehicle, Operating Machinery, Engaging in Hazardous Activities: Usually no restrictions. Be alert to the possible occurrence of nausea, diarrhea or dizziness.
Aviation Note: The use of this drug *may be a disqualification* for the piloting of aircraft. Consultation with a designated Aviation Medical Examiner is advised.
Exposure to Sun: No restrictions.

Special Storage Instructions
Capsules: keep in tightly closed container at room temperature.
Oral Solution: keep refrigerated.

Observe the Following Expiration Times
Do not take the oral solution of this drug if it is older than 3 days—when kept
at room temperature; 14 days—when kept refrigerated.

CODEINE

Year Introduced: 1886

Brand Names

USA	Canada
No brand names for codeine as a single entity drug product. Many brand names for combination drug products containing codeine.	Paveral (Desbergers) (Many brand names for combination drug products containing codeine)

Common Synonyms ("Street Names"):   Painkiller, pain reliever, robo, schoolboy, syrup

Drug Class: Analgesic, Mild (Narcotic)

Prescription Required: Yes (Controlled Drug, U.S. Schedule II)*

Available for Purchase by Generic Name: Yes

Available Dosage Forms and Strengths
Tablets — 15 mg., 30 mg., 60 mg.
Syrup — 10 mg. per ml.
Injection — 15 mg., 30 mg., 60 mg. per ml.

Tablet May Be Crushed or Capsule Opened for Administration: Yes

How This Drug Works
Intended Therapeutic Effect(s)
Relief of moderate pain.
Control of coughing.
Location of Drug Action(s)
Those areas of the brain and spinal cord involved in the perception of pain.
Those areas of the brain and spinal cord involved in the cough reflex.

*See Schedules of Controlled Drugs inside back cover.

Method of Drug Action(s): Not completely established. It is thought that this drug affects tissue sites that react specifically with opium and its derivatives to relieve pain and cough.

Principal Uses of This Drug
As a Single Drug Product: This opium derivative is used primarily to (1) relieve moderate to severe pain; (2) control cough; and (3) control diarrhea. Its widest use is as an ingredient in analgesic preparations and cough remedies. Its constipating effect is sometimes used in the treatment of diarrhea, though better drugs are now available for this purpose.

As a Combination Drug Product [CD]: Codeine is commonly combined with other milder analgesics to enhance their effectiveness, notably aspirin and acetaminophen. It is frequently added to cough mixtures containing antihistamines, decongestants, and expectorants to make these "shotgun" preparations more effective in reducing the frequency and severity of cough.

THIS DRUG SHOULD NOT BE TAKEN IF
—you have had an allergic reaction to any dosage form of it previously.

INFORM YOUR PHYSICIAN BEFORE TAKING THIS DRUG IF
—you are taking sedatives, other analgesics, sleep-inducing drugs, tranquilizers, antidepressants, or narcotic drugs of any kind.
—you have impaired liver or kidney function.
—you have underactive thyroid function.
—you plan to have surgery under general anesthesia in the near future.

Time Required for Apparent Benefit
Usually 15 to 30 minutes when taken orally.

Possible Side-Effects *(natural, expected, and unavoidable drug actions)*
Drowsiness, lightheadedness, constipation.

Possible Adverse Effects *(unusual, unexpected, and infrequent reactions)*
IF ANY OF THE FOLLOWING DEVELOP, DISCONTINUE DRUG AND NOTIFY YOUR PHYSICIAN AS SOON AS POSSIBLE

Mild Adverse Effects
  Allergic Reactions: Skin rashes, hives, itching.
  Other Reactions
    Nausea, vomiting.
    Dizziness, sensation of drunkenness.
Serious Adverse Effects
  None reported.

Precautions for Use by Those over 60 Years of Age
The aim of treatment should be to provide the maximal relief of pain consistent with minimal risk and the preservation of ability to function. Dosage should be low at the beginning with adjustment upward according to individual response.
The use of this drug should be limited to short-term treatment only.

You may be more susceptible to the development of dizziness, drowsiness, and constipation.

Advisability of Use During Pregnancy

Pregnancy Category: C (tentative). See Pregnancy Code inside back cover. Animal reproduction studies in hamsters reveal significant birth defects due to this drug.

Information from studies in pregnant women indicates no significant increase in defects in 2522 exposures to this drug.

It is advisable to avoid use of this drug during first 3 months.

Ask physician for guidance.

Advisability of Use While Nursing Infant

Drug is known to be present in milk and may have a depressant effect on infant. Ask physician for guidance.

Habit-Forming Potential

This drug can produce psychological and physical dependence (see Glossary) when used in large doses for an extended period of time.

Effects of Overdosage

With Moderate Overdose: Marked drowsiness, nausea, vomiting, restlessness, agitation.

With Large Overdose: Stupor progressing to deep sleep, convulsions, cold and clammy skin, slow and shallow breathing.

Possible Effects of Extended Use

Psychological and physical dependence.

Suggested Periodic Examinations While Taking This Drug (at physician's discretion)

None.

While Taking This Drug, Observe the Following

Foods: No restrictions.

Beverages: No restrictions.

Alcohol: Use with extreme caution until combined effects have been determined. Codeine can intensify the intoxicating effects of alcohol, and alcohol can intensify the depressant effects of codeine on brain function, breathing, and circulation.

Tobacco Smoking: No interactions expected.

Marijuana Smoking

Occasional (once or twice weekly):   Mild and transient increase in drowsiness and relief of pain.

Daily: Significant increase in drowsiness, relief of pain, and impairment of mental and physical performance.

Other Drugs

Codeine may *increase* the effects of

• all sedatives, analgesics, sleep-inducing drugs, tranquilizers, antidepressants, and other narcotic drugs.

Codeine *taken concurrently* with
- chlordiazepoxide (Librium), may cause extreme sedation and coma.

The following drugs may *increase* the effects of codeine:
- aspirin increases the analgesic action of codeine.
- chloramphenicol (Chloromycetin) increases the analgesic action of codeine.
- phenothiazines increase the sedative action of codeine (see Drug Class, Section Three).
- tricyclic antidepressants increase the sedative action of codeine (see Drug Class, Section Three).
- mono-amine oxidase (MAO) inhibitor drugs increase the sedative action of codeine (see Drug Class, Section Three).

Driving a Vehicle, Operating Machinery, Engaging in Hazardous Activities: This drug can impair mental alertness, judgment, reaction time, and physical coordination. Avoid hazardous activities.

Aviation Note: The use of this drug *is a disqualification* for the piloting of aircraft. Consultation with a designated Aviation Medical Examiner is advised.

Exposure to Sun: No restrictions.

Discontinuation: If it has been necessary to use codeine for an extended period of time, ask physician for guidance regarding dosage reduction and withdrawal.

Special Storage Instructions
Keep in a dry, tightly closed, light-resistant container.

COLCHICINE

Year Introduced: 1763

Brand Names

USA	Canada
ColBENEMID [CD] (Merck Sharp & Dohme) (No single entity brand names)	Novocolchine (Novopharm)

Common Synonyms ("Street Names"): None

Drug Class: Anti-gout

Prescription Required: USA: Yes   Canada: No

Available for Purchase by Generic Name: Yes

Available Dosage Forms and Strengths
Tablets — 0.432 mg., 0.5 mg., 0.6 mg.
Granules — 0.5 mg. per packet.
Injection — 0.5 mg. per ml. (in 2 ml. ampule).

Tablet May Be Crushed or Capsule Opened for Administration: Yes

How This Drug Works
Intended Therapeutic Effect(s):
Relief of joint pain, inflammation, and swelling associated with acute gout. Reduction in the frequency and intensity of recurring attacks of acute gout. Prevention of attacks of familial Mediterranean fever.

Location of Drug Action(s):   The tissues that comprise the linings of joint spaces and body cavities.

Method of Drug Action(s):   Not completely established. It is thought that by decreasing the acidity of joint tissues, this drug reduces the deposit of uric acid crystals which cause acute inflammation and pain. (Colchicine does not lower the level of uric acid in the blood, or increase the level of uric acid in the urine.)

Principal Uses of This Drug
As a Single Drug Product: This drug is used primarily to relieve the pain, swelling, and inflammation associated with acute attacks of gout. It is also used in smaller doses to prevent recurrence of gout attacks. An infrequent use of this drug is the prevention and control of attacks of familial Mediterranean fever.

As a Combination Drug Product [CD]:   Colchicine is combined with probenecid to enhance its ability to prevent recurrent attacks of gout. While colchicine is most effective in relieving the symptoms of acute gout, it has some effect in preventing recurrent and chronic discomfort. The action of probenecid is to increase the elimination of uric acid by the kidneys and thereby reduce the blood level of uric acid to a point where acute episodes of gout will not occur. This dual action is more effective than either drug alone in the long-term management of gout.

THIS DRUG SHOULD NOT BE TAKEN IF
—you have had an allergic reaction to it previously.
—you have an active stomach or duodenal ulcer.
—you have active ulcerative colitis.

INFORM YOUR PHYSICIAN BEFORE TAKING THIS DRUG IF
—you have a history of peptic ulcer disease or ulcerative colitis.
—you have any type of heart disease.
—you have impaired liver or kidney function.
—you plan to have surgery under general anesthesia in the near future.

Time Required for Apparent Benefit
Pain and inflammation begin to subside within 12 hours, and usually disappear completely within 48 to 72 hours. Swelling may persist for several days more.

Possible Side-Effects *(natural, expected, and unavoidable drug actions)*
Nausea, vomiting, abdominal cramping, and diarrhea.

Possible Adverse Effects *(unusual, unexpected, and infrequent reactions)*

IF ANY OF THE FOLLOWING DEVELOP, DISCONTINUE DRUG AND NOTIFY YOUR PHYSICIAN AS SOON AS POSSIBLE

Mild Adverse Effects
Allergic Reactions: Skin rash, hives, fever.
Other Reactions: None with short-term use.

Serious Adverse Effects
Allergic Reactions: Anaphylactic reaction (see Glossary).
Other Reactions
Loss of hair.
Bone marrow depression (see Glossary)—fatigue, weakness, fever, sore throat, unusual bleeding or bruising.
Peripheral neuritis (see Glossary)—numbness, tingling, pain, weakness first noted in hands and/or feet.
Inflammation of colon with bloody diarrhea.
Liver damage.

Possible Delayed Adverse Effects
Interference with production of sperm, possibly resulting in birth defects of child (conceived while father was taking this drug).

CAUTION
1. If this drug causes vomiting and/or diarrhea before relief of joint pain, discontinue it and inform your physician.
2. Try to limit each course of treatment for acute gout to 4 to 8 mg. Do not exceed 3 mg. per 24 hours or a total dose of 10 mg. per course.
3. Omit drug for 3 days between courses to avoid toxicity.
4. Carry this drug with you while traveling if you are subject to attacks of acute gout.
5. It is advisable to take colchicine preventively prior to and following surgery if you have recurrent gout. (Surgery often precipitates acute attacks of gout.)

Precautions for Use by Those over 60 Years of Age
This drug has a very narrow margin of safety. Because the total dosage required to relieve the pain of acute gout often causes vomiting and/or diarrhea, extreme caution is advised when this drug is used by anyone with heart or circulatory disorders, reduced liver or kidney function, or general debility.

Advisability of Use During Pregnancy
Pregnancy Category: C (tentative). See Pregnancy Code inside back cover.
Animal reproduction studies in hamsters and rabbits reveal significant birth defects due to this drug.
Information from adequate studies in pregnant women is not available.
Avoid completely during first 3 months.
Ask physician for guidance.

Advisability of Use While Nursing Infant
Presence of drug in milk is not known. Ask physician for guidance.

Habit-Forming Potential
None.

Effects of Overdosage
With Moderate Overdose: Nausea, vomiting, abdominal cramping, diarrhea.

With Large Overdose: Severe abdominal pain, profuse watery and bloody diarrhea, burning sensation in throat and skin, weak and rapid pulse, cold and clammy skin, progressive paralysis, inability to breathe, scant bloody urine.

Possible Effects of Extended Use
Aplastic anemia (see Glossary).
Peripheral neuritis (see Glossary).
Loss of hair.

Suggested Periodic Examinations While Taking This Drug (at physician's discretion)
Complete blood cell counts.
Uric acid blood levels to monitor status of gout.
Sperm analysis for quantity and condition.
Liver function tests.

While Taking This Drug, Observe the Following
Foods: Follow physician's advice regarding the need for a low purine diet. This drug may be taken with food or immediately after eating to reduce nausea or stomach irritation.

Beverages: It is advisable to drink no less than 3 quarts of liquids every 24 hours. This drug may be taken with milk. Some "herbal teas" (promoted as being beneficial for arthritis) contain phenylbutazone and other potentially toxic ingredients. Avoid "herbal teas" if you are not certain of their source, content, and medicinal effects.

Alcohol: No interactions expected with this drug. However, alcohol may impair the successful management of gout.

Tobacco Smoking: No interactions expected.

Marijuana Smoking
Occasional (once or twice weekly): No significant interactions expected.
Daily: Possible increase in blood uric acid level.

Other Drugs
Colchicine may *increase* the effects of
• all sedatives, sleep-inducing drugs, tranquilizers, analgesics, and narcotic drugs, and produce oversedation.
• stimulants such as amphetamine, ephedrine, epinephrine (Adrenalin, etc.).

Colchicine may *decrease* the effects of
• anticoagulant drugs (Coumadin, etc.), and make it necessary to adjust their dosages.

• anti-hypertensive drugs, and make it necessary to adjust their dosages.

Colchicine *taken concurrently* with

• allopurinol (Zyloprim), probenecid (Benemid), or sulfinpyrazone (Anturane) can prevent attacks of acute gout that often occur when treatment with these drugs is first started.

Driving a Vehicle, Operating Machinery, Engaging in Hazardous Activities: Usually no restrictions when taken continuously in small (preventive) dosage. Be alert to the possible occurrence of nausea, vomiting and/or diarrhea when taken in larger (treatment) dosage; restrict activities accordingly.

Aviation Note: The use of this drug *may be a disqualification* for the piloting of aircraft. Consultation with a designated Aviation Medical Examiner is advised.

Exposure to Sun: No restrictions.

Exposure to Heat: No restrictions.

Exposure to Cold: This drug can lower body temperature. Use caution to prevent excessive lowering (hypothermia), especially if you are over 60 years of age.

Heavy Exercise or Exertion: No restrictions.

Occurrence of Unrelated Illness: Inform your physician if you are injured, or if you develop any new illness or disorder. During periods of such stress you may be subject to acute attacks of gout, and it may be necessary to adjust your medication schedules.

Discontinuation: This drug should be discontinued as soon as joint pain begins to subside or when vomiting and/or diarrhea begin—whichever occurs first. Keep your physician informed of your response to the drug.

Special Storage Instructions

Keep in a dry, tightly closed container. Protect from light.

CYCLANDELATE

Year Introduced: 1952

Brand Names

USA	Canada
Cyclospasmol (Ives)	Cyclospasmol (Wyeth)

Common Synonyms ("Street Names"): Circulation medicine

Drug Class: Vasodilator

Prescription Required: USA: Yes   Canada: No

Available for Purchase by Generic Name: USA: Yes   Canada: No

Available Dosage Forms and Strengths
Tablets — 100 mg.
Capsules — 200 mg., 400 mg.

Tablet May Be Crushed or Capsule Opened for Administration: Yes

How This Drug Works
Intended Therapeutic Effect(s):   Relief of symptoms associated with
• impaired circulation of blood in the extremities.
• impaired circulation of blood within the brain (in carefully selected cases).
Location of Drug Action(s):   The muscles in the walls of blood vessels. The
principal therapeutic action is on the small arteries (arterioles).
Method of Drug Action(s):   By causing direct relaxation and expansion of
blood vessel walls, this drug increases the volume of blood flowing through
the vessels. The resulting increase in oxygen and nutrients relieves the
symptoms attributable to deficient circulation. The mechanism responsible
for the direct relaxation of muscle is not known.

Principal Uses of This Drug
As a Single Drug Product: Used primarily in the treatment of disorders that
require the improvement of blood flow through dilated arterial vessels.
These include arteriosclerotic disorders of the brain and extremities, Raynaud's phenomena, thrombophlebitis with associated arterial spasm, and
nocturnal leg cramps.

THIS DRUG SHOULD NOT BE TAKEN IF
—you have had an allergic reaction to any dosage form of it previously.

INFORM YOUR PHYSICIAN BEFORE TAKING THIS DRUG IF
—you have glaucoma.
—you have had a heart attack or a stroke.
—you suffer from poor circulation to the brain or heart (angina).

Time Required for Apparent Benefit
Continuous use on a regular schedule for several weeks is needed to determine this drug's effectiveness. Beneficial results from short-term use are
unlikely.

Possible Side-Effects *(natural, expected, and unavoidable drug actions)*
Flushing and warm sensation, tingling of face and extremities, sweating.

Possible Adverse Effects *(unusual, unexpected, and infrequent reactions)*

IF ANY OF THE FOLLOWING DEVELOP, DISCONTINUE DRUG AND NOTIFY YOUR PHYSICIAN AS SOON AS POSSIBLE

Mild Adverse Effects
Stomach irritation, heartburn, nausea.
Headache, dizziness, weakness.
Heart palpitation (rapid heart action).
Serious Adverse Effects
None reported.

CAUTION
Individuals with extensive or severe impairment of circulation to the brain or heart may respond unfavorably to this drug. Observe closely until the true nature of the response has been determined. Discontinue drug if condition worsens.

Precautions for Use by Those over 60 Years of Age
It is not possible to predict in advance the nature of your response to this drug. It may relieve your symptoms, have no significant effect, or make your symptoms worse. Dosage must be carefully individualized.

Advisability of Use During Pregnancy
Pregnancy Category: C (tentative). See Pregnancy Code inside back cover.
Animal reproduction studies: No data available.
Information from adequate studies in pregnant women is not available. Ask physician for guidance.

Advisability of Use While Nursing Infant
Safety not established. Ask physician for guidance.

Habit-Forming Potential
None.

Effects of Overdosage
Headache, dizziness, flushed and hot face, nausea and vomiting.

Possible Effects of Extended Use
None reported.

Suggested Periodic Examinations While Taking This Drug (at physician's discretion)
Measurement of internal eye pressure (if glaucoma is present).

While Taking This Drug, Observe the Following
Foods: No restrictions of food selection. Drug may be taken with or immediately following meals to reduce stomach irritation or nausea.

Beverages: No restrictions.

Alcohol: No interactions expected.

Tobacco Smoking: Nicotine can reduce this drug's ability to dilate blood vessels and to improve circulation. Follow physician's advice regarding smoking.

Marijuana Smoking: No interactions expected.

Other Drugs: No significant drug interactions reported.

Driving a Vehicle, Operating Machinery, Engaging in Hazardous Activities: Usually no restrictions. Be alert to the possible occurrence of dizziness and/or weakness.

Aviation Note: Serious circulatory disorders *are a disqualification* for the piloting of aircraft. Consultation with a designated Aviation Medical Examiner is advised.

Exposure to Sun: No restrictions.

Exposure to Heat: Use caution. This drug may cause excessive sweating in hot environments.

Exposure to Cold: Avoid as much as possible. This drug may be less effective in cold environments or with the handling of cold objects.

Heavy Exercise or Exertion: No restrictions.

Special Storage Instructions

Keep in a dry, tightly closed container. Protect from light and excessive heat.

CYCLOBENZAPRINE

Year Introduced: 1977

Brand Names

USA	Canada
Flexeril (Merck Sharp & Dohme)	Flexeril (Merck Sharp & Dohme)

Common Synonyms ("Street Names"):   Muscle relaxer

Drug Class: Skeletal Muscle Relaxant

Prescription Required: Yes

Available for Purchase by Generic Name: No

Available Dosage Forms and Strengths

Tablets — 10 mg.

Tablet May Be Crushed or Capsule Opened for Administration: Yes

How This Drug Works

Intended Therapeutic Effect(s):   Relief of discomfort and limitation of motion resulting from spasm of voluntary muscles.

Location of Drug Action(s):   Not completely established. This drug is thought to act on those nerve pathways in the brain stem and spinal cord that are involved in the reflex activity of voluntary muscles.

Method of Drug Action(s):   Not completely established. It is thought that this drug may relieve muscle spasm and pain by blocking the transmission of nerve impulses over reflex pathways and by producing a sedative effect that decreases the perception of pain.

Principal Uses of This Drug

As a Single Drug Product: Used primarily to relieve the pain and stiffness associated with spasm of voluntary muscles, such as that resulting from accidental injury to musculoskeletal structures. It is often necessary to supplement the use of this drug with other treatment measures, such as rest, support, and physiotherapy.

THIS DRUG SHOULD NOT BE TAKEN IF
—you have had an allergic reaction to it previously.
—you have taken any mono-amine oxidase (MAO) inhibitor drug within the past 14 days (see Mono-amine Oxidase Inhibitor Drug Class, Section Three).
—you are recovering from a recent myocardial infarction (heart attack).
—you have congestive heart failure.
—you have hyperthyroidism (overactive thyroid gland function).

INFORM YOUR PHYSICIAN BEFORE TAKING THIS DRUG IF
—you have a history of heart disease or a disturbance of heart rhythm.
—you have experienced any adverse effects from any of the tricyclic anti-depressant drugs (see Drug Class, Section Three).
—you are currently taking any tranquilizers, sedatives, sleep-inducing drugs, pain-relieving drugs, or antihistamines. (Excessive sedation may result if cyclobenzaprine is added.)
—you are currently taking any atropine-like drugs (see Drug Class, Section Three).
—you have glaucoma, or a tendency to increased internal eye pressure.
—you have an enlarged prostate gland with impaired urination (prostatism).
—you intend to pilot aircraft.

Time Required for Apparent Benefit
Drug action usually begins in 30 to 60 minutes and reaches its peak in 2 to 3 hours.
Continuous use on a regular schedule for 3 to 5 days is usually necessary to determine this drug's effectiveness in relieving the discomfort associated with muscle spasm.

Possible Side-Effects *(natural, expected, and unavoidable drug actions)*
Drowsiness (40%),* dizziness (11%), dry mouth (28%), constipation.

Possible Adverse Effects *(unusual, unexpected, and infrequent reactions)*

IF ANY OF THE FOLLOWING DEVELOP, DISCONTINUE DRUG AND NOTIFY YOUR PHYSICIAN AS SOON AS POSSIBLE
Mild Adverse Effects
   Allergic Reactions: Skin rash, hives, swelling of face and tongue.
   Other Reactions
      Headache, fatigue, weakness, numbness, blurred vision, slurred speech, unsteadiness.
      Nausea, indigestion, unpleasant taste.
Serious Adverse Effects
   Euphoria, disorientation, confusion, hallucinations.
   Impaired urination (urine retention).

CAUTION
1. This drug should not be used continuously for more than 3 weeks.
2. Allow an interval of 14 days between the discontinuation of any mono-amine oxidase (MAO) inhibitor drug and the initiation of this drug.

*The percentage figures represent the frequency of occurrence of the respective adverse reaction in patients using this drug to date.

Precautions for Use by Infants and Children

Safety and effectiveness in children below the age of 15 years have not been established.

Precautions for Use by Those over 60 Years of Age

You may be more sensitive to the sedative effects of this drug. Small doses are advisable until your individual response has been determined.

You may be more susceptible to the development of drowsiness, dizziness, muscular weakness, unsteadiness, and falling.

This drug can increase the degree of impaired urination associated with prostate gland enlargement (prostatism).

Advisability of Use During Pregnancy

Pregnancy Category: B (tentative). See Pregnancy Code inside back cover.

Animal reproduction studies reveal no birth defects due to this drug.

Information from adequate studies in pregnant women is not available.

Ask physician for guidance.

Advisability of Use While Nursing Infant

This drug is probably present in the mother's milk. It is advisable to avoid use of this drug or to refrain from breast-feeding.

Habit-Forming Potential

None.

Effects of Overdosage

With Moderate Overdose: Excessive drowsiness, confusion, impaired concentration, visual disturbances, vomiting.

With Large Overdose: Stupor progressing to coma, convulsions, low blood pressure, weak and rapid pulse, low body temperature.

Possible Effects of Extended Use

None reported.

Suggested Periodic Examinations While Taking This Drug (at physician's discretion)

Measurement of internal eye pressure if glaucoma is present.

While Taking This Drug, Observe the Following

Foods: No restrictions. Timing of Drug and Food: May be taken with or following food to prevent stomach irritation.

Beverages: No restrictions. This drug may be taken with milk.

Alcohol: Use with caution until the combined effect has been determined. This drug may add to the depressant action of alcohol on the brain.

Tobacco Smoking: No interactions expected.

Marijuana Smoking

Occasional (once or twice weekly):   Transient increase in drowsiness likely for 2 to 6 hours.

Daily: Marked increase in drowsiness and significant impairment of intellectual and physical performance. All hazardous activities should be avoided.

Other Drugs

Cyclobenzaprine may *increase* the effects of
- all atropine-like drugs (see Drug Class, Section Three).
- all tranquilizers, sedatives, sleep-inducing drugs, pain-relievers, and antihistamines, causing excessive sedation.

Cyclobenzaprine may *decrease* the effects of
- guanethidine (Esimil, Ismelin).
- reserpine (Serpasil, Ser-Ap-Es, etc.).

Cyclobenzaprine *taken concurrently* with
- mono-amine oxidase (MAO) inhibitor drugs may cause high fever, convulsions, and death.

The following drugs may *increase* the effects of cyclobenzaprine:
- all drugs with a sedative effect (see above).

Driving a Vehicle, Operating Machinery, Engaging in Hazardous Activities: This drug may cause drowsiness, dizziness, and incoordination in susceptible individuals. Avoid hazardous activities if these drug effects occur.

Aviation Note: The use of this drug *is a disqualification* for the piloting of aircraft. Consultation with a designated Aviation Medical Examiner is advised.

Exposure to Sun: Use caution until sensitivity to sun has been determined. Other drugs closely related to this drug can cause photosensitivity (see Glossary).

Exposure to Heat: Use caution in hot environments. This drug may increase the risk of heat stroke.

Exposure to Cold: The elderly may be more susceptible to the development of hypothermia, and should dress warmly.

Heavy Exercise or Exertion: Ask physician for guidance.

Discontinuation: If this drug is not clearly beneficial after 1 week of use, it should be discontinued. If effective, its use should be limited to 3 weeks.

Special Storage Instructions

Keep in a dry, tightly closed container.

CYCLOPHOSPHAMIDE

Year Introduced: 1959

Brand Names

USA	Canada
Cytoxan (Mead Johnson)	Cytoxan (Bristol)
Neosar (Adria)	Procytox (Horner)

Common Synonyms ("Street Names"):   None

Drug Class: Anti-cancer (Antineoplastic); Anti-immunity (Immunosuppressive)*

Prescription Required: Yes

Available for Purchase by Generic Name: No

Available Dosage Forms and Strengths
Tablets — 25 mg., 50 mg.
Injection — 200 mg., 500 mg., 1000 mg., 2000 mg. per vial.

Tablet May Be Crushed or Capsule Opened for Administration: Yes

How This Drug Works
Intended Therapeutic Effect(s):   The cure or control of certain types of cancer.
Location of Drug Action(s):   The principal site of action appears to be the nucleus of the cancer cell, wherever the cancer may occur in body tissues.
Method of Drug Action(s):   Not completely known. Because of its ability to kill cancer cells during all phases of their development and reproduction, this drug can suppress the primary growth and secondary spread (metastasis) of certain types of cancer throughout the body.

Principal Uses of This Drug
As a Single Drug Product: Used primarily in the treatment of various forms of cancer, notably malignant lymphomas, multiple myeloma, leukemias, and cancers of the breast and ovary. Because this drug exerts a suppressant effect on the immune system, it is also used to prevent rejection in organ transplantations.

THIS DRUG SHOULD NOT BE TAKEN IF
—you have had an allergic reaction to any dosage form of it previously.
—you now have an active infection of any kind.
—you now have bloody urine for any reason.

*This drug is being used investigationally in the treatment of rheumatoid arthritis, lupus erythematosus, and organ transplantation. This usage is not yet sanctioned by the U.S. Food and Drug Administration.

INFORM YOUR PHYSICIAN BEFORE TAKING THIS DRUG IF
—you have impaired liver or kidney function.
—you have impaired bone marrow function and deficient blood cell production.
—you have had previous chemotherapy or X-ray therapy for any type of cancer.
—you are now taking, or have taken in the past year, any cortisone-like drug (adrenal corticosteroids).
—you have diabetes.
—you plan to have surgery under general anesthesia in the near future.

Time Required for Apparent Benefit

Drug action begins in 1 hour and reaches its peak in 2 to 3 hours. Significant reduction in white blood cell formation is usually apparent in 7 to 10 days. Continuous use on a regular schedule is required to achieve and maintain a significant remission of the cancer under treatment.

Possible Side-Effects (natural, expected, and unavoidable drug actions)

Bone marrow depression (see Glossary)—impaired production primarily of white blood cells, and, to a lesser degree, red blood cells and blood platelets (see Glossary). Possible effects include fever, sore throat, fatigue, weakness, unusual bleeding, and bruising.
Impairment of natural resistance (immunity) to infection.

Possible Adverse Effects (unusual, unexpected, and infrequent reactions)

IF ANY OF THE FOLLOWING DEVELOP, DISCONTINUE DRUG AND NOTIFY YOUR PHYSICIAN AS SOON AS POSSIBLE

Mild Adverse Effects
Allergic Reactions: Skin rash (rare).
Other Reactions
Headache, dizziness.
Loss of scalp hair (50%),* darkening of skin and fingernails, transverse ridging of nails.
Loss of appetite, nausea (30%), vomiting (25%), ulceration of mouth, diarrhea (may be bloody).

Serious Adverse Effects
Idiosyncratic Reactions: Hemolytic anemia (see Glossary).
Other Reactions
Liver damage with jaundice—yellow eyes and skin, dark-colored urine, light-colored stools.
Kidney damage—impaired kidney function, reduced urine volume, bloody urine.
Severe inflammation of bladder (10%)—painful urination, bloody urine.
Impairment and suppression of ovarian function—irregular menstrual pattern or cessation of menstruation.
Impairment and suppression of testicular function—reduction or cessation of sperm production.

*The percentage figures represent the frequency of occurrence of the respective adverse reaction in patients using this drug to date.

Possible Delayed Adverse Effects

The development of other types of cancer (secondary malignancies). The development of severe cystitis with bleeding from the bladder wall. (May occur many months after last dose.)

CAUTION

1. This drug may interfere with the normal healing of wounds.
2. This drug can cause significant changes (mutations) in the chromosome structure of both sperm and eggs (ova). Any man or woman taking this drug should understand its potential for causing serious defects in children that are conceived during or following the course of medication.
3. This drug can suppress natural resistance (immunity) to infection, resulting in life-threatening illness.

Precautions for Use by Those over 60 Years of Age

To reduce the risk of developing a serious chemical cystitis, it is advisable to maintain a copious volume of urine. This may accentuate the problem of urinary retention in the bladder of the man with an enlarged prostate gland. Ask physician for guidance.

Advisability of Use During Pregnancy

Pregnancy Category: D (tentative). See Pregnancy Code inside back cover. Animal reproduction studies in mice, rats, and rabbits reveal significant birth defects due to this drug.

Information from studies in pregnant women indicates that this drug can cause serious birth defects or fetal death.

Avoid completely during first 3 months.

Ask physician for guidance regarding use during last 6 months.

Advisability of Use While Nursing Infant

This drug is known to be present in milk. Avoid drug or refrain from nursing.

Habit-Forming Potential

None.

Effects of Overdosage

With Moderate Overdose: Nausea, vomiting, diarrhea, bloody urine, water retention (edema), weight gain.

With Large Overdose: Severe bone marrow depression (see Glossary), aplastic anemia (see Glossary), severe infections, heart muscle damage.

Possible Effects of Extended Use

Development of abnormal fibrous tissue in lungs.

Suggested Periodic Examinations While Taking This Drug (at physician's discretion)

Complete blood cell counts, every 2 to 4 days during initial treatment; then every 3 to 4 weeks during maintenance treatment.

Liver function tests.

Kidney function tests.

Urinalyses for blood.

Thyroid function tests (if symptoms warrant).

While Taking This Drug, Observe the Following

Foods: No specific restrictions. It is preferable to take the tablets on an empty stomach. However, if nausea or indigestion occurs, the drug may be taken with or following food.

Beverages: No specific restrictions. Total liquid intake should be no less than 2 quarts every 24 hours to reduce the risk of chemical cystitis.

Alcohol: No interactions expected.

Tobacco Smoking: No interactions expected.

Marijuana Smoking

Occasional (once or twice weekly): No interactions expected.

Daily: Additional impairment of immunity due to this drug.

Other Drugs

Cyclophosphamide may *increase* the effects of
- oral anti-diabetic drugs, and cause hypoglycemia (see Glossary).
- insulin, and cause hypoglycemia.

Cyclophosphamide *taken concurrently* with
- allopurinol (Zyloprim) causes an increase in bone marrow depression.

The following drug may *increase* the effects of cyclophosphamide:
- phenobarbital (Luminal, etc.), by increasing the blood levels of its active forms.

Driving a Vehicle, Operating Machinery, Engaging in Hazardous Activities: Use caution if dizziness occurs.

Aviation Note: The use of this drug *may be a disqualification* for the piloting of aircraft. Consultation with a designated Aviation Medical Examiner is advised.

Exposure to Sun: No restrictions.

Exposure to Heat: No restrictions.

Exposure to Cold: No restrictions.

Heavy Exercise or Exertion: No restrictions.

Occurrence of Unrelated Illness: Report promptly the development of any indications of infection—fever, chills, sore throat, cough, "flu"-like symptoms. It may be advisable to discontinue this drug until the infection is eliminated. Consult your physician.

Discontinuation: Consult your physician for guidance regarding the need to readjust the dosage schedule of other drugs taken concurrently.

Special Storage Instructions

Keep in tightly closed, light-resistant containers, between 36° and 90° F. (2° and 32° C.). Avoid excessive heat. Liquid preparations for oral administration should be refrigerated.

Observe the Following Expiration Times

Liquid dosage forms for oral administration should be used within 14 days after preparation.

CYPROHEPTADINE

Year Introduced: 1961

Brand Names

USA	Canada
Periactin (Merck Sharp & Dohme)	Periactin (MSD) Vimicon (Frosst)

Common Synonyms ("Street Names"):   None

Drug Class: Anti-itching (Antipruritic), Antihistamines

Prescription Required: USA: Yes   Canada: No

Available for Purchase by Generic Name: USA: Yes   Canada: No

Available Dosage Forms and Strengths
Tablets — 4 mg.
Syrup — 2 mg. per teaspoonful (5 ml.)

Tablet May Be Crushed or Capsule Opened for Administration: Yes

How This Drug Works
Intended Therapeutic Effect(s):   Relief of symptoms associated with hay-fever (allergic rhinitis) and with allergic reactions in the skin, such as itching, swelling, hives, and rash.

Location of Drug Action(s):   Those hypersensitive tissues that release excessive histamine as part of an allergic reaction. The principal tissue sites are the eyes, the nose, and the skin.

Method of Drug Action(s):   This drug reduces the intensity of the allergic response by blocking the action of histamine after it has been released from sensitized tissue cells.

Principal Uses of This Drug
As a Single Drug Product: While this drug is a classical antihistamine and is effective for the treatment of common allergic disorders (allergic rhinitis and conjunctivitis, hives, etc.), it also counteracts the effects of excessive serotonin in the body. For this reason it is effective in certain conditions which are unresponsive to other antihistamines. These include cold urticaria (hives induced by exposure to cold), Cushing's disease, and the diarrhea associated with carcinoid tumors.

THIS DRUG SHOULD NOT BE TAKEN IF
—you have had an allergic reaction to any dosage form of it previously.
—you are subject to acute attacks of asthma.
—you have glaucoma (narrow-angle type).
—you have difficulty emptying the urinary bladder.
—you are taking, or have taken during the past 2 weeks, any mono-amine oxidase (MAO) inhibitor drugs (see Drug Class, Section Three).
—it has been prescribed for a newborn infant.

INFORM YOUR PHYSICIAN BEFORE TAKING THIS DRUG IF
—you have had an unfavorable reaction to any antihistamine drug in the past.
—you have a history of peptic ulcer disease.
—you plan to have surgery under general anesthesia in the near future.

Time Required for Apparent Benefit
Drug action begins in approximately 30 minutes, reaches a maximum in 1 hour, and subsides in 4 to 6 hours.

Possible Side-Effects *(natural, expected, and unavoidable drug actions)*
Drowsiness, sense of weakness, dryness of nose, mouth, and throat, constipation.

Possible Adverse Effects *(unusual, unexpected, and infrequent reactions)*

IF ANY OF THE FOLLOWING DEVELOP, DISCONTINUE DRUG AND NOTIFY YOUR PHYSICIAN AS SOON AS POSSIBLE

Mild Adverse Effects
Allergic Reactions: Skin rash, hives.
Other Reactions
  Headache, dizziness, inability to concentrate, nervousness, blurring of vision, double vision, difficulty in urination.
  Nausea, vomiting, diarrhea.
Serious Adverse Effects
Idiosyncratic Reactions: Behavioral disturbances—confusion, delirium, excitement, hallucinations.

Precautions for Use by Those over 60 Years of Age
You may be more susceptible to the development of drowsiness, dizziness, and lethargy and to the impairment of thinking, judgment, and memory.
This drug can increase the degree of impaired urination associated with prostate gland enlargement (prostatism).

Advisability of Use During Pregnancy
Pregnancy Category: B (tentative). See Pregnancy Code inside back cover. Animal reproduction studies in rats reveal no birth defects due to this drug. Information from adequate studies in pregnant women is not available. Ask physician for guidance.

Advisability of Use While Nursing Infant
This drug may impair milk formation and make nursing difficult. In addition, the drug is known to be present in milk. Ask physician for guidance.

Habit-Forming Potential
None.

Effects of Overdosage
With Moderate Overdose: Marked drowsiness, confusion, incoordination, unsteady gait, muscle tremors. In children: excitement, hallucinations, overactivity, convulsions.
With Large Overdose: Stupor progressing to coma, fever, flushed face, dilated pupils, weak pulse, shallow breathing.

Possible Effects of Extended Use
None reported.

Suggested Periodic Examinations While Taking This Drug (at physician's discretion)
Complete blood cell counts.

While Taking This Drug, Observe the Following

Foods: No restrictions. Stomach irritation can be reduced if drug is taken after eating.

Beverages: Coffee and tea may help to reduce the drowsiness caused by most antihistamines.

Alcohol: Use with extreme caution until combined effect has been determined. The combination of alcohol and antihistamines can cause rapid and marked sedation.

Tobacco Smoking: No interactions expected.

Marijuana Smoking

Occasional (once or twice weekly):   Mild increase in drowsiness and dryness of mouth.

Daily: Moderate to marked increase in drowsiness and dryness of mouth; possible accentuation of impaired thinking.

Other Drugs

Cyproheptadine may *increase* the effects of

• sedatives, sleep-inducing drugs, tranquilizers, antidepressants, pain relievers, and narcotic drugs, and result in oversedation. Careful dosage adjustments are necessary.

• atropine and drugs with atropine-like action (see Drug Class, Section Three).

The following drugs may *increase* the effects of cyproheptadine:

• all sedatives, sleep-inducing drugs, tranquilizers, pain relievers, and narcotic drugs may exaggerate its sedative action and cause oversedation.

• mono-amine oxidase (MAO) inhibitor drugs (see Drug Class, Section Three) may delay its elimination from the body, thus exaggerating and prolonging its action.

The following drugs may *decrease* the effects of cyproheptadine

• amphetamines (Benzedrine, Dexedrine, Desoxyn, etc.) may reduce the drowsiness caused by most antihistamines.

Driving a Vehicle, Operating Machinery, Engaging in Hazardous Activities: This drug may impair mental alertness, judgment, physical coordination, and reaction time. Avoid hazardous activities until full sedative effect has been determined.

Aviation Note: The use of this drug *may be a disqualification* for the piloting of aircraft. Consultation with a designated Aviation Medical Examiner is advised.

Exposure to Sun: No restrictions.

Special Storage Instructions
Keep in a dry, tightly closed container.

DEMECLOCYCLINE

Year Introduced: 1959

Brand Names

USA	Canada
Declomycin (Lederle)	Declomycin (Lederle)

Common Synonyms ("Street Names"): None

Drug Class: Antibiotic (Anti-infective), Tetracyclines

Prescription Required: Yes

Available for Purchase by Generic Name: No

Available Dosage Forms and Strengths
Tablets — 150 mg., 300 mg.
Capsules — 150 mg.

Tablet May Be Crushed or Capsule Opened for Administration: Yes

How This Drug Works
   Intended Therapeutic Effect(s): The elimination of infections responsive to the action of this drug.
   Location of Drug Action(s): Any body tissue or fluid in which sufficient concentration of the drug can be achieved.
   Method of Drug Action(s): This drug prevents the growth and multiplication of susceptible bacteria by interfering with their formation of essential proteins.

Principal Uses of This Drug
   As a Single Drug Product: This member of the tetracycline drug class is used primarily to (1) treat a broad range of infections caused by susceptible bacteria and protozoa, and (2) treat the syndrome of inappropriate secretion of antidiuretic hormone, a condition that reduces the normal production of urine.

THIS DRUG SHOULD NOT BE TAKEN IF
—you are allergic to any tetracycline drug (see Drug Class, Section Three).
—you are pregnant or breast feeding.

INFORM YOUR PHYSICIAN BEFORE TAKING THIS DRUG IF
—you have a history of liver or kidney disease.
—you have systemic lupus erythematosus.
—you are taking any penicillin drug.
—you are taking any anticoagulant drug.
—you plan to have surgery under general anesthesia in the near future.
—it is prescribed for a child under 9 years of age.

Time Required for Apparent Benefit
   Varies with nature of infection under treatment; usually 2 to 5 days.

Possible Side-Effects *(natural, expected, and unavoidable drug actions)*
Superinfections (see Glossary), often due to yeast organisms. These can occur in the mouth, intestinal tract, rectum, and/or vagina, resulting in rectal and vaginal itching.

Possible Adverse Effects *(unusual, unexpected, and infrequent reactions)*

IF ANY OF THE FOLLOWING DEVELOP, DISCONTINUE DRUG AND NOTIFY YOUR PHYSICIAN AS SOON AS POSSIBLE

Mild Adverse Effects

Allergic Reactions: Skin rash (various kinds), hives, itching of hands and feet, swelling of face or extremities.

Photosensitivity (see Glossary) Reactions: Exaggerated sunburn or skin irritation occurs commonly with some tetracyclines.

Other Reactions

Loss of appetite, nausea, vomiting, diarrhea.

Irritation of mouth or tongue, "black tongue," sore throat, abdominal pain or cramping.

Serious Adverse Effects

Allergic Reactions: Anaphylactic reaction (see Glossary), asthma, fever, painful swollen joints, unusual bleeding or bruising, jaundice (see Glossary).

Other Reactions: Permanent discoloration and/or malformation of teeth when taken under 9 years of age, including unborn child and infant.

CAUTION

1. Antacids, dairy products, and iron preparations will prevent adequate absorption of this drug and reduce its effectiveness significantly.
2. Troublesome and persistent diarrhea can develop in sensitive individuals. If diarrhea persists more than 24 hours, discontinue this drug and consult your physician for guidance.
3. If your kidney function is reduced significantly, dosage schedule must be adjusted accordingly.
4. If surgery under general anesthesia is planned while taking this drug, the choice of anesthetic agent must be considered carefully to prevent serious kidney damage.

Precautions for Use by Those over 60 Years of Age

The natural decline in kidney function that occurs after 60 may require significant reduction in dosage and lengthening of dosage intervals. Dosage must be carefully individualized and based upon measurements of kidney function.

Natural changes in the skin after 60 may predispose to severe and prolonged itching reactions in the genital and anal regions. This reaction should be reported promptly.

Advisability of Use During Pregnancy

Pregnancy Category: D (tentative). See Pregnancy Code inside back cover.

Animal reproduction studies reveal significant birth defects due to this drug.

Information from studies in pregnant women indicates that this drug can cause impaired development and discoloration of teeth and other developmental defects.

It is advisable to avoid this drug completely during entire pregnancy.

Ask physician for guidance.

Advisability of Use While Nursing Infant

Tetracyclines can be present in milk and can have adverse effects on infant. Avoid use or avoid nursing.

Habit-Forming Potential

None.

Effects of Overdosage

Possible nausea, vomiting, diarrhea.

Acute liver damage (rare).

Possible Effects of Extended Use

Impairment of bone marrow, liver, or kidney function (all rare).

Superinfections.

Suggested Periodic Examinations While Taking This Drug (at physician's discretion)

Complete blood cell counts.

Liver and kidney function tests.

During extended use, sputum and stool examinations may detect early superinfections due to yeast organisms.

While Taking This Drug, Observe the Following

Foods: Dairy products can interfere with absorption. Tetracyclines should be taken 1 hour before or 2 hours after eating.

Beverages: Avoid milk for 1 hour before and after each dose of a tetracycline.

Alcohol: Avoid while taking a tetracycline if you have a history of liver disease.

Tobacco Smoking: No interactions expected.

Marijuana Smoking: No interactions expected.

Other Drugs

Tetracyclines may *increase* the effects of
• oral anticoagulants, and make it necessary to reduce their dosage.

Tetracyclines may *decrease* the effects of
• the penicillins, and impair their effectiveness in treating infections.

The following drugs may *decrease* the effects of tetracyclines
• antacids may reduce drug absorption.
• iron and mineral preparations may reduce drug absorption.

Driving a Vehicle, Operating Machinery, Engaging in Hazardous Activities: Usually no restrictions. Be alert to the possible occurrence of nausea and/or diarrhea; restrict activities accordingly.

Aviation Note: The use of this drug *may be a disqualification* for the piloting of aircraft. Consultation with a designated Aviation Medical Examiner is advised.

Exposure to Sun: Avoid as much as possible. Photosensitivity (see Glossary) is common with some tetracyclines.

Special Storage Instructions

Keep in a tightly closed, light-resistant container.

DESIPRAMINE

Year Introduced: 1964

Brand Names

USA	Canada
Norpramin (Merrell-National)	Norpramin (Merrell)
Pertofrane (USV)	Pertofrane (Geigy)

Common Synonyms ("Street Names"):   None

Drug Class: Antidepressant, Tricyclic

Prescription Required: Yes

Available for Purchase by Generic Name: No

Available Dosage Forms and Strengths

Tablets — 25 mg., 50 mg., 75 mg., 100 mg., 150 mg.
Capsules — 25 mg., 50 mg.

Tablet May Be Crushed or Capsule Opened for Administration: Yes

How This Drug Works

Intended Therapeutic Effect(s):   Gradual improvement of mood and relief of emotional depression.

Location of Drug Action(s):   Those areas of the brain that determine mood and emotional stability.

Method of Drug Action(s):   Not established. Present thinking is that this drug slowly restores to normal levels certain constituents of brain tissue (such as norepinephrine) that transmit nerve impulses.

Principal Uses of This Drug

As a Single Drug Product: To relieve the symptoms associated with spontaneous (endogenous) depression, and to initiate the restoration of normal mood. This drug should be used only when a diagnosis of a true, primary depression of significant degree has been established. It should *not* be used to treat the symptoms of mild and transient (reactive) depression that may be associated with many life situations in the absence of a bona fide affective illness.

THIS DRUG SHOULD NOT BE TAKEN IF
—you have had an allergic reaction to any dosage form of it previously.
—you are taking or have taken within the past 14 days any mono-amine oxidase (MAO) inhibitor drug (see Drug Class, Section Three).
—you are recovering from a recent heart attack.
—you have glaucoma (narrow-angle type).
—it is prescribed for a child under 12 years of age.

INFORM YOUR PHYSICIAN BEFORE TAKING THIS DRUG IF
—you are allergic or sensitive to any other tricyclic antidepressant (see Drug Class, Section Three).
—you have a history of any of the following: diabetes, epilepsy, glaucoma, heart disease, prostate gland enlargement, or overactive thyroid function.
—you plan to have surgery under general anesthesia in the near future.

Time Required for Apparent Benefit
Some benefit may be apparent within the first 1 to 2 weeks. Adequate response may require continuous treatment for 4 to 6 weeks.

Possible Side-Effects *(natural, expected, and unavoidable drug actions)*
Drowsiness, blurring of vision, dryness of mouth, constipation, impaired urination.

Possible Adverse Effects *(unusual, unexpected, and infrequent reactions)*

IF ANY OF THE FOLLOWING DEVELOP, DISCONTINUE DRUG AND NOTIFY YOUR PHYSICIAN AS SOON AS POSSIBLE

Mild Adverse Effects
Allergic Reactions: Skin rash, hives, swelling of face or tongue, drug fever.
Other Reactions
Nausea, indigestion, irritation of tongue or mouth, peculiar taste.
Headache, dizziness, weakness, fainting, unsteady gait, tremors.
Swelling of testicles, breast enlargement, milk formation.
Fluctuation of blood sugar levels.
Serious Adverse Effects
Allergic Reactions: Hepatitis with jaundice (see Glossary).
Other Reactions
Confusion (especially in the elderly), hallucinations, agitation, restlessness, nightmares.
Heart palpitation and irregular rhythm.
Bone marrow depression (see Glossary)—fatigue, weakness, fever, sore throat, unusual bleeding or bruising.
Numbness, tingling, pain, loss of strength in arms and legs.
Parkinson-like disorders (see Glossary)—usually mild and infrequent; more likely to occur in the elderly.

Precautions for Use by Those over 60 Years of Age

During the first 2 weeks of treatment observe for the development of confusional reactions—restlessness, agitation, forgetfulness, disorientation, delusions, and hallucinations. Reduction of dosage or discontinuation may be necessary.

Observe for incoordination and instability in stance and gait which may predispose to falling and injury.

This drug can increase the degree of impaired urination associated with prostate gland enlargement (prostatism).

Advisability of Use During Pregnancy

Pregnancy Category: C (tentative). See Pregnancy Code inside back cover. Animal reproduction studies in rats and rabbits reveal significant birth defects due to this drug.

Information from adequate studies in pregnant women is not available. Ask physician for guidance.

Advisability of Use While Nursing Infant

This drug may be present in milk in small quantities. Ask physician for guidance.

Habit-Forming Potential

Psychological or physical dependence is rare and unexpected.

Effects of Overdosage

With Moderate Overdose: Confusion, hallucinations, extreme drowsiness, drop in body temperature, heart palpitation, dilated pupils, tremors.

With Large Overdose: Stupor, deep sleep, coma, convulsions.

Possible Effects of Extended Use

None reported.

Suggested Periodic Examinations While Taking This Drug (at physician's discretion)

Complete blood cell counts.

Liver function tests.

Serial blood pressure readings and electrocardiograms.

While Taking This Drug, Observe the Following

Foods: No restrictions.

Beverages: No restrictions.

Alcohol: Avoid completely. This drug can increase markedly the intoxicating effects of alcohol and accentuate its depressant action on brain function.

Tobacco Smoking: No interactions expected.

Marijuana Smoking

Occasional (once or twice weekly):   Transient increase in drowsiness and dryness of mouth.

Daily: Persistent drowsiness, increased dryness of mouth; possible reduced effectiveness of this drug.

Other Drugs

Desipramine may *increase* the effects of
- atropine and drugs with atropine-like actions (see Drug Class, Section Three).
- sedatives, sleep-inducing drugs, tranquilizers, antihistamines, and narcotic drugs, and cause oversedation. Dosage adjustments may be necessary.
- levodopa (Dopar, Larodopa, etc.), in its control of Parkinson's disease.

Desipramine may *decrease* the effects of
- guanethidine, and reduce its effectiveness in lowering blood pressure.
- other commonly used anti-hypertensive drugs. Ask physician for guidance regarding the need to monitor blood pressure readings and to adjust dosage of anti-hypertensive medications. (The action of Aldomet is not decreased by tricyclic antidepressants.)

Desipramine *taken concurrently* with
- thyroid preparations, may cause impairment of heart rhythm and function. Ask physician for guidance regarding thyroid dosage adjustment.
- ethchlorvynol (Placidyl), may cause delirium.
- quinidine, may cause impairment of heart rhythm and function. Avoid the combined use of these two drugs.
- mono-amine oxidase (MAO) inhibitor drugs (see Drug Class, Section Three), may cause high fever, delirium, and convulsions.

The following drugs may *increase* the effects of Desipramine
- thiazide diuretics (see Drug Class, Section Three) may slow its elimination from the body. Overdosage may occur.

Driving a Vehicle, Operating Machinery, Engaging in Hazardous Activities: This drug may impair mental alertness, judgment, physical coordination, and reaction time. Avoid hazardous activities.

Aviation Note: The use of this drug *is a disqualification* for the piloting of aircraft. Consultation with a designated Aviation Medical Examiner is advised.

Exposure to Sun: Use caution until sensitivity to sun has been determined. This drug may cause photosensitivity (see Glossary).

Discontinuation: If it has been necessary to use this drug for an extended period of time, do not discontinue it abruptly. Ask physician for guidance regarding dosage reduction and withdrawal. It may be necessary to adjust the dosage of other drugs taken concurrently.

Special Storage Instructions
Keep in a dry, tightly closed container.

DEXAMETHASONE

Year Introduced: 1958

Brand Names

USA	Canada
Decadron (Merck Sharp & Dohme)	Decadron (MSD)
Decadron Turbinaire (Merck Sharp & Dohme)	Deronil (Schering)
	Dexasone (ICN)
	Hexadrol (Organon)
Dexone (Rowell)	Maxidex (Alcon)
Hexadrol (Organon)	
SK-Dexamethasone (Smith Kline & French)	

Common Synonyms ("Street Names"):   Cortisone medicine

Drug Class: Cortisone-like Drug, Adrenocortical Steroids

Prescription Required: Yes

Available for Purchase by Generic Name: USA: Yes   Canada: No

Available Dosage Forms and Strengths

Tablets — 0.25 mg., 0.5 mg., 0.75 mg., 1.5 mg., 2 mg., 4 mg., 6 mg.

Elixir — 0.5 mg. per teaspoonful (5 ml.)

Aerosol inhaler — 0.084 mg. per spray

Aerosol skin spray — 0.01%

Cream — 0.04%, 0.1%

Eye ointment and solution — 0.05%

Gel — 0.1%

Tablet May Be Crushed or Capsule Opened for Administration: Yes

How This Drug Works

Intended Therapeutic Effect(s):   The symptomatic relief of inflammation (swelling, redness, heat and pain) in any tissue, and from many causes. (Cortisone-like drugs do not correct the underlying disease process.)

Location of Drug Action(s):   Significant biological effects occur in most tissues throughout the body. The principal actions of therapeutic doses occur at sites of inflammation and/or allergic reaction, regardless of the nature of the causative injury or illness.

Method of Drug Action(s):   Not completely established. Present thinking is that cortisone-like drugs probably inhibit several mechanisms within the tissues that induce inflammation. Well-regulated dosage aids the body in restoring normal stability. However, prolonged use or excessive dosage can impair the body's defense mechanisms against infectious disease.

Principal Uses of This Drug

As a Single Drug Product: This potent drug of the cortisone class is used in the treatment of a wide variety of allergic and inflammatory conditions. It is used most commonly in the management of serious skin disorders, asthma, regional enteritis and ulcerative colitis, and all types of major rheumatic disorders including bursitis, tendinitis, and most forms of arthritis.

THIS DRUG SHOULD NOT BE TAKEN IF
—you have had an allergic reaction to any dosage form of it previously.
—you have an active peptic ulcer (stomach or duodenum).
—you have an active infection of the eye caused by the herpes simplex virus (ask your eye doctor for guidance).
—you have active tuberculosis.

INFORM YOUR PHYSICIAN BEFORE TAKING THIS DRUG IF
—you have had an unfavorable reaction to any cortisone-like drug in the past.
—you have a history of tuberculosis.
—you have diabetes or a tendency to diabetes.
—you have a history of peptic ulcer disease.
—you have glaucoma or a tendency to glaucoma.
—you have a deficiency of thyroid function (hypothyroidism).
—you have high blood pressure.
—you have myasthenia gravis.
—you have a history of thrombophlebitis.
—you plan to have surgery of any kind in the near future, especially if under general anesthesia.

Time Required for Apparent Benefit

Evidence of beneficial drug action is usually apparent in 24 to 48 hours. Dosage must be individualized to give reasonable improvement. This is usually accomplished in 4 to 10 days. It is unwise to demand complete relief of all symptoms. The effective dose varies with the nature of the disease and with the patient. During long-term use it is essential that the smallest effective dose be determined and maintained.

Possible Side-Effects *(natural, expected, and unavoidable drug actions)*

Increased appetite, weight gain.
Increased susceptibility to infections.
Retention of salt and water. This occurs less frequently than with other cortisone-like drugs.

Possible Adverse Effects *(unusual, unexpected, and infrequent reactions)*

IF ANY OF THE FOLLOWING DEVELOP, DISCONTINUE DRUG AND NOTIFY YOUR PHYSICIAN AS SOON AS POSSIBLE

Mild Adverse Effects
Allergic Reactions: Skin rash.
Other Reactions
Headache, dizziness, insomnia.
Acid indigestion, abdominal distention.

Muscle cramping and weakness.

Irregular menstrual periods.

Acne, excessive growth of facial hair.

Serious Adverse Effects

Mental and emotional disturbances of serious magnitude.

Reactivation of latent tuberculosis.

Development of peptic ulcer.

Increased blood pressure.

Development of inflammation of the pancreas.

Thrombophlebitis (inflammation of a vein with the formation of blood clot) —pain or tenderness in thigh or leg, with or without swelling of the foot, ankle, or leg.

Pulmonary embolism (movement of blood clot to the lung)—sudden shortness of breath, pain in the chest, coughing, bloody sputum.

CAUTION

1. It is advisable to carry a card of personal identification with a notation that you are taking this drug if your course of treatment is to exceed 1 week (see Table 19 and Section Six).
2. Do not discontinue this drug abruptly.
3. While taking this drug, immunization procedures should be given with caution. If vaccination against measles, smallpox, rabies, or yellow fever is required, discontinue this drug 72 hours before vaccination and do not resume for at least 14 days after vaccination.

Precautions for Use by Those over 60 Years of Age

The "cortisone-related" drugs should be used very sparingly after 60, and only when the disorder under treatment is unresponsive to adequate trials of non-cortisone drugs. Prolonged use should be avoided.

The continuous use of this drug (even in small doses) can increase the severity of diabetes, enhance fluid retention, raise the blood pressure, weaken resistance to infection, induce stomach ulcer, and accelerate the development of cataract and softening of the bones (osteoporosis).

In sensitive individuals, cortisone-related drugs can cause serious emotional disturbance and disruptive behavior.

Advisability of Use During Pregnancy

Pregnancy Category: C (tentative). See Pregnancy Code inside back cover.

Animal reproduction studies in mice, rats, and rabbits reveal significant birth defects due to this drug.

Information from adequate studies in pregnant women is not available.

Avoid completely during first 3 months.

If use of this drug is considered necessary, limit dosage and duration of use as much as possible. Following birth, the infant should be examined for possible defective function of the adrenal glands (deficiency of adrenal cortical hormones).

Ask physician for guidance.

Advisability of Use While Nursing Infant
Drug is known to be present in milk. Ask physician for guidance.

Habit-Forming Potential
Use of this drug to suppress symptoms over an extended period of time may produce a state of functional dependence (see Glossary). In the treatment of conditions like rheumatoid arthritis and asthma, it is advisable to try alternate-day drug administration to keep the daily dose as small as possible and to attempt drug withdrawal after periods of reasonable improvement. Such procedures may reduce the degree of "steroid rebound"—the return of symptoms as the drug is withdrawn.

Effects of Overdosage
With Moderate Overdose: Fatigue, muscle weakness, stomach irritation, acid indigestion, excessive sweating.

With Large Overdose: Marked flushing of the face, increased blood pressure, retention of fluid with swelling of extremities, muscle cramping, marked emotional and behavioral disturbances.

Possible Effects of Extended Use
Development of increased blood sugar, possibly diabetes.

Increased fat deposits on the trunk of the body ("buffalo hump"), rounding of the face ("moon face"), and thinning of the arms and legs.

Thinning and fragility of the skin, easy bruising.

Loss of texture and strength of the bones, resulting in spontaneous fractures.

Development of increased internal eye pressure, possibly glaucoma.

Development of cataracts.

Retarded growth and development in children.

Suggested Periodic Examinations While Taking This Drug (at physician's discretion)
Measurement of blood potassium levels.

Measurement of blood sugar levels 2 hours after eating.

Measurement of blood pressure at regular intervals.

Complete eye examination at regular intervals.

Chest X-ray if history of previous tuberculosis.

Determination of the rate of development of the growing child to detect retardation of normal growth.

While Taking This Drug, Observe the Following
Foods: No interactions. Ask physician regarding need to restrict salt intake or to eat potassium-rich foods. During long-term use of this drug it is advisable to have a high protein diet.

Beverages: No restrictions.

Alcohol: No interactions expected.

Tobacco Smoking: Nicotine increases the blood levels of naturally produced cortisone and related hormones. Heavy smoking may add to the expected actions of this drug and requires close observation for excessive effects.

Marijuana Smoking
Occasional (once or twice weekly):   No interactions expected.
Daily: Additional impairment of immunity.

Other Drugs
Dexamethasone may *increase* the effects of
- barbiturates and other sedatives and sleep-inducing drugs, causing oversedation.

Dexamethasone may *decrease* the effects of
- insulin and oral anti-diabetic drugs, by raising the level of blood sugar. Doses of anti-diabetic drugs may have to be raised.
- anticoagulants of the coumarin class. Monitor prothrombin times closely and adjust doses accordingly.
- choline-like drugs (Mestinon, pilocarpine, Prostigmin), by reducing their effectiveness in treating glaucoma and myasthenia gravis.

Dexamethasone *taken concurrently* with
- thiazide diuretics, may cause excessive loss of potassium. Monitor blood levels of potassium on physician's advice.
- atropine-like drugs, may cause increased internal eye pressure and initiate or aggravate glaucoma (see Drug Class, Section Three).
- digitalis preparations, requires close monitoring of body potassium stores to prevent digitalis toxicity.
- stimulant drugs (adrenalin, amphetamines, ephedrine, etc.), may increase internal eye pressure and initiate or aggravate glaucoma.

The following drugs may *increase* the effects of Dexamethasone:
- indomethacin (Indocin, Indocid)
- aspirin

The following drugs may *decrease* the effects of dexamethasone:
- barbiturates
- phenytoin (Dantoin, Dilantin, etc.)
- antihistamines (some)
- chloral hydrate (Noctec, Somnos)
- glutethimide (Doriden)
- phenylbutazone (Azolid, Butazolidin, etc.) may reduce its effectiveness following a brief, initial increase in effectiveness.
- Propranolol (Inderal)

Driving a Vehicle, Operating Machinery, Engaging in Hazardous Activities:
Usually no restrictions. Be alert to the rare occurrence of dizziness; restrict activities accordingly.

Aviation Note: The use of this drug *may be a disqualification* for the piloting of aircraft. Consultation with a designated Aviation Medical Examiner is advised.

Exposure to Sun: No restrictions.

Occurrence of Unrelated Illness

This drug may decrease natural resistance to infection. Notify your physician if you develop an infection of any kind.

This drug may reduce your body's ability to respond appropriately to the stress of acute illness, injury, or surgery. Keep your physician fully informed of any significant changes in your state of health.

Discontinuation

If you have been taking this drug for an extended period of time, do not discontinue it abruptly. Ask physician for guidance regarding gradual withdrawal.

For a period of 2 years after discontinuing this drug, it is essential in the event of illness, injury, or surgery that you inform attending medical personnel that you used this drug in the past. The period of inadequate response to stress following the use of cortisone-like drugs may last for 1 to 2 years.

Special Storage Instructions

Keep in a tightly closed container. Protect from light.

DEXTROAMPHETAMINE

Year Introduced: 1944

Brand Names

USA	Canada
Dexedrine (Smith Kline & French)	Dexedrine (SK&F)
Biphetamine [CD] (Pennwalt)	

Common Synonyms ("Street Names"):   "A," black beauties, brain pills, browns, coast-to-coast, dex, dexies, eye-openers, lid poppers, oranges, rippers, speed, spots, uppers, ups, wedges; dextroamphetamine with amobarbital: Christmas trees, greenies, hearts

Drug Class: Stimulant, Appetite Suppressant, Amphetamines

Prescription Required: Yes (Controlled Drug, U.S. Schedule II)*

Available for Purchase by Generic Name: USA: Yes   Canada: No

Available Dosage Forms and Strengths

Tablets — 5 mg., 10 mg.

Capsules — 15 mg.

Prolonged-action capsules — 5 mg., 10 mg., 15 mg.

Elixir — 5 mg. per teaspoonful (5 ml.)

*See Schedules of Controlled Drugs inside back cover.

Tablet May Be Crushed or Capsule Opened for Administration
Tablets — Yes

Prolonged-action capsules — No

Dexedrine spansules — Yes, but do not crush or chew contents

How This Drug Works
Intended Therapeutic Effect(s)
Prevention or reduction in the frequency of episodes of sleep epilepsy (narcolepsy)—sudden attacks of sleep occurring at irregular intervals.

Reduction of restlessness, distractability, and impulsive behavior characteristic of the abnormally hyperactive child (as seen with minimal brain dysfunction).

Suppression of appetite in the management of weight reduction using low-calorie diets.

Location of Drug Action(s)
The wake-sleep center within the brain.

Areas within the outer layer (cortex) of the brain that are responsible for higher mental functions and behavioral reactions.

The appetite-regulating center within the hypothalamus of the brain.

Method of Drug Action(s)
By increasing the release of the nerve impulse transmitter norepinephrine, this drug produces wakefulness and accelerated mental activity.

The increased availability of norepinephrine may also improve alertness, concentration, and attention span. (The primary action that calms the overactive child is not known.)

By altering the chemical control of nerve impulse transmission within the appetite-regulating center, this drug can temporarily reduce or abolish hunger.

Principal Uses of This Drug
As a Single Drug Product: This most commonly used amphetamine is prescribed primarily in the treatment of three conditions: (1) narcolepsy, a variant of epilepsy that causes unpredictable episodes of drowsiness and sleep; (2) the "hyperactive child" syndrome associated with minimal brain damage; (3) obesity associated with excessive appetite and compulsive eating. While sometimes effective in treating the first two disorders, this drug loses its ability to suppress the appetite after a few weeks of continuous use.

THIS DRUG SHOULD NOT BE TAKEN IF
—you have had an allergic reaction to any dosage form of it previously. A combination drug [CD] should not be taken if you are allergic to *any* of its ingredients.

—you have advanced hardening of the arteries.

—you have heart disease that requires treatment.

—you are being treated for high blood pressure.

—you have glaucoma.

—you have an overactive thyroid disorder (hyperthyroidism).

—you have severe anxiety or nervous tension.

—you are taking, or have taken within the past 14 days, any mono-amine oxidase (MAO) inhibitor drug (see Drug Class, Section Three).

—it is prescribed for a child under 3 years of age.

INFORM YOUR PHYSICIAN BEFORE TAKING THIS DRUG IF

—you have a history of high blood pressure, heart disease, or stroke.

—you have diabetes.

—you have experienced any form of drug dependence (see Glossary) in the past.

Time Required for Apparent Benefit

Drug action begins in 30 to 60 minutes and persists for 4 to 6 hours. The effects of the prolonged-action capsule may persist for 10 to 14 hours.

Possible Side-Effects *(natural, expected, and unavoidable drug actions)*

Nervousness, increased heart rate, insomnia.

Possible Adverse Effects *(unusual, unexpected, and infrequent reactions)*

IF ANY OF THE FOLLOWING DEVELOP, DISCONTINUE DRUG AND NOTIFY YOUR PHYSICIAN AS SOON AS POSSIBLE

Mild Adverse Effects

Allergic Reactions: Hives.

Other Reactions

Headache, dizziness, overstimulation, tremor, euphoria.

Dryness of the mouth, unpleasant taste.

Heart palpitation, rapid and/or irregular heart action.

Serious Adverse Effects

Alteration of insulin requirements in the management of diabetes.

Increased blood pressure.

Changes in libido, sexual impotence.

Behavioral disturbances, psychotic episodes.

CAUTION

1. To reduce the possibility of insomnia, do not take this drug within 6 hours of retiring.
2. It is advisable to determine the lowest effective dose for each individual and to maintain dosage at this level.
3. The appetite-suppressing action of this drug may disappear after several weeks of continuous use, regardless of the size of the dose. *Do not increase the dose* beyond that prescribed.

Precautions for Use by Those over 60 Years of Age

You may be more sensitive to the stimulant effects of this drug. Small doses are advisable until your individual response has been determined.

You may be more susceptible to the development of nervousness, agitation, insomnia, high blood pressure, disturbance of heart rhythm, or angina.

Advisability of Use During Pregnancy

Pregnancy Category: C (tentative). See Pregnancy Code inside back cover.
Animal reproduction studies reveal significant birth defects due to this
drug.
Information from adequate studies in pregnant women is not available.
Avoid completely during first 3 months.
Ask physician for guidance.

Advisability of Use While Nursing Infant

This drug is known to be present in milk in very small amounts. Ask physician
for guidance.

Habit-Forming Potential

This drug can cause severe psychological dependence (see Glossary; this is the
most serious problem related to the use of amphetamines). Avoid large doses
and prolonged use if possible. Observe closely for indications of developing
dependence.

Effects of Overdosage

With Moderate Overdose: Nervous irritability, overactivity, insomnia, personality changes, tremor, rapid heart rate, headache.

With Large Overdose: Nausea, vomiting, diarrhea, dizziness, dilated pupils,
blurred vision, confusion, high fever, gasping respirations, profuse sweating, hallucinations, convulsions, coma.

Possible Effects of Extended Use

With low dosage, excessive weight loss.
With moderate to high dosage (chronic intoxication), skin eruptions, insomnia, excitability, personality changes, severe mental disturbances resembling schizophrenia.
Severe psychological dependence.

Suggested Periodic Examinations While Taking This Drug (at physician's discretion)

Observation for evidence of developing dependence.
Measurement of blood pressure to detect any tendency to abnormal elevation.

While Taking This Drug, Observe the Following

Foods: When used to suppress appetite, take this drug 30 to 60 minutes
before eating. Follow weight reduction diet as prescribed. Avoid foods rich
in tyramine (see Glossary). This drug in combination with tyramine may
cause excessive rise in blood pressure.

Beverages: Avoid beverages prepared from meat or yeast extracts. Avoid
sour cream.

Alcohol: Avoid beer (unpasteurized), Chianti, and vermouth wines.

Tobacco Smoking: No interactions expected.

Marijuana Smoking

Occasional (once or twice weekly):   Mild and transient increased heart
rate; mild reduction of stimulant effect and appetite suppressant effect
of this drug.

Daily: Persistent rapid heart rate; possible heart rhythm disturbance (in sensitive individuals); significant reduction of stimulant effect of this drug.

Other Drugs

Dextroamphetamine may *increase* the effects of
• meperidine (pethidine, Demerol).

Dextroamphetamine may *decrease* the effects of
• bethanidine (Esbaloid).
• guanethidine (Ismelin).
• hydralazine (Apresoline).
• methyldopa (Aldomet).
• reserpine (Serpasil, Ser-Ap-Es, etc.).

Dextroamphetamine *taken concurrently* with
• mono-amine oxidase (MAO) inhibitor drugs, may cause acute, severe rise in blood pressure that could be dangerous (see Drug Class, Section Three).

The following drugs may *increase* the effects of dextroamphetamine:
• acetazolamide (Diamox)
• antacids containing sodium bicarbonate (see ANTACIDS Drug Profile)
• thiazide diuretics (see Drug Class, Section Three)
• tricyclic antidepressants (see Drug Class, Section Three)

The following drugs may *decrease* the effects of dextroamphetamine:
• amantadine (Symmetrel)
• methenamine (Mandelamine)
• phenothiazines (see Drug Class, Section Three)
• Vitamin C, in large doses

Driving a Vehicle, Operating Machinery, Engaging in Hazardous Activities: This drug may impair the ability to engage safely in hazardous activities. Use caution until full effect has been determined.

Aviation Note: The use of this drug *is a disqualification* for the piloting of aircraft. Consultation with a designated Aviation Medical Examiner is advised.

Exposure to Sun: No restrictions.

Exposure to Heat: No restrictions.

Heavy Exercise or Exertion: Use caution if you have high blood pressure. Ask your physician for guidance.

Discontinuation: Abrupt withdrawal of this drug after prolonged use at moderate to high dosage may cause extreme fatigue and mental depression. Ask your physician for guidance regarding gradual reduction and discontinuation.

Special Storage Instructions

Keep tablets and capsules in a dry, tightly closed container.
Keep elixir in a tightly closed, light-resistant container.

DEXTROMETHORPHAN

Year Introduced: 1954

Brand Names

USA

Benylin DM Cough
Syrup (Parke-Davis)
Hold 4 Hour
(Beecham)
Romilar Children's
Cough Syrup
(Block)
Romilar CF 8 Hour
Cough Formula
(Block)
Cheracol-D [CD]
(Upjohn)
Children's Hold [CD]
(Beecham)
Coricidin Cough
Syrup [CD]
(Schering)
Cosanyl DM [CD]
(Parke-Davis)
Dristan Cough
Formula [CD]
(Whitehall)
Endotussin-NN [CD]
(Endo)

Formula 44-D [CD]
(Vick)
Nyquil [CD] (Vick)
Pertussin [CD]
(Chesebrough-
Pond)
Robitussin-CF [CD]
(Robins)
Robitussin-DM [CD]
(Robins)
Romilar III [CD]
(Block)
Trind-DM [CD]
(Mead Johnson)
Tussagesic [CD]
(Dorsey)
Vicks Cough Syrup
[CD] (Vick)
(Numerous other
brand names)

Canada

Balminil D.M. Syrup
(Rougier)
Broncho-Grippol-DM
(Charton)
Contratuss (Eri)
Demo-Cineol
Antitussive Syrup
(Sabex)
DM Syrup (P.D. &
Co.)
Koffex Syrup
(Rougier)
Neo DM (Neolab)
Robidex (Robins)
Sedatuss (Trianon)
Benylin-DM [CD]
(P.D. & Co.)
Robitussin-DM [CD]
(Robins)

Common Synonyms ("Street Names"): Cough medicine

Drug Class: Cough Suppressant (Antitussives)

Prescription Required: No

Available for Purchase by Generic Name: Yes

Available Dosage Forms and Strengths
Available in a wide variety of single drug and combination drug preparations
of varying strengths. Dosage forms include tablets, capsules, lozenges, elixirs,
and syrups. Read the product label to learn the identity and strength of each
drug in the preparation.

Tablet May Be Crushed or Capsule Opened for Administration: Yes

How This Drug Works
Intended Therapeutic Effect(s):   Reduction in the frequency, severity, and
duration of coughing associated with allergic or infectious disorders of the
windpipe (trachea) and/or the bronchial tubes.

Location of Drug Action(s): The principal action occurs in the cough control center located in the brain stem.

Method of Drug Action(s): By reducing the sensitivity of the cough control center to the reflex stimulation from irritated lower respiratory passages, this drug suppresses the tendency to cough.

Principal Uses of This Drug

As a Single Drug Product: This drug is used for one purpose only—to reduce the frequency of coughing.

As a Combination Drug Product [CD]: Commonly combined with expectorants and antihistamines in syrup form and marketed as cough remedies.

THIS DRUG SHOULD NOT BE TAKEN IF
—you have had an allergic reaction to it previously.

INFORM YOUR PHYSICIAN BEFORE TAKING THIS DRUG IF
—you are taking any mono-amine oxidase (MAO) inhibitor drug (see Drug Class, Section Three).

—you are subject to attacks of bronchial asthma. (This drug may intensify asthma.)

—you have impaired liver function.

Time Required for Apparent Benefit
Drug action begins in 15 to 30 minutes.

Possible Side-Effects *(natural, expected, and unavoidable drug actions)*
Mild drowsiness in sensitive individuals.

Possible Adverse Effects *(unusual, unexpected, and infrequent reactions)*

IF ANY OF THE FOLLOWING DEVELOP, DISCONTINUE DRUG AND NOTIFY YOUR PHYSICIAN AS SOON AS POSSIBLE

Mild Adverse Effects
Allergic Reactions: Skin rash, itching.
Other Reactions: Dizziness, nausea, indigestion (all rare).
Serious Adverse Effects
None reported.

CAUTION
1. The total dosage should not exceed 120 mg. per 24 hours.
2. Avoid the concurrent use of this drug with any mono-amine oxidase (MAO) inhibitor drug.

Precautions for Use by Those over 60 Years of Age
If this drug is used to control coughing, be sure that other treatment measures are used as needed to liquefy accumulations of thick mucus in the bronchial tubes.

Observe for any tendency to develop constipation, excessive drowsiness, or unsteadiness in stance or gait. Consult your physician if such effects occur.

Advisability of Use During Pregnancy

Pregnancy Category: C (tentative). See Pregnancy Code inside back cover. Animal reproduction studies: No data available.

Information from adequate studies in pregnant women is not available. Ask physician for guidance.

Advisability of Use While Nursing Infant

The presence of this drug in milk is not known. Ask physician for guidance.

Habit-Forming Potential

This drug does not produce physical dependence. However, excessive use by a predisposed individual may lead to psychological dependence (see Glossary).

Effects of Overdosage

With Moderate Overdose: Euphoria, overactivity, sense of intoxication.

With Large Overdose: Visual and auditory hallucinations, incoordination, staggering gait, stupor, suppressed breathing.

Possible Effects of Extended Use

None reported.

Suggested Periodic Examinations While Taking This Drug (at physician's discretion)

None.

While Taking This Drug, Observe the Following

Foods: No restrictions.

Beverages: No restrictions.

Alcohol: No interactions expected.

Tobacco Smoking: No interactions expected. However, continued smoking may reduce this drug's effectiveness as a cough suppressant.

Marijuana Smoking: No interactions expected.

Other Drugs

Dextromethorphan *taken concurrently* with

- mono-amine oxidase (MAO) inhibitor drugs may cause confusion, disorientation, high fever, drop in blood pressure, and loss of consciousness.

Driving a Vehicle, Operating Machinery, Engaging in Hazardous Activities: Use caution if this drug causes drowsiness or dizziness.

Aviation Note: The use of this drug *is a disqualification* for the piloting of aircraft. Consultation with a designated Aviation Medical Examiner is advised.

Exposure to Sun: No restrictions.

Exposure to Heat: No restrictions.

Exposure to Cold: Observe for intensification of cough and need for increased dose of drug.

Heavy Exercise or Exertion: Observe for intensification of cough and need for increased dose of drug.

Special Storage Instructions

Keep all dosage forms in tightly closed containers. Protect from light.

DIAZEPAM

Year Introduced: 1963

Brand Names

USA		**Canada**
Valium (Roche)	Apo-Diazepam	Rival (Riva)
Valrelease (Roche)	(Apotex)	Stress-Pam (Sabex)
	E-Pam (ICN)	Valium (Roche)
	Meval (Medic)	Vivol (Horner)
	Neo-Calme (Neo)	
	Novodipam	
	(Novopharm)	

Common Synonyms ("Street Names"):   Downs, nerve pills, tranks

Drug Class: Tranquilizer, Mild (Anti-anxiety), Skeletal Muscle Relaxant, Benzodiazepines

Prescription Required: Yes (Controlled Drug, U.S. Schedule IV)*

Available for Purchase by Generic Name: USA: No   Canada: Yes

Available Dosage Forms and Strengths

Tablets — 2 mg., 5 mg., 10 mg.
Capsules (prolonged action) — 15 mg.
Injection — 5 mg. per ml.

Tablet May Be Crushed or Capsule Opened for Administration: Yes

How This Drug Works

Intended Therapeutic Effect(s):   Relief of mild to moderate anxiety and nervous tension, without significant sedation.

Location of Drug Action(s):   Thought to be the limbic system of the brain, one of the centers that influence emotional stability.

Method of Drug Action(s):   Not established. Present thinking is that this drug may reduce the activity of certain parts of the limbic system.

Principal Uses of This Drug

As a Single Drug Product: This drug is used primarily as a mild tranquilizer to relieve mild to moderate anxiety and nervous tension. While it is less sedative than the barbiturates, it may also be used at bedtime to produce a calming effect that permits natural sleep. Another major use is the treatment of voluntary muscle spasm associated with such conditions as musculoskeletal injury, cerebral palsy, and "stiff-man" syndrome.

THIS DRUG SHOULD NOT BE TAKEN IF

—you are allergic to any of the drugs bearing the brand names listed above.
—you have glaucoma (narrow-angle type).
—you have myasthenia gravis.
—it is prescribed for an infant under 6 months of age.

*See Schedules of Controlled Drugs inside back cover.

INFORM YOUR PHYSICIAN BEFORE TAKING THIS DRUG IF

—you are allergic to any drugs chemically related to diazepam: chlordiazepoxide, clorazepate, flurazepam, oxazepam (see Drug Profiles for brand names).
—you have diabetes.
—you have glaucoma (open-angle type).
—you have epilepsy.
—you are taking sedative, sleep-inducing, tranquilizer, or anti-convulsant drugs of any kind.
—you plan to have surgery under general anesthesia in the near future.

Time Required for Apparent Benefit

Approximately 1 to 2 hours. For severe symptoms of some duration, benefit may require regular medication for several days.

Possible Side-Effects (natural, expected, and unavoidable drug actions)

Drowsiness, lethargy, unsteadiness in stance and gait.
Increase in the level of blood sugar in some cases of diabetes.

Possible Adverse Effects (unusual, unexpected, and infrequent reactions)

IF ANY OF THE FOLLOWING DEVELOP, DISCONTINUE DRUG AND NOTIFY YOUR PHYSICIAN AS SOON AS POSSIBLE

Mild Adverse Effects
Allergic Reactions: Skin rashes (various kinds).
Other Reactions: Dizziness, fainting, blurred vision, double vision, slurred speech, nausea, menstrual irregularity.

Serious Adverse Effects
Allergic Reactions: Jaundice (see Glossary), impaired resistance to infection manifested by fever and/or sore throat.
Paradoxical Reactions: Acute excitement, hallucinations, rage.
Other Reactions: Eye pain, possibly glaucoma, emotional depression.

CAUTION

This drug is transformed by the liver into long-acting forms (active metabolites) that can persist in the body for 24 hours or longer. With continuous use of this drug on a daily basis, these active drug forms accumulate and produce increasing sedation. If this drug is taken at bedtime to induce sleep, observe carefully for "hangover" effects throughout the following day. Avoid driving and all other hazardous activities if you feel drowsy or sluggish.

Precautions for Use by Infants and Children

After continuous use for several weeks or months, this drug may lose its effectiveness in the management of seizure disorders.
If this drug is used concurrently with a narcotic analgesic, the initial dose of the narcotic should be reduced by one third.

Precautions for Use by Those over 60 Years of Age

Natural changes in body functions increase the duration of this drug's action. It is necessary to use smaller doses with longer intervals between doses to avoid excessive accumulation of the drug in body tissues. Dosage must be carefully individualized and limited to the smallest effective amount.

You may be more susceptible to the development of lightheadedness, impaired thinking and memory, confusion, lethargy, drowsiness, incoordination, unsteady gait and balance, impaired bladder control, and constipation.

Be alert to the possibility of paradoxical responses consisting of excitement, agitation, anger, hostility, and rage.

Advisability of Use During Pregnancy

Pregnancy Category: C (tentative). See Pregnancy Code inside back cover.

Animal reproduction studies in mice and rats reveal significant birth defects due to this drug.

Information from adequate studies in pregnant women is not available.

The findings of some recent studies suggest a possible association between the use of this drug during early pregnancy and the occurrence of birth defects, such as cleft lip. It is advisable to avoid this drug completely during the first 3 months of pregnancy.

Ask physician for guidance.

Advisability of Use While Nursing Infant

With recommended dosage, drug is present in milk and can affect infant. Ask physician for guidance.

Habit-Forming Potential

This drug can produce psychological and/or physical dependence (see Glossary) if used in large doses for an extended period of time.

Effects of Overdosage

With Moderate Overdose: Marked drowsiness, weakness, feeling of drunkenness, staggering gait, tremor.

With Large Overdose: Stupor progressing to deep sleep or coma.

Possible Effects of Extended Use

Psychological and/or physical dependence.

Reduction of white blood cells.

Impairment of liver function.

Suggested Periodic Examinations While Taking This Drug (at physician's discretion)

Blood cell counts and liver function tests during long-term use.

Blood sugar measurements (in presence of diabetes).

While Taking This Drug, Observe the Following

Foods: No restrictions.

Beverages: Large intake of coffee, tea, or cola drinks (because of their caffeine content) may reduce the calming action of this drug.

Alcohol: Use with extreme caution until the combined effect is determined. Alcohol may increase the sedative effects of diazepam. Diazepam may increase the intoxicating effects of alcohol. Avoid alcohol completely—throughout the day and night—if you find it necessary to drive or to engage in *any* hazardous activity.

Tobacco Smoking: Heavy smoking may reduce the calming action of diazepam.

Marijuana Smoking

Occasional (once or twice weekly):   Mild increase in sedative effect of this drug.

Daily: Marked increase in sedative effect of this drug.

Other Drugs

Diazepam may *increase* the effects of

- other sedatives, sleep-inducing drugs, tranquilizers, antidepressants, and narcotic drugs. Use these only under supervision of a physician. Careful dosage adjustment is necessary.
- oral anticoagulants of the coumarin family; ask physician for guidance regarding need for dosage adjustment to prevent bleeding.
- anti-hypertensives, and produce excessive lowering of the blood pressure.

Diazepam *taken concurrently* with

- anti-convulsants, may cause an increase in the frequency or severity of seizures; an increase in the dose of the anti-convulsant may be necessary.
- mono-amine oxidase (MAO) inhibitor drugs (see Drug Class, Section Three), may cause extreme sedation, convulsions, or paradoxical excitement or rage.

The following drugs may *increase* the effects of diazepam

- cimetidine (Tagamet) may delay the elimination of diazepam and cause excessive sedation.
- disulfiram (Antabuse) may delay the elimination of diazepam.
- tricyclic antidepressants (see Drug Class, Section Three) may increase the sedative effects of diazepam.

Driving a Vehicle, Operating Machinery, Engaging in Hazardous Activities: This drug can impair mental alertness, judgment, physical coordination, and reaction time. Avoid hazardous activities.

Aviation Note: The use of this drug *is a disqualification* for the piloting of aircraft. Consultation with a designated Aviation Medical Examiner is advised.

Exposure to Sun: No restrictions.

Exposure to Heat: Use caution until effect of excessive perspiration is determined. Because of reduced urine volume, diazepam may accumulate in the body and produce effects of overdosage.

Heavy Exercise or Exertion: No restrictions in cool or temperate weather.

Discontinuation: If it has been necessary to use this drug for an extended period of time do not discontinue it abruptly. Ask physician for guidance regarding dosage reduction and withdrawal. The dosage of other drugs taken concurrently with diazepam may also require adjustment.

Special Storage Instructions

Keep in a dry, tightly closed, light-resistant container.

DICYCLOMINE

Year Introduced: 1952

Brand Names

USA	Canada
Bentyl (Merrell-Dow)	Bentylol (Merrell)
Nospaz (Reid-Provident)	Formulex (ICN)
	Lomine (Riva)
	Protylol (ProDoc)
	Spasmoban (Trianon)
	Viscerol (Medic)

Common Synonyms ("Street Names"):   Stomach relaxer

Drug Class: Antispasmodic, Atropine-like Drug

Prescription Required: USA: Yes   Canada: No

Available for Purchase by Generic Name: USA: Yes   Canada: No

Available Dosage Forms and Strengths
    Tablets — 20 mg.
    Capsules — 10 mg., 20 mg.
        Syrup — 10 mg. per teaspoonful (5 ml.)
    Injection — 10 mg. per ml.

Tablet May Be Crushed or Capsule Opened for Administration: Yes

How This Drug Works
  Intended Therapeutic Effect(s):   Relief of discomfort resulting from muscle
    spasm of the gastrointestinal tract (esophagus, stomach, intestine, and
    colon).
  Location of Drug Action(s):   The muscles of the gastrointestinal tract.
  Method of Drug Action(s):   Not completely established. It has been sug-
    gested that this drug may relax gastrointestinal muscle by means of a local
    anesthetic action that blocks reflex activity responsible for contraction and
    motility.

Principal Uses of This Drug
  As a Single Drug Product: This drug is used primarily for its atropine-like
    antispasmodic effect in the management of functional disorders of the
    gastrointestinal tract, notably the irritable bowel syndrome (spastic colon).
    It is also used to relieve cramping and pain in infant colic.

THIS DRUG SHOULD NOT BE TAKEN IF
—you have had an allergic reaction to any dosage form of it previously.
—you are unable to empty the urinary bladder completely.
—your stomach cannot empty properly into the intestine (pyloric obstruction).
—you have ulcerative colitis.
—you have myasthenia gravis.

INFORM YOUR PHYSICIAN BEFORE TAKING THIS DRUG IF
—you have glaucoma.
—you have a history of peptic ulcer disease.
—you have enlargement of the prostate gland.
—you have a history of liver or kidney disease.

Time Required for Apparent Benefit
Drug action begins in 1 to 2 hours and persists for approximately 4 hours.

Possible Side-Effects *(natural, expected, and unavoidable drug actions)*
Dryness of the mouth, blurred vision, constipation, rapid pulse.

Possible Adverse Effects *(unusual, unexpected, and infrequent reactions)*

IF ANY OF THE FOLLOWING DEVELOP, DISCONTINUE DRUG AND NOTIFY YOUR PHYSICIAN AS SOON AS POSSIBLE

Mild Adverse Effects
Allergic Reactions: Skin rash, hives.
Other Reactions
Reduced appetite, nausea, vomiting.
Headache, dizziness, drowsiness, weakness.
Difficult urination, reduced sexual function.
Serious Adverse Effects
Allergic Reactions: Anaphylactic reaction (see Glossary).
Idiosyncratic Reactions: Excitement, confusion, disturbed behavior.
Other Reactions: Increased internal eye pressure (dangerous in glaucoma).

CAUTION
Many over-the-counter medications (see OTC drugs in Glossary) for allergies, colds, and coughs contain drugs that can interact unfavorably with this drug. Ask your physician or pharmacist for guidance before using any such medication.

Precautions for Use by Those over 60 Years of Age
You may be more sensitive to all of the actions of this drug. Small doses are advisable until your individual response has been determined.
This drug can increase the degree of impaired urination associated with prostate gland enlargement (prostatism).

Advisability of Use During Pregnancy
Pregnancy Category: C (tentative). See Pregnancy Code inside back cover.
Animal reproduction studies reveal no birth defects due to this drug.
Information from adequate studies in pregnant women is not available.
Ask physician for guidance.

Advisability of Use While Nursing Infant
This drug may impair milk formation and make nursing difficult. Safety for infant not established. Ask physician for guidance.

Habit-Forming Potential

None.

Effects of Overdosage

With Moderate Overdose: Headache, dizziness, nausea, dryness of the mouth, difficulty in swallowing.

With Large Overdose: Dilated pupils, hot and dry skin, fever, excitement, restlessness.

Possible Effects of Extended Use

None reported.

Suggested Periodic Examinations While Taking This Drug (at physician's discretion)

Measurements of internal eye pressure (in presence of glaucoma or suspected glaucoma).

While Taking This Drug, Observe the Following

Foods: No interactions. Drug is more effective if taken one-half to 1 hour before eating. Follow prescribed diet.

Beverages: No interactions. As allowed by prescribed diet.

Alcohol: No interactions expected with this drug. Follow physician's advice regarding use of alcohol (based upon its effect on the disease under treatment).

Tobacco Smoking: No interactions expected. Follow physician's advice regarding smoking.

Marijuana Smoking

Occasional (once or twice weekly):   Mild increase in drowsiness and dryness of mouth.

Daily: Moderate to marked increase in drowsiness and dryness of mouth.

Other Drugs

Dicyclomine may *increase* the effects of

- all other drugs having atropine-like actions (see Drug Class, Section Three).

Dicyclomine may *decrease* the effects of

- pilocarpine eye drops, and reduce their effectiveness in lowering internal eye pressure (in the treatment of glaucoma).

The following drugs may *increase* the effects of dicyclomine:

- tricyclic antidepressants
- antihistamines
- meperidine (Demerol, pethidine)
- methylphenidate (Ritalin)
- orphenadrine (Disipal, Norflex)
- phenothiazines

Driving a Vehicle, Operating Machinery, Engaging in Hazardous Activities:
This drug may produce blurred vision, drowsiness, or dizziness. Avoid hazardous activities if these drug effects occur.

Aviation Note: The use of this drug and the disorder for which this drug is prescribed *may be disqualifications* for the piloting of air-craft. Consultation with a designated Aviation Medical Examiner is advised.

Exposure to Sun: No restrictions.

Exposure to Heat: Use extreme caution. The use of this drug in hot environ-ments may increase the risk of heat stroke.

Heavy Exercise or Exertion: Use caution in hot or warm environments. This drug may impair normal perspiration and interfere with the regulation of body temperature.

Special Storage Instructions

Keep in a tightly closed container. Protect from light.

DIETHYLPROPION

Year Introduced: 1958

Brand Names

USA	Canada
Tenuate (Merrell-Dow)	Dietec (Pharbec)
Tenuate Dospan (Merrell-Dow)	Nobesine - 75 (Nadeau)
	Propion (ProDoc)
Tepanil (Riker)	Regibon (Medic)
Tepanil Ten-Tab (Riker)	Tenuate (Merrell)

Common Synonyms ("Street Names"):   Diet pills

Drug Class: Appetite Suppressant (Anorexiant), Amphetamine-like Drug

Prescription Required: Yes (Controlled Drug, U.S. Schedule IV)*

Available for Purchase by Generic Name: USA: Yes   Canada: No

Available Dosage Forms and Strengths

Tablets — 25 mg.
Prolonged-action tablets — 75 mg.

Tablet May Be Crushed or Capsule Opened for Administration

Regular Tablets — Yes
Prolonged-Action Tablets — No

How This Drug Works

Intended Therapeutic Effect(s):   The suppression of appetite in the manage-ment of weight reduction using low-calorie diets.

Location of Drug Action(s):   Not completely established. The site of thera-peutic action is thought to be the appetite-regulating center located in the hypothalamus of the brain.

*See Schedules of Controlled Drugs inside back cover.

Method of Drug Action(s): Not established. This drug is thought to resemble the amphetamines in its action, diminishing hunger by altering the chemical control of nerve impulse transmission in the brain center which regulates appetite.

Principal Uses of This Drug

As a Single Drug Product: This drug is used for one purpose only—the control of appetite in weight reduction treatment programs. Because of its limited period of effectiveness as an appetite suppressant, its use should not exceed 6 to 12 weeks. It is most effective when combined with other weight control measures, such as diet adjustment and regular exercise.

THIS DRUG SHOULD NOT BE TAKEN IF

—you have had an allergic reaction to any dosage form of it previously.
—you have glaucoma.
—you are taking, or have taken during the past 2 weeks, any mono-amine oxidase (MAO) inhibitor drug (see Drug Class, Section Three).
—it is prescribed for a child under 12 years of age.

INFORM YOUR PHYSICIAN BEFORE TAKING THIS DRUG IF

—you have had an unfavorable reaction to any amphetamine-like drug in the past.
—you have high blood pressure or any form of heart disease.
—you have an overactive thyroid gland (hyperthyroidism).
—you have a history of serious anxiety or nervous tension.
—you have epilepsy.

Time Required for Apparent Benefit

Drug action begins in approximately 1 hour and persists for 3 to 4 hours (the regular tablet) or for 10 to 14 hours (the prolonged-action tablet).

Possible Side-Effects *(natural, expected, and unavoidable drug actions)*

Nervousness, insomnia.

Possible Adverse Effects *(unusual, unexpected, and infrequent reactions)*

IF ANY OF THE FOLLOWING DEVELOP, DISCONTINUE DRUG AND NOTIFY YOUR PHYSICIAN AS SOON AS POSSIBLE

Mild Adverse Effects
Allergic Reactions: Skin rashes, hives, bruising.
Other Reactions
Headache, dizziness, restlessness, tremor.
Dryness of the mouth, nausea, vomiting, diarrhea.
Fast, forceful, and irregular heart action (heart palpitation).
Menstrual irregularities, impaired sexual function.

Serious Adverse Effects
Idiosyncratic Reactions: Overstimulation, anxiety, euphoria, erratic behavior.
Other Reactions
Increased frequency of epileptic seizures.
Bone marrow depression (see Glossary).

CAUTION

The appetite-suppressing action of this drug may disappear after several weeks of continuous use, regardless of the size of the dose. *Do not increase the dose* beyond that prescribed.

Precautions for Use by Those over 60 Years of Age

You may be more sensitive to the stimulant effects of this drug. Small doses are advisable until your individual response has been determined.

You may be more susceptible to the development of nervousness, agitation, insomnia, high blood pressure, disturbance of heart rhythm, or angina.

Advisability of Use During Pregnancy

Pregnancy Category: B (tentative). See Pregnancy Code inside back cover. Animal reproduction studies in rats reveal no birth defects due to this drug. Information from adequate studies in pregnant women is not available. Ask physician for guidance.

Advisability of Use While Nursing Infant

Presence of drug in milk is not known. Safety for infant not established. Ask physician for guidance.

Habit-Forming Potential

This drug is related to amphetamine and can cause severe psychological dependence (see Glossary). Avoid large doses and prolonged use.

Effects of Overdosage

With Moderate Overdose: Nervous irritability, overactivity, insomnia, personality change, tremor.

With Large Overdose: Initial excitement, dilated pupils, rapid pulse, confusion, disorientation, bizarre behavior, hallucinations, convulsions, coma.

Possible Effects of Extended Use

Severe psychological dependence.
Skin eruptions.

Suggested Periodic Examinations While Taking This Drug (at physician's discretion)

Complete blood cell counts.

While Taking This Drug, Observe the Following

Foods: Avoid foods rich in tyramine (see Glossary). This drug in combination with tyramine may cause excessive rise in blood pressure.

Beverages: Avoid beverages prepared from meat or yeast extracts; avoid chocolate drinks.

Alcohol: Avoid beer, Chianti wines, and vermouth.

Tobacco Smoking: No interactions expected.

Marijuana Smoking

Occasional (once or twice weekly):   Mild and transient increased heart rate; mild reduction of stimulant effect and appetite suppressant effect of this drug.

Daily: Persistent rapid heart rate; possible heart rhythm disturbance (in sensitive individuals); significant reduction of stimulant effect of this drug.

Other Drugs

Diethylpropion may *decrease* the effects of

- the major anti-hypertensive drugs, impairing their ability to lower blood pressure. The drugs most affected are: guanethidine (Ismelin), hydralazine (Apresoline), methyldopa (Aldomet), and reserpine (Serpasil, etc.).

Diethylpropion *taken concurrently* with

- mono-amine oxidase (MAO) inhibitor drugs (see Drug Class, Section Three), may cause a dangerous rise in blood pressure. Withhold the use of diethylpropion for a minimum of 2 weeks after discontinuing any MAO inhibitor drug.

Driving a Vehicle, Operating Machinery, Engaging in Hazardous Activities: This drug may impair the ability to safely engage in hazardous activities. Use caution until full effect has been determined.

Aviation Note: The use of this drug *is a disqualification* for the piloting of aircraft. Consultation with a designated Aviation Medical Examiner is advised.

Exposure to Sun: No restrictions.

Discontinuation: If this drug has been used for an extended period of time, do not discontinue it suddenly. Ask physician for guidance regarding gradual reduction and withdrawal.

Special Storage Instructions

Keep in a dry, tightly closed container.

DIETHYLSTILBESTROL
(DES, Stilbestrol)

Year Introduced: 1941

Brand Names

USA	Canada
Stilphostrol (Dome)	Honvol (Horner)
Tylosterone [CD] (Lilly)	Stibilium (Desbergers)

Common Synonyms ("Street Names"): None

Drug Class: Female Sex Hormones, Estrogens

Prescription Required: Yes

Available for Purchase by Generic Name: Yes

Available Dosage Forms and Strengths
Tablets — 0.1 mg., 0.25 mg., 0.5 mg., 1.0 mg., 5 mg., 50 mg.
Enteric-coated tablets — 0.1 mg., 0.25 mg., 0.5 mg., 1.0 mg., 5 mg.
Suppositories — 0.1 mg., 0.5 mg., 0.7 mg.
Injection — 250 mg. per 5 ml.
Creams — 0.01%, 0.625 mg. per g., 1.5 mg. per g.

Tablet May Be Crushed or Capsule Opened for Administration
Regular tablets — Yes
Enteric-coated tablets — No

How This Drug Works
Intended Therapeutic Effect(s):   Principal uses include
- relief of symptoms ("hot flashes," sweats, etc.) associated with the menopause.
- replacement therapy in known estrogen deficiency states.
- suppression of breast engorgement and milk production following childbirth.
- control of selected cases of cancer of the breast.
- control of advanced, inoperative cancer of the prostate gland.

Location of Drug Action(s):   Principal actions occur in
- a major control center in the brain known as the hypothalamus.
- the pituitary gland.
- the female reproductive organs (the ovaries, uterus, and vagina).
- the breast tissues.

Method of Drug Action(s)

Estrogen preparations, taken to restore normal tissue levels, (1) reduce the frequency and intensity of menopausal symptoms, and (2) correct tissue abnormalities that are due to estrogen deficiency.

By inhibiting certain functions of the pituitary gland, this drug suppresses normal milk production by the breasts.

The mechanism of action responsible for control of some cases of breast cancer is not known.

By suppressing the production of the male sex hormones (androgens), this drug (an estrogen) retards the growth and spread of cancer of the prostate gland.

Principal Uses of This Drug
As a Single Drug Product: While this synthetic estrogen-like compound is as potent and effective as the natural estrogens, it is seldom used for estrogen replacement. Its primary use today is in the treatment of advanced cancer of the prostate gland. Though quite effective in suppressing the production of androgens initially, it loses its effectiveness after 1 to 2 years of continuous use, and the cancer "escapes" further control by the use of this drug.

As a Combination Drug Product [CD]:   This drug is available in combination with methyltestosterone, a synthetic androgen-like compound with actions similar to natural male sex hormone. The combination of male and female sex hormone effects is used to treat menopausal "hot flashes" that are of greater than usual degree and that fail to respond to the use of estrogen alone.

THIS DRUG SHOULD NOT BE TAKEN IF
—you have had an allergic reaction to any dosage form of it previously.
—you are, or think you may be, pregnant.
—you have active liver disease.
—you have active thrombophlebitis.
—you have had a recent pulmonary embolism.
—you have had a recent stroke or heart attack.

INFORM YOUR PHYSICIAN BEFORE TAKING THIS DRUG IF
—you have a history of cancer of the breast, ovary, uterus, or vagina.
—you have a family history of breast cancer.
—you have abnormal or unexplained vaginal bleeding.
—you have a history of thrombophlebitis, pulmonary embolism, stroke, or heart attack.
—you have cystic breast disease (cystic mastitis).
—you have endometriosis.
—you have fibroid tumors of the uterus.
—you have high blood pressure.
—you have migraine headaches or epilepsy.
—you have diabetes, or reduced sugar tolerance.
—you have impaired liver or kidney function.
—you have a high blood level of calcium.
—you plan to have major surgery in the near future.

Time Required for Apparent Benefit
Continuous use on a regular schedule for 10 to 20 days may be needed to determine the degree of effectiveness in relieving symptoms of the menopause.
In the treatment of breast cancer, favorable response can occur after 4 weeks of continuous use.
In the treatment of prostate cancer, favorable response can occur after 1 to 2 weeks of continuous use.

Possible Side-Effects *(natural, expected, and unavoidable drug actions)*
Retention of fluid, gain in weight, "breakthrough" bleeding (spotting in middle of menstrual cycle), change in menstrual flow, resumption of menstrual flow (bleeding from the uterus) after a period of natural cessation (postmenopausal bleeding). There may be an increased susceptibility to yeast infection of the genital tissues.
With larger doses (as in treatment of prostate cancer), enlargement and tenderness of the breasts often occur; atrophy of the testicles results in loss of sexual potency. Impairment of natural resistance (immunity) to infections (rare).

Possible Adverse Effects *(unusual, unexpected, and infrequent reactions)*

IF ANY OF THE FOLLOWING DEVELOP, DISCONTINUE DRUG AND NOTIFY YOUR PHYSICIAN AS SOON AS POSSIBLE

Mild Adverse Effects
Allergic Reactions: Skin rashes (various kinds), itching.
Other Reactions

Headache, dizziness, nervousness.

Tannish-brown pigmentation of face, loss of scalp hair.

Nausea, vomiting, abdominal cramping, bloating, diarrhea.

Abnormal vaginal bleeding, frequent and painful urination.

Serious Adverse Effects

Idiosyncratic Reactions: Episodes of porphyria (see Glossary.)

Other Reactions

Thrombophlebitis (inflammation of a vein with the formation of blood clot)—pain or tenderness in thigh or leg, with or without swelling of the foot, ankle, or leg.

Pulmonary embolism (movement of blood clot to the lung)—sudden shortness of breath, pain in the chest, coughing, bloody sputum.

Stroke (blood clot in the brain)—headaches, blackouts, sudden weakness or paralysis of any part of the body, severe dizziness, double vision, slurred speech, inability to speak.

Retinal thrombosis (blood clot in eye vessels)—sudden impairment or loss of vision.

Heart attack (blood clot in coronary artery)—sudden pain in chest, neck, jaw, or arm, accompanied by weakness, sweating, or nausea.

Rise in blood pressure in susceptible individuals.

Jaundice (see Glossary).

Emotional depression in susceptible individuals.

Accelerated growth of fibroid tumors of the uterus.

Development of nearsightedness (myopia).

Inability to tolerate contact lenses.

Possible Delayed Adverse Effects

The development of cancer of the vagina and/or cervix in the daughters of mothers who took this drug during early pregnancy and thus exposed their daughters to the drug at a critical time of their fetal development. This cancer usually develops in the late teens, following puberty. The risk is now estimated to be from 1.4 per 1000 exposures to as low as 1.4 per 10,000 exposures.

CAUTION

1. Advice to young women exposed to this and related drugs:* If you are past puberty and you know or suspect that you were exposed to diethylstilbestrol (or a similar drug) during your fetal development (in your mother's uterus), consult a gynecologist or other qualified physician for a thorough examination of the vagina, uterus, and ovaries. Such examinations should be repeated annually and whenever there is development of pelvic discomfort, vaginal discharge, or abnormal vaginal bleeding.

2. If this drug is being used to relieve the symptoms of the menopause, it is advisable to take the smallest effective dose, to omit it every fourth week (3 weeks on and 1 week off medication), and to evaluate with your physician the need for continuation of treatment every 3 to 6 months.

*See list of DES-Type Drugs at the end of this Drug Profile.

3. If abnormal vaginal bleeding occurs, discontinue this drug and inform your physician promptly.
4. If you experienced jaundice during pregnancy, you may develop jaundice while taking this drug. Observe for yellowish discoloration of the eyes and skin, dark-colored urine, or light-colored stools.

Precautions for Use by Those over 60 Years of Age
The natural changes in blood vessels that accompany aging require that this drug be used under close medical supervision. Report promptly any indications of impaired circulation—speech disturbances, altered vision, sudden hearing loss, vertigo, sudden weakness or paralysis, angina, or leg pains.

Advisability of Use During Pregnancy
Pregnancy Category: X (tentative). See Pregnancy Code inside back cover. Animal reproduction studies in rats reveal significant birth defects due to this drug.

Information from studies in pregnant women indicates that this drug can masculinize the female fetus and feminize the male fetus during development. In addition, it can predispose the female child to development of cancer of the vagina or cervix following puberty.

Avoid completely during entire pregnancy.

Advisability of Use While Nursing Infant
This drug is known to be present in milk and may affect the infant. It may also impair the formation of milk. Ask physician for guidance.

Habit-Forming Potential
None.

Effects of Overdosage
With Moderate Overdose: Nausea, vomiting, fluid retention, breast enlargement and discomfort, abnormal vaginal bleeding.

With Large Overdose: No serious or dangerous effects reported.

Possible Effects of Extended Use
Increased growth of fibroid tumors of the uterus.

Recent reports suggest a possible association between the use of estrogens and the development of cancer in the lining of the uterus. Further studies are needed to establish a definite cause-and-effect relationship. Prudence dictates that women with uterus intact should use estrogens only when symptoms justify it.

Prolonged use of estrogens has been reported to increase the risk of developing gall bladder disease.

Suggested Periodic Examinations While Taking This Drug (at physician's discretion)
Examination of the breasts (men and women), vagina, uterus, and ovaries—including a "Pap" smear (cervical cytology)—every 6 to 12 months.

Blood pressure measurement on a regular basis.

While Taking This Drug, Observe the Following

Foods: No restrictions. Ask physician for guidance regarding salt intake if you experience fluid retention.

Beverages: No restrictions.

Alcohol: No interactions expected.

Tobacco Smoking: Recent reports strongly suggest that heavy smoking in association with the use of estrogens may significantly increase the risk of abnormal blood clots leading to stroke (cerebral thrombosis) or heart attack (coronary thrombosis). Refrain from smoking while taking this drug.

Marijuana Smoking: No interactions expected.

Other Drugs

Diethylstilbestrol may *decrease* the effects of

- oral anticoagulants (Coumadin, etc.) by increasing the blood level of prothrombin.

Diethylstilbestrol *taken concurrently* with

- anti-diabetic drugs, may cause unpredictable fluctuations in blood sugar levels. Estrogens can cause an increase in blood sugar; they can also increase the effects of oral anti-diabetics (Diabinese, Dymelor, Orinase, Tolinase). Monitor blood sugar closely and adjust dosages for best diabetic control.

The following drugs may *decrease* the effects of diethylstilbestrol:

- meprobamate (Equanil, Miltown, etc.)
- phenobarbital

Driving a Vehicle, Operating Machinery, Engaging in Hazardous Activities: Usually no restrictions. Consult your physician for assessment of individual risk and for guidance regarding specific restrictions.

Aviation Note: The use of this drug *may be a disqualification* for the piloting of aircraft. Consultation with a designated Aviation Medical Examiner is advised.

Exposure to Sun: Use caution until full effect is known. This drug may cause photosensitivity (see Glossary).

Exposure to Heat: No restrictions.

Discontinuation: This drug should be discontinued immediately if you experience any indication of impaired circulation: severe headache, unusual disturbance of vision or hearing, sudden vertigo, difficulty with speech, weakness or paralysis of any part of the body, numbness or tingling, loss of consciousness. Inform your physician promptly.

Special Storage Instructions

Keep in a dry, tightly closed container. Protect from light. Keep suppositories in a cool place.

DES-TYPE DRUGS THAT MAY HAVE BEEN PRESCRIBED TO PREGNANT WOMEN*

Nonsteroidal Estrogens

Benzestrol
Chlorotrianisene
Comestrol
Cyren A
Cyren B
Delvinal
DES
DesPlex
Dethylstilbenediol
Dibestil
Dienestrol
Dienoestrol
Diestryl
Diethylstilbestrol
  Dipalmitate
Diethylstilbestrol
  Diphosphate
Diethylstilbestrol
  Dipropionate
Digestil
Domestrol
Estilben
Estrobene
Estrobene DP

Estrosyn
Fonatol
Gynben
Gyneben
H-Bestrol
Hexestrol
Hexoestrol
Menocrin
Meprane
Mestibol
Methallenestril
Microest
Mikarol
Mikarol forti
Milestrol
Monomestrol
Neo-Oestranol I
Neo-Oestranol II
Nulabort
Oestrogenine
Oestromenin
Oestromon
Orestol
Pabestrol D

Palestrol
Restrol
Stilbal
Stilbestrol
Stilbestronate
Stilbetin
Stilbinol
Stilboestroform
Stilboestrol
Stilboestrol DP
Stilestrate
Stilpalmitate
Stilphostrol
Stil-Rol
Stilronate
Stilrone
Stils
Synestrin
Synestrol
Synthoestrin
Tace
Vallestril
Willestrol

Nonsteroidal Estrogen-Androgen Combinations

Amperone
Di-Erone
Estan
Metystil

Teserene
Tylandril
Tylosterone

Nonsteroidal Estrogen-Progesterone Combination

Progravidium

Vaginal Cream-Suppositories with Nonsteroidal Estrogens

AVC cream with Dienestrol
Dienestrol cream

*Some of the brand name products in this list are no longer available.

DIGITOXIN

Year Introduced: 1945

Brand Names

USA	Canada
Crystodigin (Lilly)	None
Purodigin (Wyeth)	

Common Synonyms ("Street Names"):   Digitalis, heart pills

Drug Class: Digitalis Preparations

Prescription Required: USA: Yes   Canada: No

Available for Purchase by Generic Name: Yes

Available Dosage Forms and Strengths
Tablets — 0.05 mg., 0.1 mg., 0.15 mg., 0.2 mg.
Injection — 0.2 mg. per ml.

Tablet May Be Crushed or Capsule Opened for Administration: Yes

How This Drug Works
Intended Therapeutic Effect(s)
Improvement of the contraction force of the heart muscle, of benefit in the treatment of congestive heart failure.
Correction of certain heart rhythm disorders.
Location of Drug Action(s)
The heart muscle.
The pacemaker and tissues that comprise the electrical conduction system of the heart.
Method of Drug Action(s)
By increasing the availability of calcium within the heart muscle, this drug improves the efficiency of the conversion of chemical energy to mechanical energy, thus increasing the force of muscular contraction.
By slowing the activity of the pacemaker and delaying the transmission of electrical impulses through the conduction system of the heart, this drug assists in restoring normal heart rate and rhythm.

Principal Uses of This Drug
As a Single Drug Product: This drug has two primary uses: (1) the treatment of congestive heart failure; and (2) the restoration of normal heart rate and rhythm in such disorders as atrial fibrillation, atrial flutter, and atrial/supraventricular tachycardia. Since it is not eliminated by the kidney, it is most useful in those with impaired kidney function.

THIS DRUG SHOULD NOT BE TAKEN IF
—you have had an allergic reaction to any dosage form of it previously.

INFORM YOUR PHYSICIAN BEFORE TAKING THIS DRUG IF
—you have experienced any unfavorable reaction to a digitalis preparation in the past.
—you have taken any digitalis preparation within the past 2 weeks.
—you are now taking (or have recently taken) any diuretic (urine-producing) drugs.
—you have impaired liver or kidney function.
—you have a history of thyroid deficiency (hypothyroidism).

Time Required for Apparent Benefit
Drug action begins in 1 to 2 hours, reaches a maximum between 4 and 12 hours, and persists for 48 to 72 hours. (Some activity may persist for as long as 2 to 3 weeks.) Continuous use of this drug on a regular schedule (with careful, individualized dosage adjustment) is needed to achieve full benefit.

Possible Side-Effects *(natural, expected, and unavoidable drug actions)*
This drug may produce enlargement and/or sensitivity of the male breast tissue (rare). This is due to an estrogen-like (female hormone) action of certain digitalis preparations.

Possible Adverse Effects *(unusual, unexpected, and infrequent reactions)*

IF ANY OF THE FOLLOWING DEVELOP, DISCONTINUE DRUG AND NOTIFY YOUR PHYSICIAN AS SOON AS POSSIBLE

Mild Adverse Effects
Allergic Reactions: Skin rashes (various kinds), hives.
Other Reactions: Drowsiness, lethargy, changes in vision ("halo" effect, yellow-green vision, blurring, "spots," double vision), confusion, headache.

Serious Adverse Effects
Allergic Reactions: Abnormal bruising due to allergic destruction of blood platelets (see Glossary).
Other Reactions: Confusion, disorientation (usually in the elderly).

CAUTION
1. This drug has a narrow margin of safe use. Adhere strictly to prescribed dosage. Do not raise or lower the dose without first consulting your physician.
2. It is advisable to carry a card of personal identification that includes a notation that *you are taking this drug* (see Table 19 and Section Six).

Precautions for Use by Those over 60 Years of Age
The natural decline in kidney function that occurs after 60 requires smaller doses to initiate and maintain desired blood levels. Other natural changes in body function tend to reduce even further the very narrow margin between the correct therapeutic level and the toxic level.
You may be more susceptible to the development of reduced appetite, nausea, vomiting, diarrhea, blurred or yellow vision, or irregular heart rhythm.
Often the earliest indication of overdose (toxicity) will be development of confusion, emotional depression, and delusions. These should warn of a need to assess current dosage.

Advisability of Use During Pregnancy
Pregnancy Category: C (tentative). See Pregnancy Code inside back cover.
Animal reproduction studies: No data available.
Information from adequate studies in pregnant women is not available.
Ask physician for guidance.

Advisability of Use While Nursing Infant
Drug is probably present in milk. Safety for infant not established. Ask physician for guidance.

Habit-Forming Potential
None.

Effects of Overdosage
With Moderate Overdose: Loss of appetite, excessive saliva, nausea, vomiting, diarrhea. (These effects are usually the earliest indicators of an overdosage.)
With Large Overdose: Serious disturbance of heart rhythm and rate, intestinal bleeding, drowsiness, headache, confusion, delirium, hallucinations, convulsions.

Possible Effects of Extended Use
None reported.

Suggested Periodic Examinations While Taking This Drug (at physician's discretion)
Complete blood cell counts.
Electrocardiograms.
Measurement of blood potassium level.

While Taking This Drug, Observe the Following
Foods: No interactions with drug. Follow prescribed diet.
Beverages: It is advisable to use caffeine-containing beverages (coffee, tea, cola) sparingly.
Alcohol: No interactions expected. Follow physician's advice.
Tobacco Smoking: Follow physician's advice regarding smoking. Nicotine can cause irritability of the heart muscle and may confuse interpretation of your response to this drug.
Marijuana Smoking
Occasional (once or twice weekly):   No effect to mild and transient change in heart status.
Daily.   Possible accentuation of heart failure; reduced digitalis effect; possible change in electrocardiogram, confusing interpretation.
Other Drugs
Digitoxin *taken concurrently* with
• ephedrine or epinephrine (adrenaline), may cause serious disturbance of heart rhythm.
• cortisone and related drugs, may lead to digitalis toxicity (due to excessive loss of potassium from the body).

- diuretics (other than spironolactone and triamterene), may cause serious digitalis toxicity (due to excessive loss of potassium).
- reserpine, may cause additional slowing of the heart and may increase the possibility of digitalis toxicity.
- thyroid preparations, require that the combined effect be monitored very closely to prevent digitalis toxicity.

The following drugs may *increase* the effects of digitoxin
- phenytoin (Dantoin, Dilantin, etc.) may cause overdosage effects initially and reduced effects later.
- guanethidine may cause additional slowing of the heart.
- propranolol (Inderal) may cause additional slowing of the heart. Use this drug in small doses and very cautiously.
- quinidine must be used cautiously and in small doses.

The following drugs may *decrease* the effects of digitoxin
- antacids may interfere with drug absorption.
- laxatives may hasten drug's elimination and cause reduced absorption.
- phenobarbital may hasten drug's elimination and reduce effectiveness.
- phenylbutazone (Azolid, Butazolidin, etc.) may hasten drug's elimination and reduce effectiveness.

Driving a Vehicle, Operating Machinery, Engaging in Hazardous Activities: Usually no restrictions. Be alert to the possible occurrence of nausea, drowsiness and/or visual disturbance; restrict activities accordingly.

Aviation Note: Heart function disorders *are a disqualification* for the piloting of aircraft. Consultation with a designated Aviation Medical Examiner is advised.

Exposure to Sun: No restrictions.

Occurrence of Unrelated Illness: Any illness that causes vomiting, diarrhea, dehydration, or liver impairment (such as jaundice) can seriously disturb the proper control of this drug's action. Notify physician immediately so corrective action can be taken.

Discontinuation: This drug must be continued indefinitely (possibly for life). Do not discontinue it without consultation with your physician.

Special Storage Instructions
Keep in a tightly closed container. Protect from light.

DIGOXIN

Year Introduced: 1934

Brand Names

USA	Canada
Lanoxicaps (Burroughs Wellcome)	Lanoxin (B.W. Inc.)
	Natigoxine (Sabex)
Lanoxin (Burroughs Wellcome)	Novodigoxin (Novopharm)

Common Synonyms ("Street Names"):   Digitalis, heart pills

Drug Class: Digitalis Preparations

Prescription Required: USA: Yes   Canada: No

Available for Purchase by Generic Name: Yes

Available Dosage Forms and Strengths
Tablets — 0.125 mg., 0.25 mg., 0.5 mg.
Capsules — 0.05 mg., 0.1 mg., 0.2 mg.
Pediatric elixir — 0.05 mg. per ml.
Injection — 0.1 mg. per ml., 0.25 mg. per ml.

Tablet May Be Crushed or Capsule Opened for Administration: Yes

How This Drug Works
Intended Therapeutic Effect(s)
Improvement of the contraction force of the heart muscle, of benefit in the treatment of congestive heart failure.
Correction of certain heart rhythm disorders.

Location of Drug Action(s)
The heart muscle.
The pacemaker and tissues that comprise the electrical conduction system of the heart.

Method of Drug Action(s)
By increasing the availability of calcium within the heart muscle, this drug improves the efficiency of the conversion of chemical energy to mechanical energy, thus increasing the force of muscular contraction.
By slowing the activity of the pacemaker and delaying the transmission of electrical impulses through the conduction system of the heart, this drug assists in restoring normal heart rate and rhythm.

Principal Uses of This Drug
As a Single Drug Product: This drug has two primary uses: (1) the treatment of congestive heart failure and (2) the restoration of normal heart rate and rhythm in such disorders as atrial fibrillation, atrial flutter, and atrial/supraventricular tachycardia.

THIS DRUG SHOULD NOT BE TAKEN IF
—you have had an allergic reaction to any dosage form of it previously.

INFORM YOUR PHYSICIAN BEFORE TAKING THIS DRUG IF
—you have experienced any unfavorable reaction to a digitalis preparation in
the past.
—you have taken any digitalis preparation within the past 2 weeks.
—you are now taking (or have recently taken) any diuretic (urine-producing)
drugs.
—you have impaired liver or kidney function.
--you have a history of thyroid deficiency (hypothyroidism).

Time Required for Apparent Benefit
Drug action begins in 1 hour, reaches a maximum in 6 to 7 hours, and persists
for approximately 3 days. Elimination from the body is usually complete in
6 days.

Possible Side-Effects *(natural, expected, and unavoidable drug actions)*
This drug may produce enlargement and/or sensitivity of the male breast
tissue (rare). This is due to an estrogen-like (female hormone) action of some
digitalis preparations.

Possible Adverse Effects *(unusual, unexpected, and infrequent reactions)*

**IF ANY OF THE FOLLOWING DEVELOP, DISCONTINUE DRUG AND NOTIFY
YOUR PHYSICIAN AS SOON AS POSSIBLE**

Mild Adverse Effects
Allergic Reactions: Skin rashes (various kinds), hives.
Other Reactions: Drowsiness, lethargy, changes in vision ("halo" effect,
yellow-green vision, blurring, "spots," double vision), confusion, head-
ache.
Serious Adverse Effects
Confusion, disorientation (usually in the elderly).

CAUTION
1. This drug has a narrow margin of safe use. Adhere strictly to prescribed
dosage. Do not raise or lower the dose without first consulting your physician.
2. It is advisable to carry a card of personal identification that includes a
notation that *you are taking this drug* (see Table 19 and Section Six).

Precautions for Use by Those over 60 Years of Age
The natural decline in kidney function that occurs after 60 requires smaller
doses to initiate and maintain desired blood levels. Other natural changes
in body function tend to reduce even further the very narrow margin
between the current therapeutic level and the toxic level.
You may be more susceptible to the development of reduced appetite, nausea, vomiting, diarrhea, blurred or yellow vision, or irregular heart rhythm.
Often the earliest indication of overdose (toxicity) will be the development
of confusion, emotional depression, and delusions. These should warn of a
need to assess correct dosage.

Advisability of Use During Pregnancy
Pregnancy Category:　C (tentative). See Pregnancy Code inside back cover.
Animal reproduction studies: No data available.
Information from adequate studies in pregnant women is not available.
Ask physician for guidance.

Advisability of Use While Nursing Infant
Drug is known to be present in milk. Safety for infant not established. Ask
physician for guidance.

Habit-Forming Potential
None.

Effects of Overdosage
With Moderate Overdose:　Loss of appetite, excessive saliva, nausea, vomiting, diarrhea. (These effects are usually the earliest indicators of an overdosage.)
With Large Overdose:　Serious disturbance of heart rhythm and rate, intestinal bleeding, drowsiness, headache, confusion, delirium, hallucinations,
convulsions.

Possible Effects of Extended Use
None reported.

Suggested Periodic Examinations While Taking This Drug (at physician's discretion)
Electrocardiograms.
Measurement of blood potassium level.

While Taking This Drug, Observe the Following
Foods:　No interactions with drug. Follow prescribed diet.
Beverages:　It is advisable to use caffeine-containing beverages (coffee, tea,
cola) sparingly.
Alcohol:　No interactions expected. Follow physician's advice.
Tobacco Smoking:　Follow physician's advice regarding smoking. Nicotine
can cause irritability of the heart muscle and may confuse interpretation
of your response to this drug.
Marijuana Smoking
Occasional (once or twice weekly):　No effect to mild and transient change
in heart status.
Daily:　Possible accentuation of heart failure; reduced digitalis effect; possible change in electrocardiogram, confusing interpretation.
Other Drugs
Digoxin *taken concurrently* with
• ephedrine or epinephrine (adrenaline), may cause serious disturbance of
heart rhythm.
• cortisone and related drugs, may lead to digitalis toxicity (due to excessive
loss of potassium from the body).
• diuretics (other than spironolactone and triamterene), may cause serious
digitalis toxicity (due to excessive loss of potassium).

- reserpine, may cause additional slowing of the heart and may increase the possibility of digitalis toxicity.
- thyroid preparations, require that the combined effect be monitored very closely to prevent digitalis toxicity.

The following drugs may *increase* the effects of digoxin
- phenytoin (Dantoin, Dilantin, etc.) may cause overdosage effects initially and reduced effects later.
- guanethidine may cause additional slowing of the heart.
- propranolol (Inderal) may cause additional slowing of the heart. Use this drug in small doses and very cautiously.
- quinidine must be used cautiously and in small doses.

The following drugs may *decrease* the effects of digoxin
- antacids may interfere with drug absorption.
- laxatives may hasten drug's elimination and cause reduced absorption.
- phenobarbital may hasten drug's elimination and reduce effectiveness.
- phenylbutazone (Azolid, Butazolidin, etc.) may hasten drug's elimination and reduce effectiveness.

Driving a Vehicle, Operating Machinery, Engaging in Hazardous Activities: Usually no restrictions. Be alert to the possible occurrence of nausea, drowsiness and/or visual disturbances; restrict activities accordingly.

Aviation Note: Heart function disorders *are a disqualification* for the piloting of aircraft. Consultation with a designated Aviation Medical Examiner is advised.

Exposure to Sun: No restrictions.

Occurrence of Unrelated Illness: Any illness that causes vomiting, diarrhea, dehydration, or liver impairment (such as jaundice) can seriously disturb the proper control of this drug's action. Notify physician immediately so corrective action can be taken.

Discontinuation: This drug must be continued indefinitely (possibly for life). Do not discontinue it without consultation with your physician.

Special Storage Instructions
Keep in a tightly closed container. Protect from light.

DILTIAZEM

Year Introduced: 1982

Brand Names

USA	Canada
Cardizem (Marion)	Cardizem (Marion)

Common Synonyms ("Street Names"): Angina pills, heart pills.

Drug Class: Anti-anginal, Calcium Channel Blocker

Prescription Required: Yes

Available for Purchase by Generic Name: No

Available Dosage Forms and Strengths
Tablets — 30 mg., 60 mg.

Tablet May Be Crushed or Capsule Opened for Administration: Yes

How This Drug Works

Intended Therapeutic Effect(s):   Reduction in the frequency and severity of pain associated with angina pectoris (coronary artery insufficiency).

Location of Drug Action(s):   Principal sites include
- the muscular tissue in the walls of the coronary arteries in the heart and the walls of peripheral arterioles.
- the pacemaker and tissues that comprise the electrical conduction system of the heart.
- the heart muscle.

Method of Drug Action(s):   Not completely established. It is thought that by blocking the normal passage of calcium through certain cell walls (which is necessary for the function of nerve and muscle tissue), this drug slows the spread of electrical activity through the conduction system of the heart and inhibits the contraction of the coronary arteries and peripheral arterioles. As a result of these combined effects, this drug
- prevents spontaneous spasm of the coronary arteries (Prinzmetal's type of angina).
- reduces the rate and contraction force of the heart during exertion, thus lowering the oxygen requirement of the heart muscle; this reduces the occurrence of effort-induced angina (classical angina pectoris).
- reduces the degree of contraction of peripheral arterial walls, resulting in their relaxation and consequent lowering of the blood pressure. This further reduces the work load of the heart during exertion, and contributes to the prevention of angina.

Principal Uses of This Drug

As a Single Drug Product: Used primarily to treat (1) Angina pectoris due to coronary artery spasm (Prinzmetal's variant angina) that occurs spontaneously and is not associated with exertion; and (2) Classical angina-of-effort (due to atherosclerotic disease of the coronary arteries) in individuals who have not responded to or cannot tolerate the nitrates and "beta-blocker" drugs customarily used to treat this disorder.

THIS DRUG SHOULD NOT BE TAKEN IF

—you have had an allergic reaction to it previously.

—you have a "sick sinus" syndrome (and are not wearing an artificial pacemaker).

—you have been told you have a second-degree or third-degree heart block.

—you have constitutionally low blood pressure—systolic pressure below 90.

INFORM YOUR PHYSICIAN BEFORE TAKING THIS DRUG IF
—you have had an unfavorable response to any "calcium-blocker" drug in the past.
—you are currently taking any "beta-blocker" drug or any form of digitalis (see Drug Class, Section Three).
—you have a history of congestive heart failure.
—you have impaired liver or kidney function.
—you have a history of a drug-induced liver injury.

Time Required for Apparent Benefit
Drug action usually begins in 30 to 60 minutes and reaches its peak in 2 to 3 hours.
Continuous use on a regular schedule for 2 to 4 weeks is usually necessary to determine this drug's effectiveness in reducing the frequency and severity of angina.

Possible Side-Effects *(natural, expected, and unavoidable drug actions)*
Fatigue, lightheadedness.
Heart rate and rhythm changes in predisposed individuals.

Possible Adverse Effects *(unusual, unexpected, and infrequent reactions)*

IF ANY OF THE FOLLOWING DEVELOP, DISCONTINUE DRUG AND NOTIFY YOUR PHYSICIAN AS SOON AS POSSIBLE

Mild Adverse Effects
Allergic Reactions: Skin rash, hives, itching.
Other Reactions: Headache, drowsiness, dizziness, nervousness, insomnia, depression, confusion, hallucinations.
Flushing, palpitations, fainting, slow heart rate, low blood pressure.
Nausea, indigestion, heartburn, vomiting, diarrhea, constipation.

Serious Adverse Effects
Fluid retention (edema), serious disturbances of heart rate and/or rhythm, congestive heart failure.
Drug-induced liver injury (very rare).

CAUTION
1. Be sure to inform all physicians you consult that you are taking this drug. Note the use of this drug on your card of personal identification (see Section Six and Table 19).
2. You may use nitroglycerin and other nitrate drugs as needed to relieve episodes of angina pain. However, if you detect that your angina attacks are becoming more frequent or more intense, notify your physician immediately.

Precautions for Use by Those over 60 Years of Age
You may be more susceptible to the development of weakness, dizziness, fainting, and falling. Take necessary precautions to prevent injury.
Report promptly any changes in your pattern of thirst and urination.

Advisability of Use During Pregnancy
Pregnancy Category: C (tentative). See Pregnancy Code inside back cover.
Animal reproduction studies in mice, rats, and rabbits reveal embryo and
fetal deaths and skeletal defects.
Information from adequate studies in pregnant women is not available.
Avoid this drug completely during the first 3 months.
Use this drug only if clearly necessary. Ask your physician for guidance.

Advisability of Use While Nursing Infant
Presence of drug in human milk is not known. Avoid drug or refrain from
nursing.

Habit-Forming Potential
None.

Effects of Overdosage
With Moderate Overdose: Weakness, lightheadedness, low blood pressure,
fainting.
With Large Overdose: Slow pulse, marked drop in blood pressure, congestive heart failure, shortness of breath, loss of consciousness.

Suggested Periodic Examinations While Taking This Drug (at physician's discretion)
Evaluations of heart function, including electrocardiograms.
Liver function tests.

While Taking This Drug, Observe the Following
Foods: No restrictions. Avoid excessive salt intake.
It is advisable to take this drug before meals.
Beverages: No restrictions. May be taken with milk.
Alcohol: Use with caution until the combined effects have been deter-
mined. Alcohol may exaggerate the drop in blood pressure experienced by
some sensitive individuals.
Tobacco Smoking: Nicotine may reduce the effectiveness of this drug. Fol-
low your physician's advice regarding smoking.
Marijuana Smoking
Occasional (once or twice weekly): No interactions expected.
Daily: Possible reduced effectiveness of this drug; mild to moderate increase in angina; possible changes in the electrocardiogram, confusing
interpretation.
Other Drugs
Diltiazem *taken concurrently* with
• "beta-blockers" and digitalis preparations may affect heart rate and
rhythm adversely. Careful monitoring by your physician is necessary if
these drugs are taken concurrently.
Driving a Vehicle, Operating Machinery, Engaging in Hazardous Activities:
Usually no restrictions. Before engaging in any hazardous activity, determine that this drug will not cause you to have drowsiness, dizziness, or
lightheadedness.

Aviation Note: Coronary artery disease *is a disqualification* for the piloting of aircraft. Consultation with a designated Aviation Medical Examiner is advised.

Exposure to Sun: Use caution until your sensitivity has been determined. This drug can cause photosensitivity (see Glossary).

Exposure to Heat: Caution advised. Hot environments can exaggerate the blood pressure-lowering effects of this drug. Observe for lightheadedness or weakness.

Exposure to Cold: Caution advised. Cold environments may reduce the effectiveness of this drug.

Heavy Exercise or Exertion: This drug may improve your ability to be more active without resulting angina pain. Use caution and avoid excessive exertion that could impair heart function in the absence of warning pain.

Special Storage Instructions

Keep tablets in a dry, tightly closed container at room temperature. Protect from light.

DIMENHYDRINATE

Year Introduced: 1949

Brand Names

USA	Canada
Dramamine (Searle)	Apo-Dimenhydrinate
Reidamine	(Apotex)
(Reid-Provident)	Dramamine (Searle)
(Numerous other brand	Gravol (Horner)
names)	Nauseatol (Sabex)
	Novodimenate
	(Novopharm)
	Travamine (ICN)

Common Synonyms ("Street Names"): Seasick pills

Drug Class: Anti-motion sickness (Anti-emetic), Antihistamines

Prescription Required: USA: For most tablets and liquid—No
For injection—Yes
Canada: No

Available for Purchase by Generic Name: Yes

Available Dosage Forms and Strengths

Tablets — 50 mg.
Liquid — 12.5 mg. per teaspoonful (5 ml.)
Injection — 50 mg. per ml.

Tablet May Be Crushed or Capsule Opened for Administration: Yes

How This Drug Works

Intended Therapeutic Effect(s):   Prevention and management of the nausea, vomiting, and dizziness associated with motion sickness.

Location of Drug Action(s):   The nerve pathways connecting the organ of equilibrium (the labyrinth) in the inner ear with the vomiting center in the brain.

Method of Drug Action(s):   This drug reduces the sensitivity of the nerve endings in the labyrinth and blocks the transmission of excessive nerve impulses to the vomiting center.

Principal Uses of This Drug

As a Single Drug Product: This antihistamine is used primarily for the prevention and treatment of dizziness, nausea, and vomiting. It is most frequently prescribed for motion sickness and for certain disorders of the inner ear, such as labyrinthitis and Meniere's disease.

THIS DRUG SHOULD NOT BE TAKEN IF

—you have had an allergic reaction to any dosage form of it previously.

—you are taking, or have taken during the past 2 weeks, any mono-amine oxidase (MAO) inhibitor drugs (see Drug Class, Section Three).

—it has been prescribed for a newborn infant.

INFORM YOUR PHYSICIAN BEFORE TAKING THIS DRUG IF

—you have had an unfavorable reaction to any antihistamine drug in the past.

Time Required for Apparent Benefit

Drug action begins in 30 to 60 minutes and persists for approximately 4 hours.

Possible Side-Effects *(natural, expected, and unavoidable drug actions)*

Drowsiness, lassitude, dry mouth.

Possible Adverse Effects *(unusual, unexpected, and infrequent reactions)*

IF ANY OF THE FOLLOWING DEVELOP, DISCONTINUE DRUG AND NOTIFY YOUR PHYSICIAN AS SOON AS POSSIBLE

Mild Adverse Effects

Allergic Reactions: Skin rash.

Other Reactions: Nausea.

Serious Adverse Effects

None reported.

Precautions for Use by Those over 60 Years of Age

You may be more susceptible to the development of drowsiness, dizziness, and lethargy and to impairment of thinking, judgment, and memory.

This drug can increase the degree of impaired urination associated with prostate gland enlargement (prostatism).

Advisability of Use During Pregnancy

Pregnancy Category: B (tentative). See Pregnancy Code inside back cover. Animal reproduction studies reveal no birth defects due to this drug. Information from adequate studies in pregnant women is not available. Ask physician for guidance.

Advisability of Use While Nursing Infant

Presence of drug in milk is not known. Ask physician for guidance.

Habit-Forming Potential

None.

Effects of Overdosage

With Moderate Overdose: Marked drowsiness, dizziness, delirium, vomiting.

With Large Overdose: Stupor progressing to coma, convulsions, slow and shallow breathing.

Possible Effects of Extended Use

None reported.

Suggested Periodic Examinations While Taking This Drug (at physician's discretion)

None required.

While Taking This Drug, Observe the Following

Foods: No restrictions.

Beverages: No restrictions.

Alcohol: Use caution until combined effects have been determined. Alcohol in combination with some antihistamines can cause rapid and marked sedation.

Tobacco Smoking: No interactions expected.

Marijuana Smoking

Occasional (once or twice weekly):   Mild increase in drowsiness and dryness of mouth.

Daily: Moderate to marked increase in drowsiness and dryness of mouth; possible accentuation of impaired thinking.

Other Drugs: No significant drug interactions reported.

Driving a Vehicle, Operating Machinery, Engaging in Hazardous Activities: This drug may produce drowsiness that could impair mental alertness, coordination, and reaction time. Avoid hazardous activities until sedative effect has been determined.

Aviation Note: The use of this drug *is a disqualification* for the piloting of aircraft. Consultation with a designated Aviation Medical Examiner is advised.

Exposure to Sun: No restrictions.

Special Storage Instructions

Keep in a dry, tightly closed container.

DIPHENHYDRAMINE

Year Introduced: 1945

Brand Names

USA	Canada
Benadryl (Parke-Davis)	Allerdryl (ICN)
Benylin Cough Syrup (Parke-Davis)	Benadryl (P.D. & Co.)
	Insomnal (Welker-Lyster)
SK-Diphenhydramine (Smith Kline & French)	Somnifere (Albern)
	Ambenyl Expectorant [CD] (P.D. & Co.)
Ambenyl Expectorant [CD] (Parke-Davis)	Benylin Decongestant Cough Syrup [CD] (P.D. & Co.)
(Numerous other brand and combination brand names)	

Common Synonyms ("Street Names"):   Allergy pills

Drug Class: Sleep Inducer (Hypnotic), Antihistamines

Prescription Required: USA: Yes (Ambenyl is a Controlled   Canada: No
Drug, U.S. Schedule V)*

Available for Purchase by Generic Name: USA: Yes   Canada: No

Available Dosage Forms and Strengths
Tablets — 50 mg.
Capsules — 25 mg., 50 mg.
Elixir — 12.5 mg. per teaspoonful (5 ml.)
Syrup — 12.5 mg. per teaspoonful (5 ml.)
Injection — 10 mg. per ml., 50 mg. per ml.

Tablet May Be Crushed or Capsule Opened for Administration: Yes

How This Drug Works
Intended Therapeutic Effect(s):   Relief of symptoms associated with hay-fever (allergic rhinitis) and with allergic reactions in the skin, such as itching, swelling, hives, and rash.
Location of Drug Action(s):   Those hypersensitive tissues that release excessive histamine as part of an allergic reaction. The principal tissue sites are the eyes, the nose, and the skin.
Method of Drug Action(s):   This drug reduces the intensity of the allergic response by blocking the action of histamine after it has been released from sensitized tissue cells.

*See Schedules of Controlled Drugs inside back cover.

Principal Uses of This Drug

As a Single Drug Product: This versatile antihistamine has several uses. These include (1) the safe and effective induction of sleep (mild to moderate sedation); (2) the prevention and treatment of motion sickness (control of dizziness, nausea, and vomiting); (3) the relief of symptoms associated with Parkinson's disease; and (4) the treatment of parkinsonian drug reactions, especially in children and the elderly.

As a Combination Drug Product [CD]:   This drug may have a mild suppressant effect on coughing, but its true effectiveness is questionable. It has been combined with expectorants and either codeine or dextromethorphan and marketed as cough syrup.

THIS DRUG SHOULD NOT BE TAKEN IF

—you have had an allergic reaction to any dosage form of it previously.
—you are subject to acute attacks of asthma.
—you have glaucoma (narrow-angle type).
—you have difficulty emptying the urinary bladder.
—you are taking, or have taken during the past 2 weeks, any mono-amine oxidase (MAO) inhibitor drugs (see Drug Class, Section Three).
—it has been prescribed for a newborn infant.

INFORM YOUR PHYSICIAN BEFORE TAKING THIS DRUG IF

—you have had an unfavorable reaction to any antihistamine drug in the past.
—you have a history of peptic ulcer disease.
—you plan to have surgery under general anesthesia in the near future.

Time Required for Apparent Benefit

Drug action begins in approximately 30 minutes, reaches a maximum in 1 hour, and subsides in 4 to 6 hours.

Possible Side-Effects *(natural, expected, and unavoidable drug actions)*

Drowsiness, sense of weakness, dryness of nose, mouth, and throat, constipation.

Possible Adverse Effects *(unusual, unexpected, and infrequent reactions)*

IF ANY OF THE FOLLOWING DEVELOP, DISCONTINUE DRUG AND NOTIFY YOUR PHYSICIAN AS SOON AS POSSIBLE

Mild Adverse Effects
Allergic Reactions: Skin rash, hives.
Other Reactions
Headache, dizziness, inability to concentrate, nervousness, blurring of vision, double vision, difficulty in urination.
Nausea, vomiting, diarrhea.
Reduced tolerance for contact lenses.

Serious Adverse Effects
Allergic Reactions: Anaphylactic reaction (see Glossary).
Idiosyncratic Reactions
Behavioral disturbances—confusion, excitement, insomnia.
Hemolytic anemia (see Glossary).

Other Reactions: Blood platelet destruction (see Glossary)—unusual bleeding or bruising.

Precautions for Use by Those over 60 Years of Age

You may be more susceptible to the development of drowsiness, dizziness, and lethargy and to impairment of thinking, judgment, and memory.

This drug can increase the degree of impaired urination associated with prostate gland enlargement (prostatism).

Advisability of Use During Pregnancy

Pregnancy Category: B (tentative). See Pregnancy Code inside back cover. Animal reproduction studies in rats and rabbits reveal no birth defects due to this drug.

Information from studies in pregnant women indicates no significant increase in defects in 2948 exposures to this drug.

Ask physician for guidance.

Advisability of Use While Nursing Infant

This drug may impair milk formation and make nursing difficult. In addition, the drug is known to be present in milk. Ask physician for guidance.

Habit-Forming Potential

None.

Effects of Overdosage

With Moderate Overdose: Marked drowsiness, confusion, incoordination, unsteady gait, muscle tremors. In children: excitement, hallucinations, overactivity, convulsions.

With Large Overdose: Stupor progressing to coma, fever, flushed face, dilated pupils, weak pulse, shallow breathing.

Possible Effects of Extended Use

Hemolytic anemia (see Glossary).

Suggested Periodic Examinations While Taking This Drug (at physician's discretion)

Complete blood cell counts.

While Taking This Drug, Observe the Following

Foods: No restrictions. Stomach irritation can be reduced if drug is taken after eating.

Beverages: Coffee and tea may help to reduce the drowsiness caused by most antihistamines.

Alcohol: Use with extreme caution until combined effect has been determined. The combination of alcohol and antihistamines can cause rapid and marked sedation.

Tobacco Smoking: No interactions expected.

Marijuana Smoking

Occasional (once or twice weekly):   Mild increase in drowsiness and dryness of mouth.

Daily: Moderate to marked increase in drowsiness and dryness of mouth; possible accentuation of impaired thinking.

Other Drugs

Diphenhydramine may *increase* the effects of

- sedatives, sleep-inducing drugs, tranquilizers, antidepressants, pain relievers, and narcotic drugs, and result in oversedation. Careful dosage adjustments are necessary.
- atropine and drugs with atropine-like action (see Drug Class, Section Three).

Diphenhydramine may *decrease* the effects of

- oral anticoagulants, and reduce their protective action. Consult physician regarding prothrombin time testing and dosage adjustment.
- cortisone and related drugs (see Drug Class, Section Three).

Diphenhydramine *taken concurrently* with

- phenytoin (Dantoin, Dilantin, etc.), may change the pattern of epileptic seizures. Dosage adjustments may be necessary for proper control of epilepsy.

The following drugs may *increase* the effects of diphenhydramine

- all sedatives, sleep-inducing drugs, tranquilizers, pain relievers, and narcotic drugs may exaggerate its sedative action and cause oversedation.
- mono-amine oxidase (MAO) inhibitor drugs (see Drug Class, Section Three) may delay its elimination from the body, thus exaggerating and prolonging its action.

The following drugs may *decrease* the effects of diphenhydramine

- the amphetamines (Benzedrine, Dexedrine, Desoxyn, etc.) may reduce the drowsiness caused by most antihistamines.

Driving a Vehicle, Operating Machinery, Engaging in Hazardous Activities: This drug may impair mental alertness, judgment, physical coordination, and reaction time. Avoid hazardous activities until full sedative effect has been determined.

Aviation Note: The use of this drug *is a disqualification* for the piloting of aircraft. Consultation with a designated Aviation Medical Examiner is advised.

Exposure to Sun: Use caution until sensitivity has been determined. This drug may cause photosensitivity (see Glossary).

Special Storage Instructions

Keep in a dry, tightly closed, light-resistant container.

DIPHENOXYLATE

Year Introduced: 1960

Brand Names

USA	Canada
Lomotil [CD] (Searle)	Lomotil (Searle)
SK-Diphenoxylate [CD] (Smith, Kline & French)	

Common Synonyms ("Street Names"):   Diarrhea medicine

Drug Class: Anti-diarrheal

Prescription Required: Yes (Controlled Drug, U.S. Schedule V)*

Available for Purchase by Generic Name: USA: Yes   Canada: No

Available Dosage Forms and Strengths
Tablets — 2.5 mg. (+ 0.025 mg. atropine)
Liquid — 2.5 mg. (+ 0.025 mg. atropine) per teaspoonful (5 ml.)

Tablet May Be Crushed or Capsule Opened for Administration: Yes

How This Drug Works
Intended Therapeutic Effect(s):   Relief of intestinal cramping and diarrhea.
Location of Drug Action(s):   The nerve fibers in the wall of the stomach, the small intestine, and the colon.
Method of Drug Action(s):   Not completely established. It is thought that this drug acts directly on the nerve supply of the gastrointestinal tract to reduce its motility and propulsive contractions, thus relieving cramping and diarrhea.

Principal Uses of This Drug
As a Single Drug Product: Because of its potential for abuse, this drug is not marketed as a single entity. Its primary use is for the control of overactivity of the intestinal tract and diarrhea.
As a Combination Drug Product [CD]:   This drug, in therapeutically effective dosage, is combined with a small amount of atropine to discourage abusive overdosage. The accumulative effects of atropine overdosage would make the combination intolerable.

THIS DRUG SHOULD NOT BE TAKEN IF
—you are allergic to either component of this drug.
—you have active jaundice.
—it is prescribed for a child under 2 years of age.

INFORM YOUR PHYSICIAN BEFORE TAKING THIS DRUG IF
—you have a history of liver disease or impaired liver function.
—you have ulcerative colitis.

*See Schedules of Controlled Drugs inside back cover.

Time Required for Apparent Benefit
Repeated dosage may be necessary for 12 to 24 hours to control diarrhea. Duration of effect may approach 30 hours.

Possible Side-Effects *(natural, expected, and unavoidable drug actions)*
Drowsiness, constipation.

Possible Adverse Effects *(unusual, unexpected, and infrequent reactions)*
IF ANY OF THE FOLLOWING DEVELOP, DISCONTINUE DRUG AND NOTIFY YOUR PHYSICIAN AS SOON AS POSSIBLE

Mild Adverse Effects
Allergic Reactions: Skin rash, hives, localized swellings, itching.
Other Reactions
Headache, dizziness, weakness, euphoria.
Reduced appetite, nausea, vomiting, bloating.
Serious Adverse Effects
None reported.

CAUTION
Do not exceed recommended doses. Observe children closely for indications of atropine overdose (see ATROPINE Drug Profile).

Precautions for Use by Those over 60 Years of Age
You may be more sensitive to the sedative and constipating effects of this drug. Small doses are advisable until your individual response has been determined.

Advisability of Use During Pregnancy
Pregnancy Category: C (tentative). See Pregnancy Code inside back cover.
Animal reproduction studies: No data available.
Information from adequate studies in pregnant women is not available. Ask physician for guidance.

Advisability of Use While Nursing Infant
Both components of this drug are present in milk and can affect the nursing infant. Ask physician for guidance regarding safe dosage.

Habit-Forming Potential
Because of its similarity to meperidine (pethidine), this drug may cause physical and/or psychological dependence (see Glossary) if used in large doses over an extended period of time.

Effects of Overdosage
With Moderate Overdose: Marked drowsiness, lethargy, depression, numbness in arms and legs.
With Large Overdose: Dryness of skin and mouth, flushing, fever, rapid pulse, slow and shallow breathing, stupor progressing to coma.

Possible Effects of Extended Use
Physical and/or psychological dependence (see Glossary) is a remote possibility.

Suggested Periodic Examinations While Taking This Drug (at physician's discretion)
None required.

While Taking This Drug, Observe the Following
Foods: No restrictions. Follow prescribed diet.
Beverages: No restrictions. As allowed in prescribed diet.
Alcohol: Use with extreme caution until combined effect has been determined. This drug may increase the depressant action of alcohol on the brain.
Tobacco Smoking: No interactions expected.
Marijuana Smoking: No interactions expected.
Other Drugs
Diphenoxylate may *increase* the effects of
- sedatives, tranquilizers, and sleep-inducing drugs, and cause excessive sedation. Dosage adjustments may be necessary.

Diphenoxylate *taken concurrently* with
- mono-amine oxidase (MAO) inhibitor drugs (see Drug Class, Section Three), will require close observation of the blood pressure to detect any tendency to excessive rise.

Driving a Vehicle, Operating Machinery, Engaging in Hazardous Activities: This drug may cause drowsiness. Avoid hazardous activities until full effect has been determined.
Aviation Note: The use of this drug *is a disqualification* for the piloting of aircraft. Consultation with a designated Aviation Medical Examiner is advised.
Exposure to Sun: No restrictions.

Special Storage Instructions
Keep in a dry, tightly closed container.

DIPYRIDAMOLE

Year Introduced: 1962

Brand Names

USA	Canada
Persantine (Boehringer Ingelheim)	Persantine (Boehringer)

Common Synonyms ("Street Names"):   None

Drug Class: Anti-anginal (Vasodilator, Coronary), Antiplatelet (Platelet Inhibitor)

Prescription Required: USA: Yes   Canada: No

Available for Purchase by Generic Name: USA: Yes   Canada: No

Available Dosage Forms and Strengths
    Tablets — 25 mg., 50 mg., 75 mg.

Tablet May Be Crushed or Capsule Opened for Administration: Yes

How This Drug Works
    Intended Therapeutic Effect(s)
        Reduction in the frequency and intensity of acute attacks of angina pecto-
        ris; *not* intended for the relief of pain during the acute attack.
        Reduction in the need for nitroglycerin.
        Prevention of unwanted blood clotting (thrombosis) and embolism follow-
        ing heart surgery.
        Note: This use has not yet been sanctioned by the U.S. Food and Drug
        Administration.* Informed consent advised.
    Location of Drug Action(s):   Therapeutic actions are thought to occur in
        • the small vessels of the coronary artery system.
        • the blood platelets (see Glossary).
    Method of Drug Action(s):   Not completely established. It is thought that
        • by selectively dilating the small coronary arteries, this drug may increase
        the flow of blood and the supply of oxygen to the working heart muscle.
        • by preventing blood platelet (see Glossary) aggregation, this drug may
        reduce the tendency to blood clot formation in coronary artery disease
        and following heart valve surgery.

Principal Uses of This Drug
    As a Single Drug Product: This drug is used primarily for the long-term
        treatment of symptomatic coronary artery disease with angina pectoris. Its
        beneficial effects develop quite slowly, but its low toxicity permits continu-
        ous use for extended periods of time. It is usually necessary to supplement
        this drug with promptly acting nitrates (such as nitroglycerin) to relieve
        episodes of angina until the full benefit of this drug becomes apparent.

THIS DRUG SHOULD NOT BE TAKEN IF
—you have had an allergic reaction to it previously.
—you have just experienced an acute heart attack (coronary thrombosis, myocardial infarction).

INFORM YOUR PHYSICIAN BEFORE TAKING THIS DRUG IF
—you have low blood pressure.
—you have impaired liver function.

Time Required for Apparent Benefit
    Continuous use on a regular schedule for 3 months is needed to determine
    this drug's effectiveness in the treatment of chronic angina pectoris. Signifi-
    cant reduction in platelet aggregation is thought to occur in 1 week.

*This use is approved in Canada.

Possible Side-Effects *(natural, expected, and unavoidable drug actions)*
Lightheadedness, flushing, weakness.

Possible Adverse Effects *(unusual, unexpected, and infrequent reactions)*

IF ANY OF THE FOLLOWING DEVELOP, DISCONTINUE DRUG AND NOTIFY YOUR PHYSICIAN AS SOON AS POSSIBLE

Mild Adverse Effects
Allergic Reactions: Skin rash.
Other Reactions
   Headache, dizziness, fainting.
   Stomach irritation, nausea, diarrhea.
Serious Adverse Effects
None reported.

CAUTION
1. Occasionally this drug may cause an *increase* in the frequency and/or intensity of angina pectoris during the initial trial of treatment. If this response occurs, discontinue this drug promptly.
2. Anyone with a tendency to low blood pressure should avoid large doses of this drug.

Precautions for Use by Those over 60 Years of Age
It is advisable to begin treatment with small doses so that the full effect of this drug on blood pressure can be determined. Avoid doses that lower the blood pressure excessively.

Advisability of Use During Pregnancy
Pregnancy Category: C (tentative). See Pregnancy Code inside back cover.
Animal reproduction studies: No data available.
Information from adequate studies in pregnant women is not available. Ask physician for guidance.

Advisability of Use While Nursing Infant
The presence of this drug in milk is not known. Ask physician for guidance.

Habit-Forming Potential
None

Effects of Overdosage
With Moderate Overdose: Nausea, vomiting, abdominal cramping, diarrhea, weakness.
With Large Overdose: Marked drop in blood pressure resulting in weak and rapid pulse, cold and clammy skin, collapse.

Possible Effects of Extended Use
No serious effects reported.

Suggested Periodic Examinations While Taking This Drug (at physician's discretion)
None required.

While Taking This Drug, Observe the Following

Foods: This drug is most effective if taken 1 hour before meals. No specific food restrictions.

Beverages: Take with milk to reduce stomach irritation.

Alcohol: Use with caution until the combined effect has been determined. Alcohol may enhance the ability of this drug to lower the blood pressure.

Tobacco Smoking: Nicotine may reduce the effectiveness of this drug. Follow physician's advice regarding smoking, based upon its effect on the condition under treatment and its possible interaction with this drug.

Marijuana Smoking

Occasional (once or twice weekly): No interactions expected.

Daily: Possible reduced effectiveness of this drug; mild to moderate increase in angina; possible changes in electrocardiogram, confusing interpretation.

Other Drugs

Dipyridamole may *increase* the effects of

• oral anticoagulants, and improve their effectiveness in preventing embolization of blood clots following heart valve surgery. However, bleeding tendency increases and careful dosage adjustments are necessary.

• antihypertensive drugs, and cause excessive lowering of the blood pressure. Dosage adjustments may be necessary.

Dipyridamole *taken concurrenty* with

• aspirin, makes it possible to reduce the dose of pyridamole and thus lessen any side-effects that may occur.

Driving a Vehicle, Operating Machinery, Engaging in Hazardous Activities: Use caution if this drug causes lightheadedness or dizziness.

Aviation Note: Coronary artery disease *is a disqualification* for the piloting of aircraft. Consultation with a designated Aviation Medical Examiner is advised.

Exposure to Sun: No restrictions.

Exposure to Cold: Use caution. The combined effects of this drug with prolonged exposure to cold can cause excessive lowering of body temperature (hypothermia) in older individuals.

Heavy Exercise or Exertion: This drug may improve your ability to be more active without resulting angina pain. Use caution and avoid excessive exertion that could cause heart injury in the absence of warning pain.

Discontinuation: If this drug has been effective in reducing the frequency and/or intensity of angina pain, it should not be discontinued abruptly. Consult your physician if you plan to discontinue it for any reason.

Special Storage Instructions

Keep in a dry, tightly closed container.

DISOPYRAMIDE

Year Introduced: 1969

Brand Names

USA	Canada
Norpace (Searle)	Norpace (Searle)
	Rythmodan (Roussel)

Common Synonyms ("Street Names"):   Heart regulator

Drug Class: Heart Rhythm Regulator (Anti-arrhythmic)

Prescription Required: Yes

Available for Purchase by Generic Name: No

Available Dosage Forms and Strengths
Capsules — 100 mg., 150 mg.

Tablet May Be Crushed or Capsule Opened for Administration: Yes

How This Drug Works
Intended Therapeutic Effect(s):   Correction of certain heart rhythm disorders.
Location of Drug Action(s):   The heart muscle and the tissues that comprise the electrical conduction system of the heart.
Method of Drug Action(s):   By slowing the activity of the pacemaker and delaying the transmission of electrical impulses through the conduction system and muscle of the heart, this drug assists in restoring normal heart rate and rhythm.

Principal Uses of This Drug
As a Single Drug Product: This drug is classified as a Type 1 anti-arrhythmic agent, similar to procainamide and quinidine in its actions. It is used primarily to abolish and prevent the recurrence of premature beats arising in the ventricle (lower chamber) of the heart. It is also useful in the treatment and prevention of abnormally rapid heart rates (tachycardia) that originate in the ventricle.

THIS DRUG SHOULD NOT BE TAKEN IF
—you have had an allergic reaction to it previously.
—you have a second-degree or third-degree heart block (determined by the electrocardiogram.)

INFORM YOUR PHYSICIAN BEFORE TAKING THIS DRUG IF
—you have had any unfavorable reactions to other anti-arrhythmic drugs in the past.
—you have a history of heart disease of any kind, especially "heart block."
—you have a history of low blood pressure.
—you have a history of liver disease or impaired liver function.
—you have glaucoma, or a family history of glaucoma.

—you have an enlarged prostate gland with difficult urination (prostatism).
—you have myasthenia gravis.
—you are taking any form of digitalis.
—you are taking any diuretic drug that can cause excessive loss of body potassium: acetazolamide, chlorthalidone, ethacrynic acid, furosemide, metolazone, and the thiazides (see Drug Class, Section Three).

Time Required for Apparent Benefit

Drug action usually begins in 30 to 60 minutes and reaches its peak in 2 to 3 hours.

Continuous use on a regular schedule for 5 to 7 days is usually necessary to determine this drug's effectiveness in reducing the frequency of premature heart contractions and maintaining a more normal rhythm.

Possible Side-Effects *(natural, expected, and unavoidable drug actions)*

Drop in blood pressure in susceptible individuals.

Dry mouth (32%),* constipation (11%), blurred vision (3%–9%), reduced ability to urinate (14%).

Possible Adverse Effects *(unusual, unexpected, and infrequent reactions)*

IF ANY OF THE FOLLOWING DEVELOP, DISCONTINUE DRUG AND NOTIFY YOUR PHYSICIAN AS SOON AS POSSIBLE

Mild Adverse Effects
Allergic Reactions: Skin rashes (1%–3%), itching.
Other Reactions
  Headache, nervousness, fatigue, muscular weakness, mild aches.
  Loss of appetite, indigestion, nausea, vomiting, diarrhea.
  Lowered blood sugar level (hypoglycemia).

Serious Adverse Effects
Idiosyncratic Reactions: Acute psychotic behavior (rare).
Other Reactions
  Severe drop in blood pressure (hypotension).
  Progressive heart weakness (congestive heart failure).
  Inability to empty bladder (urinary retention 2%).
  Sexual impotence.
  Jaundice (see Glossary).
  Abnormally low white blood cells (rare).

Adverse Effects That May Mimic Natural Diseases or Disorders
Reversible jaundice (rare) may suggest the possibility of viral hepatitis.

Natural Diseases or Disorders That May Be Activated by This Drug

Glaucoma, myasthenia gravis.

CAUTION

1. Thorough evaluation of your heart function (including electrocardiograms) is necessary prior to using this drug.

*The percentage figures represent the frequency of occurrence of the respective adverse reaction in patients using this drug to date.

2. Periodic evaluation of your heart function is necessary to determine your response to this drug. Some individuals may experience a worsening of their heart rhythm disorder (increase in premature beats), and/or a deterioration of heart function. Ask your physician for guidance regarding the monitoring of your heart rate, rhythm, and overall performance.
3. Dosage must be determined carefully for each individual. Do not change your dosage without the knowledge and supervision of your physician.
4. *Do not* take any other anti-arrhythmic drug while taking this drug unless directed to do so by your physician.

Precautions for Use by Infants and Children
Safety and effectiveness have not been established.
Use not recommended.

Precautions for Use by Those over 60 Years of Age
The natural decline in kidney function that occurs after 60 may require reduction in dosage and/or lengthening of dosage intervals.
This drug can increase the degree of impaired urination associated with prostate gland enlargement (prostatism), and can also increase the tendency to constipation. Ensure good bowel management.
You may be more susceptible to the blood pressure–lowering effects of this drug. Report promptly the development of lightheadedness, dizziness, weakness or sense of impending faint. Use caution to prevent falls.

Advisability of Use During Pregnancy
Pregnancy Category: B (tentative). See Pregnancy Code inside back cover.
Animal reproduction studies in rats and rabbits reveal no birth defects due to this drug.
Information from adequate studies in pregnant women is not available.
Ask physician for guidance.

Advisability of Use While Nursing Infant
This drug is known to be present in the mother's milk.
It is advisable to avoid use of this drug or to refrain from breast-feeding.

Habit-Forming Potential
None.

Effects of Overdosage
With Moderate Overdose: Lowered blood pressure, dryness of eyes, nose, mouth, and throat, increasing difficulty with urination, increased constipation.
With Large Overdose: Marked drop in blood pressure, increased disturbance of heart rhythm, congestive heart failure, heart arrest.

Possible Effects of Extended Use
None reported.

Suggested Periodic Examinations While Taking This Drug (at physician's discretion)
Electrocardiograms.
Complete blood cell counts.
Measurements of potassium blood levels.

While Taking This Drug, Observe the Following

Foods: No restrictions beyond those advised by your physician. Ask for specific guidance regarding your use of salt. Timing of Drug and Food: May be taken immediately after eating to reduce stomach irritation if necessary.

Nutritional Support: Ask for specific guidance regarding your need for potassium-rich foods.

Beverages: No restrictions beyond those advised by your physician. This drug may be taken with milk.

Alcohol: Use caution until the combined effects have been determined. Alcohol may increase the blood pressure–lowering effects of this drug.

Tobacco Smoking: No interactions expected. It is advisable to discontinue all smoking in the presence of serious heart rhythm disorders. Follow your physician's advice.

Marijuana Smoking
Occasional (once or twice weekly):   No interactions expected.
Daily: Interactions with this drug are unpredictable. Marijuana may reduce its effectiveness. Use with caution and monitor heart rhythm and rate closely.

Other Drugs
Disopyramide may *increase* the effects of
• anti-hypertensive drugs, and cause excessive lowering of the blood pressure.
• atropine-like drugs (see Drug Class, Section Three).
• warfarin (Coumadin, etc.), and make it necessary to adjust the dosage of the anticoagulant.
Disopyramide may *decrease* the effects of
• ambenonium (Mytelase).
• neostigmine (Prostigmin).
• pyridostigmine (Mestinon).

The beneficial effect of these three drugs in the treatment of myasthenia gravis may be reduced.

The following drugs may *decrease* the effects of disopyramide:
• all diuretics that promote potassium loss from the body. (It is advisable to monitor the blood level of potassium and to correct any deficiency.)

Driving a Vehicle, Operating Machinery, Engaging in Hazardous Activities: Usually no restrictions. However, it is advisable to observe for the possible occurrence of blurred vision or dizziness and to restrict activities accordingly.

Aviation Note: The use of this drug *may be a disqualification* for the piloting of aircraft. Consultation with a designated Aviation Medical Examiner is advised.

Exposure to Sun: No restrictions.

Exposure to Heat: Use caution. The use of this drug in hot environments may increase the risk of heat stroke.

Heavy Exercise or Exertion: Use caution in warm or hot environments. This drug may impair normal perspiration (heat loss) and interfere with the regulation of body temperature.

Occurrence of Unrelated Illness: In the event of a new illness, injury, or need for surgery, notify *all* your attending physicians that you have been taking this drug. Dosage adjustments may be necessary.

Discontinuation: If you have been using this drug on a regular basis, avoid discontinuing it abruptly if possible. Consult your physician for guidance regarding the proper withdrawal schedule.

Special Storage Instructions
Keep capsules in a dry, tightly closed container at room temperature.

DISULFIRAM

Year Introduced: 1948

Brand Names

USA	Canada
Antabuse (Ayerst)	Antabuse (Ayerst)

Common Synonyms ("Street Names"):   None

Drug Class: Anti-alcoholism (Alcohol-drinking Deterrent)

Prescription Required: Yes

Available for Purchase by Generic Name: USA: Yes   Canada: No

Available Dosage Forms and Strengths
Tablets — 250 mg., 500 mg.

Tablet May Be Crushed or Capsule Opened for Administration: Yes

How This Drug Works
Intended Therapeutic Effect(s):   To deter the drinking of alcohol (in the management of alcoholism).

Location of Drug Action(s):   Specific enzyme systems within the liver.

Method of Drug Action(s): Following the ingestion of alcohol, this drug interrupts normal liver enzyme activity after the conversion of alcohol to acetaldehyde. This causes excessive accumulation of acetaldehyde, a highly toxic substance that produces the disulfiram (Antabuse) reaction (see Glossary).

Principal Uses of This Drug
As a Single Drug Product: This drug is used for one purpose only—to deter the abusive drinking of alcoholic beverages. It does not abolish the craving or impulse to drink. It is of value in the treatment of alcoholism because of the psychological reinforcement it provides by reminding the patient of the dire consequences of ingesting alcohol.

THIS DRUG SHOULD NOT BE TAKEN IF
—you have experienced a severe allergic reaction to disulfiram in the past. (The reaction of disulfiram and alcohol is *not* an allergic reaction.)

—you have used alcohol in any amount or in any form within the past 12 hours.

—you are taking (or have taken recently) metronidazole (Flagyl).

—you have heart disease.

INFORM YOUR PHYSICIAN BEFORE TAKING THIS DRUG IF
—you have used disulfiram in the past.

—you do *not* intend to avoid alcohol completely while taking this drug.

—you have not been given a full explanation of the reaction you will experience if you drink alcohol while taking this drug.

—you have a history of diabetes, epilepsy, liver, or kidney disease.

—you are currently taking oral anticoagulants, digitalis, isoniazid, phenytoin (Dantoin, Dilantin, etc.).

—you plan to have surgery under general anesthesia while taking this drug.

Time Required for Apparent Benefit
Full effectiveness usually requires 3 weeks.

Possible Side-Effects *(natural, expected, and unavoidable drug actions)*
None.

Possible Adverse Effects *(unusual, unexpected, and infrequent reactions)*

IF ANY OF THE FOLLOWING DEVELOP, DISCONTINUE DRUG AND NOTIFY YOUR PHYSICIAN AS SOON AS POSSIBLE
Mild Adverse Effects
Allergic Reactions: Skin rashes (various kinds), hives.
Other Reactions
Drowsiness, lethargy, headache, tremor, dizziness.
Metallic or garlic-like taste, indigestion. (These usually appear during the first 2 weeks and then gradually subside.)
Serious Adverse Effects
Peripheral neuritis (see Glossary)—numbness or tingling, pain, weakness in arms or legs.
Optic neuritis—impaired vision.

CAUTION
1. This drug should *never* be given to an individual who is in a state of alcoholic intoxication.
2. The patient should be fully informed regarding the purpose and actions of this drug *before* treatment is started.

Precautions for Use by Those over 60 Years of Age
You may be more sensitive to the sedative effects of this drug. Small doses are advisable until your individual response has been determined.

Advisability of Use During Pregnancy
Pregnancy Category: B (tentative). See Pregnancy Code inside back cover.

Animal reproduction studies in rats and hamsters reveal no birth defects due to this drug.

Information from adequate studies in pregnant women is not available. Ask physician for guidance.

Advisability of Use While Nursing Infant
Safety not established. Ask physician for guidance.

Habit-Forming Potential
None.

Effects of Overdosage
With Moderate Overdose: Marked lethargy, impaired memory, behavioral disturbances.

With Large Overdose: Headache, stomach pain, nausea, vomiting, diarrhea, confusion, impaired stance and gait, muscle weakness, temporary paralysis.

Possible Effects of Extended Use
No significant effects reported.

Suggested Periodic Examinations While Taking This Drug (at physician's discretion)
Complete blood cell counts.
Liver function tests.

While Taking This Drug, Observe the Following
Foods: Avoid all foods prepared with alcohol, including sauces, marinades, vinegars, desserts, etc. (Inquire when dining out regarding the use of alcohol in food preparation.)

Beverages: Avoid all punches, fruit drinks, etc., that may contain alcohol.

Alcohol: Avoid completely in all forms while taking this drug and for 14 days following the last dose. The combination of disulfiram and alcohol—even in small amounts—produces the "disulfiram (Antabuse) reaction." This begins within 5 to 10 minutes after ingesting alcohol and consists of intense flushing and warming of the face, a severe throbbing headache, shortness of breath, chest pains, nausea, repeated vomiting, sweating, and weakness. If the amount of alcohol ingested is large enough, the reaction may progress to blurred vision, vertigo, confusion, marked drop in blood pressure, and loss of consciousness. Severe reactions may lead to convulsions and death. The reaction may last from 30 minutes to several hours, depending upon the amount of alcohol in the body. As the symptoms subside, the individual is exhausted and usually sleeps for several hours.

Tobacco Smoking: No interactions expected.

Marijuana Smoking: No interactions expected.

Other Drugs

Disulfiram may *increase* the effects of

- oral anticoagulants, and cause abnormal bleeding; dosage adjustments may be necessary.
- barbiturates, and cause oversedation (see Drug Class, Section Three).
- chlordiazepoxide, and cause oversedation.
- diazepam, and cause oversedation.
- phenytoin (Dantoin, Dilantin, etc.), and cause toxic effects on the brain; dosage adjustments may be necessary.

Disulfiram *taken concurrently* with

- isoniazid (INH, etc.), may cause unsteady gait and acute mental disturbance, making it necessary to discontinue treatment.
- metronidazole (Flagyl), may cause acute mental and behavioral disturbances, making it necessary to discontinue treatment.
- OTC cough syrups, tonics, etc., containing alcohol, may cause a disulfiram (Antabuse) reaction (see OTC in Glossary).

Driving a Vehicle, Operating Machinery, Engaging in Hazardous Activities: No restrictions if drowsiness and dizziness do not occur.

Aviation Note: Alcoholism *is a disqualification* for the piloting of aircraft. Consultation with a designated Aviation Medical Examiner is advised.

Exposure to Sun: No restrictions.

Discontinuation: Treatment with disulfiram is only part of your total treatment program. Do *not* discontinue this drug without the knowledge and agreement of your physician.

Special Storage Instructions

Keep in a dry, tightly closed container.

DOXEPIN

Year Introduced: 1969

Brand Names

USA	Canada
Adapin (Pennwalt)	Sinequan (Pfizer)
Sinequan (Pfizer)	

Common Synonyms ("Street Names"):   None

Drug Class: Antidepressant, Tricyclic

Prescription Required: Yes

Available for Purchase by Generic Name: No

Available Dosage Forms and Strengths
        Capsules — 10 mg., 25 mg., 50 mg., 75 mg., 100 mg., 150 mg.
  Oral concentrate — 10 mg. per ml.

Tablet May Be Crushed or Capsule Opened for Administration: Yes

How This Drug Works
  Intended Therapeutic Effect(s):   Gradual improvement of mood and relief
  of emotional depression.
  Location of Drug Action(s):   Those areas of the brain that determine mood
  and emotional stability.
  Method of Drug Action(s):   Not established. Present thinking is that this
  drug slowly restores to normal levels certain constituents of brain tissue
  (such as norepinephrine) that transmit nerve impulses.

Principal Uses of This Drug
  As a Single Drug Product: To relieve the symptoms associated with spontaneous (endogenous) depression, and to initiate the restoration of normal
  mood. This drug should be used only when a diagnosis of a true, primary
  depression of significant degree has been established. It should *not* be used
  to treat the symptoms of mild and transient (reactive) depression that
  may be associated with many life situations in the absence of a bona fide
  affective illness.

THIS DRUG SHOULD NOT BE TAKEN IF
—you have had an allergic reaction to any dosage form of it previously.
—you are taking or have taken within the past 14 days any mono-amine oxidase
  (MAO) inhibitor drug (see Drug Class, Section Three).
—you are recovering from a recent heart attack.
—you have glaucoma (narrow-angle type).
—it is prescribed for a child under 12 years of age.

INFORM YOUR PHYSICIAN BEFORE TAKING THIS DRUG IF
—you are allergic or sensitive to any other tricyclic antidepressant (see Drug
  Class, Section Three).
—you have a history of any of the following: diabetes, epilepsy, glaucoma, heart
  disease, prostate gland enlargement, or overactive thyroid function.
—you plan to have surgery under general anesthesia in the near future.

Time Required for Apparent Benefit
  Some benefit may be apparent within the first 2 weeks. Maximal response
  may require continuous treatment for 3 to 4 weeks.

Possible Side-Effects *(natural, expected, and unavoidable drug actions)*
  Drowsiness, blurring of vision, dryness of mouth, constipation, impaired urination.

Possible Adverse Effects *(unusual, unexpected, and infrequent reactions)*

**IF ANY OF THE FOLLOWING DEVELOP, DISCONTINUE DRUG AND NOTIFY
YOUR PHYSICIAN AS SOON AS POSSIBLE**

Mild Adverse Effects
Allergic Reactions: Skin rash, hives, swelling of face or tongue, drug fever.
Other Reactions
Nausea, indigestion, irritation of tongue or mouth, peculiar taste.
Headache, dizziness, weakness, fainting, unsteady gait, tremors.
Swelling of testicles, breast enlargement, milk formation.
Fluctuation of blood sugar levels.

Serious Adverse Effects
Allergic Reactions: Hepatitis with jaundice (see Glossary).
Other Reactions
Bone marrow depression (see Glossary)—fatigue, fever, sore throat,
unusual bleeding or bruising.
Parkinson-like disorders (see Glossary).
Confusion, hallucinations, agitation, and restlessness (especially in the
elderly).

Precautions for Use by Those over 60 Years of Age
During the first 2 weeks of treatment observe for the development of confusional reactions—restlessness, agitation, forgetfulness, disorientation, delusions, and hallucinations. Reduction of dosage or discontinuation may be
necessary.
Observe for incoordination and instability in stance and gait which may
predispose to falling and injury.
This drug can increase the degree of impaired urination associated with
prostate gland enlargement (prostatism).

Advisability of Use During Pregnancy
Pregnancy Category: B (tentative). See Pregnancy Code inside back cover.
Animal reproduction studies in rats, rabbits, dogs, and monkeys reveal no
birth defects due to this drug.
Information from adequate studies in pregnant women is not available.
Ask physician for guidance.

Advisability of Use While Nursing Infant
Presence of drug in milk is not known. Safety has not been established. Ask
physician for guidance.

Habit-Forming Potential
None

Effects of Overdosage
With Moderate Overdose: Confusion, hallucinations, extreme drowsiness,
drop in body temperature, heart palpitation, dilated pupils, tremors.
With Large Overdose: Stupor, deep sleep, coma, convulsions.

Possible Effects of Extended Use
None reported.

Suggested Periodic Examinations While Taking This Drug (at physician's discretion)
Complete blood cell counts.
Liver function tests.
Serial blood pressure readings and electrocardiograms.

While Taking This Drug, Observe the Following
Foods: No restrictions.

Beverages: No restrictions.

Alcohol: Avoid completely. This drug can increase markedly the intoxicating effects of alcohol and accentuate its depressant action on brain function.

Tobacco Smoking: No interactions expected.

Marijuana Smoking

Occasional (once or twice weekly):   Transient increase in drowsiness and dryness of mouth.

Daily: Persistent drowsiness, increased dryness of mouth; possible reduced effectiveness of this drug.

Other Drugs

Doxepin may *increase* the effects of

- atropine and drugs with atropine-like actions (see Drug Class, Section Three).
- sedatives, sleep-inducing drugs, tranquilizers, antihistamines, and narcotic drugs, and cause oversedation. Dosage adjustments may be necessary.
- levodopa (Dopar, Larodopa, etc.), in its control of Parkinson's disease.

Doxepin *taken concurrently* with

- thyroid preparations, may cause impairment of heart rhythm and function. Ask physician for guidance regarding thyroid dosage adjustment.
- ethchlorvynol (Placidyl), may cause delirium.
- quinidine, may cause impairment of heart rhythm and function. Avoid the combined use of these two drugs.
- mono-amine oxidase (MAO) inhibitor drugs (see Drug Class, Section Three), may cause high fever, delirium, and convulsions.

The following drugs may *increase* the effects of doxepin

- diuretics of the thiazide family (see Drug Class, Section Three), may slow its elimination from the body. Overdosage may occur.

Driving a Vehicle, Operating Machinery, Engaging in Hazardous Activities:
This drug may impair mental alertness, judgment, physical coordination, and reaction time. Avoid hazardous activities.

Aviation Note: The use of this drug *is a disqualification* for the piloting of aircraft. Consultation with a designated Aviation Medical Examiner is advised.

Exposure to Sun: Use caution until sensitivity to sun has been determined. This drug may cause photosensitivity (see Glossary).

Discontinuation: If it has been necessary to use this drug for an extended period of time, do not discontinue it abruptly. Ask physician for guidance regarding dosage reduction and withdrawal. It may be necessary to adjust the dosage of other drugs taken concurrently.

Special Storage Instructions
Keep in a dry, tightly closed container.

DOXYCYCLINE

Year Introduced: 1967

Brand Names

USA	Canada
Doxychel (Rachelle)	Vibramycin (Pfizer)
Vibramycin (Pfizer)	
Vibra Tabs (Pfizer)	

Common Synonyms ("Street Names"): None

Drug Class: Antibiotic (Anti-infective), Tetracyclines

Prescription Required: Yes

Available for Purchase by Generic Name: USA: Yes   Canada: No

Available Dosage Forms and Strengths

Tablets — 100 mg.
Capsules — 50 mg., 100 mg.
Syrup — 50 mg. per teaspoonful (5 ml.)
Oral suspension — 25 mg. per teaspoonful (5 ml.)
Injection — 100 mg., 200 mg. per vial.

Tablet May Be Crushed or Capsule Opened for Administration: Yes

How This Drug Works
Intended Therapeutic Effect(s): The elimination of infections responsive to the action of this drug.

Location of Drug Action(s): Any body tissue or fluid in which sufficient concentration of the drug can be achieved.

Method of Drug Action(s): This drug prevents the growth and multiplication of susceptible bacteria by interfering with their formation of essential proteins.

Principal Uses of This Drug

As a Single Drug Product: This member of the tetracycline drug class is used primarily to (1) treat a broad range of infections caused by susceptible bacteria and protozoa, and (2) treat and prevent "traveler's diarrhea." It is often used to treat acute and chronic sinusitis and bronchitis.

THIS DRUG SHOULD NOT BE TAKEN IF
—you are allergic to any tetracycline drug (see Drug Class, Section Three).
—you are pregnant or breast feeding.

INFORM YOUR PHYSICIAN BEFORE TAKING THIS DRUG IF
—you have a history of liver or kidney disease.
—you have systemic lupus erythematosus.
—you are taking any penicillin drug.
—you are taking any anticoagulant drug.
—you plan to have surgery under general anesthesia in the near future.
—it is prescribed for a child under 9 years of age.

Time Required for Apparent Benefit
Varies with nature of infection under treatment; usually 2 to 5 days.

Possible Side-Effects *(natural, expected, and unavoidable drug actions)*
Superinfections (see Glossary), often due to yeast organisms. These can occur in the mouth, intestinal tract, rectum, and/or vagina, resulting in rectal and vaginal itching.

Possible Adverse Effects *(unusual, unexpected, and infrequent reactions)*

IF ANY OF THE FOLLOWING DEVELOP, DISCONTINUE DRUG AND NOTIFY YOUR PHYSICIAN AS SOON AS POSSIBLE

Mild Adverse Effects
Allergic Reactions: Skin rashes (various kinds), hives, itching of hands and feet, swelling of face or extremities.
Photosensitivity (see Glossary) Reactions: Exaggerated sunburn or skin irritation occurs commonly with some tetracyclines.
Other Reactions
Loss of appetite, nausea, vomiting, diarrhea.
Irritation of mouth or tongue, "black tongue," sore throat, abdominal pain or cramping.

Serious Adverse Effects
Allergic Reactions: Anaphylactic reaction (see Glossary), asthma, fever, painful swollen joints, unusual bleeding or bruising, jaundice (see Glossary).
Other Reactions: Permanent discoloration and/or malformation of teeth when taken under 9 years of age, including unborn child and infant.

CAUTION
1. Troublesome and persistent diarrhea can develop in sensitive individuals. If diarrhea persists more than 24 hours, discontinue this drug and consult your physician for guidance.

2. If surgery under general anesthesia is planned while taking this drug, the choice of anesthetic agent must be considered carefully to prevent serious kidney damage.

Precautions for Use by Those over 60 Years of Age
Natural changes in the skin after 60 may predispose to severe and prolonged itching reactions in the genital and anal regions. This reaction should be reported promptly.

Advisability of Use During Pregnancy
Pregnancy Category: D (tentative). See Pregnancy Code inside back cover.
Animal reproduction studies reveal significant birth defects due to this drug.
Information from studies in pregnant women indicates that this drug can cause impaired development and discoloration of teeth and other developmental defects.
It is advisable to avoid this drug completely during entire pregnancy.
Ask physician for guidance.

Advisability of Use While Nursing Infant
Tetracyclines can be present in milk and can have adverse effects on infant.
Avoid use or avoid nursing.

Habit-Forming Potential
None.

Effects of Overdosage
Possible nausea, vomiting, diarrhea.
Acute liver damage (rare).

Possible Effects of Extended Use
Impairment of bone marrow, liver, or kidney function (all rare).
Superinfections.

Suggested Periodic Examinations While Taking This Drug (at physician's discretion)
Complete blood cell counts.
Liver and kidney function tests.
During extended use, sputum and stool examinations may detect early superinfections due to yeast organisms.

While Taking This Drug, Observe the Following
Foods: Dairy products can interfere with absorption. Tetracyclines should be taken 1 hour before or 2 hours after eating.
Beverages: Avoid milk for 1 hour before and after each dose of a tetracycline.
Alcohol: Avoid while taking a tetracycline if you have a history of liver disease.
Tobacco Smoking: No interactions expected.
Marijuana Smoking: No interactions expected.

Other Drugs
Tetracyclines may *increase* the effects of
- oral anticoagulants, and make it necessary to reduce their dosage.

Tetracyclines may *decrease* the effects of
- the penicillins, and impair their effectiveness in treating infections.

The following drugs may *decrease* the effects of tetracyclines:
- antacids may reduce drug absorption.
- iron and mineral preparations may reduce drug absorption.

Driving a Vehicle, Operating Machinery, Engaging in Hazardous Activities: Usually no restrictions. Be alert to the possible occurrence of nausea and/or diarrhea; restrict activities accordingly.

Aviation Note: The use of this drug *may be a disqualification* for the piloting of aircraft. Consultation with a designated Aviation Medical Examiner is advised.

Exposure to Sun: Avoid as much as possible. Photosensitivity (see Glossary) is common with some tetracyclines.

Special Storage Instructions
Keep in a tightly closed, light-resistant container.

EPHEDRINE

Year Introduced: 1924 (Crude form in use in China for 5000 years)

Brand Names

USA		Canada
Bronkaid [CD] (Winthrop)	Quibron Plus [CD] (Mead Johnson)	Amesec [CD] (Lilly)
Bronkotabs [CD] (Breon)	Tedral [CD] (Parke-Davis)	Marax [CD] (Pfizer)
Marax [CD] (Roerig)	Verequad [CD] (Knoll)	Tedral [CD] (Warner/Chilcott)
Mudrane [CD] (Poythress)	(Numerous other brand and	
Nyquil [CD] (Vick)	combination brand	
Quadrinal [CD] (Knoll)	names)	
Quelidrine [CD] (Abbott)		

Common Synonyms ("Street Names"):   Asthma pills

Drug Class: Anti-asthmatic, Bronchodilator

Prescription Required: USA: For low-strength formulations—No
  For high-strength formulations—Yes
  Canada: No

Available for Purchase by Generic Name: Yes

Available Dosage Forms and Strengths
  Tablets — 25 mg.
  Capsules — 25 mg., 50 mg.
   Syrup — 4 mg. per ml., 11 mg. and 20 mg. per teaspoonful (5 ml.)
   Drops — 0.5%, 1%, 3%
  Nasal Jelly — 0.6%
Marketed generically and in a variety of combination tablets, capsules, syrups, and solutions. Strength varies according to drug product. Examine product label.

Tablet May Be Crushed or Capsule Opened for Administration: Yes

How This Drug Works
  Intended Therapeutic Effect(s)
  Prevention and symptomatic treatment of bronchial asthma.
  Relief of congestion of respiratory passages.
  Location of Drug Action(s):   This drug affects all tissues activated by the sympathetic nervous system. Its principal action sites of therapeutic importance are
   • the muscles in the walls of the bronchial tubes.
   • the small blood vessels (arterioles) in the tissues lining the respiratory passages.
  Method of Drug Action(s)
  By blocking the release of certain chemicals from sensitized tissue cells which are undergoing an allergic reaction, this drug acts to prevent the constriction of bronchial tubes which occurs as a manifestation of allergy.
  By directly producing relaxation of the bronchial muscles, this drug reverses the bronchial constriction responsible for asthma.
  By contracting the walls and thus reducing the size of the arterioles, this drug decreases the volume of blood in the tissues. This results in shrinkage of tissue mass (decongestion).

Principal Uses of This Drug
  As a Single Drug Product: This drug is seldom used as a single drug entity in treating nonhospitalized patients. It is used primarily for its bronchodilator effect in the treatment of bronchial asthma, usually in combination with other appropriate drugs.
  As a Combination Drug Product [CD]:   Usually combined with theophylline (another bronchodilator), one of the barbiturates (for its calming effect), and sometimes with an expectorant (to thin brochial mucus). In such combinations, these drugs are more effective in treating bronchial asthma and asthmatic bronchitis.

THIS DRUG SHOULD NOT BE TAKEN IF
—you have had an allergic reaction to any dosage form of it previously. A combination drug [CD] should not be taken if you are allergic to *any* of its ingredients.

INFORM YOUR PHYSICIAN BEFORE TAKING THIS DRUG IF
—you have high blood pressure or heart disease.
—you have an overactive thyroid gland (hyperthyroidism) or diabetes.
—you have difficulty emptying the urinary bladder.
—you are taking, or have taken during the past 2 weeks, any mono-amine oxidase (MAO) inhibitor drug (see Drug Class, Section Three).
—you are taking any form of digitalis (digitoxin, digoxin, etc.).
—you plan to have surgery under general anesthesia in the near future.

Time Required for Apparent Benefit
Drug action begins in 30 to 60 minutes and persists for 3 to 4 hours.

Possible Side-Effects (*natural, expected, and unavoidable drug actions*)
Nervousness, insomnia.

Possible Adverse Effects (*unusual, unexpected, and infrequent reactions*)

IF ANY OF THE FOLLOWING DEVELOP, DISCONTINUE DRUG AND NOTIFY YOUR PHYSICIAN AS SOON AS POSSIBLE

Mild Adverse Effects
Allergic Reactions: None reported when taken orally.
Other Reactions
Headache, dizziness, rapid and forceful heart action, chest discomfort, sweating.
Nausea, vomiting.
Difficult urination.
Serious Adverse Effects
None reported.

CAUTION
1. This drug may lose its effectiveness if taken too frequently on a continuous basis for 3 to 4 days. Interrupt regular use when possible to prevent or reduce the development of tolerance (see Glossary). Effectiveness is restored after several days of discontinuation.
2. Many over-the-counter (OTC) medications (see Glossary) for allergies, colds, and coughs contain drugs that may interact unfavorably with this drug. Ask your physician or pharmacist for guidance before using any such medications.

Precautions for Use by Those over 60 Years of Age
You may be more sensitive to the stimulant effects of this drug. Small doses are advisable until your individual response has been determined.
You may be more susceptible to the development of high blood pressure, disturbance of heart rhythm, angina, nervousness, or insomnia.

Advisability of Use During Pregnancy

Pregnancy Category: C (tentative). See Pregnancy Code inside back cover. Animal reproduction studies: No data available.

Information from adequate studies in pregnant women is not available. Ask physician for guidance.

Advisability of Use While Nursing Infant

Drug is known to be present in milk and to have adverse effects on the young infant. Avoid drug or discontinue nursing. Ask physician for guidance.

Habit-Forming Potential

None.

Effects of Overdosage

With Moderate Overdose: Marked nervousness, restlessness, headache, heart palpitation, sweating, nausea, vomiting.

With Large Overdose: Anxiety, confusion, delirium, muscular tremors, rapid and irregular pulse.

Possible Effects of Extended Use

None reported with normal dosage.

A toxic form of mental derangement (toxic psychosis) has resulted from long-term use of excessive doses.

Long-term use in men with prostate gland enlargement may cause increased difficulty in emptying the urinary bladder.

Suggested Periodic Examinations While Taking This Drug (at physician's discretion)

None required.

While Taking This Drug, Observe the Following

Foods: No restrictions.

Beverages: Excessive coffee or tea may add to the nervousness or insomnia caused by this drug in sensitive individuals.

Alcohol: No interactions expected.

Tobacco Smoking: No interactions expected; no restrictions unless advised otherwise by your physician.

Marijuana Smoking

Occasional (once or twice weekly):   Mild and transient increased heart rate; transient improvement in anti-asthmatic effect of this drug.

Daily: Persistent rapid heart rate; possible heart rhythm disturbance (in sensitive individuals); persistent improvement in anti-asthmatic effect of this drug.

Other Drugs

Ephedrine may *increase* the effects of

• epinephrine (Adrenalin, Bronkaid Mist, Vaponefrin, etc.), and cause excessive stimulation of the heart and an increase in blood pressure. Use caution and avoid excessive dosage.

Ephedrine may *decrease* the effects of
• anti-hypertensive drugs (see Drug Class, Section Three), and reduce their effectiveness in lowering blood pressure. Ask physician if any dosage adjustment is necessary to maintain proper blood pressure control.

Ephedrine *taken concurrently* with
• digitalis preparations (digitoxin, digoxin, etc.), may cause serious disturbances of heart rhythm.
• ergot-related preparations (Cafergot, Ergotrate, Migral, Wigraine, etc.), may cause serious increase in blood pressure.
• guanethidine, may result in reduced effectiveness of both drugs.

The following drugs may *increase* the effects of ephedrine
• mono-amine oxidase (MAO) inhibitor drugs (see Drug Class, Section Three). The combined effects may cause a dangerous increase in blood pressure.
• tricyclic antidepressants (see Drug Class, Section Three). The combined effect may cause excessive stimulation of the heart and blood pressure.

Driving a Vehicle, Operating Machinery, Engaging in Hazardous Activities: No restrictions unless dizziness occurs.

Aviation Note: The use of this drug *may be a disqualification* for the piloting of aircraft. Consultation with a designated Aviation Medical Examiner is advised.

Exposure to Sun: No restrictions.

Special Storage Instructions
Keep in a tightly closed, light-resistant container. Avoid excessive heat.

EPINEPHRINE
(Adrenaline)

Year Introduced: 1900

Brand Names

USA	Canada
Adrenalin (Parke-Davis)	Adrenalin (P.D. & Co.)
Epifrin (Allergan)	Bronkaid Mistometer
Glaucon (Alcon)	(Winthrop)
Medihaler-Epi (Riker)	Dysne-Inhal (Rougier)
Primatene Mist	Epifrin (Allergan)
(Whitehall)	Epitrate (Ayerst)
Sus-Phrine (Berlex)	Glaucon (Alcon)
Vaponefrin (Fisons)	Medihaler-Epi (Riker)
	Sus-Phrine (Pentagone)
	Vaponefrin (USV)

Common Synonyms ("Street Names"):   None

Drug Class: Anti-allergic, Anti-asthmatic (Bronchodilator), Anti-glaucoma, Decongestant

Prescription Required: USA: For nose drops and most nebulizer preparations—No
For eye drops and injection preparations—Yes
Canada: No

Available for Purchase by Generic Name: Yes

Available Dosage Forms and Strengths

Eye drops — 0.25%, 0.50%, 1.0%, 2.0%
Nose drops — 0.1%
Aerosol nebulizer — 0.16 mg., 0.20 mg., 0.25 mg. per spray
Solution for nebulizer — 1%, 2.25%
Solution for injection — 1:100,000, 1:10,000, 1:1000, 1:200

How This Drug Works
Intended Therapeutic Effect(s):   The principal uses of this drug include
- the relief of severe allergic symptoms associated with anaphylactic reaction to insect stings, allergenic extracts, other drugs, etc.
- the temporary relief of acute bronchial spasm associated with allergic asthma, asthmatic bronchitis, or emphysema.
- the reduction of internal eye pressure.
- the relief of congestion of the nose, sinuses, and throat associated with allergic disorders.

Location of Drug Action(s):   Principal sites of therapeutic actions include sympathetic nerve terminals in:
- the walls of blood vessels throughout the body.
- the walls of the bronchial tubes.
- the tissues of the eye that regulate the formation and drainage of internal eye fluids.
- the small blood vessels (arterioles) in the tissues lining the nasal passages, the sinuses, and the throat.

Method of Drug Action(s):   By stimulating certain sympathetic nerve terminals, this drug acts to:
- contract blood vessel walls and raise the blood pressure.
- inhibit the release of harmful amounts of histamine into the skin and internal organs.
- dilate those bronchial tubes that are in sustained constriction, thereby increasing the size of the airways and improving the ability to breathe.
- decrease the formation of fluid within the eye, increase its outflow from the eye, and thereby reduce the internal eye pressure.
- decrease the volume of blood in nasal tissue, thereby shrinking the tissue mass (decongestion) and expanding the nasal airway.

Principal Uses of This Drug

As a Single Drug Product: This drug is used most commonly by inhalation to relieve acute attacks of bronchial asthma. It is used less frequently as a decongestant for symptomatic relief of nasal congestion, and as eye drops in the management of glaucoma.

THIS DRUG SHOULD NOT BE TAKEN IF

—you have had an allergic reaction to any dosage form of it previously.
—you have narrow angle glaucoma.
—you have experienced a recent stroke or heart attack.

INFORM YOUR PHYSICIAN BEFORE TAKING THIS DRUG IF

—you have any degree of high blood pressure.
—you have any form of heart disease, especially coronary heart disease (with or without angina), or a heart rhythm disorder.
—you have diabetes.
—you have overactive thyroid function (hyperthyroidism).
—you have a history of stroke.
—you are taking any of the following drugs: MAO inhibitors, phenothiazines (see Drug Classes, Section Three), digitalis preparations, or quinidine.

Time Required for Apparent Benefit

By inhalation—action begins within 1 to 2 minutes.
By injection—action begins within 3 to 5 minutes.
Maximal effect usually occurs within 20 to 60 minutes.

Possible Side-Effects *(natural, expected, and unavoidable drug actions)*
In sensitive individuals—restlessness, anxiety, headache, tremor, palpitation, coldness of hands and feet, dryness of mouth and throat (with use of aerosol).

Possible Adverse Effects *(unusual, unexpected, and infrequent reactions)*

IF ANY OF THE FOLLOWING DEVELOP, DISCONTINUE DRUG AND NOTIFY YOUR PHYSICIAN AS SOON AS POSSIBLE

Mild Adverse Effects
Allergic Reactions
Skin rash.
Eye drops may cause redness, swelling and itching of the eyelids.
Other Reactions: Weakness, dizziness, pallor.

Serious Adverse Effects
Idiosyncratic Reactions: Sudden development of excessive fluid in the lungs (pulmonary edema).
Other Reactions: In predisposed individuals—excessive rise in blood pressure with resultant stroke (cerebral hemorrhage).

CAUTION
1. The frequently repeated use of this drug at short intervals can produce a condition of unresponsiveness and result in medication failure. If this develops, avoid use completely for 12 hours, at which time normal response should return.
2. Excessive use of aerosol preparations in the management of asthma has been associated with sudden death.
3. This drug can cause significant irritability of the nerve pathways and muscles of the heart, and predispose to serious disturbances of heart rhythm. If you have any form of heart disorder, consult your physician for guidance.
4. This drug can increase the blood sugar level. If you have diabetes, test your urine for sugar frequently to detect significant changes.
5. If you become unresponsive to this drug and you intend to substitute isoproterenol (Isuprel), allow an interval of 4 hours between using these two drugs.
6. *Promptly discard* all preparations of this drug at the first appearance of discoloration (pink to red to brown) or cloudiness (precipitation). Such changes indicate drug deterioration.

Precautions for Use by Those over 60 Years of Age
If you have hardening of the arteries (arteriosclerosis), heart disease, or high blood pressure, use this drug with caution. It can precipitate episodes of angina and disturbances of heart rhythm; it can cause sudden elevation of the blood pressure and induce stroke.
If you have difficulty with urination due to enlargement of the prostate gland (prostatism), this drug may increase the difficulty. Ask physician for guidance.
If you have Parkinson's disease, this drug may temporarily increase the rigidity and tremor in your extremities.

If you use this drug in the form of eye drops to treat glaucoma, report the development of "floaters" in your field of vision.

Advisability of Use During Pregnancy
Pregnancy Category: C (tentative). See Pregnancy Code inside back cover. Animal reproduction studies in mice and rats are inconclusive. Information from adequate studies in pregnant women is not available. Ask physician for guidance.

Advisability of Use While Nursing Infant
No adverse effects on milk formation or on infant.

Habit-Forming Potential
Although tolerance to this drug can develop with frequent use, neither psychological nor physical dependence (addiction) occurs (see Glossary).

Effects of Overdosage
With Moderate Overdose: Nervousness, anxiety, throbbing headache, tremor, dizziness, rapid breathing, palpitation.
With Large Overdose: Extreme increase in blood pressure, severe headache, disturbance of heart rhythm, difficult breathing, abdominal pain, vomiting of blood, reduced urine volume.

Possible Effects of Extended Use
"Epinephrine-fastness"—loss of ability to respond to the drug's bronchodilator effect.
Reduction of blood volume due to movement of water from bloodstream to body tissues.
With long-term treatment of glaucoma—pigment deposits on eyeball and eyelids, possible damage to retina, impaired vision, and blockage of the tear ducts.

Suggested Periodic Examinations While Taking This Drug (at physician's discretion)
Blood pressure measurements.
Blood and/or urine sugar measurements in presence of diabetes.
Vision testing and measurement of internal eye pressure in presence of glaucoma.

While Taking This Drug, Observe the Following
Foods: No restrictions. Be alert to the possibility that certain foods can induce allergic reactions in the form of skin rashes, hives, and asthma.
Beverages: No restrictions. Maintain adequate fluid intake (at least 1 and one-half quarts daily) during prolonged use of this drug.
Alcohol: Alcoholic beverages can increase the urinary excretion of this drug and reduce the effectiveness of the long-acting suspension given by injection.
Tobacco Smoking: No interactions expected. Follow physician's advice regarding smoking as it affects the condition under treatment.

Marijuana Smoking
   Occasional (once or twice weekly):   Mild and transient improvement in anti-asthmatic effect of this drug.
   Daily: More persistent improvement in anti-asthmatic effect of this drug.
Other Drugs
   Epinephrine may *increase* the effects of
   • ephedrine, and cause excessive stimulation of the heart and an increase in blood pressure.
   • pilocarpine, and augment its action in reducing internal eye pressure (desirable in glaucoma).

   Epinephrine may *decrease* the effects of
   • oral anti-diabetic drugs (Diabinese, Dymelor, Orinase, Tolinase).
   • insulin

   Epinephrine *taken concurrently* with
   • digitalis preparations (digitoxin, digoxin), may increase the possibility of significant heart rhythm disturbances.
   • isoproterenol (Isuprel, etc.), is potentially dangerous and should be avoided. These drugs should be given separately and at least 4 hours apart.
   • mono-amine oxidase (MAO) inhibitor drugs (see Drug Class, Section Three) is potentially dangerous and should be undertaken with extreme caution.

   The following drugs may *increase* the effects of epinephrine:
   • acetazolamide (Diamox) may augment its effect in reducing internal eye pressure.
   • chlorpheniramine (Chlor-Trimeton, etc.).
   • cocaine may increase sensitivity to epinephrine.
   • dexchlorpheniramine (Polaramine).
   • diphenhydramine (Benadryl, etc.).
   • guanethidine (Ismelin).
   • reserpine (Serpasil, etc.).
   • thyroid preparations.
   • tricyclic antidepressants (see Drug Class, Section Three).
   • tripelennamine (Pyribenzamine, etc.).

   The following drug may *decrease* the effects of epinephrine:
   • propranolol (Inderal).
Driving a Vehicle, Operating Machinery, Engaging in Hazardous Activities: No restrictions. Use caution if excessive nervousness or dizziness occurs.
Aviation Note: The use of this drug *may be a disqualification* for the piloting of aircraft. Consultation with a designated Aviation Medical Examiner is advised.
Exposure to Sun: No restrictions.
Exposure to Cold: No restrictions. Protect hands and feet from prolonged exposure to excessive cold.

Heavy Exercise or Exertion: No interactions with drug. However, excessive exertion can induce asthma in sensitive individuals.

Occurrence of Unrelated Illness: Use caution in presence of severe burns. This drug can increase drainage from burned tissue with significant loss of fluids and blood proteins.

Discontinuation: If this drug fails to provide relief after adequate trial, discontinue it and consult your physician regarding alternate drug therapy. Do not increase the dosage or the frequency of use. To do so could be dangerous.

Special Storage Instructions

Protect from exposure to air, light, and heat. Keep in a cool place, preferably in the refrigerator.

ERGOLOID MESYLATES
(formerly Ergot Alkaloids)

Year Introduced: 1949

Brand Names

USA	Canada
Circanol (Riker)	Hydergine (Sandoz)
Deapril-ST (Mead Johnson)	
Hydergine (Sandoz)	

Common Synonyms ("Street Names"):   None

Drug Class: Ergot Preparations

Prescription Required: Yes

Available for Purchase by Generic Name: Yes

Available Dosage Forms and Strengths
Tablets — 1 mg.
Sublingual tablets — 0.5 mg., 1.0 mg.
Oral liquid — 1 mg. per 1 ml.

Tablet May Be Crushed or Capsule Opened for Administration
Regular tablets — Yes

How This Drug Works

Intended Therapeutic Effect(s): Alleviation of disturbing mental symptoms commonly experienced by the elderly, such as reduced alertness, poor memory, confusion, lack of motivation, and emotional depression.

Location of Drug Action(s): Those areas of the brain that are responsible for intellect, personality, and behavior.

Method of Drug Action(s): Not completely established. Present theory is that by stimulating brain cell metabolism, this drug increases the brain's ability to utilize oxygen and nutrients. The resulting improvement in brain function is thought to contribute to the benefit seen in responsive patients.

Principal Uses of This Drug

As a Single Drug Product: The use of this drug is limited to the treatment of the aging individual with symptoms indicative of deteriorating brain function. Its benefit is unpredictable, and its use must be monitored carefully and adjusted appropriately for each individual.

THIS DRUG SHOULD NOT BE TAKEN IF
—you have had an allergic reaction to any dosage form of it previously.
—your pulse rate is below 60 beats per minute.
—your systolic blood pressure is consistently below 100.

INFORM YOUR PHYSICIAN BEFORE TAKING THIS DRUG IF
—you have a history of low blood pressure.
—you are taking any drugs for high blood pressure.
—you are taking any digitalis preparation.
—you are taking propranolol (Inderal).

Time Required for Apparent Benefit
Relief of symptoms is usually gradual. Continuous use on a regular schedule for 3 to 4 weeks may be necessary to produce improvement.

Possible Side-Effects *(natural, expected and unavoidable drug actions)*
None expected.

Possible Adverse Effects *(unusual, unexpected and infrequent reactions)*

IF ANY OF THE FOLLOWING DEVELOP, DISCONTINUE DRUG AND NOTIFY YOUR PHYSICIAN AS SOON AS POSSIBLE

Mild Adverse Effects
Allergic Reactions: Skin rashes (various kinds), drug fever (see Glossary).
Other Reactions
Headache, dizziness, flushing, blurred vision.
Nasal stuffiness, reduced appetite, nausea, vomiting, abdominal cramping.

Serious Adverse Effects
Marked drop in blood pressure, fainting.
Marked slowing of the heart rate (pulse count 40 to 50 beats per minute), accompanied by reduced activity, sluggishness, drowsiness, emotional withdrawal, and apathy.

CAUTION
Numerous studies have demonstrated that this drug can be beneficial in relieving many complaints of the elderly related to memory, intellectual performance, and social adjustment. However, it is important to remember that the causes of such symptoms are poorly understood, that they can occur whether or not drugs are being taken, and that behavioral changes in the

elderly are often frequent and unpredictable. It is therefore advisable to monitor the response to this drug very closely, and to notify the physician if any significant adverse personality changes occur. In some instances, the development of nervousness, hostility, confusion, and depression may be related to the use of the drug.

Precautions for Use by Those over 60 Years of Age
It is not possible to predict in advance the nature of your response to this drug. It may relieve your symptoms, have no significant effect, or make your symptoms worse. Dosage must be carefully individualized. See Caution.

Habit-Forming Potential
None

Effects of Overdosage
With Moderate Overdose: Headache, flushing of the face, nasal stuffiness.
With Large Overdose: Nausea, vomiting, extreme drop in blood pressure, weakness, collapse, coma.

Possible Effects of Extended Use
None reported.

Suggested Periodic Examinations While Taking This Drug (at physician's discretion)
Pulse counts and blood pressure measurements on a regular basis.

While Taking This Drug, Observe the Following
Foods: No restrictions.
Beverages: No restrictions.
Alcohol: Use with caution until combined effects have been determined. Sensitive individuals may experience an excessive drop in blood pressure.
Tobacco Smoking: No interactions expected.
Marijuana Smoking
Occasional (once or twice weekly): No interactions expected.
Daily: Possible reduced effectiveness of this drug.
Other Drugs
Ergot alkaloids may *increase* the effects of
• antihypertensive drugs, and cause excessive lowering of the blood pressure.

Ergot alkaloids *taken concurrently* with
• digitalis preparations may cause excessive slowing of the heart rate.
• propranolol (Inderal) may cause excessive slowing of the heart rate and/or excessive lowering of the blood pressure.

Driving a Vehicle, Operating Machinery, Engaging in Hazardous Activities:
No restrictions, unless dizziness or blurring of vision should occur with use of the drug.

Aviation Note: Brain function disorder *is a disqualification* for the piloting of aircraft. Consultation with a designated Aviation Medical Examiner is advised.

Exposure to Sun: No restrictions.

Exposure to Cold: Use caution. Avoid exposure that could lower body temperature and impair metabolism.

Heavy Exercise or Exertion: No restriction, if exertion is in keeping with physical condition.

Special Storage Instructions

Keep in a tightly closed container. Do not store at temperature above 86°F. (30°C.).

ERGOTAMINE

Year Introduced: 1926

Brand Names

USA		Canada
Ergomar (Fisons)	Cafergot P-B [CD]	Ergomar (Fisons)
Ergostat	(Sandoz)	Gynergen (Sandoz)
(Parke-Davis)	Wigraine [CD]	Medihaler-
Gynergen (Sandoz)	(Organon)	Ergotamine (Riker)
Medihaler-	(Several other	Bellergal [CD]
Ergotamine (Riker)	combination brand	(Sandoz)
Bellergal [CD]	names)	Cafergot [CD]
(Sandoz)		(Sandoz)
Cafergot [CD]		Ergodryl [CD] (P.D.)
(Sandoz)		Wigraine [CD]
		(Organon)

Common Synonyms ("Street Names"): Headache pills

Drug Class: Migraine Analgesic (Vasoconstrictor)

Prescription Required: Yes

Available for Purchase by Generic Name: No

Available Dosage Forms and Strengths

Tablets — 1 mg.
Sublingual tablets — 2 mg.
Aerosol inhaler — 9 mg. per ml.
Suppositories — 2 mg. (in combination with caffeine)

Tablet May Be Crushed or Capsule Opened for Administration

Regular tablets — Yes

How This Drug Works

Intended Therapeutic Effect(s): Prevention and early relief of blood vessel (vascular) headaches, such as migraine, variations of migraine, and histamine headaches.

Location of Drug Action(s):   The principal site of therapeutic action is the muscular tissue of blood vessel walls.

Method of Drug Action(s):   By directly constricting the walls of blood vessels in the head, this drug prevents or relieves the excessive expansion (dilation) responsible for the pain of migraine-like headaches.

Principal Uses of This Drug

As a Single Drug Product: This drug is used primarily in the treatment of vascular headaches, specifically migraine and "cluster" headaches. It should not be used to prevent migraine attacks, but is often effective in terminating the headache if taken within the first hour following the onset of pain. It may be used on a short-term basis in an attempt to prevent or abort "cluster" headaches during the period of their occurrence. The inhalation form provides rapid onset of action.

As a Combination Drug Product [CD]:   This drug is combined with caffeine to take advantage of caffeine's ability to enhance its absorption. This permits a smaller dose of ergotamine to be effective and reduces the risk of adverse effects with repeated use. This drug is also combined with belladonna (atropine) and one of the barbiturates to provide preparations that are useful in relieving the symptoms of premenstrual tension and the menopausal syndrome—nervousness, nausea, hot flushes, and sweating.

THIS DRUG SHOULD NOT BE TAKEN IF
—you have had an allergic reaction to any dosage form of it previously.
—you are pregnant.
—you are experiencing a severe infection.
—you have any of the following conditions:
angina pectoris
Buerger's disease
coronary artery disease
hardening of the arteries (arteriosclerosis)
high blood pressure (severe hypertension)
kidney disease (or impaired kidney function)
liver disease (or impaired liver function)
Raynaud's phenomenon
thrombophlebitis
severe itching

INFORM YOUR PHYSICIAN BEFORE TAKING THIS DRUG IF
—you have had an allergic reaction to *any* derivative of ergot in the past.

Time Required for Apparent Benefit
If taken at the onset of headache, relief is usually felt in 30 to 60 minutes. If use of the drug is delayed, larger doses and a longer period of time are needed to obtain relief.

Possible Side-Effects *(natural, expected, and unavoidable drug actions)*
Usually infrequent and mild with recommended dosage. Susceptible individuals may notice a sensation of cold hands and feet with mild numbness and tingling.

Possible Adverse Effects *(unusual, unexpected, and infrequent reactions)*

IF ANY OF THE FOLLOWING DEVELOP, DISCONTINUE DRUG AND NOTIFY YOUR PHYSICIAN AS SOON AS POSSIBLE

Mild Adverse Effects
Allergic Reactions: Localized swellings, itching.
Other Reactions
Nausea, vomiting, diarrhea.
Chest pain, numbness and tingling of fingers and toes, muscle pains in arms or legs.
Headache, dizziness, confusion, drowsiness.

Serious Adverse Effects
Gangrene of the intestine—severe abdominal pain and swelling; emergency surgery required.
Gangrene of the extremities—coldness, numbness, pain, dark discoloration, eventual loss of fingers, toes, or feet.

CAUTION
Do not exceed a total dose of 6 mg. in 24 hours or 12 mg. in 1 week. Limit use of this drug to the following:
Tablets—no more than 6 in 24 hours or 12 in 1 week.
Sublingual tablets—no more than 3 in 24 hours or 6 in 1 week.
Aerosol inhaler—no more than 6 inhalations in 24 hours or 15 in 1 week.
Suppositories—no more than 3 in 24 hours or 6 in 1 week.
Injection—no more than 12 ml. in 24 hours or 24 ml. in 1 week. (If DHE-45 is used, no more than 6 ml. in 24 hours or 12 ml. in 1 week.)

Precautions for Use by Those over 60 Years of Age
The natural changes in blood vessels and circulatory function that occur after 60 can make you more susceptible to the serious adverse effects of this drug.
See the list of diseases and disorders above which are contraindications to the use of this drug. Consult your physician for guidance.

Advisability of Use During Pregnancy
Pregnancy Category: X (tentative). See Pregnancy Code inside back cover.
Animal reproduction studies: No data available.
Information from studies in pregnant women indicates that this drug can cause abortion.
The manufacturers state that this drug is contraindicated during entire pregnancy.
Ask physician for guidance.

Advisability cf Use While Nursing Infant
Drug is known to be present in milk. Avoid use or avoid nursing. Ask physician for guidance.

Habit-Forming Potential
None.

Effects of Overdosage

With Moderate Overdose: Manifestation of "ergotism"—coldness of skin, severe muscle pains, tingling and burning pain in hands and feet, loss of blood supply to extremities resulting in tissue death (gangrene).

With Large Overdose: Ergot poisoning—nausea, vomiting, diarrhea, cold skin, rapid and weak pulse, numbness and tingling of extremities, confusion, convulsions, coma.

Possible Effects of Extended Use

Risk of developing "ergotism"—chronic overdosage (see above).

Suggested Periodic Examinations While Taking This Drug (at physician's discretion)

Evaluation of circulatory status (blood flow) to extremities.

While Taking This Drug, Observe the Following

Foods: Avoid all foods to which you are allergic. Some migraine headaches are due to food allergies. (No foods are known to interact with this drug.)

Beverages: No restrictions. Coffee may be beneficial in relieving migraine headache.

Alcohol: Best avoided while using this drug to treat a vascular (blood vessel) headache.

Tobacco Smoking: Nicotine may reduce further the restricted circulation (blood flow) produced by this drug. Follow physician's advice regarding smoking.

Marijuana Smoking

Occasional (once or twice weekly): No effect to mild and transient cooling of hands and/or feet.

Daily: More marked and persistent coldness of hands and/or feet.

Other Drugs

Ergotamine may *increase* the effects of

• amphetamines, Adrenalin, ephedrine, and pseudoephedrine, and cause a dangerous rise in blood pressure.

The following drugs may *increase* the effects of ergotamine:

• TAO (troleandomycin) may delay its elimination from the body and thus produce overdose ("ergotism").

• caffeine can add to this drug's ability to constrict blood vessels in the head and so relieve the pain of migraine headache.

Driving a Vehicle, Operating Machinery, Engaging in Hazardous Activities: Usually no restrictions. Avoid hazardous activities if drowsiness or dizziness occurs.

Aviation Note: Migraine headache *is a disqualification* for the piloting of aircraft. Consultation with a designated Aviation Medical Examiner is advised.

Exposure to Sun: No restrictions.

Exposure to Cold: Avoid as much as possible. Cold environments and handling of cold objects will reduce further the restricted circulation (blood flow) to the arms and legs which is part of this drug's normal action.

Special Storage Instructions

Keep all preparations in a cool place. Protect from light and heat. Store suppositories in a refrigerator.

ERYTHRITYL TETRANITRATE

Year Introduced: 1957

Brand Names

USA	Canada
Cardilate (Burroughs Wellcome)	Cardilate (Calmic)

Common Synonyms ("Street Names"):   Angina pills, heart pills

Drug Class: Anti-anginal, Vasodilator, Nitrates

Prescription Required: USA: Yes   Canada: No

Available for Purchase by Generic Name: No

Available Dosage Forms and Strengths
Tablets — 5 mg., 10 mg.
Chewable tablets — 10 mg.

Tablet May Be Crushed or Capsule Opened for Administration: Yes

How This Drug Works

Intended Therapeutic Effect(s):   Reduction in the frequency and severity of pain associated with angina pectoris (coronary insufficiency).

Location of Drug Action(s):   The muscular tissue in the walls of the blood vessels. The principal site of the therapeutic action is the system of coronary arteries in the heart.

Method of Drug Action(s):   This drug acts directly on the muscle cell to produce relaxation. This permits expansion of blood vessels and increases the supply of blood and oxygen to meet the needs of the working heart muscle.

Principal Uses of This Drug

As a Single Drug Product: This member of the nitrate class is used primarily in the treatment of symptomatic coronary artery disease with angina pectoris. The dosage forms available can be dissolved under the tongue or swallowed, thus permitting either rapid onset of action to relieve the pain of acute angina, or gradual and prolonged effect to prevent the development of angina during exertion. Recently the nitrates have been shown to be useful in treating selected cases of congestive heart failure that no longer respond to standard treatment with digitalis and diuretics.

THIS DRUG SHOULD NOT BE TAKEN IF
—you have had an allergic reaction to any dosage form of it previously.

INFORM YOUR PHYSICIAN BEFORE TAKING THIS DRUG IF
—you have glaucoma.
—you have had an unfavorable response to any vasodilator drug in the past.

Time Required for Apparent Benefit
The action of sublingual use (dissolved under the tongue) or chewed tablets begins in approximately 5 minutes, reaches a maximum in 30 to 45 minutes, and persists for 3 to 4 hours. The action of the swallowed tablet begins in approximately 30 minutes, reaches a maximum in 60 to 90 minutes, and persists for 3 to 4 hours.

Possible Side-Effects *(natural, expected, and unavoidable drug actions)*
Flushing, lightheadedness in upright position (see orthostatic hypotension in Glossary).

Possible Adverse Effects *(unusual, unexpected, and infrequent reactions)*

IF ANY OF THE FOLLOWING DEVELOP, DISCONTINUE DRUG AND NOTIFY YOUR PHYSICIAN AS SOON AS POSSIBLE

Mild Adverse Effects
Allergic Reactions: Skin rash.
Other Reactions
Headache (may be persistent), dizziness, fainting.
Nausea, vomiting.
Serious Adverse Effects
Allergic Reactions: Severe dermatitis with peeling of skin.

CAUTION
Many over-the-counter (OTC) medications (see Glossary) for allergies, colds, and coughs contain drugs that may counteract the desired effects of this drug. Ask your physician or pharmacist for guidance before using any such medications.

Precautions for Use by Those over 60 Years of Age
You may be more sensitive to the actions of this drug. Small doses are advisable until your individual response has been determined.
You may be more susceptible to the development of low blood pressure with associated lightheadedness, dizziness, unsteadiness, and falling.

Advisability of Use During Pregnancy
Pregnancy Category: C (tentative). See Pregnancy Code inside back cover.
Animal reproduction studies: No data available.
Information from adequate studies in pregnant women is not available. Ask physician for guidance.

Advisability of Use While Nursing Infant
Presence of drug in milk is not known. Safety for infant not established. Ask physician for guidance.

Habit-Forming Potential
None.

Effects of Overdosage
With Moderate Overdose: Headache, dizziness, marked flushing of the skin.
With Large Overdose: Vomiting, weakness, sweating, fainting, shortness of breath, coma.

Possible Effects of Extended Use
Development of tolerance (see Glossary) which may reduce the drug's effectiveness at recommended doses.
Development of abnormal hemoglobin (red blood cell pigment).

Suggested Periodic Examinations While Taking This Drug (at physician's discretion)
Measurement of internal eye pressure in those individuals with glaucoma or a tendency to glaucoma.
Red blood cell counts and hemoglobin measurements.

While Taking This Drug, Observe the Following
Foods: No restrictions. Drug is likely to be more effective if taken one-half to 1 hour before eating.
Beverages: No restrictions.
Alcohol: Use with extreme caution until combined effects have been determined. Alcohol may exaggerate the drop in blood pressure experienced by some sensitive individuals. This could be dangerous.
Tobacco Smoking: Nicotine may reduce the effectiveness of this drug. Follow physician's advice regarding smoking, based upon its effect on the condition under treatment and its possible interaction with this drug.
Marijuana Smoking
Occasional (once or twice weekly):   No interactions expected.
Daily: Possible reduced effectiveness of this drug; mild to moderate increase in angina; possible changes in electrocardiogram, confusing interpretation.
Other Drugs
Erythrityl may *increase* the effects of
• atropine-like drugs (see Drug Class, Section Three), and cause an increase in internal eye pressure.
• tricyclic antidepressants (see Drug Class, Section Three), and cause excessive lowering of the blood pressure.

Erythrityl may *decrease* the effects of
• all choline-like drugs, such as Mestinon, Mytelase, pilocarpine, Prostigmin, and Urecholine.

Erythrityl *taken concurrently* with
• anti-hypertensive drugs, may cause severe drop in blood pressure. Careful monitoring of drug response and appropriate dosage adjustments are necessary.

The following drug may *increase* the effects of erythrityl:

• propranolol (Inderal) may cause additional lowering of the blood pressure. Dosage adjustments may be necessary.

Driving a Vehicle, Operating Machinery, Engaging in Hazardous Activities: Usually no restrictions. Before engaging in hazardous activities, determine that this drug will not cause you to have orthostatic hypotension (see Glossary).

Aviation Note: Coronary artery disease *is a disqualification* for the piloting of aircraft. Consultation with a designated Aviation Medical Examiner is advised.

Exposure to Sun: No restrictions.

Exposure to Cold: Cold environment may reduce the effectiveness of this drug.

Heavy Exercise or Exertion: This drug may improve your ability to be more active without the resulting angina pain. Use caution and avoid excessive exertion that could cause heart injury in the absence of warning pain.

Special Storage Instructions

Keep in a dry, tightly closed container and in a cool place. Protect from heat and light.

ERYTHROMYCIN

Year Introduced: 1952 (Erythromycin, early forms)
1958 (Erythromycin estolate)

Brand Names

USA		Canada
Bristamycin (Bristol)	Kesso-Mycin	Apo-Erythro-S
E.E.S. (Abbott)	(McKesson)	(Apotex)
E-Mycin (Upjohn)	Pediamycin (Ross)	EES-200 (Abbott)
EryDerm (Abbott)	Pfizer-E (Pfizer)	EES-400 (Abbott)
Erypar (Parke-Davis)	Robimycin (Robins)	E-Mycin (Upjohn)
Erythrocin (Abbott)	RP-Mycin	Erythrocin (Abbott)
Ethril (Squibb)	(Reid-Provident)	Erythromid (Abbott)
Ilosone (Dista)	SK-Erythromycin	Ilosone (Lilly)
Ilotycin (Dista)	(Smith Kline &	Ilotycin (Lilly)
	French)	Novorythro
	Wyamycin (Wyeth)	(Novopharm)

Common Synonyms ("Street Names"):   None

Drug Class: Antibiotic (Anti-infective), Erythromycins

Prescription Required: USA: Yes   Canada: No

Available for Purchase by Generic Name: Yes

Available Dosage Forms and Strengths

Tablets — 125 mg., 250 mg., 400 mg., 500 mg.

Chewable tablets — 125 mg., 200 mg., 250 mg.

Enteric-coated tablets — 250 mg., 333 mg.

Capsules — 125 mg., 250 mg.

Oral suspension — 125 mg., 200 mg., 250 mg., 400 mg. per teaspoonful (5 ml.)

Pediatric suspension — 200 mg. per teaspoonful (5 ml.)

Pediatric drops — 100 mg. per 2.5 ml., 100 mg. per 1 ml.

Skin ointment — 1%

Eye ointment — 0.5%

Skin solution — 1.5%, 2%

Tablet May Be Crushed or Capsule Opened for Administration

Regular tablets and capsules — Yes

Enteric-coated tablets (E-Mycin) — No

Ilotycin tablets — No

How This Drug Works

Intended Therapeutic Effect(s):   The elimination of infections responsive to the action of this drug.

Location of Drug Action(s):   Any body tissue or fluid in which sufficient concentration of the drug can be achieved.

Method of Drug Action(s):   This drug prevents the growth and multiplication of susceptible bacteria by interfering with their formation of essential proteins.

Principal Uses of This Drug

As a Single Drug Product: This well-tolerated and versatile antibiotic is used to treat a broad variety of common infections. The more important among these are (1) skin and soft tissue infections; (2) upper and lower respiratory tract infections, including "strep" throat, diphtheria, and several types of pneumonia; (3) gonorrhea and syphilis; and (4) amebic dysentery. It is also used for the long-term prevention of recurrences of rheumatic fever. Effective use requires the precise identification of the causative organism and determination of its sensitivity to erythromycin.

THIS DRUG SHOULD NOT BE TAKEN IF

—you have had an allergic reaction to any dosage form of it previously.

—you have a history of liver disease or impaired liver function and one of the preparations of erythromycin *estolate* has been prescribed for you (Ilosone, Novorythro).

INFORM YOUR PHYSICIAN BEFORE TAKING THIS DRUG IF

—you have taken any form of erythromycin estolate in the past.

Time Required for Apparent Benefit

Varies with nature of infection under treatment; usually 2 to 5 days.

Possible Side-Effects *(natural, expected, and unavoidable drug actions)*
Superinfections (see Glossary).

Possible Adverse Effects *(unusual, unexpected, and infrequent reactions)*

IF ANY OF THE FOLLOWING DEVELOP, DISCONTINUE DRUG AND NOTIFY YOUR PHYSICIAN AS SOON AS POSSIBLE

Mild Adverse Effects
  Allergic Reactions: Skin rash, hives.
  Other Reactions: Nausea, vomiting, diarrhea (all infrequent).
Serious Adverse Effects
  Erythromycin estolate preparations (see above) can cause liver damage with jaundice (see Glossary). These forms of erythromycin should not be used for long-term treatment.

CAUTION

Troublesome and persistent diarrhea can develop in sensitive individuals. If diarrhea persists more than 24 hours, discontinue this drug and consult your physician for guidance.

Precautions for Use by Those over 60 Years of Age

Natural changes in the skin after 60 may predispose to severe and prolonged itching reactions in the genital and anal regions. This reaction should be reported promptly.

Advisability of Use During Pregnancy

Pregnancy Category: C (tentative). See Pregnancy Code inside back cover.
  Animal reproduction studies in rats are inconclusive.
  Information from adequate studies in pregnant women is not available.
  Ask physician for guidance.

Advisability of Use While Nursing Infant

Drug may be present in milk. Safety for infant not established. Ask physician for guidance.

Habit-Forming Potential

None.

Effects of Overdosage

Possible nausea, vomiting, abdominal discomfort, diarrhea.

Possible Effects of Extended Use

Superinfections (see Glossary).

Suggested Periodic Examinations While Taking This Drug (at physician's discretion)

Liver function tests if estolate form of erythromycin is used (see above).

While Taking This Drug, Observe the Following

Foods: No restrictions of food selection. Most effective if taken 1 hour before or 2 hours after eating. Estolate forms may be taken with meals.

Beverages: No restrictions.

Alcohol: Avoid if
- you have a history of liver disease.
- you are using an estolate form of erythromycin.

Tobacco Smoking: No interactions expected.

Marijuana Smoking: No interactions expected.

Other Drugs

Erythromycin may *decrease* the effects of
- clindamycin.
- lincomycin.
- the penicillins.

Driving a Vehicle, Operating Machinery, Engaging in Hazardous Activities: Usually no restrictions. Be alert to the infrequent occurrence of nausea and/or diarrhea; restrict activities accordingly.

Aviation Note: The use of this drug *may be a disqualification* for the piloting of aircraft. Consultation with a designated Aviation Medical Examiner is advised.

Exposure to Sun: No restrictions.

Discontinuation: When used to treat infections that predispose to rheumatic fever or kidney disease, take continuously in full dosage for no less than 10 days. Ask physician for guidance regarding recommended duration of therapy.

Special Storage Instructions

Keep in a dry, tightly closed, light-resistant container, at temperatures not exceeding usual room temperature. Keep liquid forms refrigerated.

Observe the Following Expiration Times

Do not take a liquid form of this drug if it is older than 14 days.

ESTROGEN
(Conjugated Estrogens, Esterified Estrogens, Estrone and Equilin)

Year Introduced: 1942

Brand Names

USA

Estrace (Mead
  Johnson)
Estratab
  (Reid-Provident)
Estrovis (Parke-Davis)
Evex (Syntex)
Menest (Beecham)
Ogen (Abbott)
Premarin (Ayerst)
Theogen (Sig:
  Pharm.)

Menrium [CD]
  (Roche)
Milprem [CD]
  (Wallace)
PMB-200 [CD]
  (Ayerst)
PMB-400 [CD]
  (Ayerst)

Canada

C.E.S. (ICN)
Climestrone (Frosst)
Delestrogen (Squibb)
Estinyl (Schering)
Estrace (Bristol)
Estromed (Medic)
Femogen (Stickley)
Oestrilin (Desbergers)
Ogen (Abbott)
Premarin (Ayerst)
Menrium [CD]
  (Roche)

Common Synonyms ("Street Names"):   None

Drug Class: Female Sex Hormones, Estrogens

Prescription Required: Yes

Available for Purchase by Generic Name: Yes

Available Dosage Forms and Strengths
    Tablets — 0.3 mg., 0.625 mg., 1 mg., 1.25 mg., 2.5 mg.
    Injection — 1 mg., 2 mg., 5 mg., 10 mg., 20 mg., 40 mg. per ml.
Vaginal cream — 0.625 mg., 1.5 mg. per gram

Tablet May Be Crushed or Capsule Opened for Administration: Yes

How This Drug Works
  Intended Therapeutic Effect(s)
    Regulation of the menstrual cycle.
    Prevention of pregnancy.
    Relief of symptoms due to the menopause.
  Location of Drug Action(s):   Principal actions occur in
    • the female reproductive tract (the Fallopian tubes, uterus, and vagina).
    • the breast tissues.
    • a major control center in the brain known as the hypothalamus.
    • the pituitary gland.
  Method of Drug Action(s)
    By cyclic increase and decrease in tissue stimulation, estrogens prepare the
      uterus for pregnancy and (in the absence of conception) induce menstru-
      ation.

When estrogens are taken in sufficient dosage and on a regular basis, their blood and tissue levels increase to resemble those that occur during pregnancy. This prevents the pituitary gland from secreting the hormones that induce ovulation.

Estrogen preparations, taken to restore normal tissue levels, reduce the frequency and intensity of menopausal symptoms.

Principal Uses of This Drug

As a Single Drug Product: This widely-used hormone is very effective when administered in proper dosage and carefully supervised. Its primary use is supplemental ("replacement" therapy) when used to treat the following conditions: (1) ovarian failure or removal in the young woman; (2) the menopausal syndrome; (3) postmenopausal atrophy of genital tissues; and (4) postmenopausal osteoporosis. It is also used in selected cases of breast cancer and prostate cancer.

As a Combination Drug Product [CD]:   Estrogen is available in combination with chlordiazepoxide and with meprobamate. These mild tranquilizers are added to provide a calming effect that makes the combination more effective in treating selected cases of the menopausal syndrome. See the Drug Profile of the Oral Contraceptives for a discussion of the combination of estrogens and progestins.

THIS DRUG SHOULD NOT BE TAKEN IF
—you are allergic to any of the drugs bearing the brand names listed above.
—you have seriously impaired liver function.
—you have a history of thrombophlebitis, embolism, stroke, or heart attack.
—you have abnormal and unexplained vaginal bleeding.

INFORM YOUR PHYSICIAN BEFORE TAKING THIS DRUG IF
—you have a history of cancer of the breast or reproductive organs.
—you have cystic disease of the breast (cystic mastitis).
—you have fibroid tumors of the uterus.
—you have a history of endometriosis.
—you have migraine headaches or epilepsy.
—you have a history of porphyria.
—you have diabetes.
—you have high blood pressure.

Time Required for Apparent Benefit
Continuous use on a regular schedule for 10 to 20 days may be needed to determine the degree of effectiveness in relieving symptoms.

Possible Side-Effects *(natural, expected, and unavoidable drug actions)*
Retention of fluid, gain in weight, "breakthrough" bleeding (spotting in middle of menstrual cycle), change in menstrual flow, resumption of menstrual flow (bleeding from the uterus) after a period of natural cessation (postmenopausal bleeding). There may be an increased susceptibility to yeast infection of the genital tissues.

Possible Adverse Effects *(unusual, unexpected, and infrequent reactions)*

IF ANY OF THE FOLLOWING DEVELOP, DISCONTINUE DRUG AND NOTIFY YOUR PHYSICIAN AS SOON AS POSSIBLE

Mild Adverse Effects
Allergic Reactions: Skin rash.
Other Reactions
Nausea, vomiting, indigestion, bloating.
Accentuation of migraine headaches.
Breast enlargement, congestion, and tenderness.

Serious Adverse Effects
Idiosyncratic Reactions: Development of cutaneous porphyria—fragility and scarring of the skin.
Other Reactions
Thrombophlebitis (inflammation of a vein with the formation of blood clot)—pain or tenderness in thigh or leg, with or without swelling of the foot, ankle, or leg.
Pulmonary embolism (movement of blood clot to the lung)—sudden shortness of breath, pain in the chest, coughing, bloody sputum.
Stroke (blood clot in the brain)—headaches, blackouts, sudden weakness or paralysis of any part of the body, severe dizziness, double vision, slurred speech, inability to speak.
Retinal thrombosis (blood clot in eye vessels)—sudden impairment or loss of vision.
Heart attack (blood clot in coronary artery)—sudden pain in chest, neck, jaw, or arm, accompanied by weakness, sweating, or nausea.
Rise in blood pressure in susceptible individuals.
Jaundice (see Glossary).
Emotional depression in susceptible individuals.

CAUTION
1. To avoid prolonged stimulation of breast tissues and uterine tissues, estrogens should be taken in cycles of 3 weeks on and 1 week off medication.
2. The estrogen in estrogen vaginal creams is absorbed systemically by the woman. It may also be absorbed through the penis during sexual intercourse and cause enlargement and tenderness of the male breast tissue.

Precautions for Use by Those over 60 Years of Age
This drug has very limited usefulness after 60. Its use in the few specific conditions for which it is beneficial should be under close medical supervision.
The natural changes in blood vessels that accompany aging require that this drug be used cautiously. Report promptly any indications of impaired circulation—speech disturbances, altered vision, sudden hearing loss, vertigo, sudden weakness or paralysis, angina, or leg pains.

Advisability of Use During Pregnancy
Pregnancy Category: X (tentative). See Pregnancy Code inside back cover.
Animal reproduction studies in mice and guinea pigs reveal significant birth defects due to this drug.

Information from studies in pregnant women indicates that this drug can masculinize the female fetus. In addition, it is known that estrogenic drugs can predispose the female child to development of cancer of the vagina or cervix following puberty.

Avoid completely during entire pregnancy.

Advisability of Use While Nursing Infant

These drugs are known to be present in milk and may affect the nursing infant. They also may impair the formation of milk. Ask physician for guidance.

Habit-Forming Potential

None.

Effects of Overdosage

With Moderate Overdose: Nausea, vomiting, fluid retention, breast enlargement and discomfort, abnormal vaginal bleeding.

With Large Overdose: No serious or dangerous effects reported.

Possible Effects of Extended Use

Increased growth of fibroid tumors of the uterus.

Recent reports suggest a possible association between the use of these drugs and the development of cancer in the lining of the uterus. Further studies are needed to establish a definite cause-and-effect relationship (see Glossary). Prudence dictates that women with uterus intact should use estrogens only when symptoms justify it.

Suggested Periodic Examinations While Taking This Drug (at physician's discretion)

Regular examinations of the breasts and reproductive organs (pelvic examination of the uterus and ovaries, including "Pap" smear).

While Taking This Drug, Observe the Following

Foods: No restrictions. Ask physician for guidance regarding salt intake if you experience fluid retention.

Beverages: No restrictions.

Alcohol: No interactions expected.

Tobacco Smoking: There are reports suggesting that heavy smoking in association with the use of estrogens may increase the risk of abnormal blood clots leading to stroke (cerebral thrombosis) or heart attack (coronary thrombosis). A cause-and-effect relationship (see Glossary) has not been established. Follow physician's advice regarding smoking.

Marijuana Smoking

Occasional (once or twice weekly):   No interactions expected.

Daily: Possible menstrual irregularities; increased breakthrough bleeding.

Other Drugs

Estrogens may *decrease* the effects of
- clofibrate (Atromid-S), and prevent the lowering of blood cholesterol or triglycerides.

Estrogens *taken concurrently* with
- anti-diabetic drugs, may cause unpredictable fluctuations in blood sugar levels. Estrogens can cause an increase in blood sugar; they can also increase the effects of oral anti-diabetics (Diabinese, Dymelor, Orinase, Tolinase). Monitor blood sugar closely and adjust dosages for best diabetic control.

The following drugs may *decrease* the effects of estrogens:
- meprobamate (Equanil, Miltown, etc.)
- phenobarbital

Driving a Vehicle, Operating Machinery, Engaging in Hazardous Activities: Usually no restrictions. Consult your physician for assessment of individual risk and for guidance regarding specific restrictions.

Aviation Note: Usually no restrictions.

Exposure to Sun: Use caution until full effect is known. These drugs may cause photosensitivity (see Glossary).

Discontinuation: It is advisable to discontinue these drugs for one week out of four, that is, 3 weeks on and 1 week off medication. In addition, it is recommended that after 3 to 6 cycles all estrogens be discontinued for a period of individual evaluation. Treatment with estrogens should be resumed only if symptoms require it.

Special Storage Instructions

Keep in a dry, tightly closed container.

ESTROGEN and the MENOPAUSE
A Perspective

The highly variable use and the alleged misuse of estrogens over the past 40 years can be attributed to the lack of a consensus in the medical community as to what constitutes a reasonable approach to the management of the menopause. Admittedly, present knowledge is incomplete, and some aspects of the management of the menopause are still controversial. However, our present understanding of the biological changes that accompany the menopause now makes it possible to devise an effective treatment program that includes the rational and prudent use of estrogen products.

The following summary and recommendations are based upon the opinions and practices of 16 clinical authorities in the disciplines of endocrinology, gynecology, and gerontology. The positions stated and the procedures outlined represent a carefully derived consensus that reflects current knowledge and understanding of menopausal physiology and the optimal use of estrogen in replacement therapy.

Estrogen should not be given routinely to the menopausal woman, but should be reserved to treat those with symptoms of estrogen deficiency. The decision to use estrogens should be made jointly by the patient and her physician after a frank discussion of the known benefits and risks. It is now generally held that for the well-informed menopausal woman who has obvious symptoms of estrogen deficiency and does not have any contraindications to its use, the benefits of estrogen replacement therapy outweigh the possible risks. The use of estrogen is considered effective and safe when prescribed appropriately and monitored properly.

CONSIDERATIONS IN THE USE OF ESTROGENS FOR TREATING THE MENOPAUSAL SYNDROME

Possible Benefits

Decrease in the frequency and/or severity of hot flushes (flashes) and night sweats with attendant insomnia

Prevention or relief of atrophic vaginitis

Prevention or relief of atrophy of the vulva and atrophic urethritis

Prevention of thinning of the skin

Prevention of osteoporosis*

Mental tonic effect

Possible Risks

Nausea, fluid retention, facial acne (for some)

Post-menopausal bleeding (requiring investigation)

Increased severity of cystic breast disease

Accelerated growth of pre-existing uterine fibroid tumors

Increased risk of gall stones (risk increased 2.5 times in one study)

Increased risk of uterine cancer†

Increased risk of breast cancer‡

Deep vein thrombophlebitis and thromboembolism§

Increased blood pressure (rare)

Decreased sugar tolerance (rare)

Principles for the Use of Estrogens in Treating Estrogen-Deficiency States

1. As each woman reaches the menopausal years (45 to 55) she should assess her own status and perceived needs. Next she should familiarize herself with the benefits and possible risks of estrogen replacement therapy. Then, if she thinks she needs medical guidance and/or treatment, she should discuss all aspects of her situation with her physician and share in the decision regarding the use of hormones.

2. A clear indication for the use of estrogen should exist. See Possible Benefits listed above. Estrogens do not retard the natural progression of general aging, and they should not be used in the hope of "preserving femininity."

3. Before estrogen therapy is started, appropriate examinations should be performed and due consideration given to the following possible contraindications to the use of estrogen:
   (1) Pregnancy
   (2) History of venous thrombosis or pulmonary embolism
   (3) Present or previous cancer of the breast

*With long-term treatment.

†Risk increased only after 3 years of continuous use; risk increases progressively with increased dosage and duration of use and ranges from four- to eightfold.

‡Existing data are controversial and contradictory. Some evidence suggests a possible increased risk but only after 3 or more years of continuous use of conjugated estrogens at a dosage of 1.25 mg. daily.

§Applies mostly to use of synthetic unconjugated steroid hormones (ethinyl estradiol and mestranol), and less likely to be related to conjugated equine estrogens, estradiol, or estriol given in customary dosage.

    (4) Cancer of the uterus
    (5) Strong family history of breast or uterine cancer
    (6) Current liver disease or previous cholestatic jaundice
    (7) Chronic gall bladder disease, with or without stones
    (8) Abnormal elevation of blood lipids (cholesterol, triglycerides, etc.)
    (9) History of porphyria
    (10) Large uterine fibroids
    (11) Any estrogen-dependent tumor
    (12) Combination of obesity, varicose veins, and cigarette smoking
    (13) Diabetes mellitus
    (14) Severe hypertension

4. In the young woman experiencing premature menopause (destruction or removal of both ovaries), the long-term use of estrogen replacement is justified, provided appropriate precautions are observed (see Guidelines, below).

5. In the menopausal woman experiencing hot flushes and/or atrophic vaginitis, the *short-term* use of estrogen therapy is generally felt to be acceptable with appropriate supervision and guidance. (Approximately 20% to 25% of menopausal women experience hot flushes of sufficient frequency and/or severity to warrant treatment.) Estrogen replacement therapy provides symptomatic relief; it is not a permanent cure for hot flushes.

6. *Long-term* estrogen therapy for *all* women after the menopause cannot be justified. Treatment must be carefully individualized (see Guidelines, below).

7. It is generally recommended that estrogens be taken cyclically. The customary schedule is from the 1st through the 25th day of each month, with no estrogen during the remaining days of the month. After 6 to 12 months of continuous use, the estrogen dose should be gradually reduced over a period of 2 to 3 months and then discontinued, to assess the individual's need for resumption of use.

8. The lowest effective daily dose of estrogen should be determined and maintained for the duration of the treatment.

9. Vaginal cream preparations of estrogen may be considered instead of orally administered estrogen if the only indication is atrophic vaginitis. However, it should be noted that these preparations allow rapid absorption of estrogen into the systemic circulation, and do not permit accurate control of dosage. They should be used intermittently and only as needed to correct the symptoms of atrophic vaginitis. (*Note:* The estrogen in vaginal creams can be absorbed through the skin of the penis and cause tenderness of the breast in men.)

10. The unnecessary prolongation of estrogen therapy should be avoided. It is advisable to use estrogens in the lowest effective dose and for only as long as necessary to relieve symptoms.

Guidelines for the Use of Estrogens in Specific Deficiency States

  I. The young woman (under 45 years of age) with both ovaries and uterus removed:

1. Choice of estrogen: A conjugated "natural" estrogen (see list of estrogen preparations, page 342).
    The lowest effective dose should be used.*
2. Dosage schedule: Once daily from the 1st through the 25th day of each month.
    Note: If the uterus is present, it is advisable to add a progestin (medroxyprogesterone), 5 to 10 mg. daily during the last 7 to 10 days of the estrogen course.†
3. Duration of use: If well tolerated, until 50 years of age, when assessment of continued need is made individually.
4. Periodic examinations:
    Base-line mammogram (low-radiation-dose xeroradiography); mammogram should be repeated only as necessary to evaluate possible breast tumor. (American Cancer Society guideline.)
    Self-examination of breasts monthly.
    Physician's examination of breasts (and uterus if present) every 6 to 12 months.

II. The woman experiencing the "menopausal syndrome" of hot flushes and sweating (usually 45 to 55 years of age):
    A. Uterus not removed
        1. Choice of hormones and recommended dosage range:
            Estrogen: Conjugated equine estrogens—0.3 to 0.625 mg. daily. (See list of alternative estrogen preparations, page 342.)
            Progestin: Medroxyprogesterone—5 to 10 mg. daily. The lowest effective dose of estrogen should be used.*
        2. Dosage schedule:
            Estrogen: Once daily from the 1st through the 25th day of each month.
            Progestin: Once daily during the last 7 to 10 days of the estrogen course.†
        3. Duration of use: 6 to 12 months, followed by gradual reduction of dose over a period of 2 to 3 months, and then discontinuation to assess the need for continued use. Treatment should be resumed only if symptoms require it. An attempt should be made to discontinue all hormones after 2 to 3 years of continuous use.
        4. Periodic examinations:
            Base-line mammogram (low-radiation-dose xeroradiography).
            Low-dose mammogram annually (over 50 years of age) during continuous use of estrogen. (American Cancer Society guideline.)
            Self-examination of breasts monthly.
            Physician's examination of breasts every 6 to 12 months.

---

*The lowest effective dose is determined by keeping a daily "flush count" to ascertain the lowest daily dose that will reduce the frequency and severity of flushes to an acceptable level.
†The use of a supplemental progestin during the last 7 to 10 days of estrogen administration is still controversial. A possible benefit is the reduced potential for uterine cancer; a possible risk is the increased potential for coronary artery disease; a possible inconvenience is withdrawal bleeding (induced menstruation). The risks of this form of long-term progestin therapy are not known.

Cervical cytology and endometrial biopsy (aspiration curettage) annually.

Blood pressure measurement every 3 to 6 months.

Two-hour blood sugar assay annually.

B. Uterus removed

1. Choice of estrogen and dose: Conjugated equine estrogens—0.3 to 0.625 mg. daily.

   The lowest effective dose should be used.*

2. Dosage schedule: Once daily from the 1st through the 25th day of each month.

3. Duration of use: 6 to 12 months, followed by gradual reduction of dose over a period of 2 to 3 months, and then discontinuation to assess the need for continued use. Treatment should be resumed only if symptoms require it. An attempt should be made to discontinue all hormones after 2 to 3 years of continuous use.

4. Periodic examinations:

   Base-line mammogram (low-radiation-dose xeroradiography).

   Low-dose mammogram annually (over 50 years of age) during continuous use of estrogen. (American Cancer Society guideline.)

   Self-examination of breasts monthly.

   Physician's examination of breasts every 6 to 12 months.

   Blood pressure measurement every 3 to 6 months.

   Two-hour blood sugar assay annually.

III. The woman in the "post-menopausal" period (usually over 55 years of age): Treatment should be individualized as follows:

1. If there are no specific symptoms of estrogen deficiency (hot flushes or atrophic vaginitis), estrogen should not be given.

2. If specific symptoms of estrogen deficiency persist to a degree requiring subjective relief, the recommendations in category II apply. However, in addition to limiting courses of estrogen to 6 to 12 months followed by gradual withdrawal, dosage might be limited to 3 times weekly on a trial basis. Estrogen should be discontinued altogether as soon as possible. If only flushes persist beyond 60 years of age, all estrogen should be discontinued. Non-hormonal drugs such as clonidine, ergot preparations, and certain sedatives may be effective for the relief of hot flushes in some women.

3. Although we do not yet have accurate and reliable predictive indicators, an attempt should be made to identify the woman who may be at high risk for the development of osteoporosis. The following features suggest the possibility of increased risk:

   (1) slender build, light-boned, Caucasian or Oriental race

   (2) a sedentary life-style, or restricted physical activity

   (3) a family history (mother or sister) of osteoporosis (reported by some investigators)

---

*The lowest effective dose is determined by keeping a daily "flush count" to ascertain the lowest daily dose that will reduce the frequency and severity of flushes to an acceptable level.

(4) a low-sodium diet (also likely to be a low-calcium diet)

(5) heavy smoking

(6) excessive use of antacids that contain aluminum

(7) long-term use of cortisone-related drugs

(8) habitual use of carbonated beverages (reported by some investigators)

(9) excessive consumption of alcohol

(10) increased urinary excretion of calcium

For the woman thought to be at increased risk for the development of osteoporosis, estrogen treatment should be started within 3 years after menstruation ceases. The following schedule of estrogen therapy may be recommended for prevention: conjugated equine estrogens—0.625 mg. daily or 3 times weekly, for the first 3 weeks of each month. Periodic examinations as outlined in category II above should be performed. Estrogen replacement therapy may continue until 65 years of age, always with appropriate supervision.

In addition to the prudent use of estrogen, regular exercise and a daily intake of 1500 mg of calcium and 400 units of vitamin D are generally thought to be beneficial in slowing the development of osteoporosis.

Conjugated Estrogens

The following conjugated estrogens are available for use in treating the menopausal syndrome. These are often called the "natural" estrogens but may be derived from natural or synthetic sources.

(1) Conjugated equine estrogens (Genisis, Premarin)

(2) Esterified estrogens (Evex, Menest)

(3) Estradiol cypionate (Depo-Estradiol Cypionate, injection)

(4) Estradiol valerate (Delestrogen, injection)

(5) Estriol (Hormonin, a mixture of estriol, estradiol, and estrone)

(6) Piperazine estrone sulfate (Ogen)

(7) Micronized 17B estradiol (Estrace)

Recommended reading: *Your Middle Years: A Doctor's Guide for Today's Woman,* by Wulf H. Utian, M.D., Ph.D., New York, Appleton-Century-Crofts, 1980.

ETHCHLORVYNOL

Year Introduced: 1956

Brand Names

USA	Canada
Placidyl (Abbott)	Placidyl (Abbott)

Common Synonyms ("Street Names"):   Dyls

Drug Class: Sleep Inducer (Hypnotic)

Prescription Required: Yes (Controlled Drug, U.S. Schedule IV)*

Available for Purchase by Generic Name: No

Available Dosage Forms and Strengths
Capsules — 100 mg., 200 mg., 500 mg., 750 mg.

Tablet May Be Crushed or Capsule Opened for Administration: No

How This Drug Works
Intended Therapeutic Effect(s):   Relief of insomnia (hypnotic effect).
Location of Drug Action(s):   Not completely established. Thought to be the wake-sleep centers of the brain, possibly the reticular activating system.
Method of Drug Action(s):   Not established.

Principal Uses of This Drug
As a Single Drug Product: Used exclusively as a bedtime sedative to induce sleep. The higher dosage forms are used on retiring to initiate sleep; the lower dosage forms are used during the night to restore sleep after untimely awakening. To prevent the development of dependence, this drug should be limited to short-term use for periods not exceeding 7 days.

THIS DRUG SHOULD NOT BE TAKEN IF
—you have had an allergic reaction to any dosage form of it previously.
—you have a history of porphyria.
—it is prescribed for a child under 12 years of age.

INFORM YOUR PHYSICIAN BEFORE TAKING THIS DRUG IF
—you are taking other sedatives, sleep-inducing drugs, tranquilizers, antihistamines, pain relievers, or narcotic drugs of any kind.
—you have a history of liver or kidney disease.

Time Required for Apparent Benefit
Usually from 30 to 60 minutes.

Possible Side-Effects (*natural, expected, and unavoidable drug actions*)
Lightheadedness in upright position, unsteadiness.

Possible Adverse Effects (*unusual, unexpected, and infrequent reactions*)
IF ANY OF THE FOLLOWING DEVELOP, DISCONTINUE DRUG AND NOTIFY YOUR PHYSICIAN AS SOON AS POSSIBLE

Mild Adverse Effects
Allergic Reactions: Hives.
Other Reactions
Dizziness, staggering gait, blurred vision.
Indigestion, nausea, vomiting.
Serious Adverse Effects
Allergic Reactions: Hepatitis with jaundice (see Glossary).

*See Schedules of Controlled Drugs inside back cover.

Idiosyncratic Reactions: Prolonged sleep, extreme muscular weakness, fainting, excitement.

Other Reactions: Reduced number of blood platelets (see Glossary), resulting in unusual bleeding or bruising.

Precautions for Use by Those over 60 Years of Age

You may be more sensitive to the actions of this drug, Small doses are advisable until your individual response has been determined.

You may be more susceptible to the "hangover" effect caused by most sleep-inducing (hypnotic) drugs.

Natural changes in body functions may make you more susceptible to the development of dizziness, confused thinking, impaired memory, incoordination, unsteady gait and balance, falling, loss of bladder control, and constipation.

Advisability of Use During Pregnancy

Pregnancy Category: C (tentative). See Pregnancy Code inside back cover.

Animal reproduction studies in rats reveal increased stillbirths.

Information from adequate studies in pregnant women is not available.

It is advisable to avoid this drug during entire pregnancy.

Ask physician for guidance.

Advisability of Use While Nursing Infant

Presence of this drug in milk is not known. If used while nursing, observe infant for unusual drowsiness. Ask physician for guidance regarding size and timing of dosage.

Habit-Forming Potential

This drug can cause both psychological and physical dependence (see Glossary). Avoid continuous use.

Effects of Overdosage

With Moderate Overdose: Excitement, delirium, incoordination, extreme drowsiness.

With Large Overdose: Deep and prolonged coma.

Possible Effects of Extended Use

Impairment of vision.

Psychological and/or physical dependence.

Suggested Periodic Examinations While Taking This Drug (at physician's discretion)

Complete blood cell counts.

Liver function tests.

Vision tests.

While Taking This Drug, Observe the Following

Foods: No restrictions.

Beverages: No restrictions.

Alcohol: Avoid completely. Alcohol can increase greatly the sedative and depressant actions of this drug on brain function.

Tobacco Smoking: No interactions expected.

Marijuana Smoking

Occasional (once or twice weekly):   Mild, transient increase in drowsiness, unsteadiness, and impairment of mental and physical performance.

Daily: Marked, prolonged drowsiness, unsteadiness, and significantly impaired mental and physical performance.

Other Drugs

Ethchlorvynol may *increase* the effects of

• all sedatives, sleep-inducing drugs, tranquilizers, antihistamines, pain relievers, and narcotic drugs. Ask physician for guidance regarding dosage adjustments.

Ethchlorvynol may *decrease* the effects of

• oral anticoagulants, and reduce their protective action. Ask physician for guidance regarding tests of prothrombin time and dosage adjustment of the anticoagulant.

Ethchlorvynol *taken concurrently* with

• amitriptyline (Elavil, etc.), may cause delirium and excessive sedation. Use caution while taking ethchlorvynol with any tricyclic antidepressant (see Drug Class, Section Three).

The following drugs may *increase* the effects of ethchlorvynol

• mono-amine oxidase (MAO) inhibitor drugs may cause oversedation (see Drug Class, Section Three). Careful dosage adjustment is necessary.

Driving a Vehicle, Operating Machinery, Engaging in Hazardous Activities: The "hangover" effects of this drug can impair mental alertness, judgment, physical coordination, and reaction time. Avoid hazardous activities until "hangover" effects have disappeared.

Aviation Note: The use of this drug *is a disqualification* for the piloting of aircraft. Consultation with a designated Aviation Medical Examiner is advised.

Exposure to Sun: No restrictions.

Discontinuation: If it has been necessary to use this drug for an extended period of time, do not discontinue it abruptly. Ask your physician for guidance regarding dosage reduction and withdrawal. Also, it may be necessary to adjust the dosage of other drugs taken concurrently with it.

Special Storage Instructions

Keep in a dry, tightly closed container.

ETHOSUXIMIDE

Note: This is an Abbreviated Drug Profile of a less frequently used but important anti-epileptic drug. It is considered to be the drug of choice by many physicians for the management of absence seizures (petit mal epilepsy). It causes serious adverse effects less frequently than other drugs used for this disorder, and it is quite effective in the presence of structural abnormalities of the brain.

Year Introduced: 1960

Brand Names

USA	Canada
Zarontin (Parke-Davis)	Zarontin (P.D. & Co.)

Common Synonyms ("Street Names"):   Epilepsy medicine

Drug Class: Anti-epilepsy (Anticonvulsant), Succinimides

Prescription Required: USA: Yes   Canada: Yes

Available for Purchase by Generic Name: USA: No   Canada: No

Available Dosage Forms and Strengths
　　Capsules — 250 mg.
　　　Syrup — 250 mg. per teaspoonful (5 ml.)

Tablet May Be Crushed or Capsule Opened for Administration: Yes

How This Drug Works
　　Intended Therapeutic Effect(s):   Reduction in the frequency of absence seizures (petit mal epilepsy).
　　Location of Drug Action(s):   Thought to be certain nerve pathways that connect the points of origin of abnormal electrical stimulation in the outer layer of the brain with deeper structures inside the brain.
　　Method of Drug Action(s):   Not established. It is thought that by altering the transmission of nerve impulses, this drug suppresses the abnormal showers of electrical activity responsible for absence seizures.

Principal Uses of This Drug
　　As a Single Drug Product: Used primarily to reduce the frequency and duration of absence seizures associated with petit mal epilepsy.

THIS DRUG SHOULD NOT BE TAKEN IF
—you are allergic to this or any other succinimide drug (see Drug Class, Section Three).
—you have active liver disease.
—you currently have a disorder affecting the production of blood cells (a blood dyscrasia).

INFORM YOUR PHYSICIAN BEFORE TAKING THIS DRUG IF
—you have a history of liver or kidney disease.
—you have a history of any type of blood cell disorder.
—you have a history of emotional depression or other mental illness.

Time Required for Apparent Benefit
Drug action usually begins in 1 hour and reaches its peak in 3 to 7 hours. Continuous use on a regular schedule for 1 to 2 weeks is usually necessary to determine this drug's effectiveness in reducing the frequency of absence seizures.

Possible Side-Effects *(natural, expected, and unavoidable drug actions)*
Drowsiness, lethargy, fatigue.

Possible Adverse Effects *(unusual, unexpected, and infrequent reactions)*

IF ANY OF THE FOLLOWING DEVELOP, DISCONTINUE DRUG AND NOTIFY YOUR PHYSICIAN AS SOON AS POSSIBLE

Mild Adverse Effects
Allergic Reactions: Skin rash, hives.
Other Reactions: Headache, dizziness, unsteadiness, impaired vision.
Loss of appetite, nausea, vomiting, stomach pain, diarrhea.
Numbness and tingling in arms and legs.
Excessive growth of hair.

Serious Adverse Effects
Allergic Reactions: Swelling of the tongue.
Other Reactions: Severe bone marrow depression; extreme fatigue and weakness, fever, sore throat, abnormal bleeding or bruising. (See Bone Marrow Depression in Glossary.)
Nervousness, hyperactivity, disturbed sleep, night terrors.
Aggravation of emotional depression and paranoid mental disorders.
Marked swelling of the gums.

Natural Diseases or Disorders That May Be Activated By This Drug
Latent psychosis. Systemic lupus erythematosus.

CAUTION
1. This drug may increase the frequency of grand mal seizures in individuals with mixed seizure disorders.
2. It is mandatory that you comply with your physician's request for periodic blood counts and any other tests that are deemed advisable.

Advisability of Use During Pregnancy
Pregnancy Category: C (tentative). See Pregnancy Code inside back cover.
Animal reproduction studies reveal bone defects in rodents.
Information from adequate studies in pregnant women is not available. Three instances of birth defects have been reported.
Avoid drug during the first 3 months. If possible, avoid drug during entire pregnancy.

Advisability of Use While Nursing Infant
This drug is present in human milk. Observe infant for drowsiness and poor feeding. If high doses are required, refrain from nursing.

Suggested Periodic Examinations While Taking This Drug (at physician's discretion)
Complete blood cell counts.
Liver and kidney function tests.

While Taking This Drug, Observe the Following
Foods: No restrictions. May be taken with food to reduce stomach irritation.
Beverages: May be taken with milk.
Alcohol: Use caution until the combined effect has been determined. This drug may increase the sedative effects of alcohol.
Driving a Vehicle, Operating Machinery, Engaging in Hazardous Activities: This drug may cause drowsiness, dizziness, unsteadiness, and impaired vision. If these drug effects occur, all hazardous activities should be avoided.
Aviation Note: The use of this drug and the disorder for which this drug is prescribed *are disqualifications* for the piloting of aircraft. Consultation with a designated Aviation Medical Examiner is advised.
Discontinuation: Do not stop taking this drug abruptly. If discontinuation is necessary, consult your physician for guidance regarding gradual reduction in dosage.

FENOPROFEN

Year Introduced: 1976

Brand Names

USA	Canada
Nalfon (Dista)	Nalfon (Lilly)

Common Synonyms ("Street Names"): Arthritis medicine, aspirin substitute

Drug Class: Analgesic, Mild, Anti-inflammatory, Fever Reducer (Antipyretic)

Prescription Required: Yes

Available for Purchase by Generic Name: No

Available Dosage Forms and Strengths
Tablets — 600 mg.
Capsules — 200 mg., 300 mg.

Tablet May Be Crushed or Capsule Opened for Administration: Yes

How This Drug Works
Intended Therapeutic Effect(s): Relief of joint pain, stiffness, inflammation, and swelling associated with arthritis.

Location of Drug Action(s):   Not completely established. This drug may act in the brain (at the level of the hypothalamus) as well as in the inflamed tissues of arthritic joints.

Method of Drug Action(s):   Not completely known. It is thought that this drug reduces the tissue concentration of prostaglandins, chemicals involved in the production of inflammation and pain.

Principal Uses of This Drug

As a Single Drug Product: This "aspirin substitute" is used in a variety of conditions to relieve pain and inflammation. While its primary use is to provide symptomatic relief in acute and chronic arthritis, including gout, it is also used to relieve the pain associated with musculo-skeletal injuries, bursitis, tendinitis, menstrual cramping, and minor surgical procedures.

THIS DRUG SHOULD NOT BE TAKEN IF

—you have had an allergic reaction to any dosage form of it previously.
—you are allergic to aspirin (hives, nasal polyps, and/or asthma caused by aspirin).
—you have a bleeding disorder.
—you have an active stomach ulcer or active ulcerative colitis.
—you have severe impairment of kidney function.
—it has been prescribed for a child under 14 years of age.

INFORM YOUR PHYSICIAN BEFORE TAKING THIS DRUG IF

—you have a history of peptic ulcer disease, ulcerative colitis, or previous stomach or intestinal bleeding.
—you are taking any kind of anticoagulant drug (see Drug Class, Section Three).
—you are presently under treatment for an active infection of any kind.

Time Required for Apparent Benefit

Drug action begins within 1 to 2 hours and persists for 3 to 5 hours. Significant improvement may require continuous use on a regular schedule for 1 to 2 weeks.

Possible Side-Effects *(natural, expected, and unavoidable drug actions)*

Drowsiness in sensitive individuals.

Possible Adverse Effects *(unusual, unexpected, and infrequent reactions)*

IF ANY OF THE FOLLOWING DEVELOP, DISCONTINUE DRUG AND NOTIFY YOUR PHYSICIAN AS SOON AS POSSIBLE

Mild Adverse Effects
  Allergic Reactions: Skin rash (various kinds), hives, itching (9%).
  Other Reactions
      Headache, dizziness, confusion, mild numbness or tingling, ringing in the ears.
      Indigestion, nausea, vomiting, constipation.

Serious Adverse Effects
Allergic Reactions
  Anaphylactic reaction (see Glossary).
  Allergic destruction of blood platelets (see Glossary). Observe for abnormal bruising or bleeding.
Other Reactions
  Stomach and/or intestinal bleeding.
  Impaired formation of white blood cells (granulocytes) with resulting reduction in resistance to infections.
  Blurred vision, impaired hearing.
Possible Delayed Adverse Effects
Mild anemia due to "silent" blood loss from the stomach (less than that caused by aspirin).

CAUTION
1. Do not exceed a dose of 3.0 grams per 24 hours.
2. The optimal dosage schedule must be determined for each person individually. Dosage should always be limited to the smallest amount that produces reasonable improvement.
3. This drug's anti-inflammatory and antipyretic effects can make it more difficult to recognize the presence of infection. If you develop any symptoms that suggest an active infection, inform your physician promptly.

Precautions for Use by Those over 60 Years of Age
It is advisable to begin treatment with small doses until individual tolerance and response have been determined. Limit dosage to the smallest amount that produces reasonable improvement.

Sudden gain in weight or the development of swelling of the feet and ankles may indicate the excessive retention of water in body tissues. Inform your physician promptly of these developments.

You may be more susceptible to the development of headache, dizziness, confusion, impairment of memory, stomach bleeding, and constipation.

Advisability of Use During Pregnancy
Pregnancy Category: C (tentative). See Pregnancy Code inside back cover.

Animal reproduction studies: No data available.

Information from adequate studies in pregnant women is not available. Ask physician for guidance.

Advisability of Use While Nursing Infant
The presence of this drug in milk is not known. Ask physician for guidance.

Habit-Forming Potential
None apparent to date.

Effects of Overdosage
With Moderate Overdose: Stomach irritation, nausea, vomiting, diarrhea.
With Large Overdose: No serious or threatening effects reported to date.

Possible Effects of Extended Use

Cataracts have been reported, but a definite cause-and-effect relationship (see Glossary) has not been established.

Suggested Periodic Examinations While Taking This Drug (at physician's discretion)

Complete blood cell counts.

Kidney function tests.

Liver function tests.

Eye examinations for possible changes in the lens.

While Taking This Drug, Observe the Following

Foods: This drug is more effective if it is taken 1 hour before or 2 hours after eating. However, it should be taken with or immediately following food if stomach irritation occurs.

Beverages: This drug may be taken with milk. No specific restrictions.

Alcohol: Use with caution. The irritant action of alcohol on the stomach lining, added to the irritant action of fenoprofen in sensitive individuals, can increase the risk of stomach bleeding and/or ulceration.

Tobacco Smoking: No interactions expected.

Marijuana Smoking

Occasional (once or twice weekly): No effect to mild increase in pain relief from this drug.

Daily: Moderate increase in pain relief from this drug.

Other Drugs

Fenoprofen may *increase* the effects of

- oral anticoagulant drugs, and increase the risk of unwanted bleeding. Consult your physician regarding the frequency of prothrombin time testing.
- oral anti-diabetic drugs, and cause hypoglycemia (see Glossary).
- phenytoin (Dilantin, etc.), and cause symptoms of overdosage.
- "sulfa" drugs, and make it advisable to reduce their dosage.

The following drugs may *decrease* the effects of fenoprofen

- aspirin and aspirin-containing compounds.
- phenobarbital.

Driving a Vehicle, Operating Machinery, Engaging in Hazardous Activities: This drug can cause dizziness and confusion in sensitive individuals. Use caution until its full effects have been determined.

Aviation Note: The use of this drug *may be a disqualification* for the piloting of aircraft. Consultation with a designated Aviation Medical Examiner is advised.

Exposure to Sun: No restrictions.

Heavy Exercise or Exertion: Follow physician's instructions.

Occurrence of Unrelated Illness: This drug may mask the usual symptoms that indicate the presence of infection. Consult your physician promptly if you suspect that you may be developing an infection of any kind.

Discontinuation: This drug may be discontinued abruptly without danger. However, it may be necessary to adjust the doses of other drugs being taken concurrently with it. Consult your physician.

Special Storage Instructions
Keep in a dry, tightly closed container.

FLUPHENAZINE

Year Introduced: 1959

Brand Names

USA	Canada
Permitil (Schering)	Apo-Fluphenazine
Prolixin (Squibb)	(Apotex)
	Modecate (Squibb)
	Moditen (Squibb)
	Permitil (Schering)

Common Synonyms ("Street Names"):   None

Drug Class: Tranquilizer, Strong (Anti-psychotic), Phenothiazines

Prescription Required: Yes

Available for Purchase by Generic Name: USA: No   Canada: Yes

Available Dosage Forms and Strengths

Tablets — 0.25 mg., 1 mg., 2.5 mg., 5 mg., 10 mg.
Prolonged-action tablets — 1 mg.
Concentrate — 5 mg. per ml. (1% alcohol)
Elixir — 2.5 mg. per teaspoonful (5 ml.) (14% alcohol)
Injection — 2.5 mg. per ml., 25 mg. per ml.

Tablet May Be Crushed or Capsule Opened for Administration

Regular tablets — Yes
Prolonged-action tablets — No

How This Drug Works
Intended Therapeutic Effect(s):   Restoration of emotional calm. Relief of severe anxiety, agitation, and psychotic behavior.

Location of Drug Action(s):   Those nerve pathways in the brain that utilize the tissue chemical dopamine for the transmission of nerve impulses.

Method of Drug Action(s):   Not completely established. Present theory is that by inhibiting the action of dopamine, this drug acts to correct an imbalance of nerve impulse transmissions that is thought to be responsible for certain mental disorders.

Principal Uses of This Drug
As a Single Drug Product: This potent "major tranquilizer" is used to treat the thought disorder and abnormal behavior that are associated with schizophrenia and related conditions. The injectable form of this drug is most useful in providing medication with an extended duration of action in patients who will not comply with daily medication taken by mouth.

THIS DRUG SHOULD NOT BE TAKEN IF
—you have had an allergic reaction to any dosage form of it previously.
—you have a history of brain damage.
—you have a history of impaired liver or kidney function.
—you have a blood or bone marrow disorder.
—it is prescribed for a child under 12 years of age.

INFORM YOUR PHYSICIAN BEFORE TAKING THIS DRUG IF
—you are allergic or sensitive to any phenothiazine drug (see Drug Class, Section Three).
—you are taking any sedatives, sleep-inducing drugs, other tranquilizers, antihistamines, antidepressants, or narcotic drugs of any kind.
—you have epilepsy.
—you have a history of asthma or emphysema.
—you have a history of peptic ulcer.
—you plan to have surgery under general or spinal anesthesia in the near future.

Time Required for Apparent Benefit
Some benefit may be apparent in first week.
Maximal benefit may require continuous use for several weeks.

Possible Side-Effects *(natural, expected, and unavoidable drug actions)*
Drowsiness (usually during the first few weeks), blurred vision.
Nasal stuffiness, dry mouth, constipation, impaired urination.

Possible Adverse Effects *(unusual, unexpected, and infrequent reactions)*

IF ANY OF THE FOLLOWING DEVELOP, DISCONTINUE DRUG AND NOTIFY YOUR PHYSICIAN AS SOON AS POSSIBLE

Mild Adverse Effects
Allergic Reactions: Skin rashes (various kinds), hives, itching.
Other Reactions
Headache, dizziness, weakness.
Excitement, restlessness, unusual dreaming.
Menstrual irregularity, breast enlargement and tenderness, milk formation.
Serious Adverse Effects
Allergic Reactions: Severe skin reaction, "silent pneumonia," anaphylactic reaction (see Glossary).
Idiosyncratic Reactions: High fever (see idiosyncrasy in Glossary).
Other Reactions
Parkinson-like disorders (see Glossary).

Spasm of the muscles of the face, neck, back, and extremities, causing rolling of the eyes, grimacing, clamping of the jaw, protrusion of the tongue, difficulty in swallowing, arching of the back, spasms of the hands and feet.

Hepatitis with jaundice (see Glossary).

Bone marrow depression (see Glossary)—fatigue, weakness, fever, sore throat, unusual bleeding or bruising.

CAUTION

1. Many over-the-counter (OTC) medications (see Glossary) for allergies, colds, and coughs contain drugs that can interact unfavorably with this drug. Ask your physician or pharmacist for guidance before using any such medications.
2. Antacids that contain aluminum and/or magnesium can prevent the absorption of this drug and reduce its effectiveness.
3. Obtain prompt evaluation of any disturbance or change in vision.

Precautions for Use by Those over 60 Years of Age

You may be more sensitive to all the actions of this drug. Small doses are advisable until your individual response has been determined.

You may be more susceptible to the development of drowsiness, lethargy, constipation, lowering of body temperature (hypothermia), and excessive drop in blood pressure on arising from a lying or sitting position (see orthostatic hypotension in Glossary).

This drug can increase the degree of impaired urination associated with prostate gland enlargement (prostatism).

You may also be more susceptible to the development of Parkinson-like disorders and/or tardive dyskinesia (see discussion of these terms in Glossary). These conditions must be recognized early since they may become unresponsive to treatment and irreversible. Consult your physician promptly if suggestive symptoms develop.

Advisability of Use During Pregnancy

Pregnancy Category: C (tentative). See Pregnancy Code inside back cover.
Animal reproduction studies in mice reveal significant birth defects due to this drug.

Information from adequate studies in pregnant women is not available.

Avoid completely during first 3 months.

Ask physician for guidance.

Advisability of Use While Nursing Infant

Safety not established. Ask physician for guidance.

Habit-Forming Potential

None

Effects of Overdosage

With Moderate Overdose: Extreme drowsiness, slow breathing, weakness.

With Large Overdose: Deep sleep, coma, perspiration, weak and rapid pulse, shallow breathing.

Possible Effects of Extended Use
Tardive dyskinesia (see Glossary).
Deposits in the cornea and lens of the eye.
Impaired liver function.

Suggested Periodic Examinations While Taking This Drug (at physician's discretion)
Complete blood cell counts, especially during the first 3 months.
Liver and kidney function tests.
Complete eye examination including vision and eye structures.
Careful inspection of tongue for the early development of fine, wave-like, rippling surface movements (involuntary) that could indicate the beginning of tardive dyskinesia.
Periodic electrocardiograms and chest X-rays.

While Taking This Drug, Observe the Following
Foods: No restrictions.
Beverages: No restrictions.
Alcohol: Use extreme caution until combined effect has been determined. Alcohol can increase the sedative action of fluphenazine and accentuate its depressant effects on brain function and blood pressure. Fluphenazine can increase the intoxicating action of alcohol.
Tobacco Smoking: No interactions expected.
Marijuana Smoking
Occasional (once or twice weekly):   No effect to mild and transient increase in drowsiness and accentuation of orthostatic hypotension (see Glossary); some risk of precipitating latent psychoses (in predisposed individuals).
Daily: Moderate increase in drowsiness, significant accentuation of orthostatic hypotension; increased risk of precipitating latent psychoses, confusing interpretation of mental status and of drug responses.
Other Drugs
Fluphenazine may *increase* the effects of
- all sedatives, sleep-inducing drugs, other tranquilizers, antidepressants, antihistamines, and narcotic drugs, and cause oversedation. Ask physician for guidance regarding dosage adjustment.
- atropine and drugs with atropine-like action (see Drug Class, Section Three).

Fluphenazine may *decrease* the effects of
- levodopa (Dopar, Larodopa, Parda, etc.), and reduce its effectiveness in the treatment of Parkinson's disease (shaking palsy).
- appetite suppressant drugs (Pre-Sate, Preludin, Benzedrine, Dexedrine, etc.).

Fluphenazine *taken concurrently* with
- anti-convulsants, may cause a change in the pattern of epileptic seizures. Ask physician for guidance regarding adjustment of anti-convulsant drug dosage.

- quinidine, may impair heart function. Avoid the combined use of these two drugs.

The following drugs may *increase* the effects of fluphenazine
- tricyclic antidepressants (see Drug Class, Section Three).

Driving a Vehicle, Operating Machinery, Engaging in Hazardous Activities: This drug may impair mental alertness, judgment, physical coordination, or reaction time. Avoid hazardous activities.

Aviation Note: The use of this drug *is a disqualification* for the piloting of aircraft. Consultation with a designated Aviation Medical Examiner is advised.

Exposure to Sun: Use caution. Drugs closely related to this drug are known to produce photosensitivity (see Glossary).   .

Exposure to Heat: Use caution until combined effect has been determined. This drug may impair the regulation of body temperature and increase the risk of heat stroke.

Heavy Exercise or Exertion: No restrictions in mild to moderate temperatures.

Discontinuation: If it has been necessary to use this drug for an extended period of time, do not discontinue it suddenly. Ask physician for guidance regarding dosage reduction and withdrawal. It may also be necessary to adjust the dosage of other drugs taken concurrently with it.

Special Storage Instructions
Keep liquid dosage forms in tightly closed, amber glass containers.

Observe the Following Expiration Times
Do not use the injectable form of this drug if its color is darker than light amber.

FLURAZEPAM

Year Introduced: 1970

Brand Names

USA	Canada
Dalmane (Roche)	Apo-Flurazepam (Apotex)
	Dalmane (Roche)
	Novoflupam (Novopharm)
	Somnol (Horner)
	Som-Pam (ICN)

Common Synonyms ("Street Names"):   Sleeping pills, tranks

Drug Class: Sleep Inducer (Hypnotic), Benzodiazepines

Prescription Required: Yes (Controlled Drug, U.S. Schedule IV)*

Available for Purchase by Generic Name: No

Available Dosage Forms and Strengths
Capsules — 15 mg., 30 mg.

Tablet May Be Crushed or Capsule Opened for Administration: Yes

How This Drug Works
Intended Therapeutic Effect(s):   Prevention of insomnia. Restoration of normal sleep pattern.
Location of Drug Action(s):   Exact site not known. Possibly the hypothalamus and limbic system of the brain.
Method of Drug Action(s):   Not established. Principal action induces sleep that closely resembles natural sleep.

Principal Uses of This Drug
As a Single Drug Product: This member of the benzodiazepine class of "minor tranquilizers" is used exclusively as a bedtime sedative to induce sleep.

THIS DRUG SHOULD NOT BE TAKEN IF
—you are allergic to flurazepam.
—it is prescribed for a child under 15 years of age.

INFORM YOUR PHYSICIAN BEFORE TAKING THIS DRUG IF
—you are allergic to any drugs chemically related to flurazepam: chlordiazepoxide, clorazepate, diazepam, oxazepam (see Drug Profiles for brand names).
—you have epilepsy.
—you have a history of acute intermittent porphyria.
—you are taking sedative, other sleep-inducing, tranquilizer, antidepressant, or anti-convulsant drugs of any kind.
—you plan to have surgery under general anesthesia in the near future.

Time Required for Apparent Benefit
Approximately 30 to 60 minutes.

Possible Side-Effects *(natural, expected, and unavoidable drug actions)*
"Hangover" effects on arising—drowsiness, lethargy, unsteadiness in stance and gait.

Possible Adverse Effects *(unusual, unexpected, and infrequent reactions)*

IF ANY OF THE FOLLOWING DEVELOP, DISCONTINUE DRUG AND NOTIFY YOUR PHYSICIAN AS SOON AS POSSIBLE
Mild Adverse Effects
Allergic Reactions: Skin rashes (various kinds), burning eyes.
Other Reactions: Dizziness, lightheadedness, staggering, blurred vision, slurred speech, headache, nausea, indigestion.

*See Schedules of Controlled Drugs inside back cover.

Serious Adverse Effects
Allergic Reactions: Jaundice (see Glossary).
Paradoxical Reactions: Restlessness, talkativeness, acute excitement, hallucinations.

CAUTION
This drug is transformed by the liver into long-acting forms (active metabolites) that can persist in the body for 24 hours or longer. With continuous use of this drug on a daily basis, these active drug forms accumulate and produce increasing sedation. If this drug is taken at bedtime to induce sleep, observe carefully for "hangover" effects throughout the following day. Avoid driving and all other hazardous activities if you feel drowsy or sluggish.

Precautions for Use by Infants and Children
Safety and effectiveness in children below the age of 15 years have not been established.

Precautions for Use by Those over 60 Years of Age
You may be more sensitive to the actions of this drug. Small doses are advisable until your individual response has been determined.

You may be more susceptible to the "hangover" effect caused by most sleep-inducing (hypnotic) drugs.

Natural changes in body functions may make you more susceptible to the development of dizziness, confused thinking, impaired memory, incoordination, unsteady gait and balance, falling, loss of bladder control and constipation.

Advisability of Use During Pregnancy
Pregnancy Category: C (tentative). See Pregnancy Code inside back cover.
Animal reproduction studies: No data available.
Information from adequate studies in pregnant women is not available.
Ask physician for guidance.

The findings of some recent studies suggest a possible association between the use of a drug closely related to flurazepam during early pregnancy and the occurrence of birth defects, such as cleft lip. It is advisable to avoid this drug completely during the first 3 months of pregnancy.

Advisability of Use While Nursing Infant
With recommended dosage, drug is probably present in milk. Ask physician for guidance.

Habit-Forming Potential
This drug is closely related to drugs that can cause psychological and/or physical dependence (see Glossary) if used in large doses for an extended period of time. Avoid continuous use.

Effects of Overdosage
With Moderate Overdose: Marked drowsiness, weakness, drunkenness, impairment of stance and gait.
With Large Overdose: Stupor, deep sleep, coma.

Possible Effects of Extended Use
Psychological and/or physical dependence.
Impairment of liver function.

Suggested Periodic Examinations While Taking This Drug (at physician's discretion)
Blood cell counts, liver and kidney function tests during long-term use.

While Taking This Drug, Observe the Following
Foods: No restrictions.

Beverages: Because of their caffeine content, large intakes of coffee, tea, or cola drinks within 4 hours of medication may reduce the sleep-inducing effect of flurazepam before, and for at least 24 hours after, the last dose.

Alcohol: Avoid completely. Alcohol can increase the sedative action of flurazepam and depress vital brain functions.

Tobacco Smoking: Heavy smoking may reduce the duration of sedative action of flurazepam.

Marijuana Smoking

Occasional (once or twice weekly):   Mild, transient increase in drowsiness, unsteadiness, and impairment of mental and physical performance.

Daily: Marked, prolonged drowsiness, unsteadiness, and significantly impaired mental and physical performance.

Other Drugs

Flurazepam *taken concurrently* with

- anti-convulsants, may cause a change in the pattern of seizures; observe closely to determine if an adjustment of the anti-convulsant dose is necessary.

The following drugs may *increase* the effects of flurazepam

- all sedatives, drugs for sleep, tranquilizers, antidepressants, anti-convulsants, and narcotic drugs may increase the sedative action of flurazepam and produce oversedation. Ask physician for guidance regarding dosage adjustment.

Driving a Vehicle, Operating Machinery, Engaging in Hazardous Activities: The "hangover" effects of this drug can impair mental alertness, judgment, and physical coordination. Avoid hazardous activities until all such drug effects have disappeared.

Aviation Note: The use of this drug *is a disqualification* for the piloting of aircraft. Consultation with a designated Aviation Medical Examiner is advised.

Exposure to Sun: No restrictions.

Discontinuation: If it has been necessary to use this drug in large doses or for an extended period of time, ask physician for guidance regarding dosage reduction and withdrawal.

Special Storage Instructions
Keep in a dry, tightly closed, light-resistant container. Avoid excessive heat.

FUROSEMIDE

Year Introduced: 1966

Brand Names

USA	**Canada**
Lasix (Hoechst-Roussel)	Apo-Furosemide (Apotex)
SK-Furosemide (Smith	Furoside (ICN)
Kline & French)	Lasix (Hoechst)
	Neo-Renal (Neolab)
	Novosemide
	(Novopharm)
	Uritol (Horner)

Common Synonyms ("Street Names"):   Water pills

Drug Class: Anti-hypertensive (Hypotensive); Diuretic

Prescription Required: Yes

Available for Purchase by Generic Name: Yes

Available Dosage Forms and Strengths
      Tablets — 20 mg., 40 mg., 80 mg.
   Oral solution — 10 mg. per ml.
      Injection — 10 mg. per ml.

Tablet May Be Crushed or Capsule Opened for Administration: Yes

How This Drug Works
  Intended Therapeutic Effect(s)
    Elimination of excessive fluid retention (edema).
    Reduction of high blood pressure.
  Location of Drug Action(s):   The tubular systems of the kidney that determine the final composition of the urine.
  Method of Drug Action(s):   By increasing the elimination of salt and water from the body (through increased urine production), this drug reduces the volume of fluid in the blood and body tissues and lowers the sodium content throughout the body. These changes may produce a lowering of blood pressure.

Principal Uses of This Drug
  As a Single Drug Product: This powerful diuretic is used primarily to increase the volume of urine and thereby relieve the body of excessive water retention (edema) that is commonly associated with congestive heart failure, liver disease, and kidney disease. It is also used in the treatment of high blood pressure, but usually in conjunction with other anti-hypertensive drugs. A less frequent use is to increase the amount of calcium excreted in the urine when the blood level of calcium is abnormally high.

THIS DRUG SHOULD NOT BE TAKEN IF
—you have had an allergic reaction to any dosage form of it previously.

INFORM YOUR PHYSICIAN BEFORE TAKING THIS DRUG IF
—you are allergic to any form of "sulfa" drug.
—you are pregnant and your physician does not know it.
—you have a history of liver or kidney disease, or impaired liver or kidney function.
—you have diabetes (or a tendency to diabetes).
—you have a history of gout.
—you have impaired hearing.
—you are taking any form of cortisone, digitalis, oral anti-diabetic drugs, or insulin.
—you plan to have surgery under general anesthesia in the near future.

Time Required for Apparent Benefit
Increased urine volume begins in 1 hour, reaches a maximum in the second hour, and gradually subsides in 6 to 8 hours. Continuous use on a regular schedule for 1 to 2 weeks may be necessary to determine this drug's effectiveness in lowering your blood pressure.

Possible Side-Effects *(natural, expected, and unavoidable drug actions)*
Lightheadedness on arising from sitting or lying position (see orthostatic hypotension in Glossary).
Increase in level of blood sugar, affecting control of diabetes.
Increase in level of blood uric acid, affecting control of gout.
Decrease in the level of blood potassium, resulting in muscle weakness and cramping.

Possible Adverse Effects *(unusual, unexpected, and infrequent reactions)*

IF ANY OF THE FOLLOWING DEVELOP, DISCONTINUE DRUG AND NOTIFY YOUR PHYSICIAN AS SOON AS POSSIBLE

Mild Adverse Effects
Allergic Reactions: Skin rashes (various kinds), hives, itching.
Other Reactions
Nausea, vomiting, diarrhea.
Dizziness, blurred vision.
Serious Adverse Effects
Allergic Reactions: Severe skin reactions.
Other Reactions: Bone marrow depression (see Glossary)—fatigue, weakness, infection manifested by fever or sore throat, unusual bleeding or bruising.

CAUTION
1. Do not exceed recommended doses. Increased dosage can cause excessive excretion of sodium and potassium with resultant loss of appetite, nausea, fatigue, weakness, confusion, and tingling in the extremities.
2. If you are also taking a digitalis preparation (digitoxin, digoxin), ensure an adequate intake of high-potassium foods to prevent potassium deficiency —a potential cause of digitalis toxicity.

Precautions for Use by Those over 60 Years of Age

You may be more sensitive to the actions of this drug. Small doses are advisable until your individual response has been determined.

You may be more susceptible to the development of impaired thinking, orthostatic hypotension, potassium loss, and elevation of blood sugar, complicating the management of diabetes.

If you are taking this drug to treat high blood pressure, remember that warm weather and fever can reduce your blood pressure and make it necessary to adjust your dosage.

Overdosage and extended use of this drug can cause excessive loss of body water, thickening of the blood, and an increased tendency of the blood to clot, predisposing to stroke, heart attack, or thrombophlebitis.

Advisability of Use During Pregnancy

Pregnancy Category: C (tentative). See Pregnancy Code inside back cover.

Animal reproduction studies reveal significant birth defects due to this drug.

Information from adequate studies in pregnant women is not available.

Ask physician for guidance.

This drug should not be used during pregnancy unless a very serious complication of pregnancy occurs for which this drug is significantly beneficial. This type of diuretic can have adverse effects on the fetus.

Advisability of Use While Nursing Infant

Reports indicate that this drug probably does appear in milk. Avoid use if possible. Ask physician for guidance.

Habit-Forming Potential

None.

Effects of Overdosage

With Moderate Overdose: Weakness, lethargy, dizziness, confusion, nausea, vomiting, leg muscle cramps, thirst.

With Large Overdose: Drowsiness progressing to stupor or deep sleep, weak and rapid pulse.

Possible Effects of Extended Use

Impaired balance of water, salt, and potassium in blood and body tissues.

Development of diabetes (in predisposed individuals).

Suggested Periodic Examinations While Taking This Drug (at physician's discretion)

Complete blood cell counts.

Measurements of blood levels of sodium, potassium, chloride, sugar and uric acid.

Liver function tests.

Kidney function tests.

While Taking This Drug, Observe the Following

Foods: It is recommended that you include in your daily diet liberal servings of foods rich in potassium (unless directed otherwise by your physician). The following foods have a high potassium content:

All-bran cereals	Fish, fresh
Almonds	Lentils
Apricots (dried)	Liver, beef
Bananas, fresh	Lonalac
Beans (navy and lima)	Milk
Beef	Peaches (dried)
Carrots (raw)	Peanut butter
Chicken	Peas
Citrus fruits, juices	Pork
Coconut	Potato, sweet
Coffee	Prunes (dried), juice
Crackers (rye)	Raisins
Dates and figs (dried)	Tomato juice

Note: Avoid licorice in large amounts while taking this drug.
Follow your physician's instructions regarding the use of salt.

Beverages: No restrictions unless directed by your physician.

Alcohol: Use with caution until the combined effect has been determined. Alcohol can exaggerate the blood pressure-lowering effect of this drug and cause orthostatic hypotension (see Glossary).

Tobacco Smoking: No interactions expected with this drug. Follow your physician's advice regarding smoking.

Marijuana Smoking

Occasional (once or twice weekly):   No effect to mild increase in thirst and/or urinary frequency.

Daily: Moderate increase in thirst and/or urinary frequency; possible accentuation of orthostatic hypotention (see Glossary).

Other Drugs

Furosemide may *increase* the effects of

- other anti-hypertensive drugs. Careful adjustment of dosages is necessary to prevent excessive lowering of the blood pressure.
- drugs of the phenothiazine family, and cause excessive lowering of the blood pressure. (The thiazides and related drugs and the phenothiazines may both cause orthostatic hypotension.)

Furosemide may *decrease* the effects of

- oral anti-diabetic drugs and insulin, by raising the level of blood sugar. Careful dosage adjustment is necessary to maintain proper control of diabetes.
- allopurinol (Zyloprim), by raising the level of blood uric acid. Careful dosage adjustment is required to maintain proper control of gout.
- probenecid (Benemid), by raising the level of blood uric acid. Careful dosage adjustments are necessary to maintain control of gout.

Furosemide *taken concurrently* with

- salicylates (aspirin, etc.), may cause aspirin poisoning by interfering with its elimination from the body and causing elevation of blood and tissue levels.
- cortisone and cortisone-related drugs, may cause excessive loss of potassium from the body.
- digitalis and related drugs, requires very careful monitoring and dosage adjustments to prevent serious disturbances of heart rhythm.
- tricyclic antidepressants (Elavil, Sinequan, etc.), may cause excessive lowering of the blood pressure.
- oral anticoagulants, requires careful monitoring of the prothrombin time and appropriate adjustment of anticoagulant dosage to prevent abnormal blood clotting.

The following drugs may *increase* the effects of furosemide

- sedatives (especially barbiturates) and narcotic drugs may exaggerate its blood pressure-lowering action.
- mono-amine oxidase (MAO) inhibitor drugs (see Drug Class, Section Three) may greatly exaggerate its blood pressure-lowering action and drop the pressure to dangerous levels.

Driving a Vehicle, Operating Machinery, Engaging in Hazardous Activities: Use caution until the possibility of orthostatic hypotension and/or impaired vision has been determined.

Aviation Note: The use of this drug *may be a disqualification* for the piloting of aircraft. Consultation with a designated Aviation Medical Examiner is advised.

Exposure to Sun: No restrictions.

Exposure to Heat: Avoid excessive perspiring which could cause additional loss of water and salt from the body.

Heavy Exercise or Exertion: Avoid exertion that produces lightheadedness, excessive fatigue, or muscle cramping. Isometric exercises—the "overload" technique for strengthening individual muscles—can raise the blood pressure significantly. Ask your physician for guidance regarding participation in this form of exercise.

Occurrence of Unrelated Illness: Illnesses which cause vomiting or diarrhea can produce a serious imbalance of important body chemistry. Discontinue this drug and ask your physician for guidance.

Discontinuation: It may be advisable to discontinue this drug approximately 5 to 7 days before major surgery. Ask your physician, surgeon, and/or anesthesiologist for guidance regarding dosage reduction or withdrawal.

Special Storage Instructions

Keep in a dry, tightly closed, light-resistant container.

GRISEOFULVIN

Year Introduced: 1959

Brand Names

USA	Canada
Fulvicin P/G (Schering)	Fulvicin P/G (Schering)
Fulvicin-U/F (Schering)	Fulvicin-U/F (Schering)
Grifulvin V (McNeil)	Grisovin-FP (Glaxo)
Grisactin (Ayerst)	
Grisactin Ultra (Ayerst)	
Grisowen (Owen)	
Gris-PEG (Sandoz)	

Common Synonyms ("Street Names"):   Fungus medicine

Drug Class: Antibiotic; Antifungal (Antimycotic)

Prescription Required: Yes

Available for Purchase by Generic Name: USA: Yes   Canada: No

Available Dosage Forms and Strengths

Tablets — 125 mg., 165 mg., 250 mg., 330 mg., 500 mg.
Capsules — 125 mg., 250 mg.
Oral suspension — 125 mg. per teaspoonful (5 ml.)

Tablet May Be Crushed or Capsule Opened for Administration: Yes

How This Drug Works

Intended Therapeutic Effect(s):   The elimination of fungus infections responsive to the action of this drug.

Location of Drug Action(s):   Those areas of the skin, the hair, and the nails infected by certain strains of fungus, and in which an adequate concentration of the drug can be achieved.

Method of Drug Action(s):   This drug prevents the growth and multiplication of susceptible strains of fungus, probably by interfering with their essential metabolic activities.

Principal Uses of This Drug

As a Single Drug Product: This drug is used solely to treat infections of the skin and nails caused by three common types of fungus. Such infections include "ringworm" of the scalp and skin, and "athlete's foot." This drug is effective only against species of fungus that are sensitive to it. It is not effective against yeast organisms, bacteria, or viruses. It should not be used for minor fungus infections that are likely to respond to local treatment with antifungal ointments or lotions.

THIS DRUG SHOULD NOT BE TAKEN IF

—you have had an allergic reaction to any dosage form of it previously.
—you have serious impairment of liver function.
—you have a history of acute intermittent porphyria.

—you have a mild or trivial fungus infection that will respond to local treatment.

INFORM YOUR PHYSICIAN BEFORE TAKING THIS DRUG IF
—you are allergic to any penicillin drug.
—you have lupus erythematosus.

Time Required for Apparent Benefit
From 2 to 10 days for skin infections; from 2 to 4 weeks for nail infections. Complete cure, however, may require continuous use for many weeks or months, depending upon nature and extent of infection.

Possible Side-Effects *(natural, expected, and unavoidable drug actions)*
Mild lowering of the blood pressure.
Superinfections (see Glossary).

Possible Adverse Effects *(unusual, unexpected, and infrequent reactions)*

IF ANY OF THE FOLLOWING DEVELOP, DISCONTINUE DRUG AND NOTIFY YOUR PHYSICIAN AS SOON AS POSSIBLE

Mild Adverse Effects
Allergic Reactions: Skin rashes (various kinds), hives, photosensitivity (see Glossary).
Other Reactions
Headache, a feeling of head fullness, lethargy, dizziness, numbness or pain in the extremities, blurred vision, insomnia.
Nausea, vomiting, diarrhea, irritation of mouth or tongue, "black tongue."

Serious Adverse Effects
Allergic Reactions: Anaphylactic reaction (see Glossary), fever, swelling of face and extremities, painful swollen joints, aching muscles, enlarged and tender lymph glands, jaundice (rare).
Other Reactions: In children: occasional enlargement of breasts, darkening of nipples and genitals.

CAUTION
Troublesome and persistent diarrhea can develop in sensitive individuals. If diarrhea persists more than 24 hours, discontinue this drug and consult your physician for guidance.

Precautions for Use by Those over 60 Years of Age
Natural changes in the skin after 60 may predispose to severe and prolonged itching reactions in the genital and anal regions. This reaction should be reported promptly.

Advisability of Use During Pregnancy
Pregnancy Category: C (tentative). See Pregnancy Code inside back cover.
Animal reproduction studies in mice, rats, cats, and dogs reveal significant birth defects due to this drug.

Information from adequate studies in pregnant women is not available. Avoid completely during first 3 months.
Ask physician for guidance.

Advisability of Use While Nursing Infant
Safety not established. Ask physician for guidance.

Habit-Forming Potential
None.

Effects of Overdosage
Possible nausea, vomiting, diarrhea.

Possible Effects of Extended Use
Superinfections, especially from yeast organisms.
Numbness and/or tingling of hands or feet (see peripheral neuritis in Glossary).

Suggested Periodic Examinations While Taking This Drug (at physician's discretion)
Complete blood cell counts weekly during first 2 months of treatment; longer if findings warrant it.
During extended use, liver and kidney function tests.

While Taking This Drug, Observe the Following
Foods: No restrictions of food selection. Absorption is improved if taken with high fat foods.

Beverages: No restrictions.

Alcohol: Use cautiously until combined effect is determined. A disulfiram-like reaction (see Glossary) can occur. In addition, for some individuals griseofulvin can increase the intoxicating effects of alcohol.

Tobacco Smoking: No interactions expected.

Marijuana Smoking: No interactions expected.

Other Drugs
Griseofulvin may *decrease* the effects of
- oral anticoagulants. Ask physician for guidance regarding prothrombin time testing and dosage adjustment.

The following drugs may *decrease* the effects of griseofulvin
- phenobarbital (and possibly other barbiturates) may reduce its absorption. (Dose of griseofulvin may have to be raised.)

Driving a Vehicle, Operating Machinery, Engaging in Hazardous Activities: No restrictions unless dizziness or impaired vision occur.

Aviation Note: The use of this drug *may be a disqualification* for the piloting of aircraft. Consultation with a designated Aviation Medical Examiner is advised.

Exposure to Sun: Use caution until sensitivity is determined. Photosensitivity can occur (see Glossary).

Discontinuation: Relatively long-term treatment is required to obtain cure. Do not discontinue drug until advised by physician.

Special Storage Instructions

Keep in a dry, tightly closed container. Store at room temperature of 59° to 86° F. (15° to 30° C.).

GUANETHIDINE

Year Introduced: 1960

Brand Names

USA	Canada
Ismelin (CIBA)	Apo-Guanethidine
Esimil [CD] (Ciba)	(Apotex)
	Ismelin (CIBA)
	Ismelin-Esidrix [CD]
	(CIBA)

Common Synonyms ("Street Names"):   Blood pressure pills

Drug Class: Anti-hypertensive (Hypotensive)

Prescription Required: Yes

Available for Purchase by Generic Name: No

Available Dosage Forms and Strengths

Tablets — 10 mg., 25 mg.

Tablet May Be Crushed or Capsule Opened for Administration: Yes

How This Drug Works

Intended Therapeutic Effect(s):   Reduction of high blood pressure.

Location of Drug Action(s):   The storage sites of the nerve impulse transmitter norepinephrine in the terminal fibers of the sympathetic nervous system that activate the muscles in blood vessel walls.

Method of Drug Action(s):   By displacing norepinephrine from its storage sites, this drug reduces the ability of the sympathetic nervous system to maintain the degree of blood vessel constriction responsible for elevation of the blood pressure. This depletion of norepinephrine results in relaxation of blood vessel walls and lowering of the blood pressure.

Principal Uses of This Drug

As a Single Drug Product: This potent anti-hypertensive drug is generally used as a "step 4" medication in conjunction with other anti-hypertensive drugs to treat moderate to severe high blood pressure.

As a Combination Drug Product [CD]: This drug is available in combination with hydrochlorothiazide, an effective diuretic. These two drugs in combination utilize three different mechanisms to lower the blood pressure: the diuretic action reduces the amount of water and sodium in the body and thereby reduces blood volume; the guanethidine provides expansion of blood vessel walls.

THIS DRUG SHOULD NOT BE TAKEN IF
—you have had an allergic reaction to any dosage form of it previously.
—you are taking or have taken within the past 2 weeks any mono-amine oxidase (MAO) inhibitor drug (see Drug Class, Section Three).
—you have a mild and uncomplicated case of high blood pressure.

INFORM YOUR PHYSICIAN BEFORE TAKING THIS DRUG IF
—you have a history of stroke, heart disease, asthma, or kidney disease.
—you have a history of peptic ulcer or chronic acid indigestion.
—you plan to have surgery under general anesthesia in the near future.

Time Required for Apparent Benefit
Continuous use on a regular schedule for several weeks may be necessary to determine this drug's effectiveness in lowering blood pressure and to establish correct dosage.

Possible Side-Effects *(natural, expected, and unavoidable drug actions)*
Lightheadedness, dizziness, weakness, feeling of impending faint in upright position (see orthostatic hypotension in Glossary).
Blurred vision, nasal congestion (stuffiness), dry mouth, water retention.

Possible Adverse Effects *(unusual, unexpected, and infrequent reactions)*

IF ANY OF THE FOLLOWING DEVELOP, DISCONTINUE DRUG AND NOTIFY YOUR PHYSICIAN AS SOON AS POSSIBLE

Mild Adverse Effects
  Allergic Reactions: Skin rash, soreness of salivary glands, loss of scalp hair.
  Other Reactions
    Drowsiness, lethargy, weakness (most apparent during early days of treatment).
    Acid indigestion, nausea, vomiting, diarrhea.
    Mild muscular aches and pains.
    Disturbance of urination. Impaired ejaculation.

Serious Adverse Effects
  Bone marrow depression (see Glossary)—fatigue, weakness, fever, sore throat, unusual bleeding or bruising.
  Activation of stomach or duodenal (peptic) ulcer.

CAUTION
1. Orthostatic hypotension can occur frequently and unexpectedly while using this drug. Avoid sudden arising from a lying or sitting position; avoid prolonged standing and excessive physical exertion. At the onset of lightheadedness, dizziness, or weakness, promptly sit down or lie down to prevent fainting. Ask your physician for guidance in adjusting dosage schedules and activities to prevent orthostatic hypotension.

2. Hot weather and the fever associated with infection can reduce the blood pressure significantly, requiring adjustment of dosage.
3. Report the development of any tendency to emotional depression.

Precautions for Use by Those over 60 Years of Age

The basic rule in treating high blood pressure after 60 is to proceed *cautiously.* The elevated systolic blood pressure often present after 60 is not necessarily a threat to health, and can serve as an adaptive and compensatory change with age that should not be altered drastically. The goals of treatment must be adjusted to the natural changes in body function that occur with aging. Unacceptably high blood pressure should be reduced without creating the risks associated with excessively low blood pressure.

It is advisable to start treatment with small doses and to monitor the blood pressure response frequently. Sudden, rapid, and excessive reduction of blood pressure can predispose to stroke or heart attack.

You may be more susceptible to the development of orthostatic hypotension with resultant lightheadedness, dizziness, unsteadiness, fainting, and falling. Report such symptoms to your physician promptly.

Advisability of Use During Pregnancy

Pregnancy Category: B (tentative). See Pregnancy Code inside back cover. Animal reproduction studies in rats reveal no birth defects due to this drug. Information from adequate studies in pregnant women is not available. Ask physician for guidance.

Advisability of Use While Nursing Infant

The presence of this drug in milk is unknown. Ask physician for guidance.

Habit-Forming Potential

None.

Effects of Overdosage

With Moderate Overdose: Marked drop in blood pressure, extreme weakness in upright position leading to falling and fainting, severe diarrhea.

With Large Overdose: Drop in blood pressure to shock levels, loss of consciousness, slow and weak pulse, cold and sweaty skin.

Possible Effects of Extended Use

Due to this drug's accumulative action, careful dosage adjustment will be necessary to prevent wide fluctuations in blood pressure and unexpected episodes of sudden drop in blood pressure accompanied by fainting.

Suggested Periodic Examinations While Taking This Drug (at physician's discretion)

Complete blood cell counts.

While Taking This Drug, Observe the Following

Foods: No restrictions with regard to drug interactions. Avoid highly seasoned and irritating foods if you are subject to acid indigestion or peptic ulcer.

Beverages: Use carbonated beverages sparingly.

Alcohol: Use sparingly and with extreme caution until combined effect has been determined. Alcohol can increase the blood pressure-lowering action of this drug and cause the development of orthostatic hypotension.

Tobacco Smoking: Nicotine can cause an elevation of blood pressure in sensitive individuals. Follow your physician's advice regarding smoking.

Marijuana Smoking

Occasional (once or twice weekly):   No effect to mild and transient accentuation of orthostatic hypotension (see Glossary).

Daily: Significant accentuation of orthostatic hypotension, requiring dosage adjustment in sensitive individuals.

Other Drugs

Guanethidine may *increase* the effects of
- other anti-hypertensives, and cause excessive lowering of the blood pressure. Careful dosage adjustments are necessary.
- insulin, and cause hypoglycemia (see Glossary).

Guanethidine *taken concurrently* with
- digitalis drugs, may cause marked reduction of heart rate. Careful monitoring and dosage adjustments are necessary.

The following drugs may *increase* the effects of guanethidine
- thiazide diuretics
- reserpine and related drugs

The following drugs may *decrease* the effects of guanethidine
- amphetamines (Benzedrine, Dexedrine, Methedrine, etc.) can reduce its blood pressure-lowering action.
- tricyclic antidepressants (Elavil, Tofranil, etc.) may completely reverse the anti-hypertensive action of guanethidine and render it ineffective. (Sinequan appears to be an exception to this interaction.)
- antihistamines may reduce its anti-hypertensive action.
- oral contraceptives significantly reduce the ability of guanethidine to lower the blood pressure.

Driving a Vehicle, Operating Machinery, Engaging in Hazardous Activities: Be alert to the possibility of orthostatic hypotension developing while engaged in hazardous activities. This drug can also cause drowsiness and impair mental alertness, coordination, and reaction time.

Aviation Note: The use of this drug and the disorder for which this drug is prescribed *are disqualifications* for the piloting of aircraft. Consultation with a designated Aviation Medical Examiner is advised.

Exposure to Sun: No restrictions.

Exposure to Heat: Hot weather and overheated environments favor the development of orthostatic hypotension. Avoid as much as possible.

Exposure to Cold: No restrictions.

Heavy Exercise or Exertion: Use caution until tolerance for physical activity and exercise are determined. Excessive exertion can induce orthostatic hypotension. Isometric exercises—the "overload" technique for strengthening individual muscles—can raise the blood pressure significantly. Ask your physician for guidance regarding participation in this form of exercise.

Discontinuation: Upon stopping this drug, the dosage schedules of other drugs taken concurrently with it will require readjustment. Ask physician for guidance.

Special Storage Instructions
Keep in a dry, tightly closed container.

HALOPERIDOL

Year Introduced: 1967

Brand Names

USA	Canada
Haldol (McNeil)	Apo-Haloperidol (Apotex)
	Haldol (McNeil)
	Peridol (Technilab)

Common Synonyms ("Street Names"):   None

Drug Class: Tranquilizer, Strong (Anti-psychotic), Butyrophenones

Prescription Required: Yes

Available for Purchase by Generic Name: No

Available Dosage Forms and Strengths
Tablets — 0.5 mg., 1 mg., 2 mg., 5 mg., 10 mg., 20 mg.
Concentrate — 2 mg. per ml.
Injection — 5 mg. per ml.

Tablet May Be Crushed or Capsule Opened for Administration: Yes

How This Drug Works
Intended Therapeutic Effect(s):   Restoration of emotional calm. Relief of severe anxiety, agitation, and psychotic behavior.

Location of Drug Action(s):   Those nerve pathways in the mesolimbic area of the brain that utilize the tissue chemical dopamine for the transmission of nerve impulses.

Method of Drug Action(s):   Not completely established. Present theory is that by inhibiting the action of dopamine, this drug acts to correct an imbalance of nerve impulse transmissions that is thought to be responsible for certain mental disorders.

Principal Uses of This Drug

As a Single Drug Product: Used primarily to control the psychotic thinking and abnormal behavior associated with acute psychosis of unknown nature, acute schizophrenia, paranoid states, and the manic phase of manic-depressive disorders. It is also used to treat the hyperactivity syndrome in children. A less frequent use is to control the tics and offensive language characteristic of Gilles de la Tourette's syndrome.

THIS DRUG SHOULD NOT BE TAKEN IF

—you have had an allergic reaction to any dosage form of it previously.
—you are experiencing mental depression at the present time.
—you have any form of Parkinson's disease.
—it is prescribed for a child under 3 years of age.

INFORM YOUR PHYSICIAN BEFORE TAKING THIS DRUG IF

—you are allergic by nature, or have a history of allergic reactions to drugs.
—you have a history of mental depression.
—you have a history of liver or kidney disease, or impaired liver or kidney function.
—you have diabetes.
—you have epilepsy.
—you have glaucoma.
—you have any form of heart disease, especially angina (coronary insufficiency).
—you have high blood pressure.
—you drink alcoholic beverages daily.
—you are taking oral anticoagulant drugs.
—you are taking sedatives, sleep-inducing drugs, tranquilizers, antidepressants, antihistamines, or narcotic drugs of any kind.
—you plan to have surgery under general or spinal anesthesia in the near future.

Time Required for Apparent Benefit

Significant benefit may occur within 3 weeks. However, maximal benefit may require continuous use on a regular basis for several months.

Possible Side-Effects *(natural, expected, and unavoidable drug actions)*

Drowsiness, lethargy, blurred vision, dryness of the mouth, impaired urination, constipation, transient drop in blood pressure.

Possible Adverse Effects *(unusual, unexpected, and infrequent reactions)*

IF ANY OF THE FOLLOWING DEVELOP, DISCONTINUE DRUG AND NOTIFY YOUR PHYSICIAN AS SOON AS POSSIBLE

Mild Adverse Effects
Allergic Reactions: Skin rashes (various kinds), loss of hair.
Other Reactions
Insomnia, restlessness, anxiety, agitation.
Headache, dizziness, weakness.
Lightheadedness or faintness in upright position, heart palpitation, rapid heart rate.

Reduced appetite, nausea, vomiting, diarrhea.

Breast fullness, tenderness, and milk production.

Serious Adverse Effects

Allergic Reactions: Jaundice (rarely; see Glossary).

Other Reactions

Parkinson-like disorders (see Glossary).

Muscle spasms affecting the jaw, neck, back, hands, or feet.

Eye-rolling, muscle twitching, convulsions.

Depression, confusion, hallucinations.

Sexual impotence.

Reduced number of red blood cells (anemia).

Fluctuations in number of white blood cells.

Fluctuations in blood sugar levels.

CAUTION

1. Many over-the-counter (OTC) medications (see Glossary) for allergies, colds, and coughs contain drugs that can interact unfavorably with this drug. Ask your physician or pharmacist for guidance before using any such medications.
2. Antacids that contain aluminum and/or magnesium can prevent the absorption of this drug and reduce its effectiveness.
3. Obtain prompt evaluation of any disturbance or change in vision.

Precautions for Use by Those over 60 Years of Age

You may be more sensitive to all of the actions of this drug. Small doses are advisable until your individual response has been determined.

You may be more susceptible to the development of drowsiness, lethargy, constipation, lowering of body temperature (hypothermia), and excessive drop in blood pressure on arising from a lying or sitting position (see orthostatic hypotension in Glossary).

This drug can increase the degree of impaired urination associated with prostate gland enlargement (prostatism).

You may also be more susceptible to the development of Parkinson-like disorders and/or tardive dyskinesia (see discussion of these terms in Glossary). These conditions must be recognized early since they may become unresponsive to treatment and irreversible. Consult your physician promptly if suggestive symptoms develop.

Advisability of Use During Pregnancy

Pregnancy Category: C (tentative). See Pregnancy Code inside back cover.

Animal reproduction studies in mice reveal significant birth defects due to this drug.

Information from adequate studies in pregnant women is not available.

It is advisable to avoid this drug during first 3 months.

Ask physician for guidance.

Advisability of Use While Nursing Infant

The presence of this drug in milk is not known. Ask your physician for guidance.

Habit-Forming Potential
None.

Effects of Overdosage
With Moderate Overdose: Marked drowsiness, weakness, muscle rigidity, tremors, confusion, dryness of mouth, blurred or double vision.
With Large Overdose: Deep sleep progressing to coma, weak and rapid pulse, shallow and slow breathing, very low blood pressure, convulsions.

Possible Effects of Extended Use
Tardive dyskinesia (see Glossary).

Suggested Periodic Examinations While Taking This Drug (at physician's discretion)
Complete blood cell counts.
Liver function tests.
Careful inspection of the tongue for early evidence of fine, involuntary, wave-like movements that could indicate the beginning of tardive dyskinesia.

While Taking This Drug, Observe the Following
Foods: No restrictions.
Beverages: No restrictions. The liquid concentrate form of this drug may be taken in water, in fruit or vegetable juices, or in milk.
Alcohol: Avoid completely. Alcohol can increase this drug's sedative action and accentuate its depressant effects on brain function. Haloperidol can increase the intoxicating effects of alcohol.
Tobacco Smoking: No interactions expected.
Marijuana Smoking
   Occasional (once or twice weekly):   No effect to mild and transient increase in drowsiness and accentuation of orthostatic hypotension (see Glossary); some risk of precipitating latent psychoses (in predisposed individuals).
   Daily: Moderate increase in drowsiness, significant accentuation of orthostatic hypotension; increased risk of precipitating latent psychoses, confusing interpretation of mental status and of drug responses.
Other Drugs
Haloperidol may *increase* the effects of
   • atropine-like drugs, and cause an increase in internal eye pressure in the presence of glaucoma.
   • sedatives, sleep-inducing drugs, other tranquilizers, antihistamines, and narcotic drugs, and cause excessive sedation.

Haloperidol may *decrease* the effects of
   • oral anticoagulants, and require adjustment of their dosage.
   • bethanidine.
   • guanethidine.
   • levodopa.

Haloperidol *taken concurrently* with
- anti-convulsant drugs, may cause a change in the pattern of seizures. Dosage adjustment of the anti-convulsant may be necessary.
- anti-hypertensive drugs (some), may cause excessive lowering of the blood pressure.
- methyldopa, may cause serious mental and behavioral abnormalities.

The following drugs may *increase* the effects of haloperidol
- barbiturates may cause excessive sedation.
- other tranquilizers may cause excessive sedation.
- tricyclic antidepressants may cause excessive sedation.

Driving a Vehicle, Operating Machinery, Engaging in Hazardous Activities: This drug can impair mental alertness, judgment, and physical coordination. Avoid all hazardous activities if you experience such drug effects.

Aviation Note: The use of this drug and the disorder for which this drug is prescribed *are disqualifications* for the piloting of aircraft. Consultation with a designated Aviation Medical Examiner is advised.

Exposure to Sun: Use caution until full effect is known. This drug can cause photosensitivity.

Special Storage Instructions
Keep all forms of this drug in airtight containers. Protect from light.

HYDRALAZINE

Year Introduced: 1952

Brand Names

USA		Canada
Apresoline (CIBA)	Ser-Ap-Es [CD]	Apresoline (CIBA)
Dralzine (Lemmon)	(CIBA)	Ser-Ap-Es [CD]
Apresazide [CD]	Serpasil-Apresoline	(CIBA)
(CIBA)	[CD] (CIBA)	Serpasil-Apresoline
Apresoline-Esidrix	Unipres [CD]	[CD] (CIBA)
[CD] (CIBA)	(Reid-Provident)	
Hydral 25/25 [CD]		
(Reid-Provident)		

Common Synonyms ("Street Names"):   Blood pressure pills

Drug Class: Anti-hypertensive (Hypotensive)

Prescription Required: Yes

Available for Purchase by Generic Name: USA: Yes   Canada: No

Available Dosage Forms and Strengths
Tablets — 10 mg., 25 mg., 50 mg., 100 mg.

Tablet May Be Crushed or Capsule Opened for Administration: Yes

How This Drug Works

Intended Therapeutic Effect(s):   Reduction of high blood pressure.

Location of Drug Action(s):   The muscles in the walls of blood vessels. The principal therapeutic action occurs in the small arteries (arterioles).

Method of Drug Action(s):   By causing direct relaxation and expansion of blood vessel walls, this drug lowers the pressure of the blood within. The mechanism of this direct action is not known.

Principal Uses of This Drug

As a Single Drug Product: This anti-hypertensive drug is used as a "step 3" medication in conjunction with other anti-hypertensive drugs in the treatment of moderate to severe high blood pressure.

As a Combination Drug Product [CD]:   This drug is available in combination with hydrochlorothiazide (a diuretic), and with reserpine (another type of anti-hypertensive). When used in combination, several different types of drug action are used concurrently to reduce the blood pressure: hydralazine relaxes and expands the blood vessel walls; the diuretic reduces the amounts of water and salt in the body; reserpine reduces the rate and contraction force of the heart and enhances the expansion of blood vessels.

THIS DRUG SHOULD NOT BE TAKEN IF

—you have had an allergic reaction to any dosage form of it previously.

—you have a history of coronary artery disease (angina, coronary insufficiency, heart attack).

—you have a history of rheumatic heart disease (consult your physician regarding specific contraindications).

INFORM YOUR PHYSICIAN BEFORE TAKING THIS DRUG IF

—you experience pain in the chest, neck, or arms on physical exertion (possible angina).

—you have a history of lupus erythematosus.

—you have had a stroke at any time.

—you have a history of kidney disease or impaired kidney function.

—you plan to have surgery under general anesthesia in the near future.

Time Required for Apparent Benefit

Continuous use on a regular schedule for several weeks may be necessary to determine this drug's effectiveness in lowering your blood pressure.

Possible Side-Effects *(natural, expected, and unavoidable drug actions)*

Lightheadedness on arising from a sitting or lying position (see orthostatic hypotension in Glossary).

Nasal congestion, constipation, difficult urination.

Possible Adverse Effects *(unusual, unexpected, and infrequent reactions)*

IF ANY OF THE FOLLOWING DEVELOP, DISCONTINUE DRUG AND NOTIFY YOUR PHYSICIAN AS SOON AS POSSIBLE

Mild Adverse Effects
Allergic Reactions: Skin rashes (various kinds), hives, itching, drug fever.
Other Reactions
Headache, dizziness, heart palpitation, flushing.
Reduced appetite, nausea, vomiting, diarrhea.
Tremors, muscle cramps.

Serious Adverse Effects
Allergic Reactions: Hepatitis with or without jaundice (see Glossary).
Other Reactions
Excessive stimulation of the heart resulting in chest pain on exertion (angina) in individuals with existing coronary artery disease.
Peripheral neuritis (see Glossary)—weakness, numbness, and tingling of the arms or legs.
Bone marrow depression (see Glossary)—weakness, fatigue, fever, sore throat, unusual bleeding or bruising.
Behavioral changes—nervousness, confusion, emotional depression.

CAUTION
1. Toxic reactions are more likely to occur with large doses. Adhere strictly to prescribed dosage schedules. Keep appointments for periodic follow-up examinations.
2. Hot weather and the fever associated with infection can reduce the blood pressure significantly, requiring adjustment of dosage.
3. Report the development of any tendency to emotional depression.

Precautions for Use by Those over 60 Years of Age
The basic rule in treating high blood pressure after 60 is to proceed *cautiously.* The elevated systolic blood pressure often present after 60 is not necessarily a threat to health, and can serve as an adaptive and compensatory change with age that should not be altered drastically. The goals of treatment must be adjusted to the natural changes in body function that occur with aging. Unacceptably high blood pressure should be reduced without creating the risks associated with excessively low blood pressure.
It is advisable to start treatment with small doses and to monitor the blood pressure response frequently. Sudden, rapid, and excessive reduction of blood pressure can predispose to stroke or heart attack.
You may be more susceptible to the development of orthostatic hypotension with resultant lightheadedness, dizziness, unsteadiness, fainting, and falling. Report such symptoms to your physician promptly.

Advisability of Use During Pregnancy
Pregnancy Category: C (tentative). See Pregnancy Code inside back cover.
Animal reproduction studies in mice reveal significant birth defects due to this drug.

Information from adequate studies in pregnant women is not available. It is advisable to avoid this drug during first 3 months. Ask physician for guidance.

Advisability of Use While Nursing Infant
This drug is known to be present in milk. Ask physician for guidance.

Habit-Forming Potential
None.

Effects of Overdosage
With Moderate Overdose: Marked lightheadedness or dizziness in upright position (orthostatic hypotension), headache, rapid heart action, generalized flushing of skin.

With Large Overdose: Collapse of circulation—extreme weakness, loss of consciousness, cold and sweaty skin, weak and rapid pulse.

Possible Effects of Extended Use
Long-term use may cause an arthritis-like illness (lupus erythematosus; see Glossary) in susceptible individuals.

Suggested Periodic Examinations While Taking This Drug (at physician's discretion)
Complete blood cell counts.
Liver function tests.
Exercise electrocardiograms.

While Taking This Drug, Observe the Following
Foods: No restrictions. Ask physician regarding the advisability of supplementing your diet with Vitamin B–6 (pyridoxine) to prevent peripheral neuritis (see Glossary).

Beverages: No restrictions.

Alcohol: Use with extreme caution until combined effect has been determined. Alcohol can exaggerate the blood pressure-lowering action of this drug and cause excessive reduction.

Tobacco Smoking: The nicotine in tobacco can contribute significantly to this drug's ability to intensify coronary insufficiency (angina) in susceptible individuals. Follow your physician's advice regarding the use of tobacco.

Marijuana Smoking
Occasional (once or twice weekly): No effect to mild and transient accentuation of orthostatic hypotension (see Glossary).
Daily: Significant accentuation of orthostatic hypotension, requiring dosage adjustment in sensitive individuals.

Other Drugs
Hydralazine may *increase* the effects of
• other anti-hypertensive drugs, and cause excessive lowering of the blood pressure. Careful dosage adjustments are necessary.

The following drugs may *increase* the effects of hydralazine
- tricyclic antidepressants (Elavil, Tofranil, Sinequan, etc.) may increase the possibility of orthostatic hypotension.
- oral diuretics (Aldactone, Dyrenium, Edecrin, Lasix, and the thiazide drug family) can significantly enhance its blood pressure-lowering action. Dosage adjustments may be necessary.
- mono-amine oxidase (MAO) inhibitor drugs may increase its blood pressure-lowering action.

The following drugs may *decrease* the effects of hydralazine
- amphetamines (Benzedrine, Dexedrine, Synatan, etc.) can impair its blood pressure-lowering action.

Driving a Vehicle, Operating Machinery, Engaging in Hazardous Activities: Avoid hazardous activities until the possibility of orthostatic hypotension has been determined.

Aviation Note: The use of this drug and the disorder for which this drug is prescribed *are disqualifications* for the piloting of aircraft. Consultation with a designated Aviation Medical Examiner is advised.

Exposure to Sun: No restrictions.

Exposure to Cold: Use caution until combined effect has been determined. Cold may increase this drug's ability to cause coronary insufficiency (angina) in susceptible individuals.

Heavy Exercise or Exertion: Use caution until combined effect has been determined. Excessive exertion can increase this drug's ability to cause coronary insufficiency (angina) in susceptible individuals. Isometric exercises—the "overload" technique for strengthening individual muscles—can raise the blood pressure significantly. Ask your physician for guidance regarding participation in this form of exercise.

Special Storage Instructions
Keep in a dry, tightly closed container.

HYDROCHLOROTHIAZIDE

Year Introduced: 1959

Brand Names

USA		**Canada**
Esidrix (CIBA)	Dyazide [CD] (Smith	ApoHydro-
HydroDIURIL	Kline & French)	chlorothiazide
(Merck Sharp &	Hydral 25/25 [CD]	(Apotex)
Dohme)	(Reid-Provident)	Diuchlor H (Medic)
Hydro Z-50	Hydro Plus [CD]	Esidrix (CIBA)
(Mayrand)	(Reid-Provident)	HydroDiuril (MSD)
Hyperetic (Elder)	Hydropres 50 [CD]	Natrimax (Trianon)
Oretic (Abbott)	(Merck Sharp &	Nefrol (Riva)
SK Hydro-	Dohme)	Neo-Codema (Neo)
chlorothiazide	Inderide [CD]	Novohydrazide
(Smith Kline &	(Ayerst)	(Novopharm)
French)	Ser-Ap-Es [CD]	Urozide (ICN)
Thiuretic	(CIBA)	Aldactazide [CD]
(Parke-Davis)	Serpasil-Esidrix [CD]	(Searle)
Zide (Tutag)	(CIBA)	Dyazide [CD] (SKF)
Aldactazide [CD]	Unipres [CD]	Hydropres 25 [CD]
(Searle)	(Reid-Provident)	(MSD)
Apresazide [CD]	(Numerous	Inderide [CD]
(CIBA)	combination brand	(Ayerst)
	names)	Ser-Ap-Es [CD]
		(CIBA)
		Serpasil Esidrix [CD]
		(CIBA)

Common Synonyms ("Street Names"):   Water pills

Drug Class: Anti-hypertensive (Hypotensive); Diuretic, Thiazides

Prescription Required: Yes

Available for Purchase by Generic Name: Yes

Available Dosage Forms and Strengths
Tablets — 25 mg., 50 mg., 100 mg.

Tablet May Be Crushed or Capsule Opened for Administration: Yes

How This Drug Works
Intended Therapeutic Effect(s)
Elimination of excessive fluid retention (edema).
Reduction of high blood pressure.
Location of Drug Action(s):   Principal actions occur in
• the tubular systems of the kidney that determine the final composition of the urine.
• the walls of the smaller arteries.

Method of Drug Action(s)

By increasing the elimination of salt and water from the body (through increased urine production), this drug reduces the volume of fluid in the blood and body tissues and lowers the sodium content throughout the body.

By relaxing the walls of the smaller arteries and allowing them to expand, this drug significantly increases the total capacity of the arterial system.

The combined effect of these two actions (reduced blood volume in expanded space) results in lowering of the blood pressure.

Principal Uses of This Drug

As a Single Drug Product: This drug is used as a mild diuretic and as the initial drug ("step 1") in the treatment of mild to moderate high blood pressure.

As a Combination Drug Product [CD]:   This drug is frequently combined with other drugs to improve its effectiveness as both a diuretic and an anti-hypertensive. Spironolactone is combined with this drug to prevent the excessive loss of potassium in the urine and to make it unecessary to take potassium supplements. Other anti-hypertensive drugs that represent "step 2" medications are combined with this drug to utilize several drug actions simultaneously for more effective control of moderate high blood pressure.

THIS DRUG SHOULD NOT BE TAKEN IF

—you are allergic to any of the drugs bearing the brand names listed above.

INFORM YOUR PHYSICIAN BEFORE TAKING THIS DRUG IF

—you are allergic to any form of "sulfa" drug.

—you are pregnant and your physician does not know it.

—you have a history of kidney disease or liver disease, or impaired kidney or liver function.

—you have diabetes (or a tendency to diabetes).

—you have a history of gout.

—you have a history of lupus erythematosus.

—you are taking any form of cortisone, digitalis, oral anti-diabetic drug, or insulin.

—you plan to have surgery under general anesthesia in the near future.

Time Required for Apparent Benefit

Increased urine volume begins in 2 hours, reaches a maximum in 4 to 6 hours, and subsides in 8 to 12 hours. Continuous use on a regular schedule will be necessary for 2 to 3 weeks to determine this drug's effectiveness in lowering your blood pressure.

Possible Side-Effects (*natural, expected, and unavoidable drug actions*)

Lightheadedness on arising from sitting or lying position (see orthostatic hypotension in Glossary).

Increase in level of blood sugar, affecting control of diabetes.

Increase in level of blood uric acid, affecting control of gout.

Decrease in level of blood potassium, resulting in muscle weakness and cramping.

Possible Adverse Effects *(unusual, unexpected, and infrequent reactions)*

IF ANY OF THE FOLLOWING DEVELOP, DISCONTINUE DRUG AND NOTIFY YOUR PHYSICIAN AS SOON AS POSSIBLE

Mild Adverse Effects
Allergic Reactions: Skin rashes (various kinds), hives, drug fever.
Other Reactions
Reduced appetite, indigestion, nausea, vomiting, diarrhea.
Headache, dizziness, yellow vision, blurred vision.

Serious Adverse Effects
Allergic Reactions
Hepatitis with jaundice (see Glossary).
Anaphylactic reaction (see Glossary).
Severe skin reactions.
Other Reactions
Inflammation of the pancreas—severe abdominal pain.
Bone marrow depression (see Glossary)—fatigue, weakness, fever, sore throat, unusual bleeding or bruising.

CAUTION
1. Do not exceed recommended doses. Increased dosage can cause excessive excretion of sodium and potassium with resultant loss of appetite, nausea, fatigue, weakness, confusion, and tingling in the extremities.
2. If you are also taking a digitalis preparation (digitoxin, digoxin), ensure an adequate intake of high-potassium foods to prevent potassium deficiency —a potential cause of digitalis toxicity.

Precautions for Use by Those over 60 Years of Age
You may be more sensitive to the actions of this drug. Small doses are advisable until your individual response has been determined.
You may be more susceptible to the development of impaired thinking, orthostatic hypotension, potassium loss, and elevation of blood sugar, complicating the management of diabetes.
If you are taking this drug to treat high blood pressure, remember that warm weather and fever can reduce your blood pressure and make it necessary to adjust your dosage.
Overdosage and extended use of this drug can cause excessive loss of body water, thickening (increased viscosity) of the blood, and an increased tendency of the blood to clot, predisposing to stroke, heart attack, or thrombophlebitis.

Advisability of Use During Pregnancy
Pregnancy Category: B (tentative). See Pregnancy Code inside back cover.
Animal reproduction studies in rats reveal no birth defects due to this drug.
Information from studies in pregnant women indicates no increased defects in 7575 exposures to this drug.

This drug should not be used during pregnancy unless a very serious complication of pregnancy occurs for which this drug is significantly beneficial. This type of diuretic can have adverse effects on the fetus.

Ask physician for guidance.

Advisability of Use While Nursing Infant
This drug is known to be present in milk. Ask physician for guidance.

Habit-Forming Potential
None.

Effects of Overdosage
With Moderate Overdose: Dryness of mouth, thirst, lethargy, weakness, muscle pain and cramping, nausea, vomiting.

With Large Overdose: Drowsiness progressing to stupor and coma, weak and rapid pulse.

Possible Effects of Extended Use
Impaired balance of water, salt, and potassium in blood and body tissues. Development of diabetes (in predisposed individuals).

Suggested Periodic Examinations While Taking This Drug (at physician's discretion)
Complete blood cell counts.

Measurements of blood levels of sodium, potassium, chloride, sugar, and uric acid.

Liver function tests.

Kidney function tests.

While Taking This Drug, Observe the Following
Foods   It is recommended that you include in your daily diet liberal servings of foods rich in potassium (unless directed otherwise by your physician). The following foods have a high potassium content:

All-bran cereals	Fish, fresh
Almonds	Lentils
Apricots (dried)	Liver, beef
Bananas, fresh	Lonalac
Beans (navy and lima)	Milk
Beef	Peaches (dried)
Carrots (raw)	Peanut butter
Chicken	Peas
Citrus fruits, juices	Pork
Coconut	Potato, sweet
Coffee	Prunes (dried), juice
Crackers (rye)	Raisins
Dates and figs (dried)	Tomato juice

Note: Avoid licorice in large amounts while taking this drug. Follow your physician's instructions regarding the use of salt.

Beverages: No restrictions unless directed by your physician.

Alcohol: Use with caution until the combined effect has been determined.

Alcohol can exaggerate the blood pressure-lowering effect of this drug and cause orthostatic hypotension.

Tobacco Smoking: No interactions expected. Follow your physician's advice regarding smoking.

Marijuana Smoking

Occasional (once or twice weekly): No effect to mild increase in thirst and/or urinary frequency.

Daily: Moderate increase in thirst and/or urinary frequency; possible accentuation of orthostatic hypotention (see Glossary).

Other Drugs

Hydrochlorothiazide may *increase* the effects of

- other anti-hypertensive drugs. Careful adjustment of dosages is necessary to prevent excessive lowering of the blood pressure.
- drugs of the phenothiazine family, and cause excessive lowering of the blood pressure. (Thiazides and related drugs and the phenothiazines both may cause orthostatic hypotension).

Hydrochlorothiazide may *decrease* the effects of

- oral anti-diabetic drugs and insulin, by raising the level of blood sugar. Careful adjustment of dosages is necessary to maintain proper control of diabetes.
- allopurinol (Zyloprim), by raising the level of blood uric acid. Careful adjustment of dosages is required to maintain proper control of gout.
- probenecid (Benemid), by raising the level of blood uric acid. Careful dosage adjustment is necessary to maintain control of gout.

Hydrochlorothiazide *taken concurrently* with

- cortisone and cortisone-related drugs, may cause excessive loss of potassium from the body.
- digitalis and related drugs, requires very careful monitoring and dosage adjustments to prevent serious disturbances of heart rhythm.
- tricyclic antidepressants (Elavil, Sinequan, etc.), may cause excessive lowering of the blood pressure.

The following drugs may *increase* the effects of hydrochlorothiazide

- barbiturates may exaggerate its blood pressure-lowering action.
- mono-amine oxidase (MAO) inhibitor drugs may increase urine volume by delaying this drug's elimination from the body.
- pain relievers (analgesics), both narcotic and non-narcotic, may exaggerate its blood pressure-lowering action.

The following drug may *decrease* the effects of hydrochlorothiazide

- cholestyramine (Cuemid, Questran) may interfere with its absorption. Take cholestyramine 30 to 60 minutes before any oral diuretic.

Driving a Vehicle, Operating Machinery, Engaging in Hazardous Activities: Use caution until the possibility of orthostatic hypotension and/or impaired vision has been determined.

Aviation Note: The use of this drug *may be a disqualification* for the piloting of aircraft. Consultation with a designated Aviation Medical Examiner is advised.

Exposure to Sun: Use caution until sensitivity has been determined. This drug can cause photosensitivity (see Glossary).

Exposure to Heat: Avoid excessive perspiring that could cause additional loss of water and salt from the body.

Heavy Exercise or Exertion: Avoid exertion that produces lightheadedness, excessive fatigue, or muscle cramping. Isometric exercises—the "overload" technique for strengthening individual muscles—can raise the blood pressure significantly. Ask your physician for guidance regarding participation in this form of exercise.

Occurrence of Unrelated Illness: Illnesses which cause vomiting or diarrhea can produce a serious imbalance of important body chemistry. Discontinue this drug and ask your physician for guidance.

Discontinuation: It may be advisable to discontinue this drug approximately 5 to 7 days before major surgery. Ask your physician, surgeon, and/or anesthesiologist for guidance regarding dosage reduction or withdrawal.

Special Storage Instructions

Keep in a dry, tightly closed container.

HYDROCODONE
(Dihydrocodeinone)

Year Introduced: 1951

Brand Names

USA		Canada
Dicodid (Knoll)	Hycotuss Expectorant	Corutol DH (Dow)
Hycodan [CD]	[CD] (DuPont)	Hycodan (Endo)
(DuPont)	Triaminic	Robidone (Robins)
Hycomine Compound	Expectorant DH	Hycodan-D [CD]
[CD] (DuPont)	[CD] (Dorsey)	(Endo)
Hycomine Pediatric	Tussend [CD] (Dow)	Hycodan-E [CD]
Syrup [CD]	Tussend Expectorant	(Endo)
(DuPont)	[CD] (Dow)	Hycomine Pediatric
Hycomine Syrup	Tussionex [CD]	Syrup [CD] (Endo)
[CD] (DuPont)	(Pennwalt)	Hycomine Syrup
		[CD] (Endo)
		Triaminic
		Expectorant DH
		[CD] (Anca)
		Tussionex [CD]
		(Pennwalt)

Common Synonyms ("Street Names"):   Cough medicine

Drug Class: Cough suppressant (Antitussives)

Prescription Required: Yes (Controlled Drug, U.S. Schedules II and III)*

Available for Purchase by Generic Name: No

Available Dosage Forms and Strengths
    Tablets — 5 mg.
    Liquid — 5 mg. per teaspoonful (5 ml.)
    Syrup — 5 mg. per teaspoonful (5 ml.)
    Note: Also available in numerous combination cough remedies of various strengths. Read the labels carefully for the strengths of individual ingredients.

Tablet May Be Crushed or Capsule Opened for Administration: Yes

How This Drug Works
    Intended Therapeutic Effect(s):   Reduction in the frequency, severity, and duration of coughing associated with allergic or infectious disorders of the windpipe (trachea) and/or the bronchial tubes.
    Location of Drug Action(s):   The principal action occurs in the cough control center located in the brain stem.
    Method of Drug Action(s):   By reducing the sensitivity of the cough control center to the reflex stimulation from irritated lower respiratory passages, this drug suppresses the tendency to cough.

Principal Uses of This Drug
    As a Single Drug Product: Used primarily to control coughing due to tracheitis and/or bronchitis of either infectious or allergic origin.
    As a Combination Drug Product [CD]:   This drug is frequently combined with other drugs in the formulation of "cough remedies." Atropine derivatives and decongestants may be added to reduce secretions in the air passages; expectorants may be added to render secretions more liquid and easier to raise with coughing; mild pain relievers and antihistamines may be combined with it to provide a sedative effect.

THIS DRUG SHOULD NOT BE TAKEN IF
—you have had an allergic reaction to any dosage form of it previously.

INFORM YOUR PHYSICIAN BEFORE TAKING THIS DRUG IF
—you have had an unfavorable reaction to any narcotic drug in the past.
—you are taking any sedatives, sleep-inducing drugs, tranquilizers, pain-relieving drugs, antihistamines, or mono-amine oxidase (MAO) inhibitor drugs (see Drug Class, Section Three).
—you have emphysema or chronic impairment of breathing.
—you have any difficulty emptying the urinary bladder.

Time Required for Apparent Benefit
    Drug action usually begins in 1 hour and persists for 4 to 8 hours.
    Continuous use on a regular schedule for 2 days is usually necessary to determine this drug's effectiveness in controlling cough.

*See Schedules of Controlled Drugs inside back cover.

Possible Side-Effects *(natural, expected, and unavoidable drug actions)*
Drowsiness, unsteadiness in stance and gait, constipation.

Possible Adverse Effects *(unusual, unexpected, and infrequent reactions)*

IF ANY OF THE FOLLOWING DEVELOP, DISCONTINUE DRUG AND NOTIFY YOUR PHYSICIAN AS SOON AS POSSIBLE

Mild Adverse Effects
  Allergic Reactions: Itching.
  Other Reactions
    Lightheadedness, dizziness, euphoria.
    Nausea, vomiting.
Serious Adverse Effects
  Idiosyncratic Reactions: Nervousness, agitation, excessive perspiration.

CAUTION
1. Maximal adult dosage should not exceed 60 mg. per 24 hours.
2. Avoid the concurrent use of this drug with any mono-amine oxidase (MAO) inhibitor drug.

Precautions for Use by Infants and Children
Young children (under 6 years of age) are especially susceptible to the depressant action of narcotic cough suppressants. Start with very small doses and monitor effects closely.

Precautions for Use by Those over 60 Years of Age
The aim of treatment should be to provide the maximal control of coughing consistent with minimal risk and the preservation of ability to function. Dosage should be low at the beginning with adjustment upward according to individual response and need.
The use of this drug should be limited to short-term treatment only.
You may be more susceptible to the development of dizziness, drowsiness, constipation, and impaired urination.

Advisability of Use During Pregnancy
Pregnancy Category: C (tentative). See Pregnancy Code inside back cover. Animal reproduction studies in hamsters reveal significant birth defects due to this drug.
Information from adequate studies in pregnant women is not available. Ask physician for guidance.

Advisability of Use While Nursing Infant
This drug is not known to be present in the mother's milk. It is advisable to proceed with breast-feeding under physician's supervision.

Habit-Forming Potential
This drug can produce both psychological and physical dependence (see Glossary). Avoid use over an extended period of time.

Effects of Overdosage
With Moderate Overdose: Marked drowsiness, staggering gait, incoordination.

With Large Overdose: Stupor progressing to coma, slow and shallow breathing, cold and clammy skin, weak and slow pulse.

Possible Effects of Extended Use
Psychological and physical dependence.

Suggested Periodic Examinations While Taking This Drug (at physician's discretion)
Observe for constipation and tendency to fecal impaction.

While Taking This Drug, Observe the Following
Foods: No restrictions. Timing of Drug and Food: May be taken with or following food to reduce stomach irritation.

Beverages: No restrictions. This drug may be taken with milk.

Alcohol: Use with extreme caution. Alcohol can increase this drug's sedative and depressant action on brain function. This drug can increase the intoxicating effect of alcohol.

Tobacco Smoking: No interactions expected. Follow your physician's advice regarding smoking.

Marijuana Smoking
Occasional (once or twice weekly): Transient increase in sedation lasting 2 to 6 hours.

Daily: Marked increase in sedation and significant impairment of intellectual and physical performance. All hazardous activities should be avoided.

Other Drugs
Hydrocodone may *increase* the effects of
- sedatives, sleep-inducing drugs, tranquilizers, pain-relieving drugs, narcotic drugs, and antihistamines. Dosage adjustments are necessary to prevent excessive sedation.

Hydrocodone *taken concurrently* with
- phenytoin (Dantoin, Dilantin, etc.), may cause excessive depression of brain function. Ask physician for guidance regarding dosage adjustment for proper control of seizures.

The following drugs may *increase* the effects of hydrocodone:
- all drugs with a sedative action: calming drugs, sleep-inducing drugs, tranquilizers, pain relievers, other narcotic drugs, antihistamines. Dosage adjustments are usually necessary to prevent excessive sedation.

Driving a Vehicle, Operating Machinery, Engaging in Hazardous Activities: This drug can impair mental alertness, judgment, physical coordination, and reaction time. Avoid hazardous activities.

Aviation Note: The use of this drug *is a disqualification* for the piloting of aircraft. Consultation with a designated Aviation Medical Examiner is advised.

Exposure to Sun: No restrictions.

Discontinuation: If it has been necessary to use this drug for an extended period of time, ask physician for guidance regarding gradual reduction and withdrawal.

Special Storage Instructions
Keep in a dry, tightly closed container. Protect from light.

HYDROFLUMETHIAZIDE

Year Introduced: 1959

Brand Names

USA	Canada
Diucardin (Ayerst)	None
Saluron (Bristol)	
Salutensin [CD] (Bristol)	
Salutensin-Demi [CD] (Bristol)	

Common Synonyms ("Street Names"):   Water pills

Drug Class: Anti-hypertensive (Hypotensive), Diuretic, Thiazides

Prescription Required: Yes

Available for Purchase by Generic Name: No

Available Dosage Forms and Strengths
Tablets — 50 mg.

Tablet May Be Crushed or Capsule Opened for Administration: Yes

How This Drug Works
Intended Therapeutic Effect(s)
  Elimination of excessive fluid retention (edema).
  Reduction of high blood pressure.
Location of Drug Action(s):   Principal actions occur in
  • the tubular systems of the kidney that determine the final composition of the urine.
  • the walls of the smaller arteries.

Method of Drug Action(s)

By increasing the elimination of salt and water from the body (through increased urine production), this drug reduces the volume of fluid in the blood and body tissues and lowers the sodium content throughout the body.

By relaxing the walls of the smaller arteries and allowing them to expand, this drug significantly increases the total capacity of the arterial system.

The combined effect of these two actions (reduced blood volume in expanded space) results in lowering of the blood pressure.

Principal Uses of This Drug

As a Single Drug Product: This member of the "thiazide" class is used primarily as a mild diuretic and to initiate treatment ("step 1") for mild to moderate high blood pressure.

As a Combination Drug Product [CD]:   It is available in combination with reserpine, another anti-hypertensive drug with a different method of action. The combination is a more effective anti-hypertensive than either drug used alone.

THIS DRUG SHOULD NOT BE TAKEN IF

—you have had an allergic reaction to any dosage form of it previously.

INFORM YOUR PHYSICIAN BEFORE TAKING THIS DRUG IF

—you are allergic to any form of "sulfa" drug.

—you are pregnant and your physician does not know it.

—you have a history of kidney disease or liver disease, or impaired kidney or liver function.

—you have diabetes (or a tendency to diabetes).

—you have a history of gout.

—you have a history of lupus erythematosus.

—you are taking any form of cortisone, digitalis, oral anti-diabetic drugs, or insulin.

—you plan to have surgery under general anesthesia in the near future.

Time Required for Apparent Benefit

Increased urine volume begins in 2 hours, reaches a maximum in 4 to 6 hours, and subsides in 8 to 12 hours. Continuous use on a regular schedule will be necessary for 2 to 3 weeks to determine this drug's effectiveness in lowering your blood pressure.

Possible Side-Effects (natural, expected, and unavoidable drug actions)

Lightheadedness on arising from sitting or lying position (see orthostatic hypotension in Glossary).

Increase in level of blood sugar, affecting control of diabetes.

Increase in level of blood uric acid, affecting control of gout.

Decrease in the level of blood potassium, resulting in muscle weakness and cramping.

Possible Adverse Effects *(unusual, unexpected, and infrequent reactions)*

IF ANY OF THE FOLLOWING DEVELOP, DISCONTINUE DRUG AND NOTIFY
YOUR PHYSICIAN AS SOON AS POSSIBLE

Mild Adverse Effects
Allergic Reactions: Skin rashes (various kinds), hives, drug fever.
Other Reactions
Reduced appetite, indigestion, nausea, vomiting, diarrhea.
Headache, dizziness, yellow vision, blurred vision.

Serious Adverse Effects
Allergic Reactions
Hepatitis with jaundice (see Glossary).
Anaphylactic reaction (see Glossary).
Severe skin reactions.
Other Reactions
Inflammation of the pancreas—severe abdominal pain.
Bone marrow depression (see Glossary)—fatigue, weakness, fever, sore
throat, unusual bleeding or bruising.

CAUTION
1. Do not exceed recommended doses. Increased dosage can cause excessive
excretion of sodium and potassium with resultant loss of appetite, nausea,
fatigue, weakness, confusion, and tingling in the extremities.
2. If you are also taking a digitalis preparation (digitoxin, digoxin, etc.), ensure
an adequate intake of high-potassium foods to prevent potassium deficiency—a potential cause of digitalis toxicity.

Precautions for Use by Those over 60 Years of Age
You may be more sensitive to the actions of this drug. Small doses are advisable until your individual response has been determined.
You may be more susceptible to the development of impaired thinking,
orthostatic hypotension, potassium loss, and elevation of blood sugar, complicating the management of diabetes.
If you are taking this drug to treat high blood pressure, remember that warm
weather and fever can reduce your blood pressure and make it necessary
to adjust your dosage.
Overdosage and extended use of this drug can cause excessive loss of body
water, thickening of the blood, and an increased tendency of the blood to
clot, predisposing to stroke, heart attack, or thrombophlebitis.

Advisability of Use During Pregnancy
Pregnancy Category: C (tentative). See Pregnancy Code inside back
cover.
Animal reproduction studies: No data available.
Information from adequate studies in pregnant women is not available.
Ask physician for guidance.
This drug should not be used during pregnancy unless a very serious com-
plication of pregnancy occurs for which this drug is significantly bene-
ficial. This type of diuretic can have adverse effects on the fetus.

Advisability of Use While Nursing Infant
This drug is known to be present in milk. Ask physician for guidance.

Habit-Forming Potential
None.

Effects of Overdosage
With Moderate Overdose: Dryness of mouth, thirst, lethargy, weakness, muscle pain and cramping, nausea, vomiting.

With Large Overdose: Drowsiness progressing to stupor and coma, weak and rapid pulse.

Possible Effects of Extended Use
Impaired balance of water, salt, and potassium in blood and body tissues. Development of diabetes (in predisposed individuals).

Suggested Periodic Examinations While Taking This Drug (at physician's discretion)
Complete blood cell counts.

Measurements of blood levels of sodium, potassium, chloride, sugar, and uric acid.

Liver function tests.

Kidney function tests.

While Taking This Drug, Observe the Following
Foods: It is recommended that you include in your daily diet liberal servings of foods rich in potassium (unless directed otherwise by your physician). The following foods have a high potassium content:

All-bran cereals	Fish, fresh
Almonds	Lentils
Apricots (dried)	Liver, beef
Bananas, fresh	Lonalac
Beans (navy and lima)	Milk
Beef	Peaches (dried)
Carrots (raw)	Peanut butter
Chicken	Peas
Citrus fruits, juices	Pork
Coconut	Potato, sweet
Coffee	Prunes (dried), juice
Crackers (rye)	Raisins
Dates and figs (dried)	Tomato Juice

Note: Avoid licorice in large amounts while taking this drug. Follow your physician's instructions regarding the use of salt.

Beverages: No restrictions unless directed by your physician.

Alcohol: Use with caution until the combined effect has been determined. Alcohol can exaggerate the blood pressure-lowering effect of this drug and cause orthostatic hypotension.

Tobacco Smoking: No interactions expected with this drug. Follow your physician's advice regarding smoking.

Marijuana Smoking
> Occasional (once or twice weekly):   No effect to mild increase in thirst and/or urinary frequency.
>
> Daily: Moderate increase in thirst and/or urinary frequency; possible accentuation of orthostatic hypotension (see Glossary).

Other Drugs
> Hydroflumethiazide may *increase* the effects of
> - other anti-hypertensive drugs. Careful adjustment of dosages is necessary to prevent excessive lowering of the blood pressure.
> - drugs of the phenothiazine family, and cause excessive lowering of the blood pressure. (The thiazides and related drugs and the phenothiazines may both cause orthostatic hypotension.)
>
> Hydroflumethiazide may *decrease* the effects of
> - oral anti-diabetic drugs and insulin, by raising the level of blood sugar. Careful dosage adjustment is necessary to maintain proper control of diabetes.
> - allopurinol (Zyloprim), by raising the level of blood uric acid. Careful dosage adjustment is required to maintain proper control of gout.
> - probenecid (Benemid), by raising the level of blood uric acid. Careful dosage adjustments are necessary to maintain control of gout.
>
> Hydroflumethiazide *taken concurrently* with
> - cortisone and cortisone-related drugs, may cause excessive loss of potassium from the body.
> - digitalis and related drugs, requires very careful monitoring and dosage adjustments to prevent serious disturbances of heart rhythm.
> - tricyclic antidepressants (Elavil, Sinequan, etc.), may cause excessive lowering of the blood pressure.
>
> The following drugs may *increase* the effects of hydroflumethiazide:
> - barbiturates may exaggerate its blood pressure-lowering action.
> - mono-amine oxidase (MAO) inhibitor drugs (see Drug Class, Section Three) may increase urine volume by delaying this drug's elimination from the body.
> - pain relievers (analgesics), both narcotic and non-narcotic, may exaggerate its blood pressure-lowering action.
>
> The following drug may *decrease* the effects of hydroflumethiazide:
> - cholestyramine (Cuemid, Questran) may interfere with its absorption. Take cholestyramine 30 to 60 minutes before any oral diuretic.

Driving a Vehicle, Operating Machinery, Engaging in Hazardous Activities: Use caution until the possibility of orthostatic hypotension and/or impaired vision has been determined.

Aviation Note: The use of this drug *may be a disqualification* for the piloting of aircraft. Consultation with a designated Aviation Medical Examiner is advised.

Exposure to Sun: Use caution until sensitivity has been determined. This drug can cause photosensitivity (see Glossary).

Exposure to Heat: Avoid excessive perspiring which could cause additional loss of water and salt from the body.

Heavy Exercise or Exertion: Avoid exertion that produces lightheadedness, excessive fatigue, or muscle cramping. Isometric exercises—the "overload" technique for strengthening individual muscles—can raise the blood pressure significantly. Ask your physician for guidance regarding participation in this form of exercise.

Occurrence of Unrelated Illness: Illnesses which cause vomiting or diarrhea can produce a serious imbalance of important body chemistry. Discontinue this drug and ask your physician for guidance.

Discontinuation: It may be advisable to discontinue this drug approximately 5 to 7 days before major surgery. Ask your physician, surgeon, and/or anesthesiologist for guidance regarding dosage reduction or withdrawal.

Special Storage Instructions

Keep in a dry, tightly closed container.

HYDROXYZINE

Year Introduced: 1956

Brand Names

USA		Canada
Atarax (Roerig)	Marax [CD] (Roerig)	Atarax (Pfizer)
Vistaril (Pfizer)	Vistrax [CD] (Pfizer)	Marax [CD] (Pfizer)
Enarax [CD] (Beecham)		

Common Synonyms ("Street Names"): Nerve pills, itch medicine

Drug Class: Tranquilizer, Mild (Anti-anxiety); Anti-itching, Antihistamines

Prescription Required: Yes

Available for Purchase by Generic Name: USA: Yes   Canada: No

Available Dosage Forms and Strengths
        Tablets — 10 mg., 25 mg., 50 mg., 100 mg.
      Capsules — 25 mg., 50 mg., 100 mg.
        Syrup — 10 mg. per teaspoonful (5 ml.)
    Suspension — 25 mg. per teaspoonful (5 ml.)
      Injection — 25 mg., 50 mg. per ml.

Tablet May Be Crushed or Capsule Opened for Administration: Yes

How This Drug Works

Intended Therapeutic Effect(s): Restoration of emotional calm, relief of anxiety, tension, apprehension, and agitation.

Location of Drug Action(s): Not established. Thought to be certain key areas of the brain that influence emotional stability.

Method of Drug Action(s): Not established. Present thinking is that this drug may reduce excessive activity in these areas of the brain. The nature of this depressant action is unknown.

Principal Uses of This Drug

As a Single Drug Product: Used primarily as a mild tranquilizer to relieve anxiety and nervous tension, whether occurring independently or in association with a physical disorder. Also used frequently to relieve itching due to allergic skin conditions.

As a Combination Drug Product [CD]: Combined with pentaerythritol tetranitrate (an anti-anginal drug), this drug relieves the anxiety that is both cause and effect of angina associated with coronary artery disease. Combined with antispasmodic drugs, this drug helps to allay the anxiety that is conducive to functional disorders of the gastro-intestinal tract. Combined with ephedrine and theophylline (bronchodilator drugs), this drug controls the anxiety that is often associated with bronchial spasm as in asthma, bronchitis, and emphysema.

THIS DRUG SHOULD NOT BE TAKEN IF
—you have had an allergic reaction to any dosage form of it previously.

INFORM YOUR PHYSICIAN BEFORE TAKING THIS DRUG IF
—you have epilepsy.
—you are taking any sedative, sleep-inducing drugs, other tranquilizers, pain relievers, or narcotic drugs of any kind.
—you plan to have surgery under general anesthesia in the near future.

Time Required for Apparent Benefit
Drug action begins in 15 to 30 minutes and persists for approximately 4 hours.

Possible Side-Effects (natural, expected, and unavoidable drug actions)
Drowsiness.

Possible Adverse Effects (unusual, unexpected, and infrequent reactions)

IF ANY OF THE FOLLOWING DEVELOP, DISCONTINUE DRUG AND NOTIFY YOUR PHYSICIAN AS SOON AS POSSIBLE

Mild Adverse Effects
Allergic Reactions: Itching.
Other Reactions: Dryness of the mouth, headache.
Serious Adverse Effects
None reported.

Precautions for Use by Those over 60 Years of Age
You may be more susceptible to the development of drowsiness, dizziness, and lethargy and to impairment of thinking, judgment, and memory.

This drug can increase the degree of impaired urination associated with prostate gland enlargement (prostatism).

Advisability of Use During Pregnancy

Pregnancy Category: C (tentative). See Pregnancy Code inside back cover. Animal reproduction studies in mice, rats, and dogs reveal significant birth defects due to this drug.

Information from adequate studies in pregnant women is not available.

The manufacturers state that this drug is *contraindicated* during the first 3 months.

Ask physician for guidance.

Advisability of Use While Nursing Infant

Drug is known to be present in milk. Ask physician for guidance.

Habit-Forming Potential

None.

Effects of Overdosage

With Moderate Overdose: Marked drowsiness, unsteady stance and gait.

With Large Overdose: Agitation, purposeless movements, tremor, convulsions.

Possible Effects of Extended Use

Reduced effectiveness due to the development of tolerance (see Glossary).

Suggested Periodic Examinations While Taking This Drug (at physician's discretion)

None required.

While Taking This Drug, Observe the Following

Foods: No restrictions.

Beverages: Large intake of coffee or tea may reduce this drug's calming action.

Alcohol: Use with extreme caution until combined effect has been determined. Alcohol can increase the sedative action of hydroxyzine. Hydroxyzine can increase the intoxicating effect of alcohol.

Tobacco Smoking: No interactions expected.

Marijuana Smoking

Occasional (once or twice weekly): Mild increase in sedative effect of this drug.

Daily: Marked increase in sedative effect of this drug.

Other Drugs

Hydroxyzine may *increase* the effects of

- sedatives, sleep-inducing drugs, other tranquilizers, and narcotic drugs. Dosage adjustments may be necessary to prevent oversedation.
- oral anticoagulants of the coumarin family (see Drug Class, Section Three), and cause abnormal bleeding or hemorrhage. Consult physician regarding prothrombin time testing and dosage adjustment.

Hydroxyzine may *decrease* the effects of
• phenytoin (Dantoin, Dilantin, etc.), by hastening its elimination from the body. It may be necessary to adjust the dose of phenytoin at any time hydroxyzine is started or stopped.

The following drugs may *increase* the effects of hydroxyzine
• all sedatives, sleep-inducing drugs, tranquilizers, antihistamines, pain relievers, and narcotic drugs. Dosage adjustments are necessary to prevent oversedation.

Driving a Vehicle, Operating Machinery, Engaging in Hazardous Activities: This drug may impair mental alertness, judgment, coordination, or reaction time. Avoid hazardous activities.

Aviation Note: The use of this drug *is a disqualification* for the piloting of aircraft. Consultation with a designated Aviation Medical Examiner is advised.

Exposure to Sun: No restrictions.

Special Storage Instructions
Keep in a tightly closed container. Protect the liquid forms from light.

IBUPROFEN

Year Introduced: 1967

Brand Names

USA	Canada
Advil (Whitehall)	Amersol (Horner)
Motrin (Upjohn)	Motrin (Upjohn)
Rufen (Boots)	
Nuprin (Upjohn)	

Common Synonyms ("Street Names"):   Arthritis medicine, aspirin substitute

Drug Class: Analgesic, Mild; Anti-inflammatory; Fever Reducer (Antipyretic)

Prescription Required: 200 mg. tablet: No
Higher strength tablets: Yes

Available for Purchase by Generic Name: No

Available Dosage Forms and Strengths
Tablets — 200 mg., 300 mg., 400 mg., 600 mg.

Tablet May Be Crushed or Capsule Opened for Administration: Yes

How This Drug Works
Intended Therapeutic Effect(s)
Relief of joint pain, stiffness, inflammation, and swelling associated with arthritis.

Relief of mild to moderate pain from any cause. Relief of menstrual cramping (dysmenorrhea).

Location of Drug Action(s):   Not completely established. It is thought that this drug acts in the brain (at the level of the hypothalamus) and in the inflamed tissues of arthritic joints; also in traumatized tissues and in the menstruating uterus.

Method of Drug Action(s)
Not completely known. It is thought that this drug reduces the tissue concentration of prostaglandins, chemicals involved in the production of inflammation and pain.

By reducing the tissue levels of prostaglandins in the muscular wall of the uterus, this drug relieves menstrual cramping.

Principal Uses of This Drug
As a Single Drug Product: This "aspirin substitute" is used in a variety of conditions to relieve pain and inflammation. Initially developed to provide symptomatic relief in acute and chronic arthritis, including gout, it is now widely used to relieve the pain associated with musculo-skeletal injuries, bursitis, tendinitis, menstrual cramping, and minor surgical procedures.

THIS DRUG SHOULD NOT BE TAKEN IF
—you have had an allergic reaction to any dosage form of it previously.
—you are allergic to aspirin (hives, nasal polyps, and/or asthma caused by aspirin).
—it has been prescribed for a child under 12 years of age.

INFORM YOUR PHYSICIAN BEFORE TAKING THIS DRUG IF
—you have a history of peptic ulcer disease.
—you have a history of gout, diabetes, high blood pressure, or heart disease.
—you have impaired kidney function.
—you have systemic lupus erythematosus.
—you are taking diuretics.

Time Required for Apparent Benefit
Drug action begins within 1 hour and persists for 3 to 5 hours. Significant improvement may require continuous use on a regular schedule for 1 to 2 weeks.

Possible Side-Effects *(natural, expected, and unavoidable drug actions)*
Fluid retention.

Possible Adverse Effects *(unusual, unexpected, and infrequent reactions)*

IF ANY OF THE FOLLOWING DEVELOP, DISCONTINUE DRUG AND NOTIFY YOUR PHYSICIAN AS SOON AS POSSIBLE

Mild Adverse Effects
Allergic Reactions: Skin rashes (various kinds), hives, itching.
Other Reactions
Nausea, vomiting, stomach irritation, heartburn, cramping, excessive gas, diarrhea.
Dizziness, lightheadedness, headache, ringing in the ears.
Altered menstrual pattern.

Serious Adverse Effects
Severe skin reactions
Blurring of vision, appearance of "colored lights," double vision.
"Allergic" meningitis (non-infectious).
Development of peptic ulcer.
Abnormally low white blood cell counts. Aplastic anemia (see Glossary).
Mild anemia due to "silent" blood loss from the stomach (less than that caused by aspirin).
Acute hepatitis-like reaction with fever, skin rash, and abnormal liver function tests.
Kidney damage, reduced kidney function.

CAUTION
1. The dosage schedule must be determined individually. It is advisable to limit dosage to the smallest amount that produces reasonable improvement. Do not exceed 2400 mg. daily.
2. This drug's anti-inflammatory and antipyretic effects can make it more difficult to recognize the presence of infection. If you develop any symptoms that suggest an active infection, inform your physician promptly.

Precautions for Use by Those over 60 Years of Age
You may be more sensitive to all of the actions of this drug. Small doses are advisable until your individual response has been determined.
You may be more susceptible to the development of headache, dizziness, confusion, stomach ulcer, stomach bleeding, diarrhea, and impaired kidney function.

Advisability of Use During Pregnancy
Pregnancy Category: B (tentative). See Pregnancy Code inside back cover.
Animal reproduction studies in rats and rabbits reveal no birth defects due to this drug.
Information from adequate studies in pregnant women is not available.
Avoid during last 3 months.
Ask physician for guidance.

Advisability of Use While Nursing Infant
Reports indicate that this drug is not present in milk. Nursing should be safe for the infant. Ask physician for guidance regarding dosage.

Habit-Forming Potential
None apparent to date.

Effects of Overdosage
With Moderate Overdose: Headache, drowsiness, possible indigestion, nausea, vomiting, stomach irritation.

With Large Overdose: Impaired breathing, depressed brain function.

Possible Effects of Extended Use
None known.

Suggested Periodic Examinations While Taking This Drug (at physician's discretion)
Complete blood cell counts.

Complete eye examinations if any change in vision occurs.

Liver and kidney function tests.

While Taking This Drug, Observe the Following
Foods: This drug should be taken with milk or food if stomach irritation occurs.

Beverages: No restrictions.

Alcohol: Use with caution. The irritant action of alcohol on the stomach lining, added to the irritant action of ibuprofen in sensitive individuals, can increase the risk of stomach bleeding or ulceration.

Tobacco Smoking: No interactions expected.

Marijuana Smoking

Occasional (once or twice weekly): No effect to mild increase in pain relief from this drug.

Daily: Moderate increase in pain relief from this drug.

Other Drugs

Ibuprofen may *decrease* the effects of

• diuretics and reduce their diuretic and antihypertensive action.

Ibuprofen *taken concurrently* with

• oral anticoagulants, requires careful monitoring of combined effects until more experience establishes a predictable pattern. The risk of bleeding may be increased.

Driving a Vehicle, Operating Machinery, Engaging in Hazardous Activities: This drug may cause dizziness, visual disturbance and/or nausea. If these drug effects occur, avoid all hazardous activities.

Aviation Note: The use of this drug *may be a disqualification* for the piloting of aircraft. Consultation with a designated Aviation Medical Examiner is advised.

Exposure to Sun: No restrictions.

Special Storage Instructions
Keep in a dry, tightly closed container.

IMIPRAMINE

Year Introduced: 1959

Brand Names

USA	Canada
Imavate (Robins)	Apo-Imipramine (Apotex)
Janimine (Abbott)	Impril (ICN)
Presamine (USV)	Novopramine
SK-Pramine (Smith Kline	(Novopharm)
& French)	Tofranil (Geigy)
Tofranil (Geigy)	

Common Synonyms ("Street Names"):   None

Drug Class: Antidepressant, Tricyclic

Prescription Required: Yes

Available for Purchase by Generic Name: Yes

Available Dosage Forms and Strengths
    Tablets — 10 mg., 25 mg., 50 mg.
    Capsules — 75 mg., 100 mg., 125 mg., 150 mg.
    Injection — 25 mg. per 2 ml.

Tablet May Be Crushed or Capsule Opened for Administration: Yes

How This Drug Works
    Intended Therapeutic Effect(s):   Gradual improvement of mood and relief
    of emotional depression.
    Location of Drug Action(s):   Those areas of the brain that determine mood
    and emotional stability.
    Method of Drug Action(s):   Not established. Present thinking is that this
    drug slowly restores to normal levels certain constituents of brain tissue
    (such as norepinephrine) that transmit nerve impulses.

Principal Uses of This Drug
    As a Single Drug Product: To relieve the symptoms associated with spon-
    taneous (endogenous) depression, and to initiate the restoration of normal
    mood. This drug should be used only when a diagnosis of a true, primary
    depression of significant degree has been established. It should not be used
    to treat the symptoms of mild and transient (reactive) depression that
    may be associated with many life situations in the absence of a bona fide
    affective illness.

THIS DRUG SHOULD NOT BE TAKEN IF
—you have had an allergic reaction to any dosage form of it previously.
—you are taking or have taken within the past 14 days any mono-amine oxidase
(MAO) inhibitor drug (see Drug Class, Section Three).
—you are recovering from a recent heart attack.

—you have glaucoma (narrow-angle type).
—it is prescribed for a child under 6 years of age.

INFORM YOUR PHYSICIAN BEFORE TAKING THIS DRUG IF
—you are allergic or sensitive to any other tricyclic antidepressant (see Drug Class, Section Three).
—you have a history of any of the following: diabetes, epilepsy, glaucoma, heart disease, prostate gland enlargement, or overactive thyroid function.
—you plan to have surgery under general anesthesia in the near future.

Time Required for Apparent Benefit
Some benefit may be apparent within 1 to 2 weeks. Adequate response may require continuous treatment for 4 to 6 weeks.

Possible Side-Effects *(natural, expected, and unavoidable drug actions)*
Drowsiness, blurring of vision, dryness of mouth, constipation, impaired urination.

Possible Adverse Effects *(unusual, unexpected, and infrequent reactions)*

IF ANY OF THE FOLLOWING DEVELOP, DISCONTINUE DRUG AND NOTIFY YOUR PHYSICIAN AS SOON AS POSSIBLE

Mild Adverse Effects
Allergic Reactions: Skin rash, hives, swelling of face or tongue, drug fever.
Other Reactions
  Nausea, indigestion, irritation of tongue or mouth, peculiar taste.
  Headache, dizziness, weakness, fainting, unsteady gait, tremors.
  Swelling of testicles, breast enlargement, milk formation.
  Fluctuation of blood sugar levels.

Serious Adverse Effects
Allergic Reactions: Hepatitis with jaundice (see Glossary).
Other Reactions
  Confusion (especially in the elderly), hallucinations, agitation, restlessness, nightmares.
  Heart palpitation and irregular rhythm.
  Bone marrow depression (see Glossary)—fatigue, weakness, fever, sore throat, unusual bleeding or bruising.
  Numbness, tingling, pain, loss of strength in arms and legs.
  Parkinson-like disorders (see Glossary)—usually mild and infrequent; more likely to occur in the elderly.

Precautions for Use by Those over 60 Years of Age
During the first 2 weeks of treatment observe for the development of confusional reactions—restlessness, agitation, forgetfulness, disorientation, delusions, and hallucinations. Reduction of dosage or discontinuation may be necessary.
Observe for incoordination and instability in stance and gait which may predispose to falling and injury.
This drug can increase the degree of impaired urination associated with prostate gland enlargement (prostatism).

Advisability of Use During Pregnancy

Pregnancy Category: C (tentative). See Pregnancy Code inside back cover.
   Animal reproduction studies are inconclusive.
   Information from adequate studies in pregnant women is not available.
   Ask physician for guidance.

Advisability of Use While Nursing Infant

This drug may be present in milk in small quantities. Ask physician for guidance.

Habit-Forming Potential

Psychological or physical dependence is rare and unexpected.

Effects of Overdosage

With Moderate Overdose: Confusion, hallucinations, extreme drowsiness, drop in body temperature, heart palpitation, dilated pupils, tremors.

With Large Overdose: Stupor, deep sleep, coma, convulsions.

Possible Effects of Extended Use

None reported.

Suggested Periodic Examinations While Taking This Drug (at physician's discretion)

Complete blood cell counts.
Liver function tests.
Serial blood pressure readings and electrocardiograms.

While Taking This Drug, Observe the Following

Foods: No restrictions.

Beverages: No restrictions.

Alcohol: Avoid completely. This drug can increase markedly the intoxicating effects of alcohol and accentuate its depressant action on brain function.

Tobacco Smoking: No interactions expected.

Marijuana Smoking

Occasional (once or twice weekly):   Transient increase in drowsiness and dryness of mouth.

Daily: Persistent drowsiness, increased dryness of mouth; possible reduced effectiveness of this drug.

Other Drugs

Imipramine may *increase* the effects of

- atropine and drugs with atropine-like actions (see Drug Class, Section Three).
- sedatives, sleep-inducing drugs, tranquilizers, antihistamines, and narcotic drugs, and cause oversedation. Dosage adjustments may be necessary.
- levodopa (Dopar, Larodopa), in its control of Parkinson's disease.

Imipramine may *decrease* the effects of

- guanethidine, and reduce its effectiveness in lowering blood pressure.

• other commonly used anti-hypertensive drugs. Ask physician for guidance regarding the need to monitor blood pressure readings and to adjust dosage of anti-hypertensive medications. (The action of Aldomet is not decreased by tricyclic antidepressants.)

Imipramine *taken concurrently* with
• thyroid preparations, may cause impairment of heart rhythm and function. Ask physician for guidance regarding thyroid dosage adjustment.
• ethchlorvynol (Placidyl), may cause delirium.
• quinidine, may cause impairment of heart rhythm and function. Avoid the combined use of these two drugs.
• mono-amine oxidase (MAO) inhibitor drugs (see Drug Class, Section Three), may cause high fever, delirium, and convulsions.

The following drugs may *increase* the effects of imipramine
• thiazide diuretics, (see Drug Class, Section Three) may slow its elimination from the body. Overdosage may occur.

Driving a Vehicle, Operating Machinery, Engaging in Hazardous Activities: This drug may impair mental alertness, judgment, physical coordination, and reaction time. Avoid hazardous activities.

Aviation Note: The use of this drug *is a disqualification* for the piloting of aircraft. Consultation with a designated Aviation Medical Examiner is advised.

Exposure to Sun: Use caution until sensitivity to sun has been determined. This drug may cause photosensitivity (see Glossary).

Discontinuation: If it has been necessary to use this drug for an extended period of time, do not discontinue it abruptly. Ask physician for guidance regarding dosage reduction and withdrawal. It may be necessary to adjust the dosage of other drugs taken concurrently.

Special Storage Instructions
Keep in a dry, tightly closed container.

INDOMETHACIN

Year Introduced: 1963

Brand Names

USA	Canada
Indocin (Merck Sharp & Dohme)	Indocid (MSD)
Indocin SR (Merck Sharp & Dohme)	Novomethacin (Novopharm)

Common Synonyms ("Street Names"): Arthritis medicine, aspirin substitute

Drug Class: Analgesic, Mild; Anti-inflammatory; Fever Reducer (Antipyretic)

Prescription Required: Yes

Available for Purchase by Generic Name: No

Available Dosage Forms and Strengths
                      Capsules — 25 mg., 50 mg.
          Capsules (prolonged action) — 75 mg.

Tablet May Be Crushed or Capsule Opened for Administration: Yes

How This Drug Works
  Intended Therapeutic Effect(s):   Relief of joint pain, stiffness, inflammation, and swelling associated with arthritis.
  Location of Drug Action(s):   Not completely established. It is thought that this drug acts in the brain (at the level of the hypothalamus) and in the inflamed tissues of arthritic joints.
  Method of Drug Action(s):   Not completely known. It is thought that this drug reduces the tissue concentration of prostaglandins, chemicals involved in the production of inflammation and pain.

Principal Uses of This Drug
  As a Single Drug Product: Used primarily to provide symptomatic relief in all forms of acute and chronic arthritis, including gout. It is also used to relieve the pain associated with bursitis, tendinitis, and capsulitis. A less frequent use is to lower the fever associated with some cases of Hodgkin's disease and other lymphomas when aspirin and acetaminophen have been ineffective.

THIS DRUG SHOULD NOT BE TAKEN IF
—you are allergic to aspirin or to any of the drugs bearing the brand names listed above.
—you have active gastritis (stomach inflammation), peptic ulcer, enteritis, ileitis, or ulcerative colitis.
—you are pregnant or nursing.
—you have had recent rectal bleeding and the suppository form of this drug has been prescribed for you.
—it is prescribed for a child under 15 years of age.

INFORM YOUR PHYSICIAN BEFORE TAKING THIS DRUG IF
—you have a history of stomach or intestinal disease, especially peptic ulcer or ulcerative colitis.
—you have a history of epilepsy, Parkinson's disease (shaking palsy), or mental illness.
—you have a history of kidney disease or impaired kidney function.

Time Required for Apparent Benefit
Some improvement may occur in 4 to 24 hours. Maximal benefit occurs within 3 weeks.

Possible Side-Effects *(natural, expected, and unavoidable drug actions)*
Because of indomethacin's ability to reduce fever and inflammation, it can
hide or mask the symptoms and indications of infection. If you suspect an
infection of any kind may be present, discontinue this drug for 48 hours and
observe. Notify physician of your action.

Possible Adverse Effects *(unusual, unexpected, and infrequent reactions)*

**IF ANY OF THE FOLLOWING DEVELOP, DISCONTINUE DRUG AND NOTIFY
YOUR PHYSICIAN AS SOON AS POSSIBLE**

Mild Adverse Effects
Allergic Reactions: Skin rashes (various kinds), hives, itching, swelling of
face and/or extremities.
Other Reactions
Headache, ringing in ears, drowsiness, lightheadedness, dizziness, feel-
ings of detachment.
Loss of appetite, nausea, vomiting, diarrhea.
Temporary loss of hair.

Serious Adverse Effects
Allergic Reactions: Asthma, shortness of breath, unusual bleeding or
bruising, irritation of mouth.
Other Reactions
Blurring of vision, confusion, depression (may be severe).
Severe indigestion, abdominal pain, heartburn, need for antacids (possi-
ble developing peptic ulcer).
Gastro-intestinal bleeding; observe stools for evidence of blood (dark red
to black discoloration).
Hepatitis and/or jaundice (see Glossary).
Bone marrow depression (see Glossary).
Numbness and/or tingling, pain, weakness in hands and/or feet.

CAUTION
This drug's anti-inflammatory and antipyretic effects can make it more difficult to recognize the presence of infection. If you develop any symptoms that
suggest an active infection, inform your physician promptly.

Precautions for Use by Those over 60 Years of Age
You may be more sensitive to all of the actions of this drug. Small doses are
advisable until your individual response has been determined.
You may be more susceptible to the development of headache, dizziness,
emotional depression, confusion, impairment of memory, stomach ulcer,
stomach bleeding, and diarrhea.

Advisability of Use During Pregnancy
Pregnancy Category: B (tentative). See Pregnancy Code inside back cover.
Animal reproduction studies in mice and rats reveal no birth defects due
to this drug.
Information from adequate studies in pregnant women is not available.
Ask physician for guidance.

Advisability of Use While Nursing Infant

Drug is known to be present in milk. Safety for infant not established. Ask physician for guidance.

Habit-Forming Potential

None.

Effects of Overdosage

With Moderate Overdose: Stomach irritation, nausea, vomiting, diarrhea, confusion, agitation.

With Large Overdose: Disorientation, incoherence, convulsions, coma, possible hemorrhage from stomach or intestine.

Possible Effects of Extended Use

Eye damage (deposits in the cornea, changes in the retina).

Suggested Periodic Examinations While Taking This Drug (at physician's discretion)

Careful and complete examinations of vision and eye structures.
Complete blood cell counts.
Liver function tests.
Urine analysis.

While Taking This Drug, Observe the Following

Foods: No restrictions of food selection. Drug should be taken with or following food to minimize stomach irritation.

Beverages: No restrictions of beverage selection. Drug may be taken with milk to minimize stomach irritation.

Alcohol: May increase the risk of stomach ulceration or bleeding.

Tobacco Smoking: No interactions expected.

Marijuana Smoking

Occasional (once or twice weekly):   No effect to mild increase in pain relief from this drug.

Daily: Moderate increase in pain relief from this drug.

Other Drugs

Indomethacin may *increase* the effects of

- oral anticoagulants of the coumarin type (see Drug Class, Section Three). Consult physician regarding dosage adjustments to prevent bleeding.
- cortisone and related drugs (see Drug Class, Section Three). Consult physician regarding dosage adjustments to prevent stomach ulceration and other effects of cortisone overdosage.

Indomethacin *taken concurrently* with

- phenylbutazone (Azolid, Butazolidin, etc.), increases the risk of stomach ulceration.
- thyroid medications, increases the risk of adverse effects on the heart and circulation.

The following drug may *increase* the effects of indomethacin

- probenecid (Benemid) may delay the elimination of indomethacin in the urine.

The following drug may *decrease* the effects of indomethacin
- aspirin may interfere with the absorption of indomethacin from the intestine.

Driving a Vehicle, Operating Machinery, Engaging in Hazardous Activities: Use caution until the occurrence of drowsiness, lightheadedness, and/or dizziness is determined.

Aviation Note: The use of this drug *may be a disqualification* for the piloting of aircraft. Consultation with a designated Aviation Medical Examiner is advised.

Exposure to Sun: No restrictions.

Discontinuation: Dosage adjustment may be necessary for any of the following drugs if taken concurrently with indomethacin: coumarin anticoagulants, cortisone and related drugs, thyroid medications.

Special Storage Instructions
Keep in a dry, tightly closed container.

INSULIN

Year Introduced: 1922

Brand Names

USA		Canada
Humulin (Lilly)	Semilente Insulin	Insulin Preparations
Iletin Preparations	Ultralente Insulin	(Connaught)
(Lilly)	Purified Insulins	Lente Insulin
Insulin Preparations	(Novo)	Neutral Insulin
(Squibb)	Actrapid	NPH Insulin
Lente Insulin	Lentard	Protamine Zinc
NPH Insulin	Monotard	Insulin
Protamine Zinc	Semitard	Semilente Insulin
Insulin	Ultratard	Ultralente Insulin
Regular Insulin		

Common Synonyms ("Street Names"):   None

Drug Class: Anti-diabetic, Injectable (Hypoglycemic)

Prescription Required: No

Available for Purchase by Generic Name: Yes

Available Dosage Forms and Strengths
Injection — 40 units per ml., 100 units per ml., 500 units per ml.

How This Drug Works
Intended Therapeutic Effect(s)   Restoration of the body's ability to use sugar normally (control of diabetes).

Location of Drug Action(s):   Principal actions occur in the tissues of voluntary muscles, the heart muscle, and the liver.

Method of Drug Action(s):   By direct action on certain cell membranes, insulin facilitates the transport of sugar through the cell wall to the interior of the cell, where it is utilized.

Principal Uses of This Drug
As a Single Drug Product: Insulin is used to "control" diabetes mellitus in those individuals whose diabetes has been shown to be insulin-dependent. Proper use involves the selection of the most appropriate type of insulin for the individual and determination of the optimal dosage schedule for the continuous regulation of blood sugar levels.

THIS DRUG SHOULD NOT BE TAKEN IF
—the need for it and its correct dosage schedule have not been established by a properly qualified physician.

INFORM YOUR PHYSICIAN BEFORE TAKING THIS DRUG IF
—you have a history of allergic reaction to any form of insulin on previous use.

—you do not know how to recognize and treat abnormally low blood sugar (see hypoglycemia in Glossary).

—you are taking any mono-amine oxidase (MAO) inhibitor drug (see Drug Class, Section Three).

Time Required for Apparent Benefit:

Insulin Preparation	Action Onset	Peak	Duration
Regular and Neutral	½–1 hour	2–3 hrs.	5–7 hrs.
Semilente	½–1 hr.	5–8 hrs.	12–16 hrs.
Globin Zinc	1–2 hrs.	6–12 hrs.	18–24 hrs.
NPH	1–3 hrs.	10–18 hrs.	18–28 hrs.
Lente	1–3 hrs.	10–18 hrs.	18–28 hrs.
Protamine Zinc	3–7 hrs.	15–22 hrs.	24–36 hrs.
Ultralente	5–8 hrs.	16–24 hrs.	28–36 hrs.

Possible Side-Effects *(natural, expected, and unavoidable drug actions)*
In the management of stable diabetes, no side-effects occur when insulin dose, diet, and physical activity are correctly balanced and maintained. In the management of unstable ("brittle") diabetes, unexpected drops in blood sugar levels can occur, resulting in periods of hypoglycemia (see Glossary).

Possible Adverse Effects *(unusual, unexpected, and infrequent reactions)*

IF ANY OF THE FOLLOWING DEVELOP, DISCONTINUE DRUG AND NOTIFY YOUR PHYSICIAN AS SOON AS POSSIBLE

Mild Adverse Effects
  Allergic Reactions
    Local redness, swelling, and itching at point of injection.
    Occasional hives.
  Other Reactions: Thinning of subcutaneous tissue (beneath the skin) at points of injection.
Serious Adverse Effects
  Allergic Reactions: Anaphylactic reaction (see Glossary).
  Other Reactions: Episodes of severe hypoglycemia (see Glossary).

CAUTION

1. It is most important that you carry with you a card of personal identification with a notation that you have diabetes and are taking insulin (see Table 19 and Section Six).
2. Be sure that you know how to recognize the onset of hypoglycemia and how to treat it. Always carry with you a readily available form of sugar such as hard candy or sugar cubes. Report episodes of hypoglycemia to your physician.
3. Improvement in vision may occur during the first several weeks of insulin treatment. It is advisable to defer examination for glasses for 6 weeks after starting insulin.
4. The rates of insulin absorption vary significantly from one anatomic site to another. Absorption is 80% greater from the abdominal wall than from the leg, and 30% greater than from the arm. Individuals with unstable diabetes may achieve better control of blood sugar levels by rotating the injection site within the same anatomic region rather than rotating from one anatomic region to another.

Precautions for Use by Those over 60 Years of Age

Insulin requirements may change with aging. Periodic evaluation of your overall status is necessary to determine your correct insulin dosage.

The aging brain adapts well to the higher blood sugar levels associated with diabetes. Attempts to achieve "normal" blood sugar levels can result in unrecognized hypoglycemia that is manifested by confusion and abnormal behavior. Repeated episodes of severe hypoglycemia in the elderly can cause brain damage.

Advisability of Use During Pregnancy

Pregnancy Category: C (tentative). See Pregnancy Code inside back cover.

Animal reproduction studies are inconclusive.

Information from adequate studies in pregnant women is not available.

Ask physician for guidance.

Diabetes may be more difficult to manage during pregnancy. To preserve the health of the mother and the welfare of the fetus, every effort must be made to establish the optimal dose of insulin and to prevent hypoglycemia.

Advisability of Use While Nursing Infant
Insulin treatment of the mother has no adverse effect on the nursing infant.

Habit-Forming Potential
None.

Effects of Overdosage
With Moderate Overdose: Fatigue, weakness, headache, nervousness, irritability, sweating, tremors, hunger, rapid pulse.

With Large Overdose: Confusion, delirium, abnormal behavior resembling drunkenness, unconsciousness, convulsions.

Possible Effects of Extended Use
None reported.

Suggested Periodic Examinations While Taking This Drug (at physician's discretion)
Monitoring of urine sugar content as a guide to adjustment of diet and insulin dose.

Measurement of blood sugar levels at intervals recommended by physician.

While Taking This Drug, Observe the Following
Foods: Follow your prescribed diabetic diet conscientiously. Do not omit snack foods in midafternoon or at bedtime if they are prescribed to prevent hypoglycemia.

Beverages: According to prescribed diabetic diet.

Alcohol: Use with caution until combined effect has been determined. Remember that alcohol has caloric value and that it tends to lower blood sugar. Used excessively, alcohol may induce severe hypoglycemia, resulting in brain damage.

Tobacco Smoking: No interactions expected. Follow physician's advice regarding smoking.

Marijuana Smoking
Occasional (once or twice weekly):   No significant interactions expected.
Daily: Possible increase in blood sugar.

Other Drugs
Insulin may *increase* the effects of
• oral anti-diabetic drugs.

Insulin *taken concurrently* with
• propranolol (Inderal), requires extreme care and attention to dosage of both drugs. Propranolol can mask the usual symptoms that indicate the development of hypoglycemia.

The following drugs may *increase* the effects of insulin
• oral anticoagulants
• isoniazid (INH) in small doses

- mono-amine oxidase (MAO) inhibitor drugs (see Drug Class, Section Three)
- oxyphenbutazone (Oxalid, Tandearil)
- phenylbutazone (Azolid, Butazolidin, etc.)
- salicylates (aspirin, sodium salicylate) in large doses
- "sulfa" drugs (see Drug Class, Section Three)
- sulfinpyrazone (Anturane)

The following drugs may *decrease* the effects of insulin
- chlorthalidone (Hygroton)
- cortisone-like drugs (see Drug Class, Section Three)
- furosemide (Lasix)
- oral contraceptives
- phenytoin (Dantoin, Dilantin, etc.)
- thiazide diuretics (see Drug Class, Section Three)
- thyroid preparations

Driving a Vehicle, Operating Machinery, Engaging in Hazardous Activities: Usually no restrictions. Be prepared to stop and take corrective action if indications of impending hypoglycemia develop.

Aviation Note: The use of this drug and the disorder for which this drug is prescribed *are disqualifications* for the piloting of aircraft. Consultation with a designated Aviation Medical Examiner is advised.

Exposure to Sun: No restrictions.

Heavy Exercise or Exertion: Use caution. Periods of unusual and unplanned heavy physical activity will hasten the burning of blood sugar and predispose to hypoglycemia.

Occurrence of Unrelated Illness: Report all illnesses that prevent regular eating. Meals omitted as a result of nausea, vomiting, or injury can lead to hypoglycemia. Consult physician for guidance regarding food intake and insulin dose.

Discontinuation: Do not discontinue this drug without consulting your physician. Diabetes that is insulin dependent requires continuous treatment on a regular basis. Omission of insulin will result in life-threatening coma.

Special Storage Instructions
Keep in refrigerator. Protect from freezing. Protect from strong light and high temperatures when not refrigerated.

Observe the Following Expiration Times
Do not take this drug if it is older than the expiration date on the vial. (Always use fresh, "within date" insulin.)

IRON

Ferrocholinate   **Ferrous sulfate**
Ferrous fumarate   **Iron dextran**
Ferrous gluconate

Year Introduced: Ferrocholinate, 1955
Ferrous fumarate, 1958
Ferrous gluconate, 1937
Ferrous sulfate, 1832
Iron dextran, 1957

Brand Names

USA

Ferrocholinate:
   None
Ferrous fumarate:
   Femiron (J.B.
   Williams)
   Fumasorb (Marion)
   Toleron
   (Mallinckrodt)
   Ferancee [CD]
   (Stuart)
   Ferro-Sequels [CD]
   (Lederle)
   Trinsicon [CD]
   (Glaxo)
   Vitron-C [CD]
   (Fisons)

Ferrous gluconate:
   Fergon (Breon)
   Simron
   (Merrell-Dow)
Ferrous sulfate:
   Feosol (Menley &
   James)
   Fer-In-Sol (Mead
   Johnson)
   Fero-Gradumet
   (Abbott)
   Fesotyme (Elder)
   Mol-Iron (Schering)
   Fero-Folic-500
   [CD] (Abbott)

Fero-Grad-500
   [CD] (Abbott)
Geritol Tablets*
   [CD] (J.B.
   Williams)
Iberet [CD]
   (Abbott)
Iberet-500 [CD]
   (Abbott)
Iberet-Folic-500
   [CD] (Abbott)
Iron dextran:
   Ferrospan
   (Imperial)
   Imferon
   (Merrell-Dow)

Canada

Ferrocholinate:
   None
Ferrous fumarate:
   Fersamal (Glaxo)
   Neo-Fer-50
   (Neolab)
   Novofumar
   (Novopharm)
   Palafer
   (Beecham)
Ferrous gluconate:
   Apo-Ferrous
   Gluconate
   (Apotex)

Fertinic
   (Desbergers)
Novoferrogluc
   (Novopharm)
Ferrous sulfate:
   Apo-Ferrous Sulfate
   (Apotex)
   Fer-In-Sol (Mead
   Johnson)
   Fero-Grad (Abbott)
   Fesofor (SKF)
   Novoferrosulfa
   (Novopharm)
   Slow-Fe (CIBA)

Fero-Folic-500
   [CD] (Abbott)
Fero-Grad-500
   [CD] (Abbott)
Iberet [CD]
   (Abbott)
Iberet-500 [CD]
   (Abbott)
Iberet-Folic-500
   [CD] (Abbott)
Iron dextran:
   Imferon (Fisons)

*The iron component in Geritol Liquid is ferrous ammonium citrate.

Common Synonyms ("Street Names"):   Iron pills

Drug Class: Iron Preparations (Hematinics)

Prescription Required: For formulations without folic acid—No
For formulations with folic acid—Yes

Available for Purchase by Generic Name: Yes

Available Dosage Forms and Strengths
Tablets
Delayed-release tablets
Chewable tablets
Enteric-coated tablets
Capsules
Delayed-release capsules
Solution (Drops)
Suspension
Syrup
Elixir
Injection
Available in a large variety of formulations and strengths. See package label for product composition and individual component strengths.

Tablet May Be Crushed or Capsule Opened for Administration
Regular tablets and capsules — Yes
Feosol tablets — No
Delayed-release tablets and capsules — No
Feosol spansule — Yes, but do not crush or chew contents
Ferro-Sequels — Yes, but do not crush or chew contents
Enteric-coated tablets — No

How This Drug Works
Intended Therapeutic Effect(s):   Sufficient supplementation of dietary iron to prevent or correct iron-deficiency anemia.
Location of Drug Action(s):   Those cellular elements in the bone marrow that are responsible for the formation of hemoglobin—the oxygen-carrying pigment of red blood cells.
Method of Drug Action(s):   Iron is absorbed by the body when iron stores are below normal and inadequate to meet the body's needs for new hemoglobin formation. When available in the bone marrow, iron is incorporated into the hemoglobin of newly formed red blood cells until the anemia is corrected.

Principal Uses of This Drug
As a Single Drug Product: Iron is used exclusively to correct or prevent anemia that is known to be due to iron deficiency.

As a Combination Drug Product [CD]:   Iron is available in a variety of combinations with Vitamin C, Vitamin B12, folic acid, and docusate. Vitamin C promotes the absorption of iron and its utilization in the production of hemoglobin. Vitamin B12 is used in the treatment and prevention of pernicious anemia. Folic acid is combined with iron to treat megaloblastic types of anemia. The stool softener docusate is combined with that form of iron that causes constipation.

THIS DRUG SHOULD NOT BE TAKEN IF
—you have acute hepatitis.
—you have hemosiderosis (excessive deposits of iron in body tissues without organ damage).
—you have hemochromatosis (excessive deposits of iron in body tissues with organ damage).
—you have a hemolytic form of anemia.

INFORM YOUR PHYSICIAN BEFORE TAKING THIS DRUG IF
—you have had stomach surgery previously.
—you have or have had peptic ulcer disease, recurrent enteritis, or ulcerative colitis.

Time Required for Apparent Benefit
Young red blood cells (reticulocytes) begin to increase in number within 3 to 7 days, and reach a peak in 7 to 14 days. Blood hemoglobin levels begin to rise after 1 week. The red blood cell count increases significantly after 3 weeks.

Possible Side-Effects *(natural, expected, and unavoidable drug actions)*
All forms of iron taken by mouth can cause gray to black discoloration of the stool.
Liquid preparations of iron can cause staining of the teeth. (Liquid dosage forms should be taken through a straw and followed by water.)
Iron given by intramuscular injection can cause staining of the skin at the injection site.

Possible Adverse Effects *(unusual, unexpected, and infrequent reactions)*

IF ANY OF THE FOLLOWING DEVELOP, DISCONTINUE DRUG AND NOTIFY YOUR PHYSICIAN AS SOON AS POSSIBLE

Mild Adverse Effects
  Allergic Reactions
    Iron by mouth: None.
    Iron by injection (iron dextran): hives, fever, joint pains, asthma.
  Other Reactions: Stomach irritation or nausea (7%), cramping or diarrhea (5%), constipation (10%).

Serious Adverse Effects
  Allergic Reactions: Iron by injection (iron dextran): anaphylactic reaction (see Glossary).
  Other Reactions: Iron by injection (iron dextran) may intensify the manifestations of rheumatoid arthritis. It may also cause abnormal depos-

its of calcium (soft tissue calcifications) at the sites of intramuscular injection.

Possible Delayed Adverse Effects
The development of sarcoma (cancer arising in muscle) at the sites of intramuscular injection of iron dextran has been reported. A definite cause-and-effect relationship (see Glossary) is inferred.

CAUTION
1. The only logical use of medicinal iron is the correction (or prevention) of iron-deficiency anemia. In the absence of such anemia, excessive iron intake only increases the iron stores of the body and does not produce an increase of the red blood cells or hemoglobin above normal levels.
2. Unneeded iron taken on a continuous basis may be hazardous. It is unwise to assume that you are "among those who need extra iron every day"—as suggested in the familiar advertising for Geritol, Femiron, and other popular iron preparations. Before initiating self-administration of iron, consult your physician to determine if you are anemic and if you need iron therapy.
3. Optimal absorption of iron requires that the total daily intake be divided into 2 or more doses, and that each dose be separated by at least 4 hours.
4. Failure of the anemia to respond to adequate iron treatment indicates need for reevaluation of the diagnosis and a careful search for causes of chronic blood loss—the major cause of iron-deficiency anemia.
5. Frequent blood donors can replenish their iron stores by taking 300 mg. of ferrous sulfate daily for 1 month after each donation of 1 pint of blood.
6. Do not take iron by mouth and by injection concurrently.
7. To avoid iron overload, do not exceed the total dose of iron needed to correct the anemia.

Precautions for Use by Those over 60 Years of Age
First be certain that iron medication is needed. Unneeded iron is stored in body tissues as "reserve iron." Excessive iron deposits (iron storage disease) can lead to the development of hemochromatosis—bronze discoloration of the skin, diabetes, heart disease, liver damage, sexual impotence.

Advisability of Use During Pregnancy
Pregnancy Category: A (tentative). See Pregnancy Code inside back cover.
Animal reproduction studies: No data available.
Studies in pregnant women reveal no fetal defects.
In the absence of anemia, iron requirements during the first half of pregnancy can usually be derived from the diet. Increased requirements during the last half should be met by supplementation with medicinal iron as recommended by your physician.

Advisability of Use While Nursing Infant
Iron should be taken while nursing only if you have an iron-deficiency anemia or an inadequate dietary intake of iron.

Habit-Forming Potential
None.

Effects of Overdosage

With Moderate Overdose: Abdominal pain, vomiting (may be bloody), diarrhea, tarry stools, drowsiness, lethargy.

With Large Overdose: Pallor, extreme weakness, collapse, weak and rapid pulse, shallow breathing, convulsions, coma.

Possible Effects of Extended Use

The unnecessary intake of iron on a continuous basis may cause iron storage disease—hemochromatosis, a disorder that may include bronze discoloration of the skin, diabetes, impaired heart function, liver damage, sexual impotence.

Suggested Periodic Examinations While Taking This Drug (at physician's discretion)

Measurements of iron and hemoglobin levels in the blood.

Red blood cell counts, with determination of red blood cell size and hemoglobin content.

While Taking This Drug, Observe the Following

Foods: For maximal absorption, iron preparations should be taken alone and preferably between meals. However, they may be taken after meals as necessary to minimize stomach irritation. Popular "whole grain" cereals (containing phytic acid) and eggs are reported to impair the absorption of iron. Avoid frequent or excessive intake of these foods.

Beverages: Liquid iron preparations should be well diluted in water, fruit juice, or vegetable juice. Do not take iron preparations with milk or antacids.

Alcohol: Use in moderation. Alcohol may increase the absorption of iron excessively. Routine iron supplements should not be used in the treatment of alcoholism. The alcohol abuser may accumulate excessive iron stores that can potentiate major organ damage.

Tobacco Smoking: No interactions expected.

Marijuana Smoking: No interactions expected.

Other Drugs

Iron preparations may *decrease* the effects of

• tetracyclines (See Drug Class, Section Three), by preventing their absorption. Iron should be given 3 hours before or 2 hours after any tetracycline.

Iron preparations *taken concurrently* with

• allopurinol (Zyloprim), may cause excessive storage of iron in the liver. (While observed in animal studies, this has not been confirmed in man.)

The following drug may *increase* the effects of iron preparations

• Vitamin C, by enhancing their absorption, and contributing to the formation of hemoglobin and red blood cells.

The following drugs may *decrease* the effects of iron preparations

• antacids, by preventing their absorption.

• chloramphenicol (Chloromycetin), by interfering with the formation of hemoglobin and red blood cells.

- cholestyramine (Cuemid, Questran), by preventing their absorption.
- clofibrate (Atromid-S), by preventing their absorption.
- dactinomycin (Cosmegen), by preventing their absorption.
- sulfasalazine (Azulfidine, etc.), by reducing iron levels in the blood.
- tetracyclines, by preventing their absorption. Iron should be given 3 hours before or 2 hours after any tetracycline.
- Vitamin E, by impairing the response to iron treatment.

Driving a Vehicle, Operating Machinery, Engaging in Hazardous Activities: No restrictions.

Aviation Note: Usually no restrictions.

Exposure to Sun: No restrictions.

Occurrence of Unrelated Illness: If you are taking medicinal iron, report the development of all infections promptly. Active infection can impair the transfer of iron to the bone marrow and the incorporation of iron into new hemoglobin and red blood cells. This "anemia of infection" does not respond to iron treatment. Medicinal iron will be ineffective until the infection is eliminated.

Discontinuation: When the causes of chronic blood loss are eliminated and the iron balance in blood and body tissues is restored to normal (usually after 3 to 6 months of continuous treatment), iron medication should be discontinued to avoid iron overload (hemosiderosis).

Special Storage Instructions
Keep in tightly closed containers. Protect tablets and capsules from air and moisture.

ISOETHARINE

Year Introduced: 1961

Brand Names

USA	Canada
Bronkometer (Breon)	None
Bronkosol (Breon)	

Common Synonyms ("Street Names"):   None

Drug Class: Anti-asthmatic, Bronchodilator

Prescription Required: Yes

Available for Purchase by Generic Name: Yes

Available Dosage Forms and Strengths
Aerosol Nebulizer — 0.61%
Solution for Nebulizer — 0.1%, 0.125%, 0.2%, 0.25%, 0.5%, 1%

How This Drug Works

Intended Therapeutic Effect(s):   Relief of difficult breathing associated with acute attacks of bronchial asthma and with other disorders characterized by spasm of the bronchial tubes, such as bronchitis and emphysema.

Location of Drug Action(s):   Those nerve terminals of the sympathetic nervous system that activate the muscles in the walls of bronchial tubes to produce dilation.

Method of Drug Action(s):   By stimulating certain sympathetic nerve terminals, this drug acts to dilate those bronchial tubes that are in sustained constriction, thereby increasing the size of the airways and improving the ability to breathe.

Principal Uses of This Drug

As a Single Drug Product: This rapid-acting bronchodilator is used exclusively to reverse spasm of the bronchial tubes. While its most common use is to provide relief during acute attacks of bronchial asthma, it may also be beneficial during bronchial spasm associated with acute or chronic bronchitis or emphysema.

THIS DRUG SHOULD NOT BE TAKEN IF

—you are allergic to any of the brand name drugs listed above.
—you have a serious heart rhythm disorder.
—you are taking, or have taken during the past 2 weeks, any mono-amine oxidase (MAO) inhibitor drug (see Drug Class, Section Three).

INFORM YOUR PHYSICIAN BEFORE TAKING THIS DRUG IF

—you are overly sensitive to drugs that stimulate the sympathetic nervous system.
—you are currently using epinephrine (Adrenalin) to relieve asthmatic breathing.
—you have high blood pressure.
—you have diabetes.
—you have a history of heart disease, especially angina (coronary insufficiency).
—you have a history of overactivity of the thyroid gland (hyperthyroidism).
—you are taking any form of digitalis.

Time Required for Apparent Benefit

Drug action begins within 1 to 2 minutes and reaches its peak in 30 to 60 minutes.

Possible Side-Effects *(natural, expected, and unavoidable drug actions)*

In sensitive individuals—nervousness, anxiety, tremor, palpitation.

Possible Adverse Effects *(unusual, unexpected, and infrequent reactions)*

IF ANY OF THE FOLLOWING DEVELOP, DISCONTINUE DRUG AND NOTIFY YOUR PHYSICIAN AS SOON AS POSSIBLE

Mild Adverse Effects
Headache, dizziness.
Nausea, vomiting.

Serious Adverse Effects
Idiosyncratic Reactions: Paradoxical spasm of the bronchial tubes and worsening of asthma—often follows excessive use.

CAUTION
1. The frequently repeated use of this drug at short intervals can produce a condition of unresponsiveness and result in medication failure. If this develops, avoid use completely for 12 hours, at which time normal response should return.
2. Excessive use of aerosol preparations in the management of asthma has been associated with sudden death.
3. Promptly discard all preparations of this drug at the first appearance of discoloration (pink to red to brown) or cloudiness (precipitation). Such changes indicate drug deterioration.

Precautions for Use by Those over 60 Years of Age
If you have hardening of the arteries (arteriosclerosis), heart disease, or high blood pressure, use this drug with caution. It can precipitate episodes of angina and disturbances of heart rhythm; it can cause sudden elevation of the blood pressure and induce stroke.

If you have difficulty with urination due to enlargement of the prostate gland (prostatism), this drug may increase the difficulty. Ask physician for guidance.

If you have Parkinson's disease, this drug may temporarily increase the rigidity and tremor in your extremities.

Advisability of Use During Pregnancy
Pregnancy Category: C (Tentative). See Pregnancy Code inside back cover.
Animal reproduction studies: No data available.
Information from adequate studies in pregnant women is not available. Ask physician for guidance.

Advisability of Use While Nursing Infant
No adverse effects on milk formation or on infant expected. Ask physician for guidance.

Habit-Forming Potential
Although tolerance to this drug can develop with frequent use, neither psychological nor physical dependence (see Glossary) occurs.

Effects of Overdosage
With Moderate Overdose: Excessive nervousness, anxiety, headache, dizziness, palpitation, tremor.
With Large Overdose: Severe palpitation, rapid heart rate, paradoxical spasm of bronchial tubes, sudden cessation of heart function (cardiac arrest).

Possible Effects of Extended Use
None reported.

Suggested Periodic Examinations While Taking This Drug (at physician's discretion)
None.

While Taking This Drug, Observe the Following
Foods: No restrictions.

Beverages: No restrictions.

Alcohol: No interactions expected.

Tobacco Smoking: No interactions expected. Follow physician's advice regarding smoking as it affects the condition under treatment.

Marijuana Smoking

Occasional (once or twice weekly):   Mild and transient improvement in anti-asthmatic effect of this drug.

Daily: More persistent improvement in anti-asthmatic effect of this drug.

Other Drugs

Isoetharine may *increase* the effects of

• ephedrine, and cause excessive stimulation of the heart.

Isoetharine *taken concurrently* with

• epinephrine (Adrenalin, etc.), may cause excessive stimulation of the heart. Avoid concurrent use.

• isoproterenol (Isuprel, etc.), may cause excessive stimulation of the heart. Avoid concurrent use.

• mono-amine oxidase (MAO) inhibitor drugs (see Drug Class, Section Three), may be dangerous. Avoid concurrent use.

The following drug may *decrease* the effects of isoetharine:

• propranolol (Inderal) may impair its effectiveness in the treatment of asthma.

Driving a Vehicle, Operating Machinery, Engaging in Hazardous Activities: Usually no restrictions. Use caution if excessive nervousness or dizziness occurs.

Aviation Note: The use of this drug *may be a disqualification* for the piloting of aircraft. Consultation with a designated Aviation Medical Examiner is advised.

Exposure to Sun: No restrictions.

Exposure to Cold: No restrictions. Protect hands and feet from prolonged exposure to excessive cold.

Heavy Exercise or Exertion: No interactions with drug. However, excessive exertion can induce asthma in sensitive individuals.

Occurrence of Unrelated Illness: The development of acute respiratory infections—head and/or chest colds—can increase the frequency and severity of asthma and reduce the effectiveness of this drug. Obtain evaluation and treatment of such illness promptly.

Discontinuation: If this drug fails to provide relief after adequate trial, discontinue it and consult your physician regarding alternate drug therapy. Do not increase the dosage or the frequency of use. To do so could be dangerous.

Special Storage Instructions

Protect from exposure to air, light, and heat. Keep in a cool place, preferably in the refrigerator.

ISONIAZID

Year Introduced: 1956

Brand Names

USA		Canada
INH (Ciba)	Rifamate [CD]	Isotamine (ICN)
Laniazid (Lannett)	(Merrell Dow)	Rimifon (Roche)
Nydrazid (Squibb)	Rimactane/INH Dual	
Teebaconin (Consol.	Pack [CD] (Ciba)	
Midland)	Teebaconin and	
Triniad (Kasar)	Vitamin B-6 [CD]	
Uniad (Kasar)	(CMC)	

Common Synonyms ("Street Names"):   TB drug

Drug Class: Antimicrobial, Anti-tuberculosis (Anti-infective)

Available for Purchase by Generic Name: USA: Yes   Canada: No

Prescription Required: Yes

Available Dosage Forms and Strengths

Tablets — 50 mg., 100 mg., 300 mg.
Injection — 100 mg. per ml.

Tablet May Be Crushed or Capsule Opened for Administration: Yes

How This Drug Works

Intended Therapeutic Effect(s):   The prevention or treatment of active tuberculosis.

Location of Drug Action(s):   Any body tissue or fluid in which adequate concentration of the drug can be achieved.

Method of Drug Action(s):   Not completely established. It is thought that the drug destroys susceptible tuberculosis organisms by interfering with several of their essential metabolic activities.

Principal Uses of This Drug

As a Single Drug Product: Used alone to prevent the development of active tuberculous infection in individuals who are considered to be at high risk by virtue of known exposure or recent conversion of a negative tuberculin skin test to positive.

As a Combination Drug Product [CD]:   This drug is available in combination with rifampin, another anti-tuberculosis drug that has a different mechanism of action. This combination is more effective than either drug used alone. Isoniazid can cause a deficiency of pyridoxine (Vitamin B-6); for this reason, a combination of the two drugs is available in tablet form.

THIS DRUG SHOULD NOT BE TAKEN IF
—you have had an allergic reaction to any dosage form of it previously.
—you have active liver disease.
—you are within the first 6 months of pregnancy.

INFORM YOUR PHYSICIAN BEFORE TAKING THIS DRUG IF
—you have serious impairment of liver or kidney function.
—you have epilepsy.
—you have diabetes.
—you have systemic lupus erythematosus.
—you plan to have surgery under general anesthesia in the near future.

Time Required for Apparent Benefit
From 3 to 6 months.

Possible Side-Effects (*natural, expected, and unavoidable drug actions*)
None.

Possible Adverse Effects (*unusual, unexpected, and infrequent reactions*)

IF ANY OF THE FOLLOWING DEVELOP, DISCONTINUE DRUG AND NOTIFY YOUR PHYSICIAN AS SOON AS POSSIBLE

Mild Adverse Effects
  Allergic Reactions: Skin rashes (various kinds), fever, swollen glands, painful muscles and joints.
  Other Reactions
  Nausea, indigestion, vomiting.
  Numbness, tingling, pain (often burning), and weakness first noted in hands and feet (see peripheral neuritis in Glossary).
Serious Adverse Effects
  Allergic Reactions: Hepatitis, with or without jaundice (see Glossary). Inform physician promptly if you develop any of the early indications of possible hepatitis—loss of appetite, nausea, fatigue, fever, itching, dark-colored urine, light-colored stools, yellow discoloration of eyes or skin.
  Other Reactions
  Acute mental and behavioral disturbance, convulsions, impaired vision.
  Increase in epileptic seizures.
  Bone marrow depression (see Glossary)—fatigue, weakness, fever, sore throat, unusual bleeding or bruising.
  Elevated blood sugar.
  Breast enlargement or discomfort.

Precautions for Use by Those over 60 Years of Age
The natural decline in kidney function that occurs after 60 may require adjustment of your dosage

You may be more susceptible to the serious adverse effects of this drug. Report promptly the development of *any* of the effects listed above.

Advisability of Use During Pregnancy

Pregnancy Category: C (tentative). See Pregnancy Code inside back cover.
Animal reproduction studies in mice, rats, and rabbits reveal no birth defects due to this drug.
Information from adequate studies in pregnant women is not available. Ask physician for guidance.
Safety not established for use during the first 6 months of pregnancy. Prudent use during the last 3 months is best determined by the physician's evaluation.

Advisability of Use While Nursing Infant

Drug may be present in milk. Safety for infant not established. Ask physician for guidance.

Habit-Forming Potential

None.

Effects of Overdosage

With Moderate Overdose: Nausea, vomiting, dizziness, blurred vision, visual hallucinations, slurred speech.
With Large Overdose: Difficult breathing, stupor, coma, convulsions.

Possible Effects of Extended Use

Nerve damage in arms or legs if a deficiency of Vitamin B-6 (pyridoxine) develops.

Suggested Periodic Examinations While Taking This Drug (at physician's discretion)

Consult physician regarding advisability of determining whether you are a "slow" or a "rapid" inactivator of isoniazid. This has a bearing on the likelihood of your developing adverse effects.
Liver function tests monthly.
Complete blood cell counts.
Careful examination of eye structures and visual acuity.

While Taking This Drug, Observe the Following

Foods: No restrictions.
Beverages: No restrictions.
Alcohol: Best avoided; alcohol can reduce effectiveness of isoniazid.
Tobacco Smoking: No interactions expected with isoniazid. Ask physician for guidance regarding smoking.
Marijuana Smoking: No interactions expected.
Other Drugs
Pyridoxine (Vitamin B-6) should be taken concurrently with isoniazid to prevent nerve damage in the extremities.

Isoniazid may *increase* the effects of
- phenytoin (Dantoin, Dilantin, etc.), to an excessive degree; dosage reduction of phenytoin may be necessary to prevent toxicity.

- disulfiram (Antabuse), causing incoordination and abnormal behavior.
- oral anticoagulants; reduced dosage may be necessary.
- oral anti-diabetic drugs; dosage may require adjustment up or down. Monitor blood and urine sugar closely.
- anti-hypertensive drugs; reduced dosage may be necessary if blood pressure falls too low.
- atropine-like drugs; caution required in presence of glaucoma.
- sedatives and narcotic drugs; caution required to avoid oversedation.
- stimulant drugs; caution required to avoid overstimulation of nervous system.

Driving a Vehicle, Operating Machinery, Engaging in Hazardous Activities: No restrictions unless dizziness occurs.

Aviation Note: The use of this drug *may be a disqualification* for the piloting of aircraft. Consultation with a designated Aviation Medical Examiner is advised.

Exposure to Sun: No restrictions.

Discontinuation: Long-term therapy required. Do not discontinue drug without physician's advice.

Special Storage Instructions
Keep in a tightly closed, light-resistant container.

ISOPROPAMIDE

Year Introduced: 1957

Brand Names

USA		Canada
Darbid (Smith Kline & French)	Combid [CD] (Smith Kline & French)	Darbid (SK&F) Combid [CD] (SK&F)

Common Synonyms ("Street Names"):   Stomach relaxer

Drug Class: Antispasmodic, Atropine-like Drugs

Prescription Required: USA: Yes   Canada: No

Available for Purchase by Generic Name: No

Available Dosage Forms and Strengths
Tablets — 5 mg.

Tablet May Be Crushed or Capsule Opened for Administration
Regular tablets — Yes
Combid capsules — Yes, but do not crush or chew contents

How This Drug Works

Intended Therapeutic Effect(s): Relief of discomfort resulting from excessive activity and spasm of the digestive tract (esophagus, stomach, intestine, and colon).

Location of Drug Action(s): The terminal nerve fibers of the parasympathetic nervous system that control the activity of the gastrointestinal tract.

Method of Drug Action(s): By blocking the action of the chemical (acetylcholine) that transmits impulses at parasympathetic nerve endings, this drug prevents stimulation of muscular contraction and glandular secretion within the organ involved. This results in reduced overall activity, including the prevention or relief of muscle spasm.

Principal Uses of This Drug

As a Single Drug Product: This drug is used as part of the overall management of peptic ulcer disease and functional disorders of the gastro-intestinal tract such as nervous stomach and the irritable bowel syndrome (spastic colon).

As a Combination Drug Product [CD]: This drug is available in combination with prochlorperazine, a phenothiazine that provides relief of anxiety and nervous tension and control of nausea and vomiting. These added drug effects render the combination drug more beneficial in treating both functional and organic disorders of the gastro-intestinal tract.

THIS DRUG SHOULD NOT BE TAKEN IF

—you have had an allergic reaction to any dosage form of it previously.
—your stomach cannot empty properly into the intestine (pyloric obstruction).
—you are unable to empty the urinary bladder completely.
—you have glaucoma (narrow-angle type).
—you have severe ulcerative colitis.

INFORM YOUR PHYSICIAN BEFORE TAKING THIS DRUG IF

—you have glaucoma (open-angle type).
—you have angina or coronary heart disease.
—you have chronic bronchitis.
—you have a hiatal hernia.
—you have enlargement of the prostate gland.
—you have myasthenia gravis.
—you have a history of peptic ulcer disease.
—you plan to have surgery under general anesthesia in the near future.

Time Required for Apparent Benefit

Drug action begins in 1 to 2 hours and persists for 10 to 12 hours.

Possible Side-Effects *(natural, expected, and unavoidable drug actions)*

Blurring of vision (impairment of focus), dryness of the mouth and throat, constipation, hesitancy in urination. (Nature and degree of side-effects depend upon individual susceptibility and drug dosage.)

Possible Adverse Effects *(unusual, unexpected, and infrequent reactions)*

IF ANY OF THE FOLLOWING DEVELOP, DISCONTINUE DRUG AND NOTIFY YOUR PHYSICIAN AS SOON AS POSSIBLE

Mild Adverse Effects
Allergic Reactions: Skin rash, hives.
Other Reactions
Dilation of pupils, causing sensitivity to light.
Flushing and dryness of the skin (reduced sweating).
Rapid heart action.
Lightheadedness, dizziness, unsteady gait.

Serious Adverse Effects
Idiosyncratic Reactions: Acute confusion, delirium, and erratic behavior.
Other Reactions: Development of acute glaucoma (in susceptible individuals).

CAUTION
Many over-the counter (OTC) medications (see Glossary) for allergies, colds, and coughs contain drugs that can interact unfavorably with this drug. Ask your physician or pharmacist for guidance before using any such medication.

Precautions for Use by Those over 60 Years of Age
You may be more sensitive to all of the actions of this drug. Small doses are advisable until your individual response has been determined.
This drug can increase the degree of impaired urination associated with prostate gland enlargement (prostatism).

Advisability of Use During Pregnancy
Pregnancy Category: C (tentative). See Pregnancy Code inside back cover.
Animal reproduction studies: No data available.
Information from studies in pregnant women indicates no increase in defects in 1071 exposures to this drug.
Ask physician for guidance.

Advisability of Use While Nursing Infant
Presence of drug in milk is not known. Safety for infant not established. Ask physician for guidance.

Habit-Forming Potential
None.

Effects of Overdosage
With Moderate Overdose: Marked dryness of the mouth, dilated pupils, blurring of near vision, rapid pulse, heart palpitation, headache, difficulty in urination.
With Large Overdose: Extremely dilated pupils, rapid pulse and breathing, hot skin, high fever, excitement, confusion, hallucinations, delirium, eventual loss of consciousness, convulsions and coma.

Possible Effects of Extended Use

Chronic constipation, severe enough to result in fecal impaction. (Constipation should be treated promptly with effective laxatives.)

Suggested Periodic Examinations While Taking This Drug (at physician's discretion)

Measurement of internal eye pressure to detect any significant increase that could indicate developing glaucoma.

While Taking This Drug, Observe the Following

Foods: No interaction with drug. Effectiveness is greater if drug is taken one-half to 1 hour before eating. Follow diet prescribed for condition under treatment.

Beverages: No interactions. As allowed by prescribed diet.

Alcohol: No interactions expected with this drug. Follow physician's advice regarding use of alcohol (based upon its effect on the condition under treatment).

Tobacco Smoking: No interactions expected. Follow physician's advice regarding smoking.

Marijuana Smoking

Occasional (once or twice weekly): Mild increase in drowsiness and dryness of mouth.

Daily: Moderate to marked increase in drowsiness and dryness of mouth.

Other Drugs

Isopropamide may *increase* the effects of

• all other drugs having atropine-like actions (see Drug Class, Section Three).

Isopropamide may *decrease* the effects of

• pilocarpine eye drops, and reduce their effectiveness in lowering internal eye pressure in the treatment of glaucoma.

Isopropamide *taken concurrently* with

• mono-amine oxidase (MAO) inhibitor drugs (see Drug Class, Section Three), may cause an exaggerated response to normal doses of atropine-like drugs. It is best to avoid atropine-like drugs for 2 weeks after the last dose of any MAO inhibitor drug.

• haloperidol (Haldol), may significantly increase internal eye pressure (dangerous in glaucoma).

The following drugs may *increase* the effects of isopropamide

• tricyclic antidepressants

• those antihistamines that have an atropine-like action

• meperidine (Demerol, pethidine)

• methylphenidate (Ritalin)

• orphenadrine (Disipal, Norflex)

• those phenothiazines that have an atropine-like action (see Drug Class, Section Three).

Driving a Vehicle, Operating Machinery, Engaging in Hazardous Activities: This drug may produce blurred vision, drowsiness, or dizziness. Avoid hazardous activities if these drug effects occur.

Aviation Note: The use of this drug and the disorder for which this drug is prescribed *may be disqualifications* for the piloting of aircraft. Consultation with a designated Aviation Medical Examiner is advised.

Exposure to Sun: No restrictions.

Exposure to Heat: Use extreme caution. The use of this drug in hot environments may significantly increase the risk of heat stroke.

Heavy Exercise or Exertion: Use caution in warm or hot environments. This drug may impair normal perspiration (heat loss) and interfere with the regulation of body temperature.

Special Storage Instructions
Keep in a tightly closed container. Protect from light.

ISOPROTERENOL
(Isoprenaline)

Year Introduced: 1948

Brand Names

USA		Canada
Isuprel (Breon)	Duo-Medihaler [CD]	Isuprel (Winthrop)
Medihaler-Iso (Riker)	(Riker)	Medihaler-Iso (Riker)
Norisodrine (Abbott)	Isuprel Compound	Duo-Medihaler [CD]
Vapo-Iso (Fisons)	Elixir [CD] (Breon)	(Riker)
		Isuprel Compound
		Elixir [CD]
		(Winthrop)
		Isuprel-Neo [CD]
		(Winthrop)

Common Synonyms ("Street Names"):   Asthma medicine

Drug Class: Anti-asthmatic, Bronchodilator

Prescription Required: Yes

Available for Purchase by Generic Name: USA: Yes   Canada: No

Available Dosage Forms and Strengths
Sublingual tablets — 10 mg., 15 mg.
Aerosol, inhalation — 0.2%, 0.25%
Powder, inhalation — 45 mcg., 110 mcg. per inhalation

Tablet May Be Crushed or Capsule Opened for Administration: No

How This Drug Works

Intended Therapeutic Effect(s):   Relief of difficult breathing associated with acute attacks of bronchial asthma and with other disorders characterized by spasm of the bronchial tubes, such as bronchitis and emphysema.

Location of Drug Action(s):   Those nerve terminals of the sympathetic nervous system that activate the muscles in the walls of bronchial tubes to produce dilation.

Method of Drug Action(s):   By stimulating certain sympathetic nerve terminals, this drug acts to dilate those bronchial tubes that are in sustained constriction, thereby increasing the size of the airway and improving the ability to breathe.

Principal Uses of This Drug

As a Single Drug Product: This rapid-acting bronchodilator is used primarily to reverse spasm of the bronchial tubes. While used most commonly to provide relief during acute attacks of bronchial asthma, it is also useful during bronchial spasm associated with acute or chronic bronchitis or emphysema.

As a Combination Drug Product [CD]:   This drug is also available in combination with phenylephrine, an effective decongestant that provides relief of excessive secretions and congestion in the bronchial passages.

THIS DRUG SHOULD NOT BE TAKEN IF

—you have had an allergic reaction to any dosage form of it previously. A combination drug [CD] should not be taken if you are allergic to *any* of its ingredients.

—you have a serious heart rhythm disorder.

—you are taking, or have taken during the past 2 weeks, any mono-amine oxidase (MAO) inhibitor drug (see Drug Class, Section Three).

INFORM YOUR PHYSICIAN BEFORE TAKING THIS DRUG IF

—you are overly sensitive to drugs that stimulate the sympathetic nervous system.

—you are currently using epinephrine (Adrenalin) to relieve asthmatic breathing.

—you have high blood pressure.

—you have diabetes.

—you have a history of heart disease, especially angina (coronary insufficiency).

—you have a history of overactivity of the thyroid gland (hyperthyroidism).

—you are taking any form of digitalis.

Time Required for Apparent Benefit

Action begins within 2 to 4 minutes and persists for 30 to 60 minutes when this drug is inhaled or dissolved under the tongue.

Possible Side-Effects *(natural, expected, and unavoidable drug action)*

Nervousness, heart palpitation.

The saliva or sputum may appear pink or red after inhalation of this drug. This is a normal response, and is not indicative of bleeding or an adverse effect of any kind.

Possible Adverse Effects *(unusual, unexpected, and infrequent reactions)*

IF ANY OF THE FOLLOWING DEVELOP, DISCONTINUE DRUG AND NOTIFY YOUR PHYSICIAN AS SOON AS POSSIBLE

Mild Adverse Effects
Headache, flushing, dizziness, tremor.
Nausea, vomiting.

Serious Adverse Effects
Intensification of angina in the presence of coronary artery insufficiency.
Slight elevation of blood sugar levels.

CAUTION

1. Do not chew or swallow the sublingual tablets. Allow them to dissolve under the tongue, and avoid swallowing until the tablet has been absorbed completely.
2. Avoid excessive use. Inhalation repeated too frequently can induce a resistance to this drug's bronchodilating action and render it ineffective. Limit use to the fewest number of inhalations necessary to produce relief.
3. The total daily dose of the sublingual tablets should not exceed 60 mg. for adults or 30 mg. for children.
4. Do not use this drug concurrently with epinephrine (Adrenalin). These two drugs may be used alternately if an interval of 4 hours is allowed between doses.

Precautions for Use by Those over 60 Years of Age

You may be more sensitive to the stimulant effects of this drug. Small doses are advisable until your individual response has been determined.

If you have hardening of the arteries (arteriosclerosis), heart disease, or high blood pressure, use this drug with caution. It can precipitate episodes of angina and disturbances of heart rhythm; if used excessively, it can cause sudden elevation of the blood pressure and induce stroke.

Advisability of Use During Pregnancy

Pregnancy Category: C (tentative). See Pregnancy Code inside back cover.
Animal reproduction studies in mice, rats, and hamsters reveal significant birth defects due to this drug.
Information from adequate studies in pregnant women is not available. Ask physician for guidance.

Advisability of Use While Nursing Infant

This drug does not appear in milk. Ask physician for guidance.

Habit-Forming Potential

None.

Effects of Overdosage

With Moderate Overdose: Excessive nervousness, heart palpitation, rapid heart rate, sweating.

With Large Overdose: Headache, tremor, vomiting, chest pain, marked drop in blood pressure, circulatory failure, irregular heart rhythm.

Possible Effects of Extended Use
Swelling of the salivary (parotid) glands.
Ulceration of the mouth, with prolonged use of the sublingual tablets.

Suggested Periodic Examinations While Taking This Drug (at physician's discretion)
Dental examinations to detect any destructive effects on teeth during extended use of sublingual tablets.

While Taking This Drug, Observe the Following
Foods: No restrictions.
Beverages: No restrictions.
Alcohol: No interactions expected.
Tobacco Smoking: No interactions expected. Follow physician's advice regarding smoking as it affects the condition under treatment.
Marijuana Smoking
Occasional (once or twice weekly):   Mild and transient improvement in anti-asthmatic effect of this drug.
Daily: More persistent improvement in anti-asthmatic effect of this drug.
Other Drugs
Isoproterenol may *increase* the effects of
• ephedrine, and cause excessive stimulation of the heart and an increase in blood pressure.
• tricyclic antidepressants (see Drug Class, Section Three).

Isoproterenol *taken concurrently* with
• epinephrine (Adrenalin), may cause serious disturbances of heart rhythm. Allow an interval of at least 4 hours between the use of these two drugs.

The following drugs may *increase* the effects of isoproterenol
• tricyclic antidepressants (see Drug Family, Section Three)

The following drug may *decrease* the effects of isoproterenol
• propranolol (Inderal)

Driving a Vehicle, Operating Machinery, Engaging in Hazardous Activities: No restrictions. Use caution if excessive nervousness or dizziness occurs.
Aviation Note: The use of this drug *is a disqualification* for the piloting of aircraft. Consultation with a designated Aviation Medical Examiner is advised.
Exposure to Sun: No restrictions.
Discontinuation: If this drug fails to provide relief after adequate trial, discontinue it and consult your physician regarding alternate drug therapy. Do not increase the dosage or the frequency of use. To do so could be dangerous.

Special Storage Instructions
Keep all forms of this drug in an airtight, nonmetallic container. Protect from light.

Observe the Following Expiration Times

Do not take any form of this drug if it has become discolored. Do not use the aerosol solution if cloudy.

ISOSORBIDE DINITRATE

Year Introduced: 1959

Brand Names

USA		Canada
Angidil (Saron)	Isordil (Ives)	Apo-ISDN (Apotex)
Dilatrate-SR (Reed &	Sorbitrate (Stuart)	Coronex (Ayerst)
Carnrick)	Sorquad (Tutag)	Isordil (Wyeth)

Common Synonyms ("Street Names"):   Angina pills, heart pills

Drug Class: Anti-anginal, Nitrates

Prescription Required: USA: Yes   Canada: No

Available for Purchase by Generic Name: USA: Yes   Canada: No

Available Dosage Forms and Strengths

Tablets — 5 mg., 10 mg., 20 mg., 30 mg., 40 mg.
Chewable tablets — 5 mg., 10 mg.
Sublingual tablets — 2.5 mg., 5 mg., 10 mg.
Prolonged-action tablets — 40 mg.
Prolonged-action capsules — 40 mg.

Tablet May Be Crushed or Capsule Opened for Administration

Regular tablets — Yes
Prolonged-action tablets and capsules — No
Isordil Tembid tablets — No
Isordil Tembid capsules — Yes, but do not crush or chew contents

How This Drug Works

Intended Therapeutic Effect(s):   Reduction in the frequency and severity of pain associated with angina pectoris (coronary insufficiency).

Location of Drug Action(s):   The muscular tissue in the walls of the blood vessels. The principal site of the therapeutic action is the system of coronary arteries in the heart.

Method of Drug Action(s):   This drug acts directly on the muscle cells to produce relaxation. This permits expansion of blood vessels and increases the supply of blood and oxygen to meet the needs of the working heart muscle.

Principal Uses of This Drug

As a Single Drug Product: The sublingual (under-the-tongue) tablets and the chewable tablets are used to prevent and to treat acute attacks of anginal pain. The longer-acting tablets and capsules are used to prevent the development of angina, but are not effective in relieving acute episodes of anginal pain.

THIS DRUG SHOULD NOT BE TAKEN IF
—you have had an allergic reaction to any dosage form of it previously.

INFORM YOUR PHYSICIAN BEFORE TAKING THIS DRUG IF
—you have glaucoma.
—you have had an unfavorable response to any vasodilator drug in the past.

Time Required for Apparent Benefit

The action of the sublingual tablet (dissolved under the tongue) begins in 2 to 5 minutes and persists for 1 to 2 hours. The action of the oral tablet (swallowed) begins in 30 to 60 minutes and persists for 4 to 6 hours.

Possible Side-Effects *(natural, expected, and unavoidable drug actions)*

Flushing, lightheadedness in upright position (see orthostatic hypotension in Glossary).

Possible Adverse Effects *(unusual, unexpected, and infrequent reactions)*

IF ANY OF THE FOLLOWING DEVELOP, DISCONTINUE DRUG AND NOTIFY YOUR PHYSICIAN AS SOON AS POSSIBLE

Mild Adverse Effects
Allergic Reactions: Skin rash.
Other Reactions
Headache (may be persistent), dizziness, fainting.
Nausea, vomiting.
Serious Adverse Effects
Allergic Reactions: Severe dermatitis with peeling of skin.

CAUTION

Many over-the-counter (OTC) medications (see Glossary) for allergies, colds, and coughs contain drugs that may counteract the desired effects of this drug. Ask your physician or pharmacist for guidance before using any such medications.

Precautions for Use by Those over 60 Years of Age

You may be more sensitive to the actions of this drug. Small doses are advisable until your individual response has been determined.

You may be more susceptible to the development of low blood pressure with associated lightheadedness, dizziness, unsteadiness, and falling.

Advisability of Use During Pregnancy

Pregnancy Category: C (tentative). See Pregnancy Code inside back cover.

Animal reproduction studies: No data available.

Information from adequate studies in pregnant women is not available. Ask physician for guidance.

Advisability of Use While Nursing Infant
Presence of drug in milk is not known. Safety for infant not established. Ask physician for guidance.

Habit-Forming Potential
None.

Effects of Overdosage
With Moderate Overdose: Headache, dizziness, marked flushing of the skin.
With Large Overdose: Vomiting, weakness, sweating, fainting, shortness of breath, coma.

Possible Effects of Extended Use
Development of tolerance (see Glossary), which may reduce the drug's effectiveness at recommended doses.
Development of abnormal hemoglobin (red blood cell pigment).

Suggested Periodic Examinations While Taking This Drug (at physician's discretion)
Measurement of internal eye pressure in those individuals with glaucoma or a tendency to glaucoma.
Red blood cell counts and hemoglobin measurements.

While Taking This Drug, Observe the Following
Foods: No restrictions. This drug is likely to be more effective if taken one-half to 1 hour before eating.
Beverages: No restrictions.
Alcohol: Use with extreme caution until combined effects have been determined. Alcohol may exaggerate the drop in blood pressure experienced by some sensitive individuals. This can be dangerous.
Tobacco Smoking: Nicotine may reduce the effectiveness of this drug. Follow physician's advice regarding smoking, based upon its effect on the condition under treatment and its possible interaction with this drug.
Marijuana Smoking
Occasional (once or twice weekly):   No interactions expected.
Daily: Possible reduced effectiveness of this drug; mild to moderate increase in angina; possible changes in electrocardiogram, confusing interpretation.
Other Drugs
Isosorbide may *increase* the effects of
- atropine-like drugs (see Drug Class, Section Three), and cause an increase in internal eye pressure.
- tricyclic antidepressants (see Drug Class, Section Three), and cause excessive lowering of the blood pressure.

Isosorbide may *decrease* the effects of
- all choline-like drugs, such as Mestinon, Mytelase, pilocarpine, Prostigmin, and Urecholine.

Isosorbide *taken concurrently* with

- anti-hypertensive drugs, may cause severe drop in blood pressure. Careful monitoring of drug response and appropriate dosage adjustments are necessary.

The following drug may *increase* the effects of isosorbide

- propranolol (Inderal) may cause additional lowering of the blood pressure. Dosage adjustments may be necessary.

Driving a Vehicle, Operating Machinery, Engaging in Hazardous Activities: Usually no restrictions. Before engaging in hazardous activities, determine that this drug will not cause you to have orthostatic hypotension (see Glossary) or dizziness.

Aviation Note: Coronary artery disease *is a disqualification* for the piloting of aircraft. Consultation with a designated Aviation Medical Examiner is advised.

Exposure to Sun: No restrictions.

Exposure to Cold: Cold environments may reduce the effectiveness of this drug.

Heavy Exercise or Exertion: This drug may improve your ability to be more active without resulting angina pain. Use caution and avoid excessive exertion that could cause heart injury in the absence of warning pain.

Special Storage Instructions

Keep in a dry, tightly closed container and in a cool place. Protect from heat and light.

ISOTRETINOIN

Note: This is an Abbreviated Drug Profile of a derivative of Vitamin A. It is highly effective in some types of severe acne that do not respond to conventional treatment. However, it can cause a variety of adverse effects, some of which are quite serious. Its use should be carefully supervised by your physician.

Year Introduced: 1979

Brand Names

USA	Canada
Accutane (Roche)	Accutane (Roche)

Common Synonyms ("Street Names"): Acne pills

Drug Class: Anti-acne, Vitamin A Derivative

Prescription Required: Yes

Available for Purchase by Generic Name: No

Available Dosage Forms and Strengths
Capsules — 10 mg., 40 mg.

Tablet May Be Crushed or Capsule Opened for Administration: No

How This Drug Works
Intended Therapeutic Effect(s):   The clearance or improvement of severe types of acne.

Location of Drug Action(s):   The sebaceous (oil) glands of the skin.

Method of Drug Action(s):   Not established. By an unknown action, this drug reduces the size of the sebaceous glands and their production of sebum (skin oil). This helps to correct the major feature of acne and its complications.

Principal Uses of This Drug
As a Single Drug Product: This drug is reserved to treat severe nodular and cystic acne (acne conglobata) that has failed to respond to all other forms of standard therapy. It should not be used to treat mild forms of acne. It is also used to treat some less common conditions of the skin that are due to disorders of keratin production.

THIS DRUG SHOULD NOT BE TAKEN IF
—you are allergic to parabens, additives that are used to preserve the drug product.

—you are pregnant, or planning pregnancy.

INFORM YOUR PHYSICIAN BEFORE TAKING THIS DRUG IF
—you have had an allergic reaction to any form of Vitamin A in the past.

—you have diabetes mellitus.

—you have a history of increased blood levels of triglycerides.

—you have a history of liver disease.

Time Required for Apparent Benefit
Continuous use on a regular schedule for 4 to 8 weeks is usually necessary to determine this drug's effectiveness in treating severe cystic acne.

Possible Side-Effects *(natural, expected, and unavoidable drug actions)*
Dryness of the nose and mouth, with inflammation of the lips. Dryness of the skin, with occasional peeling of the palms and soles.

Possible Adverse Effects *(unusual, unexpected, and infrequent reactions)*

IF ANY OF THE FOLLOWING DEVELOP, DISCONTINUE DRUG AND NOTIFY YOUR PHYSICIAN AS SOON AS POSSIBLE

Mild Adverse Effects
Skin rash, thinning of hair, conjunctivitis, muscular and joint aches, headache, fatigue, indigestion.

Serious Adverse Effects

Skin infections, worsening of arthritis.

Abnormal acceleration of bone development in children.

Development of opacities in the cornea of the eye.

Reduced red blood cell and white blood cell counts, increased blood platelet counts.

Increased pressure within the head, with associated headache, visual disturbances, nausea and vomiting.

CAUTION

1. This drug should not be used to treat mild forms of acne.
2. Do not take any other form of Vitamin A while taking this drug. (Observe content of multiple vitamin preparations.)
3. Women with potential for pregnancy should have a pregnancy test before taking this drug and should use an effective form of contraception during its use. It is recommended that contraception be continued until normal menstruation resumes after discontinuing this drug.
4. This drug may cause increased blood levels of triglycerides and cholesterol.
5. If a second course of this drug is prescribed, wait a minimum of 8 weeks before resuming medication.

Advisability of Use During Pregnancy

Pregnancy Category: X. See Pregnancy Code inside back cover.

Animal reproduction studies in rats and rabbits revealed birth defects due to this drug.

Information from adequate studies in pregnant women is not available. However, serious defects of fetal brain development, possibly related to the use of this drug, have been reported recently.

Advisability of Use While Nursing Infant

This drug should not be taken while breast-feeding.

Suggested Periodic Examinations While Taking This Drug (at physician's discretion)

Complete blood cell counts.

Measurements of blood cholesterol and triglyceride levels.

Liver and kidney function tests.

While Taking This Drug, Observe the Following

Food: This drug should be taken with meals to achieve the highest blood levels.

Other Drugs: Do not take any other forms of Vitamin A.

Exposure to Sun: This drug can increase the susceptibility to sunburn. Use caution.

ISOXSUPRINE

Year Introduced: 1955

Brand Names

USA	Canada
Vasodilan (Mead Johnson)	Vasodilan (Mead Johnson)

Common Synonyms ("Street Names"):   Circulation medicine

Drug Class: Vasodilator

Prescription Required: USA: Yes   Canada: No

Available for Purchase by Generic Name: Yes

Available Dosage Forms and Strengths
Tablets — 10 mg., 20 mg.

Tablet May Be Crushed or Capsule Opened for Administration: Yes

How This Drug Works
Intended Therapeutic Effect(s):   Relief of symptoms associated with
  • impaired circulation of blood in the extremities.
  • impaired circulation of blood within the brain (in carefully selected cases).
Location of Drug Action(s):   Those sympathetic nerve terminals in the muscles of blood vessel walls that are responsible for vessel dilation.
Method of Drug Action(s):   By stimulating the action of those nerve terminals responsible for blood vessel dilation, this drug produces expansion of vessel walls. The resulting dilation increases the volume of blood flowing through the vessels. The increase in oxygen and nutrients relieves the symptoms attributable to deficient circulation.

Principal Uses of This Drug
As a Single Drug Product: Used primarily as a blood vessel dilator to improve blood circulation through the brain and the extremities. It is given to treat conditions that are attributed to circulatory impairment, as seen with hardening of the arteries of the brain and lower limbs, and with Raynaud's disease.

THIS DRUG SHOULD NOT BE TAKEN IF
—you have had an allergic reaction to any dosage form of it previously.

INFORM YOUR PHYSICIAN BEFORE TAKING THIS DRUG IF
—you have high blood pressure.

Time Required for Apparent Benefit
Drug action begins in approximately 1 hour and persists for 3 hours.

Possible Side-Effects *(natural, expected, and unavoidable drug actions)*
Lightheadedness and lethargy (lowered blood pressure).

Possible Adverse Effects *(unusual, unexpected, and infrequent reactions)*

IF ANY OF THE FOLLOWING DEVELOP, DISCONTINUE DRUG AND NOTIFY
YOUR PHYSICIAN AS SOON AS POSSIBLE

Mild Adverse Effects
  Allergic Reactions: Severe skin rash.
  Other Reactions
    Weakness, dizziness, rapid heart action, headache.
    Nausea, vomiting.
Serious Adverse Effects
  None reported.

CAUTION
Individuals with extensive or severe impairment of circulation to the brain
or heart may respond unfavorably to this drug. Observe closely until the true
nature of the response has been determined. Discontinue drug if condition
worsens.

Precautions for Use by Those over 60 Years of Age
It is not possible to predict in advance the nature of your response to this
  drug. It may relieve your symptoms, have no significant effect, or make
  your symptoms worse. Dosage must be carefully individualized.

Advisability of Use During Pregnancy
Pregnancy Category: C (tentative). See Pregnancy Code inside back
  cover.
  Animal reproduction studies: No data available.
  Information from studies in pregnant women indicates no increase in de-
    fects in 858 exposures to this drug.
  Ask physician for guidance.

Advisability of Use While Nursing Infant
Safety not established. Ask physician for guidance.

Habit-Forming Potential
None.

Effects of Overdosage
Sudden drop in blood pressure, dizziness, heart palpitation, sense of weakness.

Possible Effects of Extended Use
None reported.

Suggested Periodic Examinations While Taking This Drug (at physician's discretion)
Measurement of blood pressure in lying, sitting, and standing positions.

While Taking This Drug, Observe the Following
Foods: No restrictions of food selection. Drug may be taken with or im-
  mediately following meals to reduce stomach irritation or nausea.
Beverages: No restrictions.

Alcohol: No interactions expected.

Tobacco Smoking: Nicotine can reduce this drug's ability to dilate blood vessels and to improve circulation. Follow physician's advice regarding smoking.

Marijuana Smoking: No interactions expected.

Other Drugs: No significant drug interactions reported.

Driving a Vehicle, Operating Machinery, Engaging in Hazardous Activities: Be alert to possible drop in blood pressure with resulting dizziness and weakness. Be prepared to stop and lie down.

Aviation Note: Serious circulatory disorders *are a disqualification* for the piloting of aircraft. Consultation with a designated Aviation Medical Examiner is advised.

Exposure to Sun: No restrictions.

Exposure to Cold: Avoid as much as possible. This drug may be less effective in cold environments or with the handling of cold objects.

Special Storage Instructions
Keep in a dry, tightly closed container.

LEVODOPA

Year Introduced: 1967

Brand Names

USA		Canada
Bendopa (ICN)	Larodopa (Roche)	Larodopa (Roche)
Dopar	Sinemet [CD] (Merck	Prolopa [CD] (Roche)
(Norwich-Eaton)	Sharp & Dohme)	Sinemet [CD] (MSD)

Common Synonyms ("Street Names"):   None

Drug Class: Anti-parkinsonism

Prescription Required: Yes

Available for Purchase by Generic Name: USA: Yes   Canada: No

Available Dosage Forms and Strengths
Tablets — 100 mg., 250 mg., 500 mg.
Capsules — 100 mg., 125 mg., 250 mg., 500 mg.

Tablet May Be Crushed or Capsule Opened for Administration: Yes

How This Drug Works
Intended Therapeutic Effect(s):   Reduction of the rigidity, tremor, sluggish movement, and gait disturbances characteristic of Parkinson's disease.

Location of Drug Action(s):   A regulating center in the brain (the corpus striatum) that governs the coordination and efficiency of bodily movements.

Method of Drug Action(s):   Not completely established. Present thinking is that levodopa enters the brain tissue and is converted to dopamine. After sufficient dosage, this corrects the deficiency of dopamine (thought to be the cause of Parkinsonism) and restores a more normal balance of the chemicals responsible for the transmission of nerve impulses.

Principal Uses of This Drug

As a Single Drug Product: Used exclusively to treat the major types of Parkinson's disease: Paralysis Agitans ("shaking palsy" of unknown cause), the type that follows encephalitis, the parkinsonism that develops with aging (associated with hardening of the brain arteries), and the forms of parkinsonism that follow poisoning by carbon monoxide or manganese.

As a Combination Drug Product [CD]:   This drug is available in combination with carbidopa, a chemical that prevents the decomposition of levodopa before it reaches its site of action in the brain. The addition of carbidopa reduces the amount of levodopa required by 75%. This combination is more effective in smaller doses and reduces the frequency and severity of adverse effects.

THIS DRUG SHOULD NOT BE TAKEN IF

—you are allergic to any of the drugs bearing the brand names listed above.
—you are taking, or have taken during the past 2 weeks, any mono-amine oxidase (MAO) inhibitor drug (see Drug Class, Section Three).
—you have glaucoma (narrow-angle type).

INFORM YOUR PHYSICIAN BEFORE TAKING THIS DRUG IF

—you have diabetes.
—you have epilepsy.
—you have a history of high blood pressure or heart or lung disease.
—you have a history of liver or kidney disease.
—you have a history of peptic ulcer disease.
—you have a history of malignant melanoma.
—you plan to have surgery under general anesthesia in the near future.

Time Required for Apparent Benefit

Improvement usually occurs in 2 to 3 weeks. Regular use for 6 weeks or longer is needed to determine this drug's maximal effectiveness. Careful dosage adjustment according to individual response is necessary.

Possible Side-Effects *(natural, expected, and unavoidable drug actions)*

Fatigue, lethargy, lightheadedness in upright position (see orthostatic hypotension in Glossary).

Pink to red coloration of urine (which turns black after exposure to air), of no significance.

Possible Adverse Effects *(unusual, unexpected, and infrequent reactions)*

IF ANY OF THE FOLLOWING DEVELOP, DISCONTINUE DRUG AND NOTIFY YOUR PHYSICIAN AS SOON AS POSSIBLE

Mild Adverse Effects
Allergic Reactions: Skin rash, itching.
Other Reactions
    Reduced appetite, nausea, vomiting.
    Headache, dizziness, faintness, unsteadiness, blurred vision.
    Heart palpitation.
    Difficulty in emptying the urinary bladder.
    Unusual, unpleasant taste sensation.
    Offensive body odor.

Serious Adverse Effects
Emotional depression, confusion, abnormal thinking and behavior.
Abnormal, purposeless movements of the head, face, arms, or legs.
Development of peptic ulcer, stomach or intestinal bleeding.
Hemolytic anemia (see Glossary).
Abnormally low white blood cell count, resulting in lowered resistance to
    infection—fever, sore throat.

CAUTION
1. To reduce the high frequency of serious adverse effects, it is advisable to begin treatment with small doses, and to increase dosage gradually until the desired response is achieved.
2. As improvement occurs, avoid excessive and hurried activity (which often causes falls and injury).

Precautions for Use by Those over 60 Years of Age
You may be more sensitive to the actions of this drug. Small doses are advisable until your individual response has been determined.
You may be more susceptible to the development of impaired thinking, confusion, agitation, nightmares, and hallucinations. Careful dosage adjustments are mandatory.

Advisability of Use During Pregnancy
Pregnancy Category: C (tentative). See Pregnancy Code inside back cover.
    Animal reproduction studies in rodents reveal significant birth defects due to this drug.
    Information from adequate studies in pregnant women is not available.
    It is advisable to avoid this drug during first 3 months.
    Ask physician for guidance.

Advisability of Use While Nursing Infant
This drug may be present in milk. Ask physician for guidance.

Habit-Forming Potential
None.

Effects of Overdosage

With Moderate Overdose: Muscle twitching, spastic closure of the eyelids, nausea, vomiting, diarrhea.

With Large Overdose: Irregular and rapid pulse, weakness, fainting, confusion, agitation, hallucinations.

Possible Effects of Extended Use

Development of involuntary, abnormal, purposeless movements of the head, face, mouth, tongue, arms, or legs. These developments are reversible and gradually disappear when the drug is discontinued.

Development of "on-off" and "wearing-off" episodes during the course of drug treatment. These consist of periods of sudden loss of drug effectiveness with a return of all features of parkinsonism. These episodes occur in approximately 40% of users.

Suggested Periodic Examinations While Taking This Drug (at physician's discretion)

Complete blood cell counts.

Liver and kidney function tests.

Regular measurement of internal eye pressure (in presence of open-angle glaucoma).

Regular measurement of blood pressure in lying, sitting, and standing positions to detect any tendency to orthostatic hypotension.

While Taking This Drug, Observe the Following

Foods: No restrictions of food selection. Drug is best taken with meals to reduce stomach irritation or nausea.

Beverages: No restrictions.

Alcohol: No interactions expected.

Tobacco Smoking: No interactions expected.

Marijuana Smoking

Occasional (once or twice weekly):   No effect to mild increase in fatigue and lethargy.

Daily: Moderate to marked increase in fatigue and lethargy; possible accentuation of orthostatic hypotension (see Glossary).

Other drugs

Levodopa may *increase* the effects of

- anti-hypertensive drugs such as methyldopa (Aldomet), reserpine preparations, and pargyline, and cause excessive lowering of the blood pressure. Dosage adjustments may be necessary.

Levodopa *taken concurrently* with

- mono-amine oxidase (MAO) inhibitor drugs (see Drug Class, Section Three) may cause a dangerous rise in blood pressure and body temperature. Do not use these drugs concurrently.

The following drugs may *increase* the effects of levodopa

- other anti-parkinsonism drugs (Artane, Cogentin, Kemadrin, etc.) may improve its effectiveness in treating Parkinsonism. Individual dosage adjustment is essential to determine the combined effect.

The following drugs may *decrease* the effects of levodopa
• haloperidol (Haldol)
• methyldopa (Aldomet)
• papaverine (Cerespan, Pavabid, Vasospan, etc.)
• phenothiazines (see Drug Class, Section Three)
• pyridoxine (Vitamin B-6) can reduce or even abolish the beneficial action of levodopa. Be sure that any vitamin preparation you are taking does not contain pyridoxine.
• reserpine (and related drugs)

Driving a Vehicle, Operating Machinery, Engaging in Hazardous Activities: Be alert to the possible occurrence of orthostatic hypotension, dizziness and/or impaired vision while engaged in hazardous activities. Be prepared to stop and lie down to prevent fainting.

Aviation Note: Parkinsonism *is a disqualification* for the piloting of aircraft. Consultation with a designated Aviation Medical Examiner is advised.

Exposure to Sun: No restrictions.

Heavy Exercise or Exertion: Use caution as ability to be more active improves. Rapid, excessive, or unrestrained activity often causes falls and serious injury.

Special Storage Instructions
Keep in a dry, tightly closed container. Protect from light.

LIOTHYRONINE
(Triiodothyronine, T–3)

Year Introduced: 1956

Brand Names

USA		Canada
Cytomel (Smith Kline & French)	Thyrolar [CD] (Armour)	Cytomel (SK&F)
Euthroid [CD] (Parke-Davis)		Tertroxin (Glaxo)
		Thyrolar [CD] (Harris)

Common Synonyms ("Street Names"):   Thyroid pills

Drug Class: Thyroid Hormones

Prescription Required: Yes

Available for Purchase by Generic Name: No

Available Dosage Forms and Strengths
Tablets — 0.005 mg., 0.025 mg., 0.05 mg., 0.1 mg., 0.125 mg., 0.15 mg., 0.175 mg., 0.2 mg., 0.3 mg.

Tablet May Be Crushed or Capsule Opened for Administration: Yes

How This Drug Works

Intended Therapeutic Effect(s): Correction of thyroid hormone deficiency (hypothyroidism) by replacement therapy.

Location of Drug Action(s): Affects the biochemical activity of all tissues throughout the body.

Method of Drug Action(s): By altering the processes of cellular chemistry that store energy in an inactive (reserve) form, this drug makes more energy available for biochemical activity and increases the rate of cellular metabolism.

Principal Uses of This Drug

As a Single Drug Product: Used solely to treat deficiency of thyroid hormone (hypothyroidism). In the absence of true thyroid deficiency, the use of this drug to reduce weight is inappropriate and possibly harmful.

As a Combination Drug Product [CD]: This thyroid hormone is available in combination with the other principal thyroid hormone, levothyroxine, in a preparation that resembles as closely as possible the natural hormone material produced by the thyroid gland.

THIS DRUG SHOULD NOT BE TAKEN IF

—you have had an allergic reaction to any dosage form of it previously.

—you are recovering from a recent heart attack (ask physician for guidance).

—you are using it to lose weight and you do not have a thyroid deficiency (your thyroid function is normal).

INFORM YOUR PHYSICIAN BEFORE TAKING THIS DRUG IF

—you have any form of heart disease.

—you have high blood pressure.

—you have diabetes.

—you have Addison's disease or a history of adrenal gland deficiency.

—you are using adrenalin, ephedrine, or isoproterenol to treat asthma.

—you are taking any anticoagulant drugs.

Time Required for Apparent Benefit

Drug action begins within the first 12 hours, reaches a maximum in 2 to 3 days, and gradually subsides within 5 days. Full effectiveness requires continuous use on a regular schedule for several weeks.

Possible Side-Effects *(natural, expected, and unavoidable drug actions)*

None if dosage is adjusted correctly.

Possible Adverse Effects *(unusual, unexpected, and infrequent reactions)*

IF ANY OF THE FOLLOWING DEVELOP, DISCONTINUE DRUG AND NOTIFY YOUR PHYSICIAN AS SOON AS POSSIBLE.

Mild Adverse Effects

Allergic Reactions: Skin rash, hives.

Other Reactions

Headache may occur in sensitive individuals even with proper dosage adjustment.

Change in menstrual pattern may occur during dosage adjustment.

Serious Adverse Effects
Increased frequency or intensity of angina in the presence of coronary artery disease.

CAUTION
1. Thyroid hormones are used to correct conditions due to thyroid deficiency and to treat thyroid gland enlargement (goiter) and thyroid cancer. They should not be used to treat obesity if diagnostic studies indicate that there is no thyroid deficiency contributing to the obesity.
2. The need for and response to thyroid hormone treatment varies greatly from person to person. Careful supervision of individual response is necessary to determine correct dosage. Do not change your dosage schedule without consulting your physician.

Precautions for Use by Those over 60 Years of Age
Natural changes in body composition and function after 60 usually increase sensitivity to thyroid hormone action. It is anticipated that you will respond well to small doses. Report promptly any indications that suggest overdosage.

Advisability of Use During Pregnancy
Pregnancy Category: C (tentative). See Pregnancy Code inside back cover.
Animal reproduction studies in guinea pigs reveal the development of fetal goiter.

Information from adequate studies in pregnant women is not available. Ask physician for guidance.

Thyroid hormones do not reach the fetus (cross the placenta) in significant amounts. This drug is safe to use in pregnancy but *only* if given to correct a true thyroid deficiency and the dosage is properly adjusted.

Advisability of Use While Nursing Infant
Thyroid hormones are present in milk. Nursing is safe when the mother's dose of thyroid hormones is correctly adjusted to maintain normal thyroid activity.

Habit-Forming Potential
None.

Effects of Overdosage
With Moderate Overdose: Sense of increased body heat, heart palpitation, nervousness, increased sweating, hand tremors, insomnia.

With Large Overdose: Rapid and irregular pulse, fever, headache, marked nervousness and irritability, diarrhea, weight loss, muscle spasm and cramping.

Possible Effects of Extended Use
None with correct dosage adjustment.

Suggested Periodic Examinations While Taking This Drug (at physician's discretion)

Physician's assessment of response to treatment, with evaluation of subjective and objective changes due to thyroid hormone activity.

Measurement of thyroid hormone levels in the blood.

While Taking This Drug, Observe the Following

Foods: To improve absorption this drug should be taken on arising and before eating. Avoid heavy use of soybean preparations because of their ability to interfere with thyroid function.

Beverages: No restrictions.

Alcohol: No interactions expected.

Tobacco Smoking: No interactions expected.

Marijuana Smoking: No interactions expected.

Other Drugs

Liothyronine may *increase* the effects of

- stimulants such as adrenalin, ephedrine, the amphetamines (Dexedrine), methylphenidate (Ritalin), etc., and cause excessive stimulation. Dosage adjustment may be necessary.
- oral anticoagulants of the coumarin family (see Drug Class, Section Three), and cause bleeding or hemorrhage. Reduction in dosage of the anticoagulant is usually necessary.
- tricyclic antidepressants (see Drug Class, Section Three).
- digitalis preparations. Careful dosage adjustment is necessary to prevent digitalis toxicity.

Liothyronine may *decrease* the effects of

- barbiturates, making larger doses necessary for effective sedation.

Liothyronine *taken concurrently* with

- all anti-diabetic drugs (insulin and oral anti-diabetic medications), may require an increase in the dosage of the anti-diabetic agent to obtain proper control of blood sugar levels. After the correct doses of both drugs have been determined, a reduction in the dose of thyroid will require a simultaneous reduction in the dose of the anti-diabetic drug to prevent hypoglycemia.
- cortisone-like drugs, requires careful dosage adjustment to prevent the development of cortisone deficiency.

The following drugs may *increase* the effects of liothyronine

- aspirin (in large doses and with continuous use)
- phenytoin (Dantoin, Dilantin, etc.)

The following drug may *decrease* the effects of liothyronine

- cholestyramine (Cuemid, Questran) may reduce its absorption. Intake of the two drugs should be 5 hours apart.

Driving a Vehicle, Operating Machinery, Engaging in Hazardous Activities: No restrictions or precautions.

Aviation Note: The use of this drug *may be a disqualification* for the piloting of aircraft. Consultation with a designated Aviation Medical Examiner is advised.

Exposure to Sun: No restrictions.

Exposure to Heat: This drug may decrease individual tolerance to warm environments, increasing the discomfort due to heat. Avoid excessive sweating.

Exposure to Cold: This drug may increase individual tolerance to cold, decreasing the discomfort due to cold.

Heavy Exercise or Exertion: Use caution in the presence of angina and known coronary artery disease. This drug may increase the frequency of angina during physical activity.

Discontinuation: This drug must be taken continuously on a regular schedule to correct thyroid deficiency. Do not discontinue it without consulting your physician.

Special Storage Instructions

Keep in a dry, tightly closed container at room temperature. Protect from light.

LITHIUM

Year Introduced: 1949

Brand Names

USA		Canada
Cibalith-S (CIBA)	Lithonate (Rowell)	Carbolith (ICN)
Eskalith (Smith Kline & French)	Lithotabs (Rowell)	Lithane (Pfizer)
	Pfi-Lith	Lithizine (Technilab)
Lithane (Miles)	(Pfipharmecs)	
Lithobid (CIBA)		

Common Synonyms ("Street Names"):   None

Drug Class: Tranquilizer, Strong (Anti-manic)

Prescription Required: Yes

Available for Purchase by Generic Name: USA: Yes   Canada: No

Available Dosage Forms and Strengths

Tablets — 300 mg.
Tablets, slow release — 300 mg.
Tablets, controlled release — 450 mg.
Capsules — 300 mg.
Syrup — 8 mEq. per teaspoonful (5 ml.)

Tablet May Be Crushed or Capsule Opened for Administration: Yes

How This Drug Works

Intended Therapeutic Effect(s):   Normalization of mood and behavior in chronic manic-depressive mental illness.

Location of Drug Action(s):   Those areas of the brain that determine mood and emotional stability.

Method of Drug Action(s):   Not established. Present thinking is that lithium may act to correct chemical imbalances in certain nerve impulse transmitters that influence emotional status and behavior.

Principal Uses of This Drug

As a Single Drug Product.   Used primarily in the management of manic-depressive disorders. While its principal use is the prompt correction of acute mania, it is also used to stabilize these disorders by reducing the frequency and severity of recurrent manic-depressive mood swings. It is also beneficial in treating the depression phase of these disorders in individuals who do not experience the manic phase. Additional uses, which are experimental for the present, include the prevention of cluster headaches and the stimulation of production of white blood cells.

THIS DRUG SHOULD NOT BE TAKEN IF
—you are allergic to any of the drugs bearing the brand names listed above.
—you have serious heart or kidney disease.
—it is prescribed for a child under 12 years of age.

INFORM YOUR PHYSICIAN BEFORE TAKING THIS DRUG IF
—you are taking any type of diuretic (urine producing) drug (see Drug Class, Section Three).
—you have diabetes.
—you have epilepsy.

Time Required for Apparent Benefit
Improvement in the manic phase may occur in 1 to 3 weeks. Improvement in the depressive phase may require continuous use for several months.

Possible Side-Effects *(natural, expected, and unavoidable drug actions)*
Increased urine volume and thirst, drowsiness or lethargy (in sensitive individuals).

Possible Adverse Effects *(unusual, unexpected, and infrequent reactions)*

IF ANY OF THE FOLLOWING DEVELOP, DISCONTINUE DRUG AND NOTIFY YOUR PHYSICIAN AS SOON AS POSSIBLE

Mild Adverse Effects

Allergic Reactions: Generalized itching, skin rash.

Other Reactions

Headache, dizziness, †drowsiness, †sluggishness, hand tremors, †muscle twitching, blurred vision.

Irregular pulse, heart palpitation.

Loss of appetite, nausea, †vomiting, †diarrhea, metallic taste.

†May be an early sign of lithium toxicity, indicating need for dosage adjustment.

Serious Adverse Effects

Severe, involuntary, spasmodic movements of arms or legs, impaired balance, staggering gait.

Blackout spells, epileptic-like seizures.

Loss of bladder or rectal control.

CAUTION

1. This drug has a very narrow margin of safe use. The level of drug required to be effective is quite close to the level that can cause adverse effects. Careful dosage adjustments based on periodic measurements of blood levels are mandatory. Follow instructions exactly regarding blood examinations and drug dosage.

2. Many over-the-counter (OTC) medications contain drugs that can interact unfavorably with this drug. Consult your physician or pharmacist before taking new medication of any kind.

Precautions for Use by Infants and Children

Initial dose should be low—not over 450 mg/24 hrs.

Increase dose at weekly intervals in steps of 600, 900, 1350, 1800 mg. per day until a blood level of 1.0 mEq/L is reached.

Maintain blood level between 0.6 and 1.2 mEq/L. Do not exceed 1.8 mEq/L.

Safety and effectiveness in children below the age of 12 years have not been established. Informed consent of parents is advised.

Precautions for Use by Those over 60 Years of Age

The natural decline in kidney function that occurs after 60 makes it advisable to begin treatment with small doses.

You may be more susceptible to the toxic effects of this drug. Coma can occur suddenly and without warning symptoms.

The use of diuretics and a low-salt diet can raise the blood levels of lithium significantly and increase the risk of lithium overdosage.

Advisability of Use During Pregnancy

Pregnancy Category: D (tentative). See Pregnancy Code inside back cover.

Animal reproduction studies in mice and rats reveal significant birth defects due to this drug.

Information from studies in pregnant women indicates the development of neonatal goiter and the presence of 11 cardiovascular defects in 143 exposures to this drug.

It is advisable to avoid this drug during entire pregnancy if possible.

Ask physician for guidance.

Advisability of Use While Nursing Infant

Lithium is known to be present in milk and in the blood of the nursing infant.

It is advisable to avoid drug or to refrain from nursing. Ask physician for guidance.

Habit-Forming Potential

None.

Effects of Overdosage

With Moderate Overdose: Drowsiness, muscular weakness, lack of coordination, nausea, vomiting, diarrhea, tremors, muscular spasms.

With Large Overdose: Blurred vision, ringing in the ears, dizziness, staggering gait, increased urine volume, slurred speech, confusion, stupor progressing to coma, convulsions.

Possible Effects of Extended Use

The development of thyroid gland enlargement (goiter), with or without reduced thyroid function (hypothyroidism).

Suggested Periodic Examinations While Taking This Drug (at physician's discretion)

Regular determinations of blood lithium levels are absolutely essential to the safe and effective use of this drug.

Periodic evaluation of thyroid gland size and functional status.

While Taking This Drug, Observe the Following

Foods: Maintain a normal diet. Do *not* restrict your use of salt.

Beverages: Drink at least 2 and one-half to 3 quarts of liquids every 24 hours.

Alcohol: Use with caution until combined effect has been determined. Avoid alcohol completely if symptoms of lithium toxicity appear (see Effects of Overdosage, above).

Tobacco Smoking: No interactions expected.

Marijuana Smoking

Occasional (once or twice weekly):   No effect to mild and transient increase in tremor; some risk of precipitating latent psychoses.

Daily: Accentuation of tremor due to this drug; increased risk of precipitating psychoses.

Other Drugs

Lithium *taken concurrently* with

• diuretics (urine promoting drugs), may cause severe lithium toxicity due to excessive loss of sodium and water and to excessive retention of lithium in the body.

The following drugs may *increase* the effects of lithium:

• tetracycline (Achromycin, Panmycin, Sumycin, etc.)

• phenylbutazone (Butazolidin, Azolid, etc.)

The following drug may *decrease* the effects of lithium:

• chlorpromazine (Thorazine, Largactil) may reduce lithium's effectiveness by hastening its excretion from the body. Dosage adjustments may be necessary.

Driving a Vehicle, Operating Machinery, Engaging in Hazardous Activities: This drug can impair mental alertness, judgment, physical coordination, and reaction time. Avoid all hazardous activities if these drug effects occur.

Aviation Note: The use of this drug *is a disqualification* for the piloting of aircraft. Consultation with a designated Aviation Medical Examiner is advised.

Exposure to Sun: No restrictions.

Exposure to Heat: Excessive sweating may cause lithium toxicity. Avoid hot environments as much as possible.

Heavy Exercise or Exertion: Use good judgment. In hot environments avoid exercise that could induce excessive sweating.

Occurrence of Unrelated Illness: Any illness that causes fever, heavy perspiration, nausea, or vomiting can greatly increase the risk of lithium toxicity. Notify your physician of all such illnesses and ask for guidance.

Special Storage Instructions
Keep in a dry, tightly closed container.

LORAZEPAM

Year Introduced: 1977

Brand Names

USA	Canada
Ativan (Wyeth)	Ativan (Wyeth)

Common Synonyms ("Street Names"):   Downs, nerve pills, tranks

Drug Class: Tranquilizer, Mild (Anti-anxiety), Benzodiazepines

Prescription Required: Yes (Controlled Drug, U.S. Schedule IV)*

Available for Purchase by Generic Name: No

Available Dosage Forms and Strengths
Tablets — 0.5 mg., 1.0 mg., 2.0 mg.

Tablet May Be Crushed or Capsule Opened for Administration: Yes

How This Drug Works
Intended Therapeutic Effect(s):   Relief of mild to moderate anxiety, nervous tension, agitation, and irritability; relief of insomnia associated with such states of nervousness.

Location of Drug Action(s):   Thought to be the limbic system of the brain, one of the centers that influence emotional stability.

Method of Drug Action(s):   Not established. Present thinking is that this drug may reduce the activity of certain parts of the limbic system.

*See Schedules of Controlled Drugs inside back cover.

Principal Uses of This Drug
As a Single Drug Product: Used primarily as a mild tranquilizer to relieve mild to moderate anxiety and nervous tension. While it is less sedative than the barbiturates, it is also used at bedtime to produce a calming effect that permits natural sleep.

THIS DRUG SHOULD NOT BE TAKEN IF
—you have had an allergic reaction to any drug of the benzodiazepine family (see Drug Class, Section Three).

—you have acute glaucoma (narrow-angle type only).

INFORM YOUR PHYSICIAN BEFORE TAKING THIS DRUG IF
—you are emotionally depressed.

—you have myasthenia gravis.

—you have impaired liver or kidney function.

—you are taking sedatives, sleep-inducing drugs, tranquilizers, antidepressants, or anticonvulsant drugs of any kind.

—it is prescribed for a child less than 12 years of age.

Time Required for Apparent Benefit
Drug action begins in approximately 30 minutes and reaches its peak in 2 to 6 hours (depending on dose). For severe symptoms of some duration, relief may require continuous medication for several days.

Possible Side-Effects *(natural, expected and unavoidable drug actions)*
Drowsiness, lethargy, unsteadiness in stance and gait.

Possible Adverse Effects *(unusual, unexpected and infrequent reactions)*

IF ANY OF THE FOLLOWING DEVELOP, DISCONTINUE DRUG AND NOTIFY YOUR PHYSICIAN AS SOON AS POSSIBLE

Mild Adverse Effects
Allergic Reactions: Skin rashes.
Other Reactions: Dizziness, blurred vision, headaches, nausea, indigestion, excessive dreaming, sweating.

Serious Adverse Effects
Allergic Reactions: None reported.
Other Reactions: Disorientation, emotional depression, agitation, disturbed sleep.

CAUTION
1. Total dosage should not exceed 10 mg. per 24 hours.
2. Do not discontinue this drug abruptly.
3. Over-the-counter preparations for allergies, colds, and sleep that contain antihistamines may cause excessive sedation when taken with lorazepam.

Precautions for Use by Those over 60 Years of Age
Initial total dosage should not exceed 0.5 to 1.0 mg. per 24 hours.

Natural changes in body functions increase the duration of this drug's action. It is necessary to use smaller doses with longer intervals between doses to avoid excessive accumulation of the drug in body tissues. Dosage must be carefully individualized and limited to the smallest effective amount.

You may be more susceptible to the development of lightheadedness, impaired thinking and memory, confusion, lethargy, drowsiness, incoordination, unsteady gait and balance, impaired bladder control, and constipation.

Be alert to the possibility of paradoxical responses consisting of excitement, agitation, anger, hostility, and rage.

Advisability of Use During Pregnancy

Pregnancy Category: C (tentative). See Pregnancy Code inside back cover. Animal reproduction studies in rabbits reveal significant birth defects due to this drug.

Information from adequate studies in pregnant women is not available. Ask physician for guidance.

The findings of some recent studies suggest a possible association between the use of a drug closely related to lorazepam during early pregnancy and the occurrence of birth defects, such as cleft lip. It is advisable to avoid this drug completely during the first 3 months of pregnancy.

Advisability of Use While Nursing Infant

With recommended dosage, drug is probably present in milk. Avoid use if possible. Ask physician for guidance.

Habit-Forming Potential

This drug can cause psychological and/or physical dependence (see Glossary) if used in large doses for an extended period of time.

Effects of Overdosage

With Moderate Overdose: Marked drowsiness, weakness, drunkenness, impairment of stance and gait.

With Large Overdose: Stupor progressing to deep sleep or coma.

Possible Effects of Extended Use

Psychological and/or physical dependence.
Impairment of blood cell production.
Impairment of liver function.
This drug is not recommended for use beyond 6 weeks without reevaluation of emotional and physical status and reassessment of continued need.

Suggested Periodic Examinations While Taking This Drug (at physician's discretion)

Complete blood cell counts and liver function tests during long-term use.

While Taking This Drug, Observe the Following

Foods: No restrictions.

Beverages: Large intake of coffee, tea, or cola drinks (because of their caffeine content) may reduce the calming action of this drug.

Alcohol: Use with extreme caution until the combined effect is determined. Alcohol may increase the sedative effects of lorazepam. Lorazepam may increase the intoxicating effects of alcohol.

Tobacco Smoking: Heavy smoking may reduce the calming action of lorazepam.

Marijuana Smoking
Occasional (once or twice weekly):   Mild increase in sedative effect of this drug.
Daily: Marked increase in sedative effect of this drug.
Other Drugs
Lorazepam may *increase* the effects of
- other sedatives, sleep-inducing drugs, tranquilizers, anticonvulsants, and narcotic drugs. Use these only under supervision of a physician. Careful dosage adjustment is necessary.

Lorazepam *taken concurrently* with
- pyrimethamine (Daraprim) may cause impairment of liver function.

Driving a Vehicle, Operating Machinery, Engaging in Hazardous Activities: This drug can impair mental alertness, judgment, physical coordination, and reaction time. Avoid hazardous activities.

Aviation Note: The use of this drug *is a disqualification* for the piloting of aircraft. Consultation with a designated Aviation Medical Examiner is advised.

Exposure to Sun: No restrictions.

Exposure to Heat: Use caution until effect of excessive perspiration is determined. Because of reduced urine volume, lorazepam may accumulate in the body and produce effects of overdosage.

Heavy Exercise or Exertion: No restrictions in cool or temperate weather.

Discontinuation: If it has been necessary to use this drug for an extended period of time do not discontinue it abruptly. Ask physician for guidance regarding dosage reduction and withdrawal.

Special Storage Instructions
Keep in a dry, tightly closed, light-resistant container.

MAPROTILINE

Year Introduced: 1974

Brand Names

USA	Canada
Ludiomil (CIBA)	Ludiomil (CIBA)

Common Synonyms ("Street Names"):   Depression pills

Drug Class: Antidepressants, Tetracyclic

Prescription Required: USA: Yes   Canada: Yes

Available for Purchase by Generic Name: USA: No   Canada: No

Available Dosage Forms and Strengths
Tablets — 25 mg., 50 mg., 75 mg.

Tablet May Be Crushed or Capsule Opened for Administration: Yes

How This Drug Works
Intended Therapeutic Effect(s):   The relief of emotional depression and the gradual improvement of mood in all types of depressive disorders.

Location of Drug Action(s):   Those areas of the brain that control mood and emotional stability.

Method of Drug Action(s):   Not established. It is thought that by increasing the availability of a certain nerve impulse transmitter (norepinephrine), this drug relieves the symptoms associated with depression.

Principal Uses of This Drug
As a Single Drug Product: To provide symptomatic relief in all types of depression, and to initiate the restoration of normal mood.

THIS DRUG SHOULD NOT BE TAKEN IF
—you have had an allergic reaction to it previously.

—you are taking or have taken within the past 14 days any mono-amine oxidase (MAO) inhibitor drug (see Drug Class, Section Three).

—you are recovering from a recent heart attack.

—it is prescribed for a child under 18 years of age.

INFORM YOUR PHYSICIAN BEFORE TAKING THIS DRUG IF
—you are allergic or abnormally sensitive to any tricyclic antidepressant drug (see Drug Class, Section Three).

—you have a history of any of the following: alcoholism, bronchial asthma, epilepsy, glaucoma, heart disease, paranoia, prostate gland enlargement, schizophrenia, or overactive thyroid function.

—you have impaired liver function.

—you plan to have surgery under general anesthesia in the near future.

Time Required for Apparent Benefit
Continuous use on a regular schedule for 14 to 21 days is usually necessary to determine this drug's effectiveness in relieving depression. However, benefit may be apparent within 7 days in some individuals.

Possible Side-Effects *(natural, expected, and unavoidable drug actions)*
Drowsiness, blurring of vision, dryness of mouth, constipation, impaired urination.

Possible Adverse Effects *(unusual, unexpected, and infrequent reactions)*
IF ANY OF THE FOLLOWING DEVELOP, DISCONTINUE DRUG AND NOTIFY YOUR PHYSICIAN AS SOON AS POSSIBLE

Mild Adverse Effects
    Allergic Reactions: Skin rash, itching.
    Other Reactions: Insomnia, nervousness, palpitations, dizziness, unsteadiness, tremors, fainting, weakness.
        Nausea, vomiting, acid indigestion, diarrhea.
    Increased sweating.

Serious Adverse Effects
Behavioral effects: anxiety, confusion, hallucinations.
Aggravation of paranoid psychosis and schizophrenia.
Aggravation of epilepsy (siezures).
Jaundice (see Glossary).

Adverse Effects That May Mimic Natural Diseases or Disorders
The development of jaundice may suggest viral hepatitis.

Natural Diseases or Disorders That May Be Activated By This Drug
Latent epilepsy, glaucoma, prostatism.

CAUTION
1. The dosage of this drug should be adjusted carefully for each person individually. This requires observation of symptom improvement and, in some instances, the measurement of drug levels in the blood.
2. Observe for early indications of toxicity: confusion, agitation, rapid heart beat.
3. It is advisable to withhold this drug if electroconvulsive therapy (ECT) is to be used.

Precautions for Use by Infants and Children
Safety and effectiveness in children below the age of 18 years have not been established.

Precautions for Use by Those over 60 Years of Age
During the first 2 weeks of treatment, observe for the development of confusional reactions—restlessness, agitation, forgetfulness, disorientation, delusions, hallucinations. Reduction of dosage or discontinuation may be necessary.

Observe for lightheadedness, dizziness, unsteadiness, and incoordination which may predispose to falling and injury.

This drug can increase the degree of impaired urination associated with prostate gland enlargement (prostatism).

It is advisable to take the total daily dose at bedtime to reduce the risks of postural hypotension (see Orthostatic Hypotension in Glossary).

Advisability of Use During Pregnancy
Pregnancy Category: B (tentative). See Pregnancy Code inside back cover.
Animal reproduction studies in mice, rats, and rabbits revealed no birth defects.
Information from adequate studies in pregnant women is not available.
Avoid completely during the first 3 months if possible.
Use this drug only if clearly needed.

Advisability of Use While Nursing Infant
This drug is present in breast milk. Nursing may be permitted with careful observation of the infant for drowsiness or failure to feed. Ask physician for guidance.

Habit-Forming Potential
None.

Effects of Overdosage

With Moderate Overdose: Marked drowsiness, unsteadiness, tremors, dilated pupils, vomiting.

With Large Overdose: Agitation, confusion, rapid heart rate, low blood pressure, stupor, coma, convulsions.

Possible Effects of Extended Use

None reported.

Suggested Periodic Examinations While Taking This Drug (at physician's discretion)

Complete blood cell counts.

Liver function tests.

Serial blood pressure readings.

While Taking This Drug, Observe the Following

Foods: No restrictions. May be taken on an empty stomach or following food to reduce stomach irritation.

Beverages: No restrictions. May be taken with milk.

Alcohol: Avoid completely. This drug can increase markedly the intoxicating effects of alcohol and accentuate its depressant action on brain function.

Tobacco Smoking: No interactions expected.

Marijuana Smoking

Occasional (once or twice weekly): Transient increase in drowsiness and dryness of the mouth.

Daily: Persistent drowsiness, increased dryness of mouth; possible reduced effectiveness of this drug.

Other Drugs

Maprotiline may *increase* the effects of

• atropine-like drugs (see Drug Class, Section Three).

• sedatives, sleep-inducing drugs, tranquilizers, antihistamines, and narcotic drugs, and cause over-sedation. Dosage adjustments may be necessary.

Maprotiline may *decrease* the effects of

• clonidine (Catapres)

• guanethidine (Ismelin)

• methyldopa (Aldomet)

• reserpine (Serpasil, Ser-Ap-Es, etc.)

Maprotiline *taken concurrently* with

• amphetamine-like drugs may cause severe high blood pressure and/or high fever (see Drug Class, Section Three).

• anti-seizure (anticonvulsant) drugs requires careful monitoring for changes in seizure patterns; dosage of the anticonvulsant may need adjustment.

• ethchlorvynol may cause delirium; avoid concurrent use.

• mono-amine oxidase (MAO) inhibitor drugs may cause high fever, delirium, and convulsions (see Drug Class, Section Three). Avoid the concurrent use of these drugs. Do not begin to take any tricyclic or tetracyclic antidepressant drug within 14 days after the last dose of any MAO inhibitor drug.

• thyroid preparations may impair heart rhythm and function; ask physician for guidance regarding adjustment of thyroid dose.

The following drugs may *decrease* the effects of maprotiline:
• estrogen.
• oral contraceptives.

Driving a Vehicle, Operating Machinery, Engaging in Hazardous Activities: This drug may impair mental alertness, judgment, physical coordination, and reaction time. Avoid hazardous activities.

Aviation Note: The use of this drug *is a disqualification* for the piloting of aircraft. Consultation with a designated Aviation Medical Examiner is advised.

Exposure to Sun: Use caution until sensitivity to sun has been determined. This drug may cause photosensitivity.

Exposure to Heat: Caution advised. This drug can inhibit sweating and impair the body's adaptation to hot environments, increasing the risk of heat stroke. Avoid saunas.

Exposure to Cold: The elderly should use caution to avoid conditions that could cause hypothermia.

Exposure to Environmental Chemicals: This drug can mask the early indications of poisoning due to organophosphorus insecticides; observe the label of any insecticides you use.

Heavy Exercise or Exertion: No restrictions in temperate environment.

Occurrence of Unrelated Illness: In any condition that tends to lower the blood pressure, this drug may exaggerate the response and cause additional reduction of pressure beyond the expected.

Discontinuation: It is advisable to discontinue this drug gradually. Sudden withdrawal after prolonged use may cause headache, malaise, and nausea. When this drug is discontinued, it may be necessary to adjust the doses of other drugs taken concurrently.

Special Storage Instructions
Keep tablets in a dry, tightly closed container at room temperature. Protect from light.

MECLIZINE

Year Introduced: 1954

Brand Names

USA	Canada
Antivert (Roerig)	Bonamine (Pfizer)
Bonine (Pfipharmecs)	Antivert [CD] (Pfizer)
Vertrol (Saron)	

Common Synonyms ("Street Names"):   Seasick pills

Drug Class: Antinausea (Anti-emetic), Antihistamines

Prescription Required: Yes
For Bonine—No

Available for Purchase by Generic Name: USA: Yes   Canada: No

Available Dosage Forms and Strengths
Tablets — 12.5 mg., 25 mg.
Chewable tablets — 25 mg.

Tablet May Be Crushed or Capsule Opened for Administration: Yes

How This Drug Works
Intended Therapeutic Effect(s):   Prevention and management of the nausea, vomiting, and dizziness associated with motion sickness.
Location of Drug Action(s):   The nerve pathways connecting the organ of equilibrium (the labyrinth) in the inner ear with the vomiting center in the brain.
Method of Drug Action(s):   This drug reduces the sensitivity of the nerve endings in the labyrinth and blocks the transmission of excessive nerve impulses to the vomiting center.

Principal Uses of This Drug
As a Single Drug Product: This antihistamine is used primarily to control dizziness and vertigo associated with disorders of the inner ear. It is also used to prevent or relieve the nausea, vomiting, and dizziness characteristic of motion sickness.
As a Combination Drug Product [CD]:   This drug is available (in Canada) in combination with niacin (nicotinic acid) which is added because of its ability to dilate blood vessels and (theoretically) improve circulation.

THIS DRUG SHOULD NOT BE TAKEN IF
—you have had an allergic reaction to any dosage form of it previously.
—you are taking, or have taken during the past 2 weeks, any mono-amine oxidase (MAO) inhibitor drug (see Drug Class, Section Three).
—you are, or think you may be, pregnant.

INFORM YOUR PHYSICIAN BEFORE TAKING THIS DRUG IF
—you have had an unfavorable reaction to any antihistamine in the past.

Time Required for Apparent Benefit
Drug action begins in approximately 1 hour and persists for 12 to 24 hours.

Possible Side-Effects *(natural, expected, and unavoidable drug actions)*
Drowsiness, dryness of nose, mouth, or throat.

Possible Adverse Effects *(unusual, unexpected, and infrequent reactions)*

IF ANY OF THE FOLLOWING DEVELOP, DISCONTINUE DRUG AND NOTIFY
YOUR PHYSICIAN AS SOON AS POSSIBLE

Mild Adverse Effects
Blurring of vision.
Serious Adverse Effects
None reported.

Precautions for Use by Those over 60 Years of Age
You may be more susceptible to the development of drowsiness, dizziness,
and lethargy and to impairment of thinking, judgment, and memory.
This drug may increase the degree of impaired urination associated with
prostate gland enlargment (prostatism).

Advisability of Use During Pregnancy
Pregnancy Category: C (tentative). See Pregnancy Code inside back
cover.
Animal reproduction studies in mice, rats, and ferrets reveal significant
birth defects due to this drug.
Information from studies in pregnant women is inconclusive. No increase
in defects in 1793 exposures. Twelve cleft lips or palates occurred in 3333
exposures. It is advisable to avoid this drug completely during first 3
months.
Ask physician for guidance.

Advisability of Use While Nursing Infant
Safety for infant not established. Ask physician for guidance.

Habit-Forming Potential
None.

Effects of Overdosage
With Moderate Overdose: Marked drowsiness, confusion, incoordination,
unsteady gait, muscle tremors. In children: excitement, hallucinations,
overactivity, convulsions.
With Large Overdose: Stupor progressing to coma, fever, flushed face,
dilated pupils, weak pulse, shallow breathing.

Possible Effects of Extended Use
None reported.

**Suggested Periodic Examinations While Taking This Drug (at physician's
discretion)**
None required.

While Taking This Drug, Observe the Following

Foods: No restrictions. Stomach irritation can be reduced if drug is taken after eating.

Beverages: Coffee and tea may help to reduce the drowsiness caused by most antihistamines.

Alcohol: Use with extreme caution until combined effect has been determined. The combination of alcohol and antihistamines can cause rapid and marked sedation.

Tobacco Smoking: No interactions expected.

Marijuana Smoking

Occasional (once or twice weekly):   Mild increase in drowsiness and dryness of mouth.

Daily: Moderate to marked increase in drowsiness and dryness of mouth; possible accentuation of impaired thinking.

Other Drugs

Meclizine may *increase* the effects of

- sedatives, sleep-inducing drugs, tranquilizers, antidepressants, pain relievers, and narcotic drugs, and result in oversedation. Careful dosage adjustments are necessary.
- atropine and drugs with atropine-like action (see Drug Class, Section Three).

The following drugs may *increase* the effects of meclizine:

- all sedatives, sleep-inducing drugs, tranquilizers, pain relievers, and narcotic drugs may exaggerate its sedative action and cause oversedation.
- mono-amine oxidase (MAO) inhibitor drugs (see Drug Class, Section Three) may delay its elimination from the body, thus exaggerating and prolonging its action.

The following drugs may *decrease* the effects of meclizine:

- amphetamines (Benzedrine, Dexedrine, Desoxyn, etc.) may reduce the drowsiness caused by most antihistamines.

Driving a Vehicle, Operating Machinery, Engaging in Hazardous Activities: This drug may impair mental alertness, judgment, physical coordination, and reaction time. Avoid hazardous activities until response has been determined.

Aviation Note: The use of this drug *is a disqualification* for the piloting of aircraft. Consultation with a designated Aviation Medical Examiner is advised.

Exposure to Sun: No restrictions.

Special Storage Instructions

Keep in a dry, tightly closed container.

MEDROXYPROGESTERONE

Year Introduced: 1959

Brand Names

USA	Canada
Amen (Carnrick)	Provera (Upjohn)
Curretab	
(Reid-Provident)	
Provera (Upjohn)	

Common Synonyms ("Street Names"):   None

Drug Class: Female Sex Hormones (Progestins)

Prescription Required: Yes

Available for Purchase by Generic Name: No

Available Dosage Forms and Strengths
Tablets — 2.5 mg., 10 mg.

Tablet May Be Crushed or Capsule Opened for Administration: Yes

How This Drug Works
Intended Therapeutic Effect(s):   Correction of menstrual disorders due to hormone imbalance. Progesterone and related drugs (progestins) are also used to prevent pregnancy.
Location of Drug Action(s)
The hypothalamus and the pituitary gland in the brain.
The lining of the uterus.
The mucus-producing glands in the neck (cervix) of the uterus.
Method of Drug Action(s)
By inducing and maintaining a lining in the uterus that resembles pregnancy, this drug can prevent uterine bleeding.
By suppressing the release of the pituitary gland hormone that induces ovulation, this drug can prevent ovulation (contraceptive effect).
By stimulating the secretion of mucus (by the uterine cervix) that resists the passage of sperm, this drug increases its contraceptive effect.

Principal Uses of This Drug
As a Single Drug Product: Used primarily to treat the lack of menstruation and abnormal menstrual bleeding associated with "hormone imbalance." The injectable form of this drug is being used to prevent pregnancy.

THIS DRUG SHOULD NOT BE TAKEN IF
—you have had an allergic reaction to any dosage form of it previously.
—you have seriously impaired liver function.
—you have a history of cancer of the breast or genital organs.
—you have a history of thrombophlebitis, embolism, or stroke.
—you have abnormal and unexplained vaginal bleeding.

INFORM YOUR PHYSICIAN BEFORE TAKING THIS DRUG IF
—you have migraine headaches.
—you have epilepsy.
—you have diabetes (or a tendency to diabetes).

Time Required for Apparent Benefit
Improvement in control of abnormal menstrual bleeding may occur in 24 to 48 hours. Long-range benefit requires regular use on a cyclic schedule adjusted to individual needs.

Possible Side-Effects *(natural, expected, and unavoidable drug actions)*
Retention of fluid, gain in weight, changes in menstrual timing and flow, spotting between periods.

Possible Adverse Effects *(unusual, unexpected, and infrequent reactions)*

IF ANY OF THE FOLLOWING DEVELOP, DISCONTINUE DRUG AND NOTIFY YOUR PHYSICIAN AS SOON AS POSSIBLE

Mild Adverse Effects
Allergic Reactions: Skin rashes, hives, itching.
Other Reactions
Breast tenderness and secretion.
Excessive hair growth.

Serious Adverse Effects
Hepatitis with jaundice (see Glossary)—yellow eyes and skin, dark-colored urine, light-colored stools.
Thrombophlebitis (inflammation of a vein with the formation of blood clot) —pain or tenderness in thigh or leg, with or without swelling of the foot, ankle, or leg.
Pulmonary embolism (movement of blood clot to the lung)—sudden shortness of breath, pain in the chest, coughing, bloody sputum.
Stroke (blood clot in the brain)—headaches, blackouts, sudden weakness or paralysis of any part of the body, severe dizziness, double vision, slurred speech, inability to speak.
Retinal thrombosis (blood clot in blood vessels of the eye)—sudden impairment or loss of vision.

Precautions for Use by Those over 60 Years of Age
No diseases or disorders occur after 60 that require the use of this drug.

Advisability of Use During Pregnancy
Pregnancy Category: X (tentative). See Pregnancy Code inside back cover.
Animal reproduction studies in rats and rabbits reveal significant birth defects due to this drug.
Information from studies in pregnant women indicates an estimated 4.7-fold increased risk of limb reduction defects. In addition, this drug can also cause masculinization of the female fetus. Avoid this drug during entire pregnancy.
Ask physician for guidance.

Advisability of Use While Nursing Infant
These drugs are known to be present in milk. Safety for the nursing infant has not been established. Ask physician for guidance.

Habit-Forming Potential
None.

Effects of Overdosage
With Moderate Overdose: Nausea, vomiting, fluid retention, breast enlargement and discomfort, abnormal vaginal bleeding.
With Large Overdose: No serious or dangerous effects reported.

Possible Effects of Extended Use
None reported.

Suggested Periodic Examinations While Taking This Drug (at physician's discretion)
Regular examinations of the breasts and reproductive organs (pelvic examination of the uterus and ovaries, including "Pap" smear).

While Taking This Drug, Observe the Following
Foods: No restrictions. If you experience fluid retention, ask physician for guidance regarding salt intake.
Beverages: No restrictions.
Alcohol: No interactions expected.
Tobacco Smoking: It is advisable to smoke lightly or not at all. Follow physician's advice.
Marijuana Smoking
Occasional (once or twice weekly): No interactions expected.
Daily: Possible menstrual irregularities; increased breakthrough bleeding.
Other Drugs
Medroxyprogesterone may *increase* the effects of
• phenothiazines.

The following drugs may *decrease* the effects of medroxyprogesterone
• antihistamines
• phenobarbital
• phenylbutazone (Azolid, Butazolidin, etc.)

Driving a Vehicle, Operating Machinery, Engaging in Hazardous Activities:
Usually no restrictions. Consult your physician for assessment of individual risk and for guidance regarding specific restrictions.

Aviation Note: The use of this drug *may be a disqualification* for the piloting of aircraft. Consultation with a designated Aviation Medical Examiner is advised.

Exposure to Sun: No restrictions.

Special Storage Instructions
Keep in a dry, tightly closed container. Protect from light.

MEPERIDINE
(Pethidine)

Year Introduced: 1939

Brand Names

USA	Canada
Demerol (Winthrop)	Demerol (Winthrop)
Demerol (APAP)[CD]	Demer-Idine (Sabex)
(Breon)	

Common Synonyms ("Street Names"):   Demies, painkiller, pain reliever

Drug Class: Analgesic, Strong (Synthetic Narcotic)

Prescription Required: Yes (Controlled Drug, U.S. Schedule II)*

Available for Purchase by Generic Name: Yes

Available Dosage Forms and Strengths
    Tablets — 50 mg., 100 mg.
        Syrup — 50 mg. per teaspoonful (5 ml.)
    Injection — 25 mg., 50 mg., 75 mg., 100 mg. per ml.

Tablet May Be Crushed or Capsule Opened for Administration: Yes

How This Drug Works
    Intended Therapeutic Effect(s):   Relief of moderate to severe pain.
    Location of Drug Action(s):   Those areas of the brain and spinal cord involved in the perception of pain.
    Method of Drug Action(s):   Not completely established. It has been suggested that the resulting increase of chemicals that transmit nerve impulses somehow contributes to the analgesic effect of this drug.

Principal Uses of This Drug
    As a Single Drug Product: This potent analgesic is used by mouth or injection to relieve moderate to severe pain.
    As a Combination Drug Product [CD]:   This drug is available in combination with acetaminophen (APAP) to create a dosage form that utilizes two pain relievers, one of which also reduces fever.

THIS DRUG SHOULD NOT BE TAKEN IF
—you have had an allergic reaction to any dosage form of it previously.
—you are taking now, or have taken within the past 14 days, any mono-amine oxidase (MAO) inhibitor drug (see Drug Class, Section Three).

INFORM YOUR PHYSICIAN BEFORE TAKING THIS DRUG IF
—you are taking sedatives, sleep-inducing drugs, tranquilizers, antidepressants, or narcotic drugs of any kind.
—you plan to have surgery under general anesthesia in the near future.

*See Schedules of Controlled Drugs inside back cover.

—you are subject to attacks of asthma.
—you have epilepsy.
—you have impaired liver or kidney function.
—you are being treated for glaucoma.

Time Required for Apparent Benefit
Usually from 15 minutes to 1 hour when taken orally.

Possible Side-Effects *(natural, expected, and unavoidable drug actions)*
Drowsiness, lightheadedness, weakness, euphoria, dryness of the mouth, constipation.

Possible Adverse Effects *(unusual, unexpected, and infrequent reactions)*

IF ANY OF THE FOLLOWING DEVELOP, DISCONTINUE DRUG AND NOTIFY YOUR PHYSICIAN AS SOON AS POSSIBLE

Mild Adverse Effects
Allergic Reactions: Skin rash, hives, itching.
Other Reactions
  Headache, dizziness, visual disturbances, agitation.
  Nausea, vomiting.
  Flushing of face, sweating, heart palpitation, faintness.

Serious Adverse Effects
Drop in blood pressure, causing severe weakness and fainting.
Disorientation, hallucinations, unstable gait, tremor, muscle twitching.
Interference with urination.

Precautions for Use by Those over 60 Years of Age
You may be more sensitive to all of the actions of this drug. Small doses are advisable until your individual response has been determined.
You may be more susceptible to the development of nausea, lightheadedness, dizziness, faintness, unsteadiness, falling, constipation, and inability to urinate (urinary retention).

Advisability of Use During Pregnancy
Pregnancy Category: C (tentative). See Pregnancy Code inside back cover.
  Animal reproduction studies in hamsters reveal significant birth defects due to this drug.
  Information from studies in pregnant women indicates no significant increase in defects in 1100 exposures to this drug.
  Ask physician for guidance.

Advisability of Use While Nursing Infant
Drug is known to be present in milk. Ask physician for guidance.

Habit-Forming Potential
This drug can produce psychological and physical dependence (see Glossary).

Effects of Overdosage
With Moderate Overdose: Marked drowsiness, confusion, tremors, convulsions, extreme weakness.

With Large Overdose: Stupor progressing to coma, cold and clammy skin, slow and shallow breathing.

Possible Effects of Extended Use
Psychological and physical dependence.

Suggested Periodic Examinations While Taking This Drug (at physician's discretion)
None.

While Taking This Drug, Observe the Following
Foods: No restrictions.

Beverages: No restrictions.

Alcohol: Use with extreme caution until combined effects have been determined. Alcohol can greatly increase the sedative effect of meperidine as well as its depressant action on breathing, heart function, and circulation.

Tobacco Smoking: No interactions expected.

Marijuana Smoking

Occasional (once or twice weekly):   Mild and transient increase in drowsiness and relief of pain.

Daily: Significant increase in drowsiness, relief of pain, and impairment of mental and physical performance.

Other Drugs

Meperidine/pethidine may *increase* the effects of

- all other sedatives, sleep-inducing drugs, tranquilizers, antidepressants, and narcotic drugs. Appropriate dosage adjustments are mandatory. Ask physician for guidance.

Meperidine/pethidine may *decrease* the effects of

- eye drops prescribed for the treatment of glaucoma. Ask physician for guidance regarding dosage adjustment.

Meperidine/pethidine *taken concurrently* with

- mono-amine oxidase (MAO) inhibitor drugs (see Drug Class, Section Three), can cause the equivalent of acute narcotic overdose—unconsciousness, severe depression of breathing, heart action, and circulation. A variation of this reaction can be excitability, convulsions, high fever, and rapid heart action.
- anti-hypertensive (anti-high blood pressure) drugs (see Drug Class, Section Three), may cause excessive lowering of the blood pressure and result in severe dizziness and fainting.

The following drugs may *increase* the effects of meperidine/pethidine

- mild and strong tranquilizers, especially the phenothiazines (see respective Drug Classes, Section Three).
- antidepressants may enhance the unfavorable effect of meperidine on glaucoma.
- nitrates (see Drug Class, Section Three) and nitrites used to treat angina and coronary heart disease can enhance the blood pressure-lowering effect of meperidine.

Driving a Vehicle, Operating Machinery, Engaging in Hazardous Activities: This drug can impair mental alertness, judgment, reaction time, and physical coordination. Avoid hazardous activities.

Aviation Note: The use of this drug *is a disqualification* for the piloting of aircraft. Consultation with a designated Aviation Medical Examiner is advised.

Exposure to Sun: No restrictions.

Discontinuation: If used for an extended period of time, ask physician for guidance regarding dosage reduction and withdrawal.

Special Storage Instructions

Keep in a dry, tightly closed container.

MEPROBAMATE

Year Introduced: 1955

Brand Names

USA		Canada
Arcoban (Arcum)	Tranmep	Apo-Meprobamate
Bamate (Century)	(Reid-Provident)	(Apotex)
Coprobate (Coastal)	Deprol [CD]	Equanil (Wyeth)
Equanil (Wyeth)	(Wallace)	Meditran (Medic)
Meprocon (CMC)	Equagesic [CD]	Meprospan-400
Meprospan (Wallace)	(Wyeth)	(Horner)
Miltown (Wallace)	Milprem [CD]	Miltown (Horner)
Pax 400 (Kenyon)	(Wallace)	Neo-Tran (Neolab)
Robamate (Robinson)	Miltrate [CD]	Novomepro
Saronil (Saron)	(Wallace)	(Novopharm)
SK-Bamate (Smith	PMB [CD] (Ayerst)	
Kline & French)		

Common Synonyms ("Street Names"):   Downs, nerve pills, tranks

Drug Class: Tranquilizer, Mild (Anti-anxiety)

Prescription Required: Yes (Controlled Drug, U.S. Schedule IV)*

Available for Purchase by Generic Name: Yes

Available Dosage Forms and Strengths

Tablets — 200 mg., 400 mg., 600 mg.

Capsules — 400 mg.

Sustained-release capsules — 200 mg., 400 mg.

*See Schedules of Controlled Drugs inside back cover.

Tablet May Be Crushed or Capsule Opened for Administration
> Regular tablets — Yes
> Sustained-release capsules — No

How This Drug Works
Intended Therapeutic Effect(s)
> Relief of mild to moderate anxiety and tension (sedative effect).
> Relief of insomnia due to anxiety and tension (hypnotic effect).

Location of Drug Action(s):   Not completely established. It is thought that this drug acts on multiple sites in the brain, including the thalamus and limbic systems.

Method of Drug Action(s):   Not known.

Principal Uses of This Drug
As a Single Drug Product: This mildly sedative drug is used primarily for the short-term symptomatic relief of anxiety and nervous tension. It is also used at bedtime to relieve recurring insomnia. Although not officially approved as a muscle relaxant, it is sometimes used in conjunction with other measures to treat skeletal muscle spasm.

As a Combination Drug Product [CD]:   This drug is used in combination with several other types of drugs in order to utilize its mild tranquilizer effect. Combined with benactyzine, a mild antidepressant, it is used to treat acute and chronic depressions of mild to moderate severity. Combined with aspirin, it is used to treat the discomfort of musculo-skeletal injury. Combined with estrogens, it is used for symptomatic relief in treating the menopausal syndrome. Combined with pentaerythritol tetranitrate, an anti-anginal drug, it is used in the management of coronary artery disease.

THIS DRUG SHOULD NOT BE TAKEN IF
—you have had an allergic reaction to any dosage form of it previously.
—you are allergic or sensitive to any chemically related drugs: carbromal, carisoprodol, tybamate (see Drug Profiles for brand names).
—you have a history of intermittent porphyria.
—it is prescribed for a child under 6 years of age.

INFORM YOUR PHYSICIAN BEFORE TAKING THIS DRUG IF
—you have epilepsy.
—you have impaired liver or kidney function.
—you are taking sedatives, sleep-inducing drugs, tranquilizers, antidepressants, or anti-convulsants.

Time Required for Apparent Benefit
Approximately 1 to 2 hours. For severe symptoms of some duration, benefit may require regular medication for several days.

Possible Side-Effects *(natural, expected, and unavoidable drug actions)*
Drowsiness, lethargy, unsteadiness in stance and gait.

Possible Adverse Effects *(unusual, unexpected, and infrequent reactions)*

IF ANY OF THE FOLLOWING DEVELOP, DISCONTINUE DRUG AND NOTIFY YOUR PHYSICIAN AS SOON AS POSSIBLE

Mild Adverse Effects

Allergic Reactions: Skin rashes (various kinds), swelling of hands or feet, swelling of glands, low-grade fever.

Other Reactions: Dizziness, slurred speech, headache, blurred vision, nausea, diarrhea, heart palpitation, fainting.

Serious Adverse Effects

Allergic Reactions: Anaphylactic reaction (see Glossary), high fever, asthmatic breathing, reduced urine formation, unusual bruising or bleeding.

Paradoxical Reactions: Excitement, overactivity.

Other Reactions

Bone marrow depression (see Glossary)—fatigue, weakness, impaired resistance to infection, fever, sore throat, unusual bleeding.

Sudden drop in blood pressure, which may be hazardous in those with heart disease and impaired circulation.

Precautions for Use by Infants and Children

Safety and effectiveness in children below the age of 6 years have not been established.

Precautions for Use by Those over 60 Years of Age

Natural changes in body functions increase the duration of this drug's action. It is necessary to use smaller doses with longer intervals between doses to avoid excessive accumulation of the drug in body tissues. Dosage must be carefully individualized and limited to the smallest effective amount.

You may be more susceptible to the development of lightheadedness, impaired thinking and memory, confusion, lethargy, drowsiness, incoordination, unsteady gait and balance, impaired bladder control, and constipation.

Be alert to the possibility of paradoxical responses consisting of excitement, agitation, anger, hostility, and rage.

Advisability of Use During Pregnancy

Pregnancy Category: C (tentative). See Pregnancy Code inside back cover.

Animal reproduction studies in mice reveal significant birth defects due to this drug.

Information from studies in pregnant women is conflicting.

Ask physician for guidance.

The findings of some recent studies suggest a possible association between the use of this drug during early pregnancy and the occurrence of birth defects, such as cleft lip. It is advisable to avoid this drug completely during the first 3 months of pregnancy.

Advisability of Use While Nursing Infant

Drug is known to be present in milk. Avoid use if possible. Ask physician for guidance.

Habit-Forming Potential

This drug can produce psychological and/or physical dependence (see Glossary) if used in large doses for an extended period of time.

Effects of Overdosage

With Moderate Overdose: Dizziness, slurred speech, impaired stance, staggering gait.

With Large Overdose: Stupor progressing to deep sleep and coma; depression of breathing and heart function.

Possible Effects of Extended Use

Psychological and/or physical dependence.
Impairment of blood cell production.

Suggested Periodic Examinations While Taking This Drug (at physician's discretion)

Complete blood cell counts during long-term use.

While Taking This Drug, Observe the Following

Foods: No restrictions.

Beverages: Large intake of coffee, tea, or cola drinks (because of their caffeine content) may reduce the calming action of this drug.

Alcohol: Use with extreme caution until combined effect is determined. Alcohol can increase the sedative effects of meprobamate. The combination can cause serious depression of vital brain functions.

Tobacco Smoking: No interactions expected.

Marijuana Smoking

Occasional (once or twice weekly):   Mild increase in sedative effect of this drug.

Daily: Marked increase in sedative effect of this drug.

Other Drugs

Meprobamate may *increase* the effects of

• other sedatives, sleep-inducing drugs, tranquilizers, antidepressants, and narcotic drugs, resulting in oversedation.

Meprobamate may *decrease* the effects of

• oral anticoagulants, making it necessary to increase their dosage to maintain their intended action.
• estrogens used in the treatment of menopause, by hastening their destruction and elimination.
• oral contraceptives, by hastening their destruction and elimination.

Meprobamate *taken concurrently* with

• anti-convulsants, may cause a change in the pattern of seizures, making it necessary to adjust the dosage of the anti-convulsant. Observe closely to determine combined effect of the two drugs.

The following drugs may *increase* the effects of meprobamate

• mono-amine oxidase (MAO) inhibitor drugs (see Drug Class, Section Three) can increase the sedative and brain-depressant effects of meprobamate. Ask physician for guidance regarding dosage adjustment.

Driving a Vehicle, Operating Machinery, Engaging in Hazardous Activities:
This drug can impair mental alertness, judgment, physical coordination,
and reaction time. Avoid hazardous activities.

Aviation Note: The use of this drug *is a disqualification* for the piloting of
aircraft. Consultation with a designated Aviation Medical Examiner is advised.

Exposure to Sun: No restrictions.

Discontinuation: If it has been necessary to use this drug for an extended
period of time, ask physician for guidance regarding reduction of dose and
withdrawal. The dosage of other drugs taken concurrently with meprobamate may also require adjustment.

Special Storage Instructions
Keep in a dry, tightly closed container.

MESORIDAZINE

Year Introduced: 1970

Brand Names

USA	Canada
Serentil (Boehringer Ingleheim)	Serentil (Sandoz)

Common Synonyms ("Street Names"): None

Drug Class: Tranquilizer, Strong (Anti-psychotic), Phenothiazines

Prescription Required: Yes

Available for Purchase by Generic Name: No

Available Dosage Forms and Strengths
Tablets — 10 mg., 25 mg., 50 mg., 100 mg.
Concentrate — 25 mg. per ml.
Injection — 25 mg. per ml.

Tablet May Be Crushed or Capsule Opened for Administration: Yes

How This Drug Works
Intended Therapeutic Effect(s): Restoration of emotional calm. Relief of
severe anxiety, agitation, and psychotic behavior.

Location of Drug Action(s): Those nerve pathways in the brain that utilize
the tissue chemical dopamine for the transmission of nerve impulses.

Method of Drug Action(s): Not completely established. Present theory is
that by inhibiting the action of dopamine, this drug acts to correct an
imbalance of nerve impulse transmissions that is thought to be responsible
for certain mental disorders.

Principal Uses of This Drug
As a Single Drug Product: This major tranquilizer is used to treat the thought disorder, abnormal behavior, anxiety and agitation associated with schizophrenia, brain damage, acute and chronic alcoholism, and certain personality disorders.

THIS DRUG SHOULD NOT BE TAKEN IF
—you have had an allergic reaction to any dosage form of it previously.
—it is prescribed for a child under 12 years of age.

INFORM YOUR PHYSICIAN BEFORE TAKING THIS DRUG IF
—you are allergic or sensitive to any phenothiazine drug (see Drug Class, Section Three).
—you are taking any sedatives, sleep-inducing drugs, other tranquilizers, antidepressants, antihistamines, or narcotic drugs of any kind.
—you have epilepsy.
—you have a history of heart disease.
—you plan to have surgery under general or spinal anesthesia in the near future.

Time Required for Apparent Benefit
Some benefit usually apparent in first week. Maximal benefit may require regular dosage for several weeks.

Possible Side-Effects *(natural, expected, and unavoidable drug actions)*
Drowsiness, lethargy, blurred vision, nasal stuffiness, dryness of the mouth, constipation, impaired urination.

Possible Adverse Effects *(unusual, unexpected, and infrequent reactions)*

IF ANY OF THE FOLLOWING DEVELOP, DISCONTINUE DRUG AND NOTIFY YOUR PHYSICIAN AS SOON AS POSSIBLE

Mild Adverse Effects
Allergic Reactions: Skin rashes (various kinds), hives, swelling of the salivary glands, fever.
Other Reactions
Headache, lightheadedness, and faintness in upright position (see orthostatic hypotension in Glossary).
Confusion, agitation, restlessness.
Breast congestion, milk formation, menstrual irregularity.
Nausea, vomiting, loss of appetite.
Serious Adverse Effects
Allergic Reactions: Hepatitis with jaundice (see Glossary), very rare with this drug.
Other Reactions
Bone marrow depression (see Glossary), usually mild.
Convulsions.
Parkinson-like disorders (see Glossary), less frequent than with other phenothiazines.

CAUTION
1. Many over-the-counter (OTC) medications (see Glossary) for allergies, colds, and coughs contain drugs that can interact unfavorably with this drug. Ask your physician or pharmacist for guidance before using any such medications.
2. Antacids that contain aluminum and/or magnesium can prevent the absorption of this drug and reduce its effectiveness.
3. Obtain prompt evaluation of any disturbance or change in vision.

Precautions for Use by Those over 60 Years of Age
You may be more sensitive to all of the actions of this drug. Small doses are advisable until your individual response has been determined.

You may be more susceptible to the development of drowsiness, lethargy, constipation, lowering of body temperature (hypothermia), and excessive drop in blood pressure on arising from a lying or sitting position (see orthostatic hypotension in Glossary).

This drug can increase the degree of impaired urination associated with prostate gland enlargement (prostatism).

You may also be more susceptible to the development of Parkinson-like disorders and/or tardive dyskinesia (see discussion of these terms in Glossary). These conditions must be recognized early since they may become unresponsive to treatment and irreversible. Consult your physician promptly if suggestive symptoms develop.

Advisability of Use During Pregnancy
Pregnancy Category: B (tentative). See Pregnancy Code inside back cover. Animal reproduction studies in rats reveal no birth defects due to this drug.

Information from adequate studies in pregnant women is not available. Ask physician for guidance.

Advisability of Use While Nursing Infant
Safety not established. Ask physician for guidance.

Habit-Forming Potential
None.

Effects of Overdosage
With Moderate Overdose: Marked drowsiness, confusion, disorientation, blurred vision, nasal congestion, marked dryness of mouth, weakness.

With Large Overdose: Deep sleep, coma, convulsions, drop in body temperature, shallow breathing.

Possible Effects of Extended Use
Tardive dyskinesia (see Glossary).

Discoloration (pigmentation) of the skin and/or surface structures of the eye.

Opacities in the cornea or lens of the eye, resembling cataracts.

Suggested Periodic Examinations While Taking This Drug (at physician's dicretion)

Complete eye examinations for changes in vision and pigment deposits in the retina.

Complete blood cell counts and liver function tests.

Periodic electrocardiograms.

Periodic examinations of the tongue for the appearance of fine, involuntary, wave-like movements that could indicate the development of tardive dyskinesia.

While Taking This Drug, Observe the Following

Foods: No restrictions.

Beverages: No restrictions.

Alcohol: Use extreme caution until combined effects have been determined. Alcohol can increase the sedative action of mesoridazine and accentuate its depressant effects on brain function. Mesoridazine may increase the intoxicating effects of alcohol.

Tobacco Smoking: No interactions expected.

Marijuana Smoking

Occasional (once or twice weekly):   No effect to mild and transient increase in drowsiness and accentuation of orthostatic hypotension (see Glossary); some risk of precipitating latent psychoses (in predisposed individuals).

Daily: Moderate increase in drowsiness, significant accentuation of orthostatic hypotension; increased risk of precipitating latent psychoses, confusing interpretation of mental status and of drug responses.

Other Drugs

Mesoridazine may *increase* the effects of

• all sedatives, sleep-inducing drugs, other tranquilizers, antidepressants, antihistamines, and narcotic drugs, and produce oversedation. Ask physician for guidance regarding dosage adjustments.

• all drugs containing atropine or having atropine-like actions (see Drug Class, Section Three).

Mesoridazine may *decrease* the effects of

• levodopa (Dopar, Larodopa, etc.), and reduce its effectiveness in the treatment of Parkinson's disease (shaking palsy).

• appetite suppressant drugs (Pre-Sate, Preludin, Benzedrine, Dexedrine, etc.).

Mesoridazine *taken concurrently* with

• quinidine may impair heart function. Avoid the use of these two drugs at the same time.

The following drugs may *increase* the effects of mesoridazine

• tricyclic antidepressants (see Drug Class, Section Three)

Driving a Vehicle, Operating Machinery, Engaging in Hazardous Activities: This drug can impair mental alertness, judgment, and physical coordination. Avoid hazardous activities.

Aviation Note: The use of this drug *is a disqualification* for the piloting of aircraft. Consultation with a designated Aviation Medical Examiner is advised.

Exposure to Sun: Use caution until sensitivity has been determined. This drug may produce photosensitivity (see Glossary).

Exposure to Heat: Use caution and avoid excessive heat. This drug may impair the regulation of body temperature and increase the risk of heat stroke.

Heavy Exercise or Exertion: Use caution and follow your physician's instructions if you have any form of heart disease.

Discontinuation: If it has been necessary to use this drug for an extended period of time, do not discontinue it suddenly. Ask physician for guidance regarding dosage reduction and withdrawal. Upon discontinuation of this drug, it may also be necessary to adjust the dosages of other drugs taken concurrently with it.

Special Storage Instructions
Store liquid concentrate in a tightly closed, amber glass container, at temperatures below 86° F. (30°C.).

METAPROTERENOL
(Orciprenaline)

Year Introduced: 1964

Brand Names

USA	Canada
Alupent (Boehringer Ingleheim)	Alupent (Boehringer)
Metaprel (Dorsey)	

Common Synonyms ("Street Names"): Asthma medicine

Drug Class: Anti-asthmatic, Bronchodilator

Prescription Required: USA: Yes   Canada: Yes

Available for Purchase by Generic Name: USA: No   Canada: No

Available Dosage Forms and Strengths
Powder for Inhalation — 0.65 mg. per inhalation
Solution for Nebulization — 5%
Syrup — 10 mg. per teaspoonful (5 ml.)
Tablets — 10 mg., 20 mg.

Tablet May Be Crushed or Capsule Opened for Administration: No

How This Drug Works

Intended Therapeutic Effect(s):   Relief of difficult breathing associated with acute attacks of bronchial asthma.

Location of Drug Action(s):   Those nerve terminals of the sympathetic nervous system that activate the muscles in the walls of bronchial tubes to produce dilation.

Method of Drug Action(s):   By stimulating certain sympathetic nerve terminals, this drug acts to dilate those bronchial tubes that are in sustained constriction, thereby increasing the size of the airway and improving the ability to breathe.

Principal Uses of This Drug

As a Single Drug Product: Used primarily to treat those conditions of difficult breathing that are due to reversible bronchospasm: asthma, bronchitis, emphysema.

THIS DRUG SHOULD NOT BE TAKEN IF

—you have had an allergic reaction to any dosage form of it previously.

—you have a serious heart rhythm disorder.

—you are taking, or have taken during the last 2 weeks, any mono-amine oxidase (MAO) inhibitor drug (see Drug Class, Section Three).

INFORM YOUR PHYSICIAN BEFORE TAKING THIS DRUG IF

—you are overly sensitive to other drugs that stimulate the sympathetic nervous system.

—you are currently using epinephrine (Adrenalin) to relieve asthmatic breathing.

—you have a history of any form of heart disease, especially angina and heart rhythm disorders.

—you have high blood pressure, diabetes, or an overactive thyroid gland (hyperthyroidism).

—you are taking any form of digitalis.

Time Required for Apparent Benefit

When administered by aerosol inhalation, drug action begins within 1 minute, reaches its peak in 1 hour, and persists for 1 to 5 hours.

When administered in the form of syrup or tablet, drug action begins in 15 minutes, reaches its peak in 1 hour, and persists for up to 4 hours.

Possible Side-Effects *(natural, expected, and unavoidable drug actions)*

Nervousness, heart palpitation, bad taste.

Possible Adverse Effects *(unusual, unexpected, and infrequent reactions)*

IF ANY OF THE FOLLOWING DEVELOP, DISCONTINUE DRUG AND NOTIFY YOUR PHYSICIAN AS SOON AS POSSIBLE

Mild Adverse Effects

Headache, dizziness, weakness, tremor.

Rapid, pounding heart beat, increased sweating, muscle cramps in arms and legs.

Nausea, vomiting.

Serious Adverse Effects

Intensification of angina in the presence of coronary artery disease. Mild elevation of blood sugar levels.

Natural Diseases or Disorders That May Be Activated By This Drug

Latent coronary artery insufficiency.

CAUTION

1. *Avoid excessive use of the aerosol inhalation.* Prolonged use can produce tolerance that requires more frequent use of larger doses to obtain relief. The accumulative effects of excessive dosage can cause cardiac arrest.
2. Do not use this drug concurrently with epinephrine (Adrenalin). These two drugs may be used alternately if an interval of 4 hours is allowed between doses.
3. If you do not respond to your usually effective dose, ask your physician for guidance. Do not increase the size or frequency of the dose without his or her approval.

Precautions for Use by Infants and Children

Dosage, safety, and effectiveness in children under 6 years of age have not been established.

Precautions for Use by Those over 60 Years of Age

You may be more sensitive to the stimulant effects of this drug. Small doses are advisable until your individual response has been determined.

If you have hardening of the arteries (arteriosclerosis), heart disease, or high blood pressure, use this drug with caution. It can precipitate episodes of angina and disturbances of heart rhythm; if used excessively, it can cause sudden elevation of blood pressure and induce stroke.

Advisability of Use During Pregnancy

Pregnancy Category: C (tentative). See Pregnancy Code inside back cover. Animal reproduction studies in rabbits reveal significant birth defects due to this drug.

Information from adequate studies in pregnant women is not available. Avoid this drug during the first 3 months.

Use only if clearly necessary. Ask physician for guidance.

Advisability of Use While Nursing Infant

The presence of this drug in human milk is not known. Avoid drug or refrain from nursing infant.

Habit-Forming Potential

None.

Effects of Overdosage

With Moderate Overdose: Excessive nervousness, heart palpitation, rapid heart rate, sweating.

With Large Overdose: Headache, tremor, chest pain, irregular heart rhythm, marked drop in blood pressure, circulatory failure.

Possible Effects of Extended Use
Development of tolerance. See CAUTION category above.

Suggested Periodic Examinations While Taking This Drug (at physician's discretion)
Heart function, blood pressure measurements.

While Taking This Drug, Observe the Following
Foods: No restrictions.

Beverages: No restrictions. Avoid excessive use of caffeine drinks if prone to nervousness.

Alcohol: No interactions expected.

Tobacco Smoking: No interactions expected. Follow your physician's advice regarding smoking as it affects the condition under treatment.

Marijuana Smoking

Occasional (once or twice weekly): Possible mild and transient improvement in the anti-asthmatic effect of this drug.

Daily: More persistent improvement in the anti-asthmatic effect of this drug.

Other Drugs
Metaproterenol may *increase* the effects of
- ephedrine, and cause excessive stimulation of the heart and an increase in blood pressure.

Metaproterenol *taken concurrently* with
- epinephrine (Adrenalin) may cause serious disturbances of heart rhythm. Allow an interval of at least 4 hours between the use of these two drugs.

The following drugs may *decrease* the effects of metaproterenol
- propranolol (Inderal), and other beta-blocker drugs (see Drug Class, Section Three).

Driving a Vehicle, Operating Machinery, Engaging in Hazardous Activities: Usually no restrictions. Use caution if excessive nervousness or dizziness occurs.

Aviation Note: The use of this drug *is a disqualification* for the piloting of aircraft. Consultation with a designated Aviation Medical Examiner is advised.

Exposure to Sun: No restrictions.

Discontinuation: If this drug fails to provide relief after a reasonable trial, discontinue it and consult your physician regarding alternative drug therapy. Do not increase the dose or the frequency of use beyond the instructions you were given.

Special Storage Instructions
Keep all forms of this drug in airtight, nonmetallic containers at room temperature. Protect from light.

METHADONE

Year Introduced: 1948

Brand Names

USA	Canada
Dolophine (Lilly)	None

Common Synonyms ("Street Names"):   Dollies, meth, painkiller, pain reliever

Drug Class: Analgesic, Strong (Synthetic Narcotic)

Prescription Required: Yes (Controlled Drug, U.S. Schedule II)*

Available for Purchase by Generic Name: Yes

Available Dosage Forms and Strengths

Tablets — 5 mg., 10 mg.
Effervescent tablets — 2.5 mg., 5 mg., 10 mg., 40 mg.
Oral solution — 1 mg. per 1 ml., 2 mg. per 1 ml. (8% alcohol)
Injection — 10 mg. per ml.

Tablet May Be Crushed or Capsule Opened for Administration: Yes

How This Drug Works

Intended Therapeutic Effect(s):   Relief of moderate to severe pain.

Location of Drug Action(s):   Those areas of the brain and spinal cord involved in the perception of pain.

Method of Drug Action(s):   Not completely established. It has been suggested that the resulting increase of chemicals that transmit nerve impulses somehow contributes to the analgesic effect of this drug.

Principal Uses of This Drug

As a Single Drug Product: This potent narcotic analgesic is used to relieve moderate to severe pain. However, its primary use today is to provide an appropriate substitute for heroin in treatment programs for drug addiction.

THIS DRUG SHOULD NOT BE TAKEN IF
—you have had an allergic reaction to any dosage form of it previously.

INFORM YOUR PHYSICIAN BEFORE TAKING THIS DRUG IF
—you are taking now, or have taken within the past 14 days, any mono-amine oxidase (MAO) inhibitor drug (see Drug Class, Section Three).
—you are taking sedatives, sleep-inducing drugs, tranquilizers, antidepressants, or other narcotic drugs of any kind.
—you plan to have surgery under general anesthesia in the near future.
—you are subject to attacks of asthma.
—you have impaired liver or kidney function.

*See Schedules of Controlled Drugs inside back cover.

Time Required for Apparent Benefit
Usually 30 minutes to 1 hour when taken orally.

Possible Side-Effects *(natural, expected, and unavoidable drug actions)*
Drowsiness, lightheadedness, weakness, euphoria, dryness of the mouth, constipation.

Possible Adverse Effects *(unusual, unexpected, and infrequent reactions)*

IF ANY OF THE FOLLOWING DEVELOP, DISCONTINUE DRUG AND NOTIFY
YOUR PHYSICIAN AS SOON AS POSSIBLE

Mild Adverse Effects
Allergic Reactions: Skin rash, hives, itching.
Other Reactions
Headache, dizziness, visual disturbances, agitation.
Nausea, vomiting.
Flushing of face, sweating, heart palpitation, faintness.
Serious Adverse Effects
Drop in blood pressure, causing severe weakness and fainting.
Disorientation, hallucinations, unstable gait, tremor, muscle twitching.
Interference with urination.

Precautions for Use by Those over 60 Years of Age
You may be more sensitive to all of the actions of this drug. Small doses are advisable until your individual response has been determined.
You may be more susceptible to the development of nausea, lightheadedness, dizziness, faintness, unsteadiness, falling, constipation, and inability to urinate (urinary retention).

Advisability of Use During Pregnancy
Pregnancy Category: C (tentative). See Pregnancy Code inside back cover.
Animal reproduction studies in mice and hamsters reveal significant birth defects due to this drug.
Information from adequate studies in pregnant women is not available.
It is advisable to avoid this drug during first 3 months if possible.
Ask physician for guidance.

Advisability of Use While Nursing Infant
Drug is known to be present in milk. Avoid use if possible. Ask physician for guidance.

Habit-Forming Potential
This drug can produce psychological and physical dependence (see Glossary).

Effects of Overdosage
With Moderate Overdose: Marked drowsiness, confusion, tremors, convulsions, extreme weakness.
With Large Overdose: Stupor progressing to coma, cold and clammy skin, slow and shallow breathing.

Possible Effects of Extended Use
Psychological and physical dependence.

Suggested Periodic Examinations While Taking This Drug (at physician's discretion)
None required.

While Taking This Drug, Observe the Following
Foods: No restrictions.

Beverages: No restrictions.

Alcohol: Use with extreme caution until combined effects have been determined. Alcohol can greatly increase the sedative effect of methadone as well as its depressant effect on breathing, heart function, and circulation.

Tobacco Smoking: No interactions expected.

Marijuana Smoking
Occasional (once or twice weekly):   Mild and transient increase in drowsiness and relief of pain.
Daily: Significant increase in drowsiness, relief of pain, and impairment of mental and physical performance.

Other Drugs
Methadone may *increase* the effects of
- all other sedatives, sleep-inducing drugs, tranquilizers, antidepressants, and narcotic drugs. Appropriate dosage adjustments are mandatory. Ask physician for guidance.

Methadone *taken concurrently* with
- pentazocine, may result in withdrawal symptoms if the methadone is being used as maintenance treatment for narcotic addiction.
- anti-hypertensive (anti-high blood pressure) drugs (see Drug Class, Section Three) may cause excessive lowering of blood pressure and result in severe dizziness and fainting.

The following drugs may *increase* the effects of methadone
- isoniazid (INH, etc.)
- mild and strong tranquilizers, especially the phenothiazines (see respective Drug Classes, Section Three)

The following drugs may *decrease* the effects of methadone
- cyproheptadine (Periactin) may interfere with its analgesic action.
- methysergide (Sansert) may interfere with its analgesic action.
- phenytoin (Dilantin, etc.) may hasten its elimination and cause withdrawal symptoms.

Driving a Vehicle, Operating Machinery, Engaging in Hazardous Activities:
This drug can impair mental alertness, judgment, reaction time, and physical coordination. Avoid hazardous activities.

Aviation Note: The use of this drug *is a disqualification* for the piloting of aircraft. Consultation with a designated Aviation Medical Examiner is advised.

Exposure to Sun: No restrictions.

Discontinuation: If used for an extended period of time, do not discontinue abruptly. Ask physician for guidance regarding dosage reduction and withdrawal.

Special Storage Instructions
Keep in a dry, tightly closed container.

METHOCARBAMOL

Year Introduced: 1957

Brand Names

USA	Canada
Robaxin (Robins)	Robaxin (Robins)
Robaxin-750 (Robins)	Robaxin-750 (Robins)
Robaxisal [CD] (Robins)	Robaxisal [CD] (Robins)
	Robaxisal-C [CD] (Robins)

Common Synonyms ("Street Names"):   For methocarbamol: None
For codeine (an ingredient of Robaxisal-C):   Robo, schoolboy, syrup
For phenobarbital (an ingredient of Robaxisal-PH):   Barbs, candy, goofballs, peanuts, phennies, purple hearts, sleepers, stoppers, stumblers

Drug Class: Muscle Relaxant

Prescription Required: USA: Yes   Canada: For Robaxin and Robaxisal
—No
For Robaxisal-C—Yes

Available for Purchase by Generic Name: USA: Yes   Canada: No

Available Dosage Forms and Strengths
Tablets — 500 mg., 750 mg.
Injection — 100 mg. per ml.

Tablet May Be Crushed or Capsule Opened for Administration: Yes

How This Drug Works
Intended Therapeutic Effect(s):   Relief of discomfort resulting from painful spasm of voluntary muscles.
Location of Drug Action(s):   Not completely established. This drug is thought to act on those nerve pathways in the brain and spinal cord that are involved in the reflex activity of voluntary muscles.
Method of Drug Action(s):   Not completely established. It is thought that this drug may relieve muscle spasm and pain by blocking the transmission of nerve impulses over reflex pathways in the spinal cord and/or by producing a sedative effect that decreases the perception of pain.

Principal Uses of This Drug

As a Single Drug Product: Used in conjunction with other treatment methods to provide relief from discomfort associated with acute, painful musculo-skeletal conditions of any nature.

As a Combination Drug Product [CD]:   This drug is available in combination with aspirin (in the USA), and with aspirin and codeine (in Canada). Aspirin and codeine are added to provide greater relief of pain.

THIS DRUG SHOULD NOT BE TAKEN IF

—you have had an allergic reaction to any dosage form of it previously.

INFORM YOUR PHYSICIAN BEFORE TAKING THIS DRUG IF

—you have experienced any unfavorable reactions to muscle relaxant drugs in the past.
—you have epilepsy.
—you have myasthenia gravis.
—you have impaired kidney function.
Note: This drug should not be given by injection if kidney function is impaired.

Time Required for Apparent Benefit

Drug action begins in 30 to 45 minutes and reaches a maximal effect in 1 to 3 hours.

Possible Side-Effects *(natural, expected, and unavoidable drug actions)*

Lightheadedness, lethargy, drowsiness.
Brown, black, green, or blue discoloration of the urine (if allowed to stand), of no significance.

Possible Adverse Effects *(Unusual, unexpected, and infrequent reactions)*

IF ANY OF THE FOLLOWING DEVELOP, DISCONTINUE DRUG AND NOTIFY YOUR PHYSICIAN AS SOON AS POSSIBLE

Mild Adverse Effects
Allergic Reactions: Skin rash, hives, itching, eye irritation, nasal congestion, fever.
Other Reactions: Headache, dizziness, blurred vision, weakness, unsteady stance and gait, flushing.
Serious Adverse Effects
Allergic Reactions: Anaphylactic reaction (see Glossary), reduced white blood cells.

CAUTION

All muscle relaxants cause some degree of sedation. Use caution if other sedatives, tranquilizers, or pain relievers are taken concurrently with this drug.

Precautions for Use by Those over 60 Years of Age

It is advisable to use small doses initially until individual tolerance and response have been determined. The impairment of thought processes, understanding, memory, and physical coordination that may accompany aging may be intensified by doses recommended for younger adults.

Advisability of Use During Pregnancy

Pregnancy Category: C (tentative). See Pregnancy Code inside back cover.

Animal reproduction studies. No data available.

Information from adequate studies in pregnant women is not available. Ask physician for guidance.

Advisability of Use While Nursing Infant

This drug is present in milk in small amounts. Ask physician for guidance.

Habit-Forming Potential

None.

Effects of Overdosage

With Moderate Overdose: Nausea, vomiting, heartburn, abdominal pain, constipation or diarrhea, unsteady gait, impaired coordination.

With Large Overdose: Extreme weakness, generalized paralysis, weak and rapid pulse, shallow breathing, cold and sweaty skin.

Possible Effects of Extended Use

None reported.

Suggested Periodic Examinations While Taking This Drug (at physician's discretion)

White blood cell counts.

While Taking This Drug, Observe the Following

Foods: No specific food restrictions. This drug may be taken with or following food.

Beverages: No restrictions. This drug may be taken with milk.

Alcohol: Use with caution until the combined effect has been determined. This drug may add to the depressant effect of alcohol on the brain.

Tobacco Smoking: No interactions expected.

Marijuana Smoking

Occasional (once or twice weekly):   No effect to mild and transient increase in drowsiness, muscle weakness, and orthostatic hypotension (see Glossary).

Daily: Moderate to marked drowsiness, muscle weakness, and incoordination, and significant accentuation of orthostatic hypotension.

Other Drugs

Methocarbamol may *increase* the effects of

• sedatives, sleep-inducing drugs, tranquilizers, pain relievers and narcotic drugs, and cause excessive sedation.

Methocarbamol may *decrease* the effects of
- pyridostigmine (Mestinon, Regonol), and reduce its effectiveness in treating myasthenia gravis.

Driving a Vehicle, Operating Machinery, Engaging in Hazardous Activities: This drug may cause drowsiness, lightheadedness, dizziness, and impaired coordination in susceptible individuals. Avoid hazardous activities if these drug effects occur.

Aviation Note: The use of this drug *is a disqualification* for the piloting of aircraft. Consultation with a designated Aviation Medical Examiner is advised.

Exposure to Sun: No restrictions.

Heavy Exercise or Exertion: Ask physician for guidance.

Occurrence of Unrelated Illness: If you require medical care by a physician other than the one who prescribed this drug, inform him/her that you are taking methocarbamol.

Discontinuation: This drug may be used in conjunction with rest, physiotherapy, and other treatment techniques. To obtain maximal benefit, do not discontinue it until advised to do so by your physician.

Special Storage Instructions
Keep in a dry, tightly closed container.

METHOTREXATE

Note: This is an Abbreviated Drug Profile of a very potent anti-cancer drug that is used primarily in the management of severe, unresponsive psoriasis and in the treatment of certain types of cancer. Because of its potential for causing serious, life-threatening adverse effects, its use should be supervised by a physician who is experienced and skilled in using this class of drugs. It is mandatory that indications of possible toxic effects be recognized and evaluated promptly and that appropriate measures be taken without delay.

Year Introduced: 1948

Brand Names

USA	Canada
Methotrexate (Lederle)	Methotrexate (Lederle)
Mexate (Bristol)	

Common Synonyms ("Street Names"):   MTX, Psoriasis pills

Drug Class: Anti-psoriasis, Anti-cancer (Antineoplastic), Folic Acid Derivative

Prescription Required: USA: Yes   Canada: Yes

Available Dosage Forms and Strengths
Tablets — 2.5 mg.

Tablet May Be Crushed or Capsule Opened for Administration: Yes

How This Drug Works
Intended Therapeutic Effect(s)
1. The symptomatic control of severe, generalized, and disabling psoriasis.
2. The control of certain types of cancer.

Location of Drug Action(s):   The rapidly multiplying cells of the skin, the bone marrow, and the membranes lining the mouth, intestinal tract, and urinary bladder; also the cells of the developing fetus, and cancerous cells.

Method of Drug Action(s):   By interfering with the normal utilization of folic acid in tissue-cell reproduction, this drug retards abnormally rapid tissue growth (as in psoriasis and cancer).

Principal Uses of This Drug
As a Single Drug Product: This drug is used primarily to treat (1) severe and widespread forms of disabling psoriasis that have failed to respond to all standard treatment procedures; (2) various types of both childhood and adult cancer. In addition, it is used to prevent rejection of transplanted bone marrow. More recently, it is being used experimentally in the treatment of connective tissue disorders such as rheumatoid arthritis, scleroderma, and related conditions.

THIS DRUG SHOULD NOT BE TAKEN IF
—you have had an allergic reaction to any form of it previously.
—you have severely impaired liver or kidney function.
—you have any impairment of bone marrow function (blood cell production).
—you are pregnant and intending to use this drug to treat psoriasis.

INFORM YOUR PHYSICIAN BEFORE TAKING THIS DRUG IF
—you have a history of bone marrow impairment of any nature, especially drug-induced bone marrow depression.
—you have a history of gout, peptic ulcer disease, or ulcerative colitis.
—you have a history of liver or kidney disease.
—you have a chronic infection of any kind.

Possible Side-Effects *(natural, expected, and unavoidable drug actions)*
The following are due to the pharmacological actions of this drug. **Report such developments to your physician promptly.**
Sores on the lips, in the mouth or throat, vomiting, intestinal cramping, diarrhea (may be bloody), painful urination, bloody urine.
Reduced resistance to infection, fatigue, weakness, fever, unusual bleeding or bruising.

Possible Adverse Effects *(unusual, unexpected, and infrequent reactions)*

IF ANY OF THE FOLLOWING DEVELOP, DISCONTINUE DRUG AND NOTIFY
YOUR PHYSICIAN AS SOON AS POSSIBLE

Mild Adverse Effects
   Allergic Reactions: Skin rash, hives, itching.
   Other Reactions:
      Headache, drowsiness, blurred vision.
      Loss of hair, loss of skin pigmentation, acne.
      Altered menstrual pattern.
Serious Adverse Effects
   Speech disturbances, paralysis, convulsions.
   Liver toxicity with jaundice (see Glossary).
   Cough, chest pain, shortness of breath (drug-induced pneumonia).
   Reduced urine volume (kidney failure).

CAUTION
1. This drug has a high potential for toxicity. Its use must be monitored carefully and continuously by a physician who is skilled in its proper administration.
2. Appropriate laboratory studies, before and during the use of this drug, are mandatory. Consult your physician.
3. Women with potential for pregnancy should have a pregnancy test before taking this drug, and should use an effective form of contraception during its use and for 8 weeks following its discontinuation.

Advisability of Use During Pregnancy
   Pregnancy Category: D (tentative). See Pregnancy Code inside back cover.
      This drug is known to cause fetal death and birth defects. Its use during pregnancy to treat psoriasis cannot be justified. If its use during pregnancy is deemed necessary to treat a type of cancer, it should be avoided during the first 3 months if possible.

Advisability of Use While Nursing Infant
   This drug is present in breast milk. Refrain from nursing.

Suggested Periodic Examinations While Taking This Drug (at physician's discretion)
   Complete blood cell counts.
   Liver and kidney function tests.
   Blood uric acid levels.
   Chest X-Ray.

While Taking This Drug, Observe the Following
   Foods: Avoid highly seasoned foods that could be irritating. May be taken with or following food to reduce stomach irritation.
   Beverages: Drink at least 3 pints of liquids daily.
      This drug may be taken with milk.
   Alcohol: Avoid completely.

Other Drugs
Methotrexate may *increase* the effects of
• oral anticoagulants (Coumadin, etc.) and cause abnormal bleeding. Monitor prothrombin times carefully.

Methotrexate may *decrease* the effects of
• anti-gout drugs (Benemid, Zyloprim) by raising the blood level of uric acid.

The following drugs may *increase* the effects of methotrexate and enhance its toxicity:
• aspirin and other salicylates.
• chloramphenicol (Chloromycetin).
• phenylbutazone (Butazolidin).
• phenytoin (Dilantin).
• probenecid (Benemid).
• sulfonamides ("sulfa" drugs) (see Drug Class, Section Three).
• tetracyclines (see Drug Class, Section Three).

Driving a Vehicle, Operating Machinery, Engaging in Hazardous Activities: Use caution. If this drug causes drowsiness, dizziness, blurring of vision, or severe abdominal distress, avoid hazardous activities.

Exposure to Sun: Use caution until skin sensitivity has been determined. This drug may cause photosensitivity. Avoid ultraviolet lamps.

METHYCLOTHIAZIDE

Year Introduced: 1960

Brand Names

USA		Canada
Aquatensen (Wallace)	Enduronyl [CD]	Duretic (Abbott)
Enduron (Abbott)	(Abbott)	
Diutensen [CD]	Enduronyl Forte	
(Wallace)	[CD] (Abbott)	
Diutensen-R [CD]		
(Wallace)		

Common Synonyms ("Street Names"):   Water pills

Drug Class: Anti-hypertensive (Hypotensive), Diuretic, Thiazides

Prescription Required: Yes

Available for Purchase by Generic Name: No

Available Dosage Forms and Strengths
Tablets — 2.5 mg., 5 mg.

Tablet May Be Crushed or Capsule Opened for Administration: Yes

How This Drug Works
Intended Therapeutic Effect(s)
Elimination of excessive fluid retention (edema).
Reduction of high blood pressure.
Location of Drug Action(s):   Principal actions occur in
- the tubular systems of the kidney that determine the final composition of the urine.
- the walls of the smaller arteries.

Method of Drug Action(s)
By increasing the elimination of salt and water from the body (through increased urine production), this drug reduces the volume of fluid in the blood and body tissues and lowers the sodium content throughout the body.
By relaxing the walls of the smaller arteries and allowing them to expand, this drug significantly increases the total capacity of the arterial system. The combined effect of these two actions (reduced blood volume in expanded space) results in lowering of the blood pressure.

Principal Uses of This Drug
As a Single Drug Product: This member of the "thiazide" class is used primarily as a mild diuretic and to initiate treatment ("step 1") for mild to moderate high blood pressure.
As a Combination Drug Product [CD]:   It is available in combination with cryptenamine, another anti-hypertensive drug with a different method of action. It is also available in combination with reserpine and with deserpidine, two closely related anti-hypertensive drugs that utilize yet another method for lowering blood pressure. The combinations of two drugs are usually more effective than either drug used alone.

THIS DRUG SHOULD NOT BE TAKEN IF
—you have had an allergic reaction to any dosage form of it previously. A combination drug [CD] should not be taken if you are allergic to *any* of its ingredients.

INFORM YOUR PHYSICIAN BEFORE TAKING THIS DRUG IF
—you are allergic to any form of "sulfa" drug.
—you are pregnant and your physician does not know it.
—you have a history of kidney disease or liver disease, or impaired kidney or liver function.
—you have diabetes (or a tendency to diabetes).
—you have a history of gout.
—you have a history of lupus erythematosus.
—you are taking any form of cortisone, digitalis, oral anti-diabetic drugs, or insulin.
—you plan to have surgery under general anesthesia in the near future.

Time Required for Apparent Benefit

Increased urine volume begins in 2 hours, reaches a maximum in 6 hours, and subsides in 24 hours. Continuous use on a regular schedule will be necessary for 2 to 3 weeks to determine this drug's effectiveness in lowering your blood pressure.

Possible Side-Effects *(natural, expected, and unavoidable drug actions)*

Lightheadedness on arising from sitting or lying position (see orthostatic hypotension in Glossary).

Increase in level of blood sugar, affecting control of diabetes.

Increase in level of blood uric acid, affecting control of gout.

Decrease in level of blood potassium, resulting in muscle weakness and cramping.

Possible Adverse Effects *(unusual, unexpected, and infrequent reactions)*

IF ANY OF THE FOLLOWING DEVELOP, DISCONTINUE DRUG AND NOTIFY YOUR PHYSICIAN AS SOON AS POSSIBLE

Mild Adverse Effects

Allergic Reactions: Skin rashes (various kinds), hives, drug fever.
Other Reactions
Reduced appetite, indigestion, nausea, vomiting, diarrhea.
Headache, dizziness, yellow vision, blurred vision.

Serious Adverse Effects

Allergic Reactions
Hepatitis with jaundice (see Glossary).
Anaphylactic reaction (see Glossary). Severe skin reactions.
Other Reactions
Inflammation of the pancreas—severe abdominal pain.
Bone marrow depression (see Glossary)—fatigue, weakness, fever, sore throat, unusual bleeding or bruising.

CAUTION

1. Do not exceed recommended doses. Increased dosage can cause excessive excretion of sodium and potassium with resultant loss of appetite, nausea, fatigue, weakness, confusion, and tingling in the extremities.
2. If you are also taking a digitalis preparation (digitoxin, digoxin), ensure an adequate intake of high-potassium foods to prevent potassium deficiency —a potential cause of digitalis toxicity.

Precautions for Use by Those over 60 Years of Age

You may be more sensitive to the actions of this drug. Small doses are advisable until your individual response has been determined.

You may be more susceptible to the development of impaired thinking, orthostatic hypotension, potassium loss, and elevation of blood sugar, complicating the management of diabetes.

If you are taking this drug to treat high blood pressure, remember that warm weather and fever can reduce your blood pressure and make it necessary to adjust your dosage.

Overdosage and extended use of this drug can cause excessive loss of body water, thickening (increased viscosity) of the blood, and an increased tendency of the blood to clot, predisposing to stroke, heart attack, or thrombophlebitis.

Advisability of Use During Pregnancy
Pregnancy Category: C (tentative). See Pregnancy Code inside back cover.
Animal reproduction studies. No data available.
Information from adequate studies in pregnant women is not available.
Ask physician for guidance.
This drug should not be used during pregnancy unless a very serious complication of pregnancy occurs for which this drug is significantly beneficial. This type of diuretic can have adverse effects on the fetus.

Advisability of Use While Nursing Infant
This drug is known to be present in milk. Ask physician for guidance.

Habit-Forming Potential
None.

Effects of Overdosage
With Moderate Overdose: Dryness of mouth, thirst, lethargy, weakness, dizziness, muscle pain and cramping, nausea, vomiting.
With Large Overdose: Drowsiness progressing to stupor and coma, weak and rapid pulse.

Possible Effects of Extended Use
Impaired balance of water, salt, and potassium in blood and body tissues.
Development of diabetes (in predisposed individuals).

Suggested Periodic Examinations While Taking This Drug (at physician's discretion)
Complete blood cell counts.
Measurement of blood levels of sodium, potassium, chloride, sugar, and uric acid.
Liver function tests.
Kidney function tests.

While Taking This Drug, Observe the Following
Foods: It is recommended that you include in your daily diet liberal servings of foods rich in potassium (unless directed otherwise by your physician). The following foods have a high potassium content:

All-bran cereals	Coconut
Almonds	Coffee
Apricots (dried)	Crackers (rye)
Bananas, fresh	Dates and figs (dried)
Beans (navy and lima)	Fish, fresh
Beef	Lentils
Carrots (raw)	Liver, beef
Chicken	Lonalac
Citrus fruits, juices	Milk

Peaches (dried)	Potato, sweet
Peanut butter	Prunes (dried), juice
Peas	Raisins
Pork	Tomato juice

Note: Avoid licorice in large amounts while taking this drug. Follow your physician's instructions regarding the use of salt.

Beverages: No restrictions unless directed by your physician.

Alcohol: Use with caution until the combined effect has been determined. Alcohol can exaggerate the blood pressure-lowering effect of this drug and cause orthostatic hypotension.

Tobacco Smoking: No interactions expected. Follow your physician's advice regarding smoking.

Marijuana Smoking

Occasional (once or twice weekly):   No effect to mild increase in thirst and/or urinary frequency.

Daily: Moderate increase in thirst and/or urinary frequency; possible accentuation of orthostatic hypotension (see Glossary).

Other Drugs

Methyclothiazide may *increase* the effects of

- other anti-hypertensive drugs. Careful adjustment of dosages is necessary to prevent excessive lowering of the blood pressure.
- drugs of the phenothiazine drug family, and cause excessive lowering of the blood pressure. (The thiazide and related drugs and the phenothiazines both may cause orthostatic hypotension).

Methyclothiazide may *decrease* the effects of

- the oral anti-diabetic drugs and insulin, by raising the level of blood sugar. Careful adjustment of dosages is necessary to maintain proper control of diabetes.
- allopurinol (Zyloprim), by raising the level of blood uric acid. Careful adjustment of dosages is required to maintain proper control of gout.
- probenecid (Benemid), by raising the level of blood uric acid. Careful dosage adjustment is necessary to maintain control of gout.

Methyclothiazide *taken concurrently* with

- cortisone and cortisone-related drugs, may cause excessive loss of potassium from the body.
- digitalis and related drugs, requires very careful monitoring and dosage adjustments to prevent serious disturbances of heart rhythm.
- tricyclic antidepressants (Elavil, Sinequan, etc.), may cause excessive lowering of the blood pressure.

The following drugs may *increase* the effects of methyclothiazide

- the barbiturates may exaggerate its blood pressure-lowering action.
- the mono-amine oxidase (MAO) inhibitor drugs may increase urine volume by delaying this drug's elimination from the body.
- the pain relievers (analgesics), both narcotic and non-narcotic, may exaggerate its blood pressure-lowering action.

The following drug may *decrease* the effects of methyclothiazide
• cholestyramine (Cuemid, Questran) may interfere with its absorption. Take cholestyramine 30 to 60 minutes before any oral diuretic.

Driving a Vehicle, Operating Machinery, Engaging in Hazardous Activities: Use caution until the possibility of orthostatic hypotension or impaired vision has been determined.

Aviation Note: The use of this drug *may be a disqualification* for the piloting of aircraft. Consultation with a designated Aviation Medical Examiner is advised.

Exposure to Sun: Use caution until sensitivity has been determined. This drug may cause photosensitivity (see Glossary).

Exposure to Heat: Avoid excessive perspiring which could cause additional loss of water and salt from the body.

Heavy Exercise or Exertion: Avoid exertion that produces lightheadedness, excessive fatigue, or muscle cramping. Isometric exercises—the "overload" technique for strengthening individual muscles—can raise the blood pressure significantly. Ask your physician for guidance regarding participation in this form of exercise.

Occurrence of Unrelated Illness: Illnesses which cause vomiting or diarrhea can produce a serious imbalance of important body chemistry. Discontinue this drug and ask your physician for guidance.

Discontinuation: It may be advisable to discontinue this drug approximately 5 to 7 days before major surgery. Ask your physician, surgeon, and/oranesthesiologist for guidance regarding dosage reduction or withdrawal.

Special Storage Instructions
Keep in a dry, tightly closed container.

METHYLDOPA

Year Introduced: 1963

Brand Names

USA		Canada
Aldomet (Merck Sharp & Dohme)	Aldoril D30 [CD] (Merck Sharp & Dohme)	Apo-Methyldopa (Apotex)
Aldoclor [CD] (Merck Sharp & Dohme)	Aldoril D50 [CD] (Merck Sharp & Dohme)	Aldomet (MSD)
Aldoril-15 [CD] (Merck Sharp & Dohme)		Dopamet (ICN)
		Medimet-250 (Medic)
		Melopa (Riva)
Aldoril-25 [CD] (Merck Sharp & Dohme)		Novomedopa (Novopharm)
		Aldoril [CD] (MSD)
		Novodoparil [CD] (Novopharm)

Common Synonyms ("Street Names"):   Blood pressure pills

Drug Class: Anti-hypertensive (Hypotensive)

Prescription Required: Yes

Available for Purchase by Generic Name: USA: No   Canada: Yes

Available Dosage Forms and Strengths
> Tablets — 125 mg., 250 mg., 500 mg.
Oral suspension — 250 mg. per teaspoonful (5 ml.)

Tablet May Be Crushed or Capsule Opened for Administration: Yes

How This Drug Works
> **Intended Therapeutic Effect(s):**   Reduction of high blood pressure.
> **Location of Drug Action(s):**   The vasomotor center in the brain that influences the control of the sympathetic nervous system over blood vessels (principally arterioles) throughout the body.
> **Method of Drug Action(s):**   By decreasing the activity of the vasomotor center, this drug reduces the ability of the sympathetic nervous system to maintain the degree of blood vessel constriction responsible for elevation of the blood pressure. This change results in relaxation of blood vessel walls and lowering of the blood pressure.

Principal Uses of This Drug
> **As a Single Drug Product:**   This anti-hypertensive drug is used as a "step 2" medication in conjunction with other anti-hypertensive drugs in the treatment of moderate to severe high blood pressure.

As a Combination Drug Product [CD]: This drug is available in combination with chlorothiazide and with hydrochlorothiazide, mild diuretics that represent "step 1" anti-hypertensive drugs. Combinations of "step 1" and "step 2" drugs are more effective and more convenient for long-term use.

THIS DRUG SHOULD NOT BE TAKEN IF
—you have had an allergic reaction to any dosage form of it previously.
—you have active liver disease.
—you have a mild and uncomplicated case of hypertension.

INFORM YOUR PHYSICIAN BEFORE TAKING THIS DRUG IF
—you have a history of liver disease or impaired liver function.
—you are taking any tricyclic antidepressant (Elavil, Tofranil, Sinequan, etc.; see Drug Class, Section Three).
—you are taking any mono-amine oxidase (MAO) inhibitor drug (Eutonyl, Marplan, Nardil, Niamid, etc.; see Drug Class, Section Three).
—you plan to have surgery under general anesthesia in the near future.

Time Required for Apparent Benefit
Continuous use with periodic dosage adjustment for 2 to 4 weeks may be necessary to determine this drug's effectiveness in controlling high blood pressure.

Possible Side-Effects (*natural, expected, and unavoidable drug actions*)
Drowsiness, lethargy, weakness, which may occur during first few weeks and then subside.
Lightheadedness in upright position (see orthostatic hypotension in Glossary).
Nasal stuffiness, dryness of the mouth.

Possible Adverse Effects (*unusual, unexpected, and infrequent reactions*)

IF ANY OF THE FOLLOWING DEVELOP, DISCONTINUE DRUG AND NOTIFY YOUR PHYSICIAN AS SOON AS POSSIBLE

Mild Adverse Effects
Allergic Reactions: Skin rash, joint and muscle discomfort, malaise, fever.
Other Reactions
Headache, dizziness.
Nausea, vomiting, irritation of tongue, diarrhea.
Water retention and weight gain.
Breast enlargement, milk production, impaired sex drive and performance.
Serious Adverse Effects
Allergic Reactions: Hepatitis with jaundice (see Glossary).
Idiosyncratic Reactions: Episodes of high fever (not due to infection)—1% of users.
Other Reactions
Bone marrow depression (see Glossary)—fatigue, weakness, fever, sore throat, unusual bleeding or bruising.
Inflammation of the pancreas—abdominal pain, fever, nausea, vomiting.

Parkinson-like disorders (see Glossary).
Behavioral changes—confusion, depression, nightmares.

CAUTION
1. Hot weather and the fever associated with infection can reduce the blood pressure significantly, requiring adjustment of dosage.
2. Report the development of any tendency to emotional depression.

Precautions for Use by Those over 60 Years of Age
The basic rule in treating high blood pressure after 60 is to proceed *cautiously.* The elevated systolic blood pressure often present after 60 is not necessarily a threat to health, and can serve as an adaptive and compensatory change with age that should not be altered drastically. The goals of treatment must be adjusted to the natural changes in body function that occur with aging. Unacceptably high blood pressure should be reduced without creating the risks associated with excessively low blood pressure.

It is advisable to start treatment with small doses and to monitor the blood pressure response frequently. Sudden, rapid, and excessive reduction of blood pressure can predispose to stroke or heart attack.

You may be more susceptible to the development of orthostatic hypotension with resultant lightheadedness, dizziness, unsteadiness, fainting, and falling. Report such symptoms to your physician promptly.

This drug can produce parkinsonism or intensify existing parkinsonism in the elderly. Report such effects promptly.

Advisability of Use During Pregnancy
Pregnancy Category: B (tentative). See Pregnancy Code inside back cover.
Animal reproduction studies in mice, rats, and rabbits reveal no birth defects due to this drug.
Information from adequate studies in pregnant women is not available.
Ask physician for guidance.

Advisability of Use While Nursing Infant
This drug's presence in milk is not known. Ask physician for guidance.

Habit-Forming Potential
None.

Effects of Overdosage
With Moderate Overdose: Marked drowsiness, weakness, sense of exhaustion, orthostatic hypotension.
With Large Overdose: Stupor, confusion, slow and weak pulse.

Possible Effects of Extended Use
Development of hemolytic anemia (see Glossary).
Retention of salt and water with gain in weight.

Suggested Periodic Examinations While Taking This Drug (at physician's discretion)
Complete blood cell counts.
Coombs' test of red blood cells.
Liver function tests.

While Taking This Drug, Observe the Following

Foods: Ask physician for guidance regarding intake of salt.

Beverages: Drink enough water to satisfy thirst and prevent constipation.

Alcohol: Use with extreme caution until combined effect has been determined. Alcohol can exaggerate this drug's sedative effect and can add to its ability to lower the blood pressure. Excessive drop in blood pressure may result from this combination.

Tobacco Smoking: Follow your physician's advice regarding the use of tobacco. Nicotine can raise the blood pressure in sensitive individuals.

Marijuana Smoking

Occasional (once or twice weekly):   No effect to mild and transient accentuation of orthostatic hypotension (see Glossary).

Daily: Significant accentuation of orthostatic hypotension, requiring dosage adjustment in sensitive individuals.

Other Drugs

Methyldopa may *increase* the effects of

- oral anticoagulants, and cause bleeding or hemorrhage. Careful dosage adjustments are necessary.
- other anti-hypertensive drugs. Careful dosage adjustments are necessary to prevent excessive drop in blood pressure.

Methyldopa may *decrease* the effects of

- levodopa (L-Dopa, Larodopa, Dopar, etc.), and reduce its effectiveness in treating Parkinson's disease.

Methyldopa *taken concurrently* with

- tricyclic antidepressants (Elavil, Tofranil, Sinequan, etc.) may cause dangerous elevation of the blood pressure. Avoid combined use.
- mono-amine oxidase (MAO) inhibitor drugs (Eutonyl, Marplan, Nardil, Niamid, etc.) may cause dangerous elevation of the blood pressure. Avoid combined use.
- digoxin (Lanoxin, etc.) may cause excessive slowing of the heart rate.

The following drugs may *increase* the effects of methyldopa

- thiazide diuretics usually enhance its blood pressure-lowering action.

The following drugs may *decrease* the effects of methyldopa

- amphetamines (Benzedrine, Dexedrine, Desoxyn, etc.) can reduce its effectiveness in lowering blood pressure.

Driving a Vehicle, Operating Machinery, Engaging in Hazardous Activities: Avoid hazardous activities until the early manifestations of drowsiness and lethargy have subsided. Be alert to the occurrence of orthostatic hypotension.

Aviation Note: The use of this drug and the disorder for which this drug is prescribed *may be disqualifications* for the piloting of aircraft. Consultation with a designated Aviation Medical Examiner is advised.

Exposure to Sun: No restrictions.

Heavy Exercise or Exertion: Use caution. Excessive physical activity may increase the possibility of orthostatic hypotension. Isometric exercises—the "overload" technique for strengthening individual muscles—can raise the blood pressure significantly. The use of this drug may intensify the hypertensive response to isometric exercises. Ask your physician for guidance.

Discontinuation: Consult physician for guidance regarding the need to readjust the dosage schedule of other drugs taken concurrently with methyldopa, such as anticoagulants and other anti-hypertensives.

Special Storage Instructions
Keep in a dry, tightly closed container.

METHYLPHENIDATE

Year Introduced: 1956

Brand Names

USA	Canada
Ritalin (CIBA)	Ritalin (CIBA)
Ritalin-SR (CIBA)	

Common Synonyms ("Street Names"): Uppers (when used by adults); nerve calmers (when used by the hyperkinetic child)

Drug Class: Stimulant, Amphetamine-like Drug

Prescription Required: Yes (Controlled Drug, U.S. Schedule II)*

Available for Purchase by Generic Name: USA: Yes   Canada: No

Available Dosage Forms and Strengths
Tablets — 5 mg., 10 mg., 20 mg.
Tablets, prolonged action — 20 mg.

Tablet May Be Crushed or Capsule Opened for Administration: Yes

How This Drug Works
Intended Therapeutic Effect(s)
Improvement of mood, confidence, initiative, and performance in states of fatigue and depression.
Reduction of restlessness, distractability, and impulsive behavior characteristic of the abnormally hyperactive child (as seen with minimal brain damage).

*See Schedules of Controlled Drugs inside back cover.

Location of Drug Action(s):   Areas within the outer layer (cortex) of the brain that are responsible for higher mental functions and behavioral reactions.

Method of Drug Action(s):   Not established. Present thinking is that this drug may increase the release of the nerve impulse transmitter, norepinephrine. The resulting stimulation of brain tissue improves alertness and concentration, and increases learning ability and attention span. (The primary action that calms the overactive child is not known.)

Principal Uses of This Drug

As a Single Drug Product: This drug is used primarily to treat (1) narcolepsy, recurrent spells of uncontrollable drowsiness and sleep; and (2) attention deficit disorders, formerly known as the hyperactive child syndrome, minimal brain damage, and minimal brain dysfunction. Additional uses include the treatment of mild to moderate depression, and the management of apathetic and withdrawal states in the elderly.

THIS DRUG SHOULD NOT BE TAKEN IF

—you are allergic to either of the drugs bearing the brand names listed above.

—you have glaucoma.

—you are experiencing a period of severe anxiety, nervous tension, or emotional depression.

—it has been prescribed for a child under 6 years of age.

INFORM YOUR PHYSICIAN BEFORE TAKING THIS DRUG IF

—you have epilepsy.

—you have high blood pressure.

—you are taking any mono-amine oxidase (MAO) inhibitor drug (see Drug Class, Section Three).

Time Required for Apparent Benefit

It is advisable to start with low dosage and increase gradually. Continuous use, with dosage adjustments, may be needed for a full month to determine this drug's effectiveness.

Possible Side-Effects *(natural, expected, and unavoidable drug actions)*

Nervousness, insomnia.

Possible Adverse Effects *(unusual, unexpected, and infrequent reactions)*

IF ANY OF THE FOLLOWING DEVELOP, DISCONTINUE DRUG AND NOTIFY YOUR PHYSICIAN AS SOON AS POSSIBLE

Mild Adverse Effects

Allergic Reactions: Skin rash, hives, drug fever, joint pains.

Other Reactions

Reduced appetite, nausea, abdominal discomfort.

Headache, dizziness, drowsiness.

Rapid and forceful heart palpitation.

Serious Adverse Effects

Allergic Reactions: Severe skin reactions, extensive bruising due to destruction of blood platelets (see Glossary).

Idiosyncratic Reactions: Abnormal patterns of behavior.
Other Reactions: Abnormally low red blood cells and white blood cells.

CAUTION
Careful dosage adjustments on an individual basis are essential. In a paradoxical reaction (see Glossary), aggravation of symptoms may occur.

Precautions for Use by Those over 60 Years of Age
You may be more sensitive to the stimulant effects of this drug. Small doses are advisable until your individual response has been determined.

You may be more susceptible to the development of nervousness, agitation, insomnia, high blood pressure, disturbance of heart rhythm, or angina.

Advisability of Use During Pregnancy
Pregnancy Category: B (tentative). See Pregnancy Code inside back cover. Animal reproduction studies in mice reveal no birth defects due to this drug.

Information from adequate studies in pregnant women is not available. Ask physician for guidance.

Advisability of Use While Nursing Infant
The presence of this drug in milk is not known. Safety for infant not established. Ask physician for guidance.

Habit-Forming Potential
This drug can produce tolerance and psychological dependence, a potentially dangerous characteristic of amphetamine-like drugs (see Drug Family, Section Three). Avoid excessive dosage and long-term use if possible.

Effects of Overdosage
With Moderate Overdose: Vomiting, agitation, tremors, muscle twitching, headache, sweating, dryness of the mouth.

With Large Overdose: High fever, rapid and irregular pulse, confusion, hallucinations, convulsions, coma.

Possible Effects of Extended Use
Suppression of growth (in weight and/or height) has been reported in children. Monitor growth carefully during long-term use of this drug.

Suggested Periodic Examinations While Taking This Drug (at physician's discretion)
Measurement of blood pressure on a regular basis to detect any tendency to abnormal elevation.

Complete blood cell counts.

While Taking This Drug, Observe the Following
Foods: Avoid foods rich in tyramine (see Glossary). This drug in combination with tyramine may cause excessive rise in blood pressure.

Beverages: Avoid beverages prepared from meat or yeast extracts; avoid chocolate drinks.

Alcohol: Avoid beer, Chianti wines and vermouth.

Tobacco Smoking: No interactions expected.

Marijuana Smoking

Occasional (once or twice weekly):   Mild and transient increased heart rate; mild reduction of stimulant effect and appetite suppressant effect of this drug.

Daily: Persistent rapid heart rate; possible heart rhythm disturbance (in sensitive individuals); significant reduction of stimulant effect of this drug.

Other Drugs

Methylphenidate may *increase* the effects of

- oral anticoagulants of the coumarin family.
- anti-convulsants such as phenobarbital, phenytoin, and primidone.
- phenylbutazone (Azolid, Butazolidin, etc.).
- tricyclic antidepressants.
- atropine-like drugs.

(Consult appropriate Drug Class, Section Three, to see if you are taking any drugs that may require reduction in dosage.)

Methylphenidate may *decrease* the effects of

- guanethidine (Ismelin), and reduce its ability to lower blood pressure.

Methylphenidate *taken concurrently* with

- anti-convulsants, may cause a significant change in the pattern of epileptic seizures. Dosage adjustments may be necessary for proper control.
- mono-amine oxidase (MAO) inhibitor drugs (see Drug Class, Section Three), may cause a dangerous rise in blood pressure. The simultaneous use of these two drugs should be avoided.

Driving a Vehicle, Operating Machinery, Engaging in Hazardous Activities: Usually no restrictions. Use caution if drowsiness or dizziness occurs.

Aviation Note: The use of this drug *is a disqualification* for the piloting of aircraft. Consultation with a designated Aviation Medical Examiner is advised

Exposure to Sun: No restrictions.

Discontinuation: If it has been necessary to use this drug for an extended period of time, do not discontinue it abruptly. Careful supervision is necessary during withdrawal to prevent severe depression and erratic behavior.

Special Storage Instructions

Keep in a dry, tightly closed container.

METHYLPREDNISOLONE

Year Introduced: 1957

Brand Names

USA	**Canada**
Medrol (Upjohn)	Medrol (Upjohn)

Common Synonyms ("Street Names"):   Cortisone medicine

Drug Class: Cortisone-like Drug, Adrenocortical Steroids

Prescription Required: Yes

Available for Purchase by Generic Name: USA: Yes   Canada: No

Available Dosage Forms and Strengths

Tablets — 2 mg., 4 mg., 8 mg., 16 mg., 24 mg., 32 mg.
Enema suspension — 40 mg.
Ointment — 0.25%, 1%

Tablet May Be Crushed or Capsule Opened for Administration: Yes

How This Drug Works

Intended Therapeutic Effect(s):   The symptomatic relief of inflammation (swelling, redness, heat and pain) in any tissue, and from many causes. (Cortisone-like drugs do not correct the underlying disease process.)

Location of Drug Action(s):   Significant biological effects occur in most tissues throughout the body. The principal actions of therapeutic doses occur at sites of inflammation and/or allergic reaction, regardless of the nature of the causative injury or illness.

Method of Drug Action(s):   Not completely established. Present thinking is that cortisone-like drugs probably inhibit several mechanisms within the tissues that induce inflammation. Well-regulated dosage aids the body in restoring normal stability. However, prolonged use or excessive dosage can impair the body's defense mechanisms against infectious disease.

Principal Uses of This Drug

As a Single Drug Product: This member of the cortisone class of drugs is used to treat a wide variety of allergic and inflammatory conditions. It is used primarily in the management of serious skin disorders, bronchial asthma, regional enteritis and ulcerative colitis, and all types of major rheumatic disorders including most forms of arthritis, bursitis, tendinitis, and related conditions.

THIS DRUG SHOULD NOT BE TAKEN IF

—you have had an allergic reaction to any dosage form of it previously.
—you have an active peptic ulcer (stomach or duodenum).

INFORM YOUR PHYSICIAN BEFORE TAKING THIS DRUG IF

—you have had an unfavorable reaction to any cortisone-like drug in the past.
—you have a history of tuberculosis.
—you have diabetes or a tendency to diabetes.

—you have a history of peptic ulcer disease.
—you have glaucoma or a tendency to glaucoma.
—you have a deficiency of thyroid function (hypothyroidism).
—you have high blood pressure.
—you have myasthenia gravis.
—you have a history of thrombophlebitis.
—you plan to have surgery of any kind in the near future, especially if under general anesthesia.

Time Required for Apparent Benefit

Evidence of beneficial drug action is usually apparent in 24 to 48 hours. Dosage must be individualized to give reasonable improvement; this is usually accomplished in 4 to 10 days. It is unwise to demand complete relief of all symptoms. The effective dose varies with the nature of the disease and with the patient. During long-term use it is essential that the smallest effective dose be determined and maintained.

Possible Side-Effects *(natural, expected, and unavoidable drug actions)*

The retention of salt and water (common with some cortisone-like drugs) is less likely to occur with this drug. Increased susceptibility to infection may occur.

Possible Adverse Effects *(unusual, unexpected, and infrequent reactions)*

IF ANY OF THE FOLLOWING DEVELOP, DISCONTINUE DRUG AND NOTIFY YOUR PHYSICIAN AS SOON AS POSSIBLE

Mild Adverse Effects
Allergic Reactions: Skin rash.
Other Reactions
Headache, dizziness, insomnia.
Acid indigestion, abdominal distention.
Muscle cramping and weakness.
Irregular menstrual periods.
Acne, excessive growth of facial hair.

Serious Adverse Effects
Mental and emotional disturbances of serious magnitude.
Reactivation of latent tuberculosis.
Development of peptic ulcer.
Increased blood pressure.
Development of inflammation of the pancreas.
Thrombophlebitis (inflammation of a vein with the formation of blood clot)
—pain or tenderness in thigh or leg, with or without swelling of the foot, ankle, or leg.
Pulmonary embolism (movement of blood clot to the lung)—sudden shortness of breath, pain in the chest, coughing, bloody sputum.

CAUTION

1. It is advisable to carry a card of personal identification with a notation that you are taking this drug if your course of treatment is to exceed 1 week (see Table 19 and Section Six).
2. Do not discontinue this drug abruptly.

3. While taking this drug, immunization procedures should be given with caution. If vaccination against measles, smallpox, rabies, or yellow fever is required, discontinue this drug 72 hours before vaccination and do not resume for at least 14 days after vaccination.

Precautions for Use by Those over 60 Years of Age

The "cortisone-related" drugs should be used very sparingly after 60, and only when the disorder under treatment is unresponsive to adequate trials of non-cortisone drugs. Prolonged use should be avoided.

The continuous use of this drug (even in small doses) can increase the severity of diabetes, enhance fluid retention, raise the blood pressure, weaken resistance to infection, induce stomach ulcer, and accelerate the development of cataract and softening of the bones (osteoporosis).

In sensitive individuals, cortisone-related drugs can cause serious emotional disturbance and disruptive behavior.

Advisability of Use During Pregnancy

Pregnancy Category: C (tentative). See Pregnancy Code inside back cover.

Animal reproduction studies in mice reveal significant birth defects due to this drug.

Information from adequate studies in pregnant women is not available.

Avoid completely during first 3 months.

Ask physician for guidance.

If use of this drug is considered necessary, limit dosage and duration of use as much as possible. Following birth, the infant should be examined for possible defective function of the adrenal glands (deficiency of adrenal cortical hormones).

Advisability of Use While Nursing Infant

Drug is known to be present in milk. Ask physician for guidance.

Habit-Forming Potential

Use of this drug to suppress symptoms over an extended period of time may produce a state of functional dependence (see Glossary). In the treatment of conditions like rheumatoid arthritis and asthma, it is advisable to try alternate-day drug administration to keep the daily dose as small as possible and to attempt drug withdrawal after periods of reasonable improvement. Such procedures may reduce the degree of "steroid rebound"—the return of symptoms as the drug is withdrawn.

Effects of Overdosage

With Moderate Overdose: Excessive fluid retention, swelling of extremities, flushing of the face, nervousness, stomach irritation, weakness.

With Large Overdose: Severe headache, convulsions, heart failure in susceptible individuals, emotional and behavioral disturbances.

Possible Effects of Extended Use

Development of increased blood sugar, possibly diabetes.

Increased fat deposits on the trunk of the body ("buffalo hump"), rounding of the face ("moon face"), and thinning of the arms and legs.

Thinning and fragility of the skin, easy bruising.
Loss of texture and strength of the bones, resulting in spontaneous fractures.
Development of increased internal eye pressure, possibly glaucoma.
Development of cataracts.
Retarded growth and development in children.

Suggested Periodic Examinations While Taking This Drug (at physician's discretion)
Measurement of blood potassium levels.
Measurement of blood sugar levels 2 hours after eating.
Measurement of blood pressure at regular intervals.
Complete eye examination at regular intervals.
Chest X-ray if history of previous tuberculosis.
Determination of the rate of development of the growing child to detect retardation of normal growth.

While Taking This Drug, Observe the Following
Foods: No interactions. Ask physician regarding need to restrict salt intake or to eat potassium-rich foods. During long-term use of this drug it is advisable to have a high protein diet.

Beverages: No restrictions.

Alcohol: No interactions expected.

Tobacco Smoking: Nicotine increases the blood levels of naturally produced cortisone and related hormones. Heavy smoking may add to the expected actions of this drug and requires close observation for excessive effects.

Marijuana Smoking
Occasional (once or twice weekly): No interactions expected.
Daily: Additional impairment of immunity due to this drug.

Other Drugs
Methylprednisolone may *increase* the effects of
- barbiturates and other sedatives and sleep-inducing drugs, causing over-sedation.

Methylprednisolone may *decrease* the effects of
- insulin and oral anti-diabetic drugs, by raising the level of blood sugar. Doses of anti-diabetic drugs may have to be raised.
- anticoagulants of the coumarin family. Monitor prothrombin times closely and adjust dosage accordingly.
- choline-like drugs (Mestinon, pilocarpine, Prostigmin), and reduce their effectiveness in treating glaucoma and myasthenia gravis.

Methylprednisolone *taken concurrently* with
- thiazide diuretics, may cause excessive loss of potassium. Monitor blood levels of potassium on physician's advice.
- atropine-like drugs, may cause increased internal eye pressure and initiate or aggravate glaucoma (see Drug Class, Section Three).
- digitalis preparations, requires close monitoring of body potassium stores to prevent digitalis toxicity.

• stimulant drugs (Adrenalin, amphetamines, ephedrine, etc.), may increase internal eye pressure and initiate or aggravate glaucoma.

The following drugs may *decrease* the effects of methylprednisolone
• indomethacin (Indocin, Indocid)
• aspirin

The following drugs may *increase* the effects of methylprednisolone
• barbiturates
• phenytoin (Dantoin, Dilantin, etc.)
• antihistamines (some)
• chloral hydrate (Noctec, Somnos)
• glutethimide (Doriden)
• phenylbutazone (Azolid, Butazolidin, etc.) may reduce its effectiveness following a brief, initial increase in effectiveness.
• propranolol (Inderal)

Driving a Vehicle, Operating Machinery, Engaging in Hazardous Activities: Usually no restrictions. Be alert to the possible occurrence of dizziness; restrict activities accordingly.

Aviation Note: The use of this drug *is a disqualification* for the piloting of aircraft. Consultation with a designated Aviation Medical Examiner is advised.

Exposure to Sun: No restrictions.

Occurrence of Unrelated Illness

This drug may decrease natural resistance to infection. Notify your physician if you develop an infection of any kind.

This drug may reduce your body's ability to respond appropriately to the stress of acute illness, injury, or surgery. Keep your physician fully informed of any significant changes in your state of health.

Discontinuation

If you have been taking this drug for an extended period of time, do not discontinue it abruptly. Ask physician for guidance regarding gradual withdrawal.

For a period of 2 years after discontinuing this drug, it is essential in the event of illness, injury, or surgery that you inform attending medical personnel that you used this drug in the past. The period of inadequate response to stress following the use of cortisone-like drugs may last for 1 to 2 years.

Special Storage Instructions

Keep in a tightly closed container. Protect from light.

METHYSERGIDE

Year Introduced: 1961

Brand Names

USA	Canada
Sansert (Sandoz)	Sansert (Sandoz)

Common Synonyms ("Street Names"):   None

Drug Class: Migraine Preventive

Prescription Required: Yes

Available for Purchase by Generic Name: No

Available Dosage Forms and Strengths
Tablets — 2 mg.

Tablet May Be Crushed or Capsule Opened for Administration: Yes

How This Drug Works
Intended Therapeutic Effect(s): Prevention of blood vessel (vascular) headaches of the migraine type, or reduction of their frequency or severity.

Location of Drug Action(s):   Those blood vessels in the head that undergo excessive constriction in response to stimulation by the tissue chemical serotonin.

Method of Drug Action(s):   Not fully established. It is thought that by blocking the action of serotonin, this drug prevents the blood vessel constriction that initiates the migraine syndrome.

Principal Uses of This Drug
As a Single Drug Product: This drug is used exclusively for the prevention of vascular type headaches, such as recurrent migraine and cluster headaches. Its use should be limited to individuals whose headaches are unusually frequent and disabling, and unresponsive to conventional treatment. This drug should not be used to treat acute headaches at their onset. It is ineffective for tension headaches.

THIS DRUG SHOULD NOT BE TAKEN IF
—you have had an allergic reaction to any dosage form of it previously
—you are pregnant.
—you are experiencing a severe infection.
—you have any of the following conditions:
angina pectoris
Buerger's disease
chronic lung disease
connective tissue (collagen) disease
coronary artery disease
hardening of the arteries (arteriosclerosis)
heart valve disease

high blood pressure (severe hypertension)
kidney disease (or impaired kidney function)
liver disease (or impaired liver function)
phlebitis of any kind
Raynaud's disease or phenomenon

INFORM YOUR PHYSICIAN BEFORE TAKING THIS DRUG IF
—you have had an allergic reaction to *any other forms of ergot.*
—you have a history of peptic ulcer disease.

Time Required for Apparent Benefit
This drug is used solely to *prevent* migraine headaches. If it has not proved to be effective after a trial of 3 weeks, it should be discontinued.

Possible Side-Effects *(natural, expected, and unavoidable drug actions)*
Weight gain, fluid retention (in some individuals).

Possible Adverse Effects *(unusual, unexpected, and infrequent reactions)*

IF ANY OF THE FOLLOWING DEVELOP, DISCONTINUE DRUG AND NOTIFY YOUR PHYSICIAN AS SOON AS POSSIBLE

Mild Adverse Effects
Allergic Reactions: Skin rashes, flushing of the face, transient loss of scalp hair.
Other Reactions
Heartburn, nausea, vomiting, diarrhea.
Drowsiness, dizziness, unsteadiness.
Transient muscle and joint pains.
Serious Adverse Effects
Idiosyncratic Reactions: Nightmares, hallucinations, acute mental disturbances.
Other Reactions
The development of cold, numb and painful hands and feet, leg cramps on walking, pain in the chest, abdomen, or back, fatigue or fever, urinary disturbance.
Abnormally low white blood cell counts.
Hemolytic anemia (see Glossary).

CAUTION
Continuous use without interruption must not exceed 6 months. There should be a drug-free period of 1 month between each 6-month course of treatment.

Precautions for Use by Those over 60 Years of Age
The natural changes in blood vessels and circulatory function that occur after 60 can make you more susceptible to the serious adverse effects of this drug.
See the list of diseases and disorders above which are contraindications to the use of this drug. Consult your physician for guidance.

Advisability of Use During Pregnancy
Pregnancy Category: X (tentative). See Pregnancy Code inside back cover.
Animal reproduction studies: No data available.
Information from adequate studies in pregnant women is not available.
The manufacturer states that this drug is contraindicated during entire
pregnancy.
Ask physician for guidance.

Advisability of Use While Nursing Infant
Drug is probably present in milk. Avoid use or avoid nursing. Ask physician
for guidance.

Habit-Forming Potential
None.

Effects of Overdosage
With Moderate Overdose: Nausea, vomiting, abdominal pain, diarrhea, incoordination.

Possible Effects of Extended Use
Formation of scar tissue inside chest cavity or abdominal cavity, on heart
valves, in lung tissue, and surrounding major blood vessels and internal
organs. (This tissue reaction is referred to as fibrosis.) The possibility of this
potentially dangerous reaction requires close and continuous medical
supervision while taking this drug.

Suggested Periodic Examinations While Taking This Drug (at physician's discretion)
Careful examination at regular intervals for scar tissue formation or circula-
tory complications.
Complete blood cell counts.
Kidney function tests.
Serial sedimentation rates (of red blood cells).

While Taking This Drug, Observe the Following
Foods: No restrictions other than foods to which you are allergic. (Some
migraine headaches are due to food allergy.) Drug should be taken with
meals.
Beverages: No restrictions.
Alcohol: No interactions expected with this drug. Observe closely to determine if alcoholic beverages can initiate a migraine-like headache.
Tobacco Smoking: Because of the constrictive action of nicotine on blood
vessels (reducing blood flow), heavy smoking should be avoided. Follow
physician's advice regarding smoking.
Marijuana Smoking: No interactions expected.
Other Drugs
Methysergide may *decrease* the effects of
• narcotic analgesics (morphine, codeine, oxycodone, meperidine, methadone, etc.), reducing their ability to relieve pain.

Driving a Vehicle, Operating Machinery, Engaging in Hazardous Activities:
Usually no restrictions. Avoid hazardous activities if drowsiness or dizziness
occurs.

Aviation Note: The use of this drug *is a disqualification* for the piloting of
aircraft. Consultation with a designated Aviation Medical Examiner is advised.

Exposure to Sun: No restrictions.

Exposure to Cold: Use caution until combined effect has been determined.
Cold environment may increase the occurrence of reduced circulation
(blood flow) to the extremities.

Discontinuation: If this drug has been used for an extended period of time,
do not discontinue it abruptly. Gradual withdrawal can prevent the occurrence of "rebound" headaches. Ask physician for instructions.

Special Storage Instructions
Keep in a dry, tightly closed container. Protect from light and heat. Store in
a cool place.

METOLAZONE

Year Introduced: 1973

Brand Names

USA	Canada
Diulo (Searle)	Zaroxolyn (Pennwalt)
Zaroxolyn (Pennwalt)	

Common Synonyms ("Street Names"):   Blood pressure pills, water pills

Drug Class: Anti-hypertensive (Hypotensive), Diuretic

Prescription Required: Yes

Available for Purchase by Generic Name: USA: No   Canada: No

Available Dosage Forms and Strengths
Tablets — 2.5 mg., 5 mg., 10 mg.

Tablet May Be Crushed or Capsule Opened for Administration: Yes

How This Drug Works
Intended Therapeutic Effect(s)
Elimination of excessive fluid retention (edema).
Reduction of high blood pressure.
Location of Drug Action(s): Principal actions occur in
• the tubular systems of the kidney that determine the final composition of
the urine.
• the walls of the smaller arteries (possibly).

Method of Drug Action(s):

By increasing the elimination of salt and water from the body (through increased urine production), this drug reduces the volume of fluid in the blood and body tissues and lowers the sodium content throughout the body.

By relaxing the walls of the smaller arteries and allowing them to expand, this drug increases the total capacity of the arterial system (a possible action).

The combined effect of these two actions (reduced blood volume in expanded space) results in lowering of the blood pressure.

Principal Uses of This Drug

As a Single Drug Product: This diuretic is used to relieve excessive fluid retention (edema) in such conditions as congestive heart failure, cirrhosis of the liver, and kidney disease. It is also used to initiate treatment ("step 1") in mild to moderate high blood pressure.

THIS DRUG SHOULD NOT BE TAKEN IF

—you are allergic to any of the drugs bearing the brand names listed above.

INFORM YOUR PHYSICIAN BEFORE TAKING THIS DRUG IF

—you are allergic to any form of "sulfa" drug, to thiazide diuretics, or to quinethazone (Hydromox).

—you are pregnant and your physician does not know it.

—you have a history of kidney disease or liver disease, or impaired kidney or liver function.

—you have diabetes (or a tendency to diabetes).

—you have a history of gout.

—you have a history of lupus erythematosus.

—you are taking any form of cortisone, digitalis, oral anti-diabetic drug, or insulin.

—you plan to have surgery under general anesthesia in the near future.

Time Required for Apparent Benefit

Drug action usually begins in 1 hour, reaches its peak in 2 to 3 hours, and persists for 12 to 24 hours.

Continuous use on a regular schedule for 3 to 4 weeks is usually necessary to determine this drug's effectiveness in maintaining a significant reduction of blood pressure.

Possible Side-Effects *(natural, expected, and unavoidable drug actions)*

Lightheadedness on arising from sitting or lying position (see orthostatic hypotension in Glossary).

Increase in level of blood sugar, affecting control of diabetes.

Increase in level of blood uric acid, affecting control of gout.

Decrease in level of blood potassium, resulting in muscle weakness and cramping.

Dryness of the mouth, thirst, constipation.

Possible Adverse Effects *(unusual, unexpected, and infrequent reactions)*

IF ANY OF THE FOLLOWING DEVELOP, DISCONTINUE DRUG AND NOTIFY
YOUR PHYSICIAN AS SOON AS POSSIBLE

Mild Adverse Effects
Allergic Reactions: Skin rashes (various kinds), hives.
Other Reactions
Headache, dizziness, drowsiness.
Reduced appetite, indigestion, nausea, vomiting, diarrhea.
Serious Adverse Effects
Allergic Reactions: Hepatitis with jaundice (see Glossary).
Other Reactions
Acute attacks of gout (in susceptible individuals).
Abnormally low white blood cells—possible fever and sore throat.
Adverse Effects That May Mimic Natural Diseases or Disorders
Jaundice may suggest the possibility of viral hepatitis.
Natural Diseases or Disorders That May Be Activated by This Drug
Diabetes, gout, systemic lupus erythematosus.

CAUTION
1. Do not exceed recommended doses. Increased dosage can cause excessive excretion of sodium and potassium with resultant loss of appetite, nausea, fatigue, weakness, confusion, and tingling in the extremities.
2. If you are also taking a digitalis preparation (digitoxin, digoxin), ensure an adequate intake of high-potassium foods to prevent potassium deficiency —a potential cause of digitalis toxicity.
3. It may be advisable to discontinue this drug during the week prior to surgery under general anesthesia. Consult your physician, surgeon or anesthesiologist.

Precautions for Use by Infants and Children
Use not recommended in children under 12 years of age.

Precautions for Use by Those over 60 Years of Age
You may be more sensitive to the actions of this drug. Small doses are advisable until your individual response has been determined.
You may be more susceptible to the development of impaired thinking, orthostatic hypotension (see Glossary), potassium loss, and elevation of blood sugar, complicating the management of diabetes.
If you are taking this drug to treat high blood pressure, remember that warm weather and fever can reduce your blood pressure and make it necessary to adjust your dosage.
Overdosage and extended use of this drug can cause excessive loss of body water, thickening (increased viscosity) of the blood, and an increased tendency of the blood to clot, predisposing to stroke, heart attack, or thrombophlebitis.

Advisability of Use During Pregnancy

Pregnancy Category: C (tentative). See Pregnancy Code inside back cover.
This drug should not be used during pregnancy unless a very serious complication of pregnancy occurs for which this drug is significantly beneficial.
This type of diuretic can have adverse effects on the fetus.

Advisability of Use While Nursing Infant

This drug is known to be present in the mother's milk. It is advisable to avoid use of this drug or to refrain from breast-feeding.

Habit-Forming Potential

None.

Effects of Overdosage

With Moderate Overdose: Dryness of mouth, thirst, lethargy, weakness, muscle pain and cramping, nausea, vomiting.
With Large Overdose: Drowsiness progressing to stupor and coma, weak and rapid pulse.

Possible Effects of Extended Use

Impaired balance of water, salt, and potassium in blood and body tissues.
Development of diabetes (in predisposed individuals).

Suggested Periodic Examinations While Taking This Drug (at physician's discretion)

Complete blood cell counts.
Measurements of blood levels of sodium, potassium, chloride, sugar, and uric acid.
Liver function tests.
Kidney function tests.

While Taking This Drug, Observe the Following

Foods: It is recommended that you include in your daily diet liberal servings of foods rich in potassium (unless directed otherwise by your physician). The following foods have a high potassium content:

All-bran cereals	Fish, fresh
Almonds	Lentils
Apricots (dried)	Liver, beef
Bananas, fresh	Lonalac
Beans (navy and lima)	Milk
Beef	Peaches (dried)
Carrots (raw)	Peanut butter
Chicken	Peas
Citrus fruits, juices	Pork
Coconut	Potato, sweet
Coffee	Prunes (dried), juice
Crackers (rye)	Raisins
Dates and figs (dried)	Tomato juice

Note: Avoid licorice in large amounts while taking this drug. Follow your physician's instructions regarding the use of salt.

Timing of Drug and Food: May be taken after eating to reduce stomach irritation.

Beverages: No restrictions unless directed by your physician. This drug may be taken with milk.

Alcohol: Use with caution until the combined effect has been determined. Alcohol can exaggerate the blood pressure-lowering effect of this drug and cause orthostatic hypotension (see Glossary).

Tobacco Smoking: No interactions expected. Follow your physician's advice regarding smoking.

Marijuana Smoking: No interactions expected.

Other Drugs

Metolazone may *increase* the effects of

- other anti-hypertensive drugs and diuretics. Careful adjustment of dosages is necessary to prevent excessive lowering of the blood pressure and/or excessive loss of salt and water.
- drugs of the phenothiazine family, and cause excessive lowering of the blood pressure. (Diuretics and the phenothiazines both may cause orthostatic hypotension.)

Metolazone may *decrease* the effects of

- oral anti-diabetic drugs and insulin, by raising the level of blood sugar. Careful adjustment of dosages is necessary to maintain proper control of diabetes.
- allopurinol (Zyloprim), by raising the level of blood uric acid. Careful adjustment of dosages is required to maintain proper control of gout.
- probenecid (Benemid), by raising the level of blood uric acid. Careful dosage adjustment is necessary to maintain control of gout.

Metolazone *taken concurrently* with

- cortisone and cortisone-related drugs, may cause excessive loss of potassium from the body.
- digitalis and related drugs, requires very careful monitoring and dosage adjustments to prevent serious disturbances of heart rhythm.
- lithium (Lithane, etc.) greatly increases the risk of lithium toxicity.
- tricyclic antidepressants (Elavil, Sinequan, etc.), may cause excessive lowering of the blood pressure.

The following drugs may *increase* the effects of metolazone:

- barbiturates may exaggerate its blood pressure-lowering action.
- mono-amine oxidase (MAO) inhibitor drugs may increase urine volume by delaying this drug's elimination from the body.
- pain relievers (analgesics), both narcotic and non-narcotic, may exaggerate its blood pressure-lowering action.

The following drugs may *decrease* the effects of metolazone:

- cholestyramine (Cuemid, Questran) may interfere with its absorption. Take cholestyramine 30 to 60 minutes before any oral diuretic.
- hydralazine (Apresoline) may impair the blood pressure-lowering effect of metolazone.

Driving a Vehicle, Operating Machinery, Engaging in Hazardous Activities: Use caution until the possibility of orthostatic hypotension and/or impaired vision has been determined.

Aviation Note: The use of this drug *may be a disqualification* for the piloting of aircraft. Consultation with a designated Aviation Medical Examiner is advised.

Exposure to Sun: Use caution until sensitivity has been determined. This drug may cause photosensitivity (see Glossary).

Exposure to Heat: Avoid excessive perspiring that could cause additional loss of water and salt from the body.

Heavy Exercise or Exertion: Avoid exertion that produces lightheadedness, excessive fatigue, or muscle cramping. Isometric exercises—the "overload" technique for strengthening individual muscles—can raise the blood pressure significantly. Ask your physician for guidance regarding participation in this form of exercise.

Occurrence of Unrelated Illness: Illnesses which cause vomiting or diarrhea can produce a serious imbalance of important body chemistry. Discontinue this drug and ask your physician for guidance.

Discontinuation: It may be advisable to discontinue this drug before major surgery. Ask your physician, surgeon, and/or anesthesiologist for guidance regarding dosage reduction or withdrawal.

Special Storage Instructions
Keep in a dry, tightly closed container at room temperature.

METOPROLOL

Year Introduced: 1975 (Europe)
1978 (USA)

Brand Names:

USA	Canada
Lopressor (Geigy)	Betaloc (ASTRA)
	Lopressor (Geigy)

Common Synonyms ("Street Names"): Blood pressure pills

Drug Class: Anti-hypertensive (Hypotensive), Beta-Adrenergic Blocker

Prescription Required: Yes

Available for Purchase by Generic Name: No

Available Dosage Forms and Strengths
Tablets — 50 mg., 100 mg.

Tablet May Be Crushed or Capsule Opened for Administration: Yes

How This Drug Works

Intended Therapeutic Effect(s):   Reduction of high blood pressure.

Location of Drug Action(s):   Principal sites of therapeutic actions include
- the heart pacemaker and tissues that comprise the electrical conduction system.
- the heart muscle.
- the vasomotor center in the brain that influences the control of the sympathetic nervous system over blood vessels (principally arterioles) throughout the body.
- sympathetic nerve terminals in blood vessel walls.

Method of Drug Action(s):   Not completely established. By blocking certain actions of the sympathetic nervous system, this drug
- reduces the rate and the contraction force of the heart, thus lowering the oxygen requirement of the heart muscle.
- prolongs the conduction time of nerve impulses through the heart.
- reduces the degree of contraction of blood vessel walls, resulting in their relaxation and expansion and lowering of the blood pressure.

Principal Uses of This Drug

As a Single Drug Product: This member of the "beta-blocker" class of drugs is used exclusively to treat high blood pressure. It may be used alone or as a "step 2" medication in conjunction with a thiazide diuretic.

THIS DRUG SHOULD NOT BE TAKEN IF

—you have had an allergic reaction to any dosage form of it previously.
—you are subject to episodes of asthma.
—you are presently experiencing seasonal hay fever.
—you are taking, or have taken within the past 2 weeks, any mono-amine oxidase (MAO) inhibitor drug (see Drug Class, Section Three).

INFORM YOUR PHYSICIAN BEFORE TAKING THIS DRUG IF

—you have a history of serious heart disease, with or without episodes of heart failure.
—you have a history of hay fever (allergic rhinitis), asthma, chronic bronchitis, or emphysema.
—you have a history of overactive thyroid function (hyperthyroidism).
—you have a history of low blood sugar (hypoglycemia).
—you have a history of impaired liver or kidney function.
—you have diabetes.
—you are taking any form of digitalis or quinidine.
—you are taking any form of reserpine.
—you play to have surgery under general anesthesia in the near future.

Time Required for Apparent Benefit

Drug action begins in 1 hour, reaches a maximum within 4 hours, and subsides in 6 to 8 hours. Full effectiveness can be determined only by continuous use on a regular schedule for several weeks, during which time dosage is carefully adjusted according to individual response (this can vary widely from person to person).

Possible Side-Effects *(natural, expected, and unavoidable drug actions)*
Lethargy and fatigability, cold hands and feet, lightheadedness in upright position (see orthostatic hypotension in Glossary).

Possible Adverse Effects *(unusual, unexpected, and infrequent reactions)*

IF ANY OF THE FOLLOWING DEVELOP, DISCONTINUE DRUG AND NOTIFY YOUR PHYSICIAN AS SOON AS POSSIBLE

Mild Adverse Effects
Allergic Reactions: Skin rashes, itching, temporary loss of hair, drug fever.
Other Reactions
Reduced appetite, indigestion, nausea, vomiting, diarrhea.
Insomnia, vivid dreaming, headache, dizziness (10%).
Serious Adverse Effects
Idiosyncratic Reactions: Acute behavioral disturbances: disorientation, confusion, hallucinations, amnesia.
Other Reactions
Reduced heart muscle strength and reserve.
Increased risk of asthma.
Emotional depression (5%).
Reduction of white blood cells resulting in fever and sore throat.
Reduction of blood platelets (see Glossary), resulting in unusual bleeding or bruising.

CAUTION
1. *Do not discontinue this drug suddenly.* Include a notation on your card of personal identification that you are taking this drug (see Table 19 and Section Six).
2. Hot weather and the fever associated with infection can reduce the blood pressure significantly, requiring adjustment of dosage.
3. Report the development of any tendency to emotional depression.

Precautions for Use by Those over 60 Years of Age
The basic rule in treating high blood pressure after 60 is to proceed *cautiously.* The elevated systolic blood pressure often present after 60 is not necessarily a threat to health, and can serve as an adaptive and compensatory change with age that should not be altered drastically. The goals of treatment must be adjusted to the natural changes in body function that occur with aging. Unacceptably high blood pressure should be reduced without creating the risks associated with excessively low blood pressure.
It is advisable to start treatment with small doses and to monitor the blood pressure response frequently. Sudden, rapid, and excessive reduction of blood pressure can predispose to stroke or heart attack.
You may be more susceptible to the development of orthostatic hypotension with resultant lightheadedness, dizziness, unsteadiness, fainting, and falling. Report such symptoms to your physician promptly.

Advisability of Use During Pregnancy

Pregnancy Category: B (tentative). See Pregnancy Code inside back cover. Animal reproduction studies reveal no birth defects due to this drug. Information from adequate studies in pregnant women is not available. Ask physician for guidance.

Advisability of Use While Nursing Infant

The presence of this drug in milk is not known. Avoid drug or refrain from nursing.

Habit-Forming Potential

None

Effects of Overdosage

With Moderate Overdose: General weakness, slow pulse, orthostatic hypotension.

With Large Overdose: Marked drop in blood pressure, fainting, weak and slow pulse, cold and sweaty skin.

Possible Effects of Extended Use

Reduced reserve of heart muscle strength, which may result from prolonged use of high doses.

Suggested Periodic Examinations While Taking This Drug (at physician's discretion)

Complete blood cell counts, including platelet counts.
Evaluation of heart function.

While Taking This Drug, Observe the Following

Foods: No interactions with drug. Follow physician's advice regarding salt and total calorie intake. Drug is absorbed best when taken before eating.

Beverages: No restrictions.

Alcohol: Use with caution until combined effect has been determined. Alcohol may exaggerate this drug's ability to lower blood pressure and may increase its mild sedative action.

Tobacco Smoking: Follow physician's advice regarding use of tobacco. Nicotine may reduce this drug's effectiveness in treating high blood pressure.

Marijuana Smoking

Occasional (once or twice weekly):   No effect to mild and transient accentuation of orthostatic hypotension (see Glossary); transient cooling of hands and/or feet.

Daily: Significant accentuation of orthostatic hypotension, requiring dosage adjustment in sensitive individuals; more marked and persistent coldness of hands and/or feet.

Other Drugs

Metoprolol may *increase* the effects of

• oral anti-diabetic drugs and insulin, causing or prolonging hypoglycemia. Careful dosage adjustments are necessary.

• other anti-hypertensive drugs, and cause excessive lowering of the blood pressure. Careful dosage adjustments are necessary.

- barbiturates and narcotic drugs, and cause dangerous oversedation.
- reserpine, and cause excessive sedation and depression.

Metoprolol may *decrease* the effects of
- antihistamines, and reduce their effectiveness in treating allergies.
- anti-inflammatory drugs, including aspirin, cortisone, phenylbutazone (Azolid, Butazolidin, etc.), oxyphenbutazone (Oxalid, Tandearil).

Metoprolol *taken concurrently* with
- digitalis preparations (digitoxin, digoxin), may cause adverse interactions —excessive slowing of heart action and reduction of digitalis effectiveness in treating heart failure. Careful dosage adjustments are necessary.
- quinidine, may cause excessive slowing of the heart. Careful dosage adjustments are necessary.

The following drugs may *increase* the effects of metoprolol:
- phenytoin (Dantoin, Dilantin, etc.) may exaggerate its sedative action on the brain.
- reserpine may cause excessive lowering of the blood pressure.

Driving a Vehicle, Operating Machinery, Engaging in Hazardous Activities: Avoid hazardous activities until the full extent of drowsiness or lethargy has been determined.

Aviation Note: The use of this drug and the disorder for which this drug is prescribed *may be disqualifications* for the piloting of aircraft. Consultation with a designated Aviation Medical Examiner is advised.

Exposure to Sun: No restrictions.

Exposure to Heat: No restrictions.

Exposure to Cold: Use caution until combined effect has been determined. If you are subject to Raynaud's phenomenon, this drug may exaggerate further the impaired circulation in hands and feet.

Heavy Exercise or Exertion: Avoid levels of exertion which produced angina prior to the use of this drug. Isometric exercises—the "overload" technique for strengthening individual muscles—can raise the blood pressure significantly. The use of this drug may intensify the hypertensive response to isometric exercises. Ask your physician for guidance.

Occurrence of Unrelated Illness: If an illness causes vomiting and interrupts the regular use of this drug, notify your physician as soon as possible.

Discontinuation: This drug must not be discontinued abruptly. Gradual withdrawal over a period of 2 or more weeks is necessary to prevent possible angina or risk of heart attack. Ask your physician for guidance.

Special Storage Instructions
Keep in a dry, tightly closed container at room temperature. Protect from moisture.

METRONIDAZOLE

Year Introduced: 1960

Brand Names

USA		Canada
Flagyl (Searle)	Flagyl (Poulenc)	Novonidazol
Protostat (Ortho)	Neo-Tric (Neolab)	(Novopharm)

Common Synonyms ("Street Names"):   None

Drug Class: Antimicrobial, Antiprotozoal (Anti-infective)

Prescription Required: Yes

Available for Purchase by Generic Name: USA: Yes   Canada: No

Available Dosage Forms and Strengths
        Tablets — 250 mg.
    Vaginal inserts — 500 mg.

Tablet May Be Crushed or Capsule Opened for Administration: Yes

How This Drug Works
    Intended Therapeutic Effect(s):   The elimination of protozoal infections responsive to the action of this drug.
    Location of Drug Action(s):   Those body tissues and fluids infected by certain protozoal microorganisms, and in which adequate concentration of the drug can be achieved.
    Method of Drug Action(s):   Not established.

Principal Uses of This Drug
    As a Single Drug Product: This anti-infective drug is used primarily to treat trichomonal infections of the vaginal canal and cervix and of the male urethra. It is also used to treat giardiasis, amebic dysentery, and serious infections caused by certain strains of anaerobic bacteria.

THIS DRUG SHOULD NOT BE TAKEN IF
—you have had an allergic reaction to any dosage form of it previously.
—you have or have had a disease of the bone marrow or blood cells (a blood dyscrasia).

INFORM YOUR PHYSICIAN BEFORE TAKING THIS DRUG IF
—you have an active disorder of the nervous system (brain or spinal cord).
—you use alcoholic beverages frequently or heavily.

Time Required for Apparent Benefit
    Drug action begins in 1 hour, reaches a maximum in 2 to 3 hours, and persists for 12 hours. Continuous treatment for up to 10 days may be needed to cure infection.

Possible Side-Effects *(natural, expected, and unavoidable drug actions)*
A sharp, metallic, unpleasant taste.
Dark discoloration of the urine (of no significance).
Superinfection (see Glossary) by yeast organisms in the mouth or vagina.

Possible Adverse Effects *(unusual, unexpected, and infrequent reactions)*

**IF ANY OF THE FOLLOWING DEVELOP, DISCONTINUE DRUG AND NOTIFY
YOUR PHYSICIAN AS SOON AS POSSIBLE**

Mild Adverse Effects
Allergic Reactions: Skin rash, hives, flushing, itching.
Other Reactions
Reduced appetite, nausea, vomiting, abdominal pain, cramping, diarrhea, altered taste, irritation of mouth or tongue.
Headache, dizziness, unsteadiness, incoordination.
Sense of numbness or abnormal sensation in the extremities.
Serious Adverse Effects
Idiosyncratic Reactions: Behavioral disturbances, irritability, confusion, depression, insomnia.
Other Reactions: Abnormally low white blood cell count.

CAUTION
1. Troublesome and persistent diarrhea can develop in sensitive individuals. If diarrhea persists more than 24 hours, discontinue this drug and consult your physician for guidance.
2. Discontinue this drug immediately if you develop any indications of toxic effects on the brain or nervous system: confusion, irritability, dizziness, incoordination, unsteady stance or gait, muscle jerking or twitching, numbness or weakness in the extremities.

Precautions for Use by Those over 60 Years of Age
Natural changes in the skin after 60 may predispose to severe and prolonged itching reactions in the genital and anal regions. This reaction should be reported promptly.

Advisability of Use During Pregnancy
Pregnancy Category: X (tentative). See Pregnancy Code inside back cover.
Animal reproduction studies reveal no birth defects due to this drug. However, other animal studies in rodents reveal that this drug can cause tumors.
Information from adequate studies in pregnant women is not available.
The manufacturers state that this drug is contraindicated during the first 3 months and that its use is very limited during the last 6 months.
Ask physician for guidance.

Advisability of Use While Nursing Infant
Drug is known to be present in milk. Avoid use or discontinue nursing. Ask physician for guidance.

Habit-Forming Potential
None.

Effects of Overdosage
With Moderate Overdose: Weakness, stomach irritation, nausea, vomiting.
With Large Overdose: Disorientation, confusion.

Possible Effects of Extended Use
None reported.

Suggested Periodic Examinations While Taking This Drug (at physician's discretion)
Complete blood cell counts.

While Taking This Drug, Observe the Following
Foods: No restrictions. Drug may be taken after eating to reduce stomach irritation or nausea.

Beverages: No restrictions.

Alcohol: Avoid completely. This drug combined with alcohol may produce a disulfiram-like reaction (see Glossary).

Tobacco Smoking: No interactions expected.

Marijuana Smoking: No interactions expected.

Other Drugs

Metronidazole may *increase* the effects of
- warfarin (Coumadin, etc.), and cause abnormal bleeding or bruising. Monitor the prothrombin time closely, especially during the first 10 days of concurrent use.

Metronidazole *taken concurrently* with
- disulfiram (Antabuse), may cause severe emotional and behavioral disturbances.

The following drug may *decrease* the effects of metronidazole
- oxytetracycline (Terramycin, etc.) may reduce its effectiveness in treating trichomonas infection.

Driving a Vehicle, Operating Machinery, Engaging in Hazardous Activities: Use caution until tolerance has been determined. Avoid hazardous activities if dizziness or incoordination occurs.

Aviation Note: The use of this drug *may be a disqualification* for the piloting of aircraft. Consultation with a designated Aviation Medical Examiner is advised.

Exposure to Sun: No restrictions.

Special Storage Instructions
Keep in a dry, tightly closed container. Protect from light.

MINOCYCLINE

Year Introduced: 1970

Brand Names

USA	Canada
Minocin (Lederle)	Minocin (Lederle)

Common Synonyms ("Street Names"):   None

Drug Class: Antibiotic (Anti-infective), Tetracycline

Prescription Required: Yes

Available for Purchase by Generic Name: No

Available Dosage Forms and Strengths
Capsules — 50 mg., 100 mg.
Oral suspension — 50 mg. per teaspoonful (5 ml.)
Tablets — 50 mg., 100 mg.

Tablet May Be Crushed or Capsule Opened for Administration: Yes

How This Drug Works
Intended Therapeutic Effect(s):   The elimination of infections responsive to the action of this drug.
Location of Drug Action(s):   Any body tissue or fluid in which sufficient concentration of the drug can be achieved.
Method of Drug Action(s):   This drug prevents the growth and multiplication of susceptible bacteria by interfering with their formation of essential proteins.

Principal Uses of This Drug
As a Single Drug Product: This drug is used to treat a wide variety of common and uncommon infections. For this drug to be effective, the infecting organism must be sensitive to the action of this form of tetracycline. Appropriate sensitivity testing may be necessary to determine the most effective drug to use for any given infection.

THIS DRUG SHOULD NOT BE TAKEN IF
—you are allergic to *any* tetracycline drug (see Drug Class, Section Three).
—you are pregnant or breast feeding.

INFORM YOUR PHYSICIAN BEFORE TAKING THIS DRUG IF
—you have a history of liver or kidney disease.
—you have systemic lupus erythematosus.
—you are taking any penicillin drug.
—you are taking any anticoagulant drug.
—you plan to have surgery under general anesthesia in the near future.
—it is prescribed for a child under 9 years of age.

Time Required for Apparent Benefit
Varies with nature of infection under treatment; usually 2 to 5 days.

Possible Side-Effects *(natural, expected, and unavoidable drug actions)*
Superinfections (see Glossary).

Possible Adverse Effects *(unusual, unexpected, and infrequent reactions)*

IF ANY OF THE FOLLOWING DEVELOP, DISCONTINUE DRUG AND NOTIFY YOUR PHYSICIAN AS SOON AS POSSIBLE

Mild Adverse Effects
Allergic Reactions: Skin rashes (various kinds), hives, itching of hands and feet, swelling of face or extremities.

Photosensitivity (see Glossary) Reactions: Exaggerated sunburn occurs with the use of some tetracyclines, but this has not been reported with minocycline.

Other Reactions

Loss of appetite, nausea, vomiting, diarrhea.

Sensation of lightheadedness or dizziness (this is relatively common and usually occurs during first 3 days).

Serious Adverse Effects
Allergic Reactions: Anaphylactic reaction (see Glossary), asthma, fever, unusual bleeding or bruising.

Other Reactions

Stomach irritation, superinfections, rectal or vaginal itching.

Permanent discoloration and/or malformation of teeth when taken under 9 years of age, including unborn child or infant.

CAUTION
1. Antacids, dairy products, and iron preparations will prevent adequate absorption of this drug and reduce its effectiveness significantly.
2. Troublesome and persistent diarrhea can develop in sensitive individuals. If diarrhea persists more than 24 hours, discontinue this drug and consult your physician for guidance.
3. If your kidney function is reduced significantly, dosage schedule must be adjusted accordingly.
4. If surgery under general anesthesia is planned while taking this drug, the choice of anesthetic agent must be considered carefully to prevent serious kidney damage.

Precautions for Use by Those over 60 Years of Age
The natural decline in kidney function that occurs after 60 may require significant reduction in dosage and lengthening of dosage intervals. Dosage must be carefully individualized and based upon measurements of kidney function.

Natural changes in the skin after 60 may predispose to severe and prolonged itching reactions in the genital and anal regions. This reaction should be reported promptly.

Advisability of Use During Pregnancy
Pregnancy Category: D (tentative). See Pregnancy Code inside back cover.
Animal reproduction studies in rats and rabbits reveal significant birth
defects due to this drug.

Information from studies in pregnant women indicates that this drug can
cause impaired development and discoloration of teeth and other developmental defects.

It is advisable to avoid this drug completely during entire pregnancy.
Ask physician for guidance.

Advisability of Use While Nursing Infant
Tetracyclines can be present in milk and can have adverse effects on infant.
Avoid use.

Habit-Forming Potential
None.

Effects of Overdosage
Possible nausea, vomiting, diarrhea, dizziness.
Acute liver damage (rare).

Possible Effects of Extended Use
Impairment of bone marrow, liver, or kidney function (all rare).
Superinfections.

Suggested Periodic Examinations While Taking This Drug (at physician's discretion)
Complete blood cell counts.
Liver and kidney function tests.
During extended use, sputum and stool examinations may detect early super-
infections due to yeast organisms.

While Taking This Drug, Observe the Following
Foods: No restrictions of food selection. Drug may be taken at any time
with relationship to eating.
Beverages: No restrictions.
Alcohol: Avoid while taking minocycline if you have a history of liver dis-
ease.
Tobacco Smoking: No interactions expected.
Marijuana Smoking: No interactions expected.
Other Drugs
Minocycline may *increase* the effects of
• oral anticoagulants, and make it necessary to reduce their dosage.

Minocycline may *decrease* the effects of
• the penicillins, and impair their effectiveness in treating infections.

The following drugs may *decrease* the effects of minocycline
• antacids may reduce drug absorption.
• iron and mineral preparations may reduce drug absorption.

Driving a Vehicle, Operating Machinery, Engaging in Hazardous Activities:
Avoid all hazardous activities if lightheaded or dizzy.

Aviation Note: The use of this drug *may be a disqualification* for the
piloting of aircraft. Consultation with a designated Aviation Medical Examiner is advised.

Exposure to Sun: Photosensitivity (see Glossary) is common with some
tetracyclines. Use caution until sensitivity is determined.

Special Storage Instructions

Keep in a tightly closed, light-resistant container. Avoid temperatures above
90°F. (32°C.). Syrup need not be refrigerated.

MINOXIDIL

Note: This is an Abbreviated Drug Profile of a potent, long-acting anti-hypertensive
drug that is reserved to treat severe high blood pressure that has failed to respond to
maximal doses of standard anti-hypertensive drugs. It is effective in approximately 75%
of such cases and has several significant advantages over other drugs commonly used
to treat high blood pressure. However, it causes an excessive growth of hair on the face,
back, arms, and legs of 80% of users after 1 to 2 months of continuous use. In addition,
it may cause excessive fluid retention, and can aggravate existing coronary artery
disease and intensify angina.

Year Introduced: 1972

Brand Names

USA	Canada
Loniten (Upjohn)	Loniten (Upjohn)

Common Synonyms ("Street Names"):   Blood pressure pills

Drug Class: Anti-hypertensives

Prescription Required: USA: Yes   Canada: Yes

Available for Purchase by Generic Name: USA: No   Canada: No

Available Dosage Forms and Strengths

Tablets — 2.5 mg., 10 mg.

Tablet May Be Crushed or Capsule Opened for Administration: Yes

How This Drug Works

Intended Therapeutic Effect(s):   Reduction of severe, unresponsive high
blood pressure.

Location of Drug Action(s):   The principal therapeutic action occurs in the
muscles within the walls of small arteries (arterioles).

Method of Drug Action(s):   By causing direct relaxation of the constricted muscles within the walls of small arteries throughout the body, this drug permits expansion of the arteries with resultant lowering of the pressure of the blood within.

Principal Uses of This Drug

As a Single Drug Product: Currently the use of this drug is limited to the treatment of severe high blood pressure that cannot be reduced by conventional therapy. Investigations are under way to determine the value of this drug when used in lotions and ointments to treat scalp baldness. These dosage forms are experimental and not available to the public at this time.

THIS DRUG SHOULD NOT BE TAKEN IF
—you have had an allergic reaction to it previously.
—you are known to have a pheochromocytoma (an adrenalin-producing tumor).
—you have pulmonary hypertension due to mitral valve stenosis.

INFORM YOUR PHYSICIAN BEFORE TAKING THIS DRUG IF
—you are pregnant or planning pregnancy.
—you have a history of coronary artery disease, or impaired heart function.
—you have had a stroke at any time in the past.
—you have impaired liver or kidney function.

Time Required for Apparent Benefit
Drug action usually begins in 30 minutes and reaches its peak in 3 to 8 hours. Continuous use on a regular schedule for 3 to 7 days is usually necessary to determine this drug's effectiveness in controlling severe high blood pressure.

Possible Side-Effects *(natural, expected, and unavoidable drug actions)*
Increased heart rate, fluid retention with weight gain (7%), excessive hair growth (80%).

Possible Adverse Effects *(unusual, unexpected, and infrequent reactions)*

IF ANY OF THE FOLLOWING DEVELOP, DISCONTINUE DRUG AND NOTIFY YOUR PHYSICIAN AS SOON AS POSSIBLE

Mild Adverse Effects
Allergic Reactions: Skin rash
Other Reactions: Headache, fatigue.
Nausea, increased thirst.
Breast tenderness (less than 1%).

Serious Adverse Effects
Idiosyncratic Reactions: Fluid formation around the heart (pericardial effusion) (3%).
Other Reactions: High blood pressure in the lung circulation (pulmonary hypertension).

Natural Diseases or Disorders That May Be Activated By This Drug
Coronary artery insufficiency with angina.

CAUTION

1. Long-term use may require the addition of other drugs to counteract the increase in heart rate and fluid retention. Take these drugs as directed on a regular schedule.
2. Consult your physician regarding the advisability of using a "no salt added" diet.

Advisability of Use During Pregnancy

Pregnancy Category: C (tentative). See Pregnancy Code inside back cover. Animal reproduction studies in rats and rabbits reveal no birth defects. However, they did reveal decreased fertility and increased fetal deaths. Information from adequate studies in pregnant women is not available. Use this drug only if clearly needed.

Advisability of Use While Nursing Infant

The presence of this drug in human milk is not known.
It is advisable to refraing from nursing while taking this drug.

While Taking This Drug, Observe the Following

Foods: Avoid excessive salt. A "no salt added" diet is recommended. May be taken with food or on an empty stomach.

Beverages: No restrictions. May be taken with milk.

Alcohol: Use extreme caution until the combined effects have been determined. Alcohol can exaggerate the blood pressure-lowering effect of this drug.

Other Drugs

Minoxidil may *increase* the effects of
- all other anti-hypertensive drugs. Careful dosage adjustments are necessary.

Minoxidil *taken concurrently* with
- guanethidine (Ismelin, Esimil) may cause severe orthostatic hypotension (see Glossary). Avoid the concurrent use of these two drugs.

Driving a Vehicle, Operating Machinery, Engaging in Hazardous Activities: Usually no restrictions. However, observe for the possible occurrence of dizziness or fatigue and restrict activities accordingly.

Aviation Note: The use of this drug and the disorder for which this drug is prescribed *are disqualifications* for the piloting of aircraft.

Discontinuation: This drug should not be stopped abruptly.
If it is to be discontinued, consult your physician regarding gradual reduction in dosage and appropriate replacement with other drugs.

NADOLOL

Year Introduced: 1980

Brand Names

USA	Canada
Corgard (Squibb)	Corgard (Squibb)
Corzide [CD] (Squibb)	

Common Synonyms ("Street Names"):   Blood pressure pills, heart pills

Drug Class: Anti-anginal, Anti-hypertensive (Hypotensive), Beta-Adrenergic Blocker

Prescription Required: Yes

Available for Purchase by Generic Name: No

Available Dosage Forms and Strengths
Tablets — 40 mg., 80 mg., 120 mg., 160 mg.

Tablet May Be Crushed or Capsule Opened for Administration: Yes

How This Drug Works
Intended Therapeutic Effect(s)
Reduction in the frequency and intensity of pain associated with angina pectoris (coronary insufficiency).
Reduction of high blood pressure.
Location of Drug Action(s):   Principal sites of therapeutic actions include
• the heart pacemaker and tissues that comprise the electrical conduction system.
• the heart muscle.
• the vasomotor center in the brain that influences the control of the sympathetic nervous system over blood vessels (principally arterioles) throughout the body.
• sympathetic nerve terminals in blood vessel walls.
Method of Drug Action(s):   Not completely established. By blocking certain actions of the sympathetic nervous system, this drug
• reduces the rate and the contraction force of the heart, thus lowering the oxygen requirement of the heart muscle. This reduces the occurrence of angina.
• prolongs the conduction time of nerve impulses through the heart.
• reduces the degree of contraction of blood vessel walls, resulting in their relaxation and expansion and lowering of the blood pressure.

Principal Uses of This Drug
As a Single Drug Product: This "beta-blocker" drug is used in the management of coronary artery disease to prevent attacks of effort-induced angina pectoris. It is also used to treat moderately high blood pressure, either alone or as a "step 2" medication in conjunction with a thiazide diuretic.

As a Combination Drug Product [CD]:   This drug is now available in combination with bendroflumethiazide, a mild diuretic "step 1" anti-hypertensive drug. This combination product is more effective and more convenient
for long-term use.

THIS DRUG SHOULD NOT BE TAKEN IF
—you have had an allergic reaction to any dosage form of it previously.
—you are subject to episodes of asthma.
—you are presently experiencing seasonal hay fever.

INFORM YOUR PHYSICIAN BEFORE TAKING THIS DRUG IF
—you have a history of serious heart disease, with or without episodes of heart
failure or heart block.
—you have a history of hay fever (allergic rhinitis), asthma, chronic bronchitis,
or emphysema.
—you have a history of overactive thyroid function (hyperthyroidism).
—you have a history of low blood sugar (hypoglycemia).
—you have a history of impaired liver or kidney function.
—you have diabetes.
—you have Raynaud's syndrome.
—you are taking any form of reserpine, digitalis, or quinidine.
—you plan to have surgery under general anesthesia in the near future.

Time Required for Apparent Benefit
Drug action usually begins in 1 hour, reaches its peak in 3 to 4 hours, and
persists for 24 hours. Continuous use on a regular schedule for several weeks
is usually necessary to determine this drug's effectiveness in relieving angina
and/or lowering the blood pressure. Dosage must be carefully adjusted according to individual response; this can vary widely.

Possible Side-Effects *(natural, expected, and unavoidable drug actions)*
Lethargy and fatigability, cold hands and feet, lightheadedness in upright
position (see orthostatic hypotension in Glossary).

Possible Adverse Effects *(unusual, unexpected, and infrequent reactions)*

**IF ANY OF THE FOLLOWING DEVELOP, DISCONTINUE DRUG AND NOTIFY
YOUR PHYSICIAN AS SOON AS POSSIBLE**

Mild Adverse Effects
Allergic Reactions: Skin rashes, itching, temporary loss of hair, drug
fever.
Other Reactions
Reduced appetite, nausea, vomiting, diarrhea, indigestion.
Insomnia, vivid dreaming, dizziness, fatigue, headache, blurred vision.
Serious Adverse Effects
Idiosyncratic Reactions: Acute behavioral disturbances, disorientation,
confusion, hallucinations, amnesia.
Other Reactions
Reduced heart muscle strength and reserve; worsening of heart failure.
Increased risk of asthma.

Emotional depression.

Reduced libido, impotence.

Reduction of white blood cells resulting in fever and sore throat.

Reduction of blood platelets (see Glossary), resulting in unusual bleeding or bruising.

Adverse Effects That May Mimic Natural Diseases or Disorders

Peyronie's disease (reported occurring with the use of other beta-adrenergic blocker drugs).

The development of drug fever (see Glossary) may suggest the presence of an infection.

Natural Diseases or Disorders That May Be Activated by This Drug

Bronchial asthma, congestive heart failure, emotional depression.

CAUTION

1. *Do not discontinue this drug suddenly if you have angina (coronary heart disease).* Include a notation on your card of personal identification that you are taking this drug (see Table 19 and Section Six).
2. Hot weather and the fever associated with infection can reduce the blood pressure significantly, requiring adjustment of dosage.
3. Report the development of any tendency to emotional depression to your physician.
4. If you have diabetes, this drug can prevent the development of the symptoms that indicate the onset of hypoglycemia. Adjust the dosage of all anti-diabetic drugs carefully.
5. The maximal dose should not exceed 240 mg. per 24 hours in the treatment of angina, or 320 mg. in the treatment of hypertension.

Precautions for Use by Infants and Children

Safety and effectiveness in children below the age of 12 years have not been established. Use is not recommended.

Precautions for Use by Those over 60 Years of Age

The basic rule in treating high blood pressure after 60 is to proceed *cautiously.* The elevated systolic blood pressure often present after 60 is not necessarily a threat to health, and can serve as an adaptive and compensatory change with age that should not be altered drastically. The goals of treatment must be adjusted to the natural changes in body function that occur with aging. Unacceptably high blood pressure should be reduced without creating the risks associated with excessively low blood pressure.

It is advisable to start treatment with small doses and to monitor the blood pressure response frequently. Sudden, rapid, and excessive reduction of blood pressure can predispose to stroke or heart attack.

You may be more susceptible to the development of orthostatic hypotension (see Glossary) with resultant lightheadedness, dizziness, unsteadiness, fainting, and falling. Report such symptoms to your physician promptly.

Advisability of Use During Pregnancy

Pregnancy Category: C (tentative). See Pregnancy Code inside back cover.
Animal reproduction studies in rabbits reveal significant toxicity due to this drug.

Information from adequate studies in pregnant women is not available. Ask physician for guidance.

Advisability of Use While Nursing Infant

This drug is not known to be present in the mother's milk.

It is advisable to avoid use of this drug or to proceed with breast-feeding under physician supervision.

Habit-Forming Potential

None.

Effects of Overdosage

With Moderate Overdose: General weakness, slow pulse, orthostatic hypotension.

With Large Overdose: Marked drop in blood pressure, fainting, weak and slow pulse, cold and sweaty skin.

Possible Effects of Extended Use

Reduced reserve of heart muscle strength, which may result from prolonged use of high doses. This may increase the risk of heart failure.

Suggested Periodic Examinations While Taking This Drug (at physician's discretion)

Complete blood cell counts, including platelet counts.
Evaluation of heart function.

While Taking This Drug, Observe the Following

Foods: No interactions with drug. Follow physician's advice regarding salt and total caloric intake. Timing of drug and food: May be taken without regard to eating.

Beverages: No restrictions. This drug may be taken with milk.

Alcohol: Use with caution until combined effect has been determined. Alcohol may exaggerate this drug's ability to lower blood pressure and may increase its mild sedative action.

Tobacco Smoking: Follow physician's advice regarding use of tobacco. Nicotine may reduce this drug's effectiveness in treating angina and high blood pressure.

Marijuana Smoking

Occasional (once or twice weekly):   No interaction expected.
Daily: A mild to moderate increase in fatigue and lethargy.

Other Drugs

Nadolol may *increase* the effects of

- oral anti-diabetic drugs and insulin, causing or prolonging hypoglycemia. Careful dosage adjustments are necessary.
- other anti-hypertensive drugs, and cause excessive lowering of the blood pressure. Careful dosage adjustments are necessary.

- barbiturates and narcotic drugs, and cause dangerous oversedation.
- reserpine, and cause excessive sedation, depression, and low blood pressure.

Nadolol may *decrease* the effects of
- antihistamines, and reduce their effectiveness in treating allergies.
- anti-inflammatory drugs, including aspirin, cortisone, phenylbutazone (Azolid, Butazolidin, etc.), oxyphenbutazone (Oxalid, Tandearil).

Nadolol *taken concurrently* with
- digitalis preparations (digitoxin, digoxin, etc.), may cause adverse interactions—excessive slowing of heart action and reduction of digitalis effectiveness in treating heart failure. Careful dosage adjustments are necessary.
- quinidine, may cause excessive slowing of the heart. Careful dosage adjustments are necessary.

The following drugs may *increase* the effects of nadolol:
- phenytoin (Dantoin, Dilantin, etc.) may exaggerate its sedative action on the brain.

Driving a Vehicle, Operating Machinery, Engaging in Hazardous Activities: Avoid hazardous activities until the full extent of drowsiness and lethargy has been determined.

Aviation Note: The use of this drug and the disorder for which this drug is prescribed *are disqualifications* for the piloting of aircraft. Consultation with a designated Aviation Medical Examiner is advised.

Exposure to Sun: No restrictions.

Exposure to Cold: Use caution until combined effect has been determined. If you are subject to Raynaud's phenomenon, this drug may exaggerate further the impaired circulation in hands and feet.

Heavy Exercise or Exertion: Avoid levels of exertion which produced severe angina prior to the use of this drug. Isometric exercises—the "overload" technique for strengthening individual muscles—can raise the blood pressure significantly. The use of this drug may intensify the hypertensive response to isometric exercises. Ask your physician for guidance.

Occurrence of Unrelated Illness: If an illness causes vomiting and interrupts the regular use of this drug, notify your physician as soon as possible. In the event of injury or of need for emergency surgery, your attending physicians must be notified that you are taking this drug.

Discontinuation: This drug must not be discontinued abruptly. Gradual withdrawal over a period of 2 or more weeks is necessary to prevent serious increase of angina or risk of heart attack. Ask your physician for guidance.

Special Storage Instructions

Keep in a dry, tightly closed container, at room temperature. Protect from light, excessive heat, and moisture.

NAFCILLIN

Year Introduced: 1961

Brand Names

USA	Canada
Nafcil (Bristol)	Unipen (Wyeth)
Unipen (Wyeth)	

Common Synonyms ("Street Names"):   None

Drug Class: Antibiotic (Anti-infective), Penicillins

Prescription Required: Yes

Available for Purchase by Generic Name: No

Available Dosage Forms and Strengths
    Tablets — 500 mg.
    Capsules — 250 mg.
  Oral solution — 250 mg. per teaspoonful (5 ml.)

Tablet May Be Crushed or Capsule Opened for Administration: Yes

How This Drug Works
  Intended Therapeutic Effect(s):   The elimination of infections responsive to
  the action of this drug.
  Location of Drug Action(s):   Any body tissue or fluid in which sufficient
  concentration of the drug can be achieved.
  Method of Drug Action(s):   This drug destroys susceptible infecting bacteria
  by interfering with their ability to produce new protective cell walls as they
  multiply and grow.

Principal Uses of This Drug
  As a Single Drug Product: This type of penicillin is used specifically to treat
  infections caused by strains of staphylococcus bacteria that are resistant to
  other penicillins.

THIS DRUG SHOULD NOT BE TAKEN IF
—you have had an allergic reaction to any dosage form of it previously.
—you are certain you are allergic to any form of penicillin.

INFORM YOUR PHYSICIAN BEFORE TAKING THIS DRUG IF
—you suspect you may be allergic to penicillin, or you have a history of a
previous "reaction" to penicillin.
—you are allergic to cephalosporin antibiotics (Ancef, Ceporan, Ceporex, Kafocin, Keflex, Keflin, Kefzol, Loridine).
—you are allergic by nature (hayfever, asthma, hives, eczema).

Time Required for Apparent Benefit
  Varies with the nature of the infection under treatment; usually from 2 to 5
  days.

Possible Side-Effects *(natural, expected, and unavoidable drug actions)*
Superinfections (see Glossary).

Possible Adverse Effects *(unusual, unexpected, and infrequent reactions)*

IF ANY OF THE FOLLOWING DEVELOP, DISCONTINUE DRUG AND NOTIFY
YOUR PHYSICIAN AS SOON AS POSSIBLE

Mild Adverse Effects
Allergic Reactions: Skin rashes (various kinds).
Other Reactions: Irritation of mouth or tongue, "black tongue," nausea,
vomiting, diarrhea, gaseous indigestion.
Serious Adverse Effects
Allergic Reactions: †Anaphylactic reaction (see Glossary), severe skin
reactions, high fever, swollen painful joints, sore throat, unusual bleeding
or bruising.

Precautions for Use by Those over 60 Years of Age
It is advisable to evaluate kidney function before and during use of this drug
to determine the need for dosage adjustment.
Natural changes in the skin after 60 may predispose to severe and prolonged
itching reactions in the genital and anal regions. This reaction should be
reported promptly.

Advisability of Use During Pregnancy
Pregnancy Category: B (tentative). See Pregnancy Code inside back cover.
Animal reproduction studies in rats and rabbits reveal no birth defects due
to this drug.
Information from studies in pregnant women indicates no increase in de-
fects in 3546 pregnancies exposed to penicillin derivatives.
Ask physician for guidance.

Advisability of Use While Nursing Infant
Drug may be present in milk and can sensitize infant to penicillin. Ask
physician for guidance.

Habit-Forming Potential
None.

Effects of Overdosage
Possible nausea, vomiting, and/or diarrhea.

Possible Effects of Extended Use
Superinfections.

**Suggested Periodic Examinations While Taking This Drug (at physician's
discretion)**
Complete blood cell counts.
Liver and kidney function tests.

†A rare but potentially dangerous reaction characteristic of penicillins.

While Taking This Drug, Observe the Following

Foods: No restrictions of food selection. Drug is most effective when taken on an empty stomach, 1 hour before or 2 hours after eating.

Beverages: No restrictions.

Alcohol: No interactions expected.

Tobacco Smoking: No interactions expected.

Marijuana Smoking: No interactions expected.

Other Drugs

The following drugs may *decrease* the effects of nafcillin

- antacids can reduce absorption of nafcillin.
- chloramphenicol (Chloromycetin, etc.)
- erythromycin (Erythrocin, E-Mycin, etc.)
- paromomycin (Humatin)
- tetracyclines (see Drug Class, Section Three)
- troleandomycin (Cyclamycin, TAO)

Driving a Vehicle, Operating Machinery, Engaging in Hazardous Activities: Usually no restrictions. Be alert to the rare occurrence of nausea and/or diarrhea; restrict activities accordingly.

Aviation Note: The use of this drug *may be a disqualification* for the piloting of aircraft. Consultation with a designated Aviation Medical Examiner is advised.

Exposure to Sun: No restrictions.

Special Storage Instructions

Keep tablets and capsules in a tightly closed container at room temperature. Refrigerate oral solution.

Observe the Following Expiration Times

Do not take the oral solution of this drug if it is older than 1 week—when kept refrigerated.

NALIDIXIC ACID

Year Introduced: 1963

Brand Names

USA	Canada
NegGram (Winthrop)	NegGram (Winthrop)

Common Synonyms ("Street Names"):   None

Drug Class: Antimicrobial (Anti-infective)

Prescription Required: Yes

Available for Purchase by Generic Name: No

Available Dosage Forms and Strengths
Tablets — 250 mg., 500 mg., 1 g.
Suspension — 250 mg. per teaspoonful (5 ml.)

Tablet May Be Crushed or Capsule Opened for Administration: Yes

How This Drug Works
Intended Therapeutic Effect(s):   The elimination of infections in the urinary tract that are responsive to the action of this drug.

Location of Drug Action(s):   Primarily within the organs of the urinary tract —the kidneys, ureters, bladder, and urethra.

Method of Drug Action(s):   This drug destroys susceptible bacteria by inhibiting the formation of essential nuclear protein (DNA).

Principal Uses of This Drug
As a Single Drug Product: Because this drug is concentrated in the urine and never attains significant levels in the blood, it is used exclusively to treat infections of the urinary tract.

THIS DRUG SHOULD NOT BE TAKEN IF
—you have had an allergic reaction to any dosage form of it previously.
—you have any type of convulsive disorder (seizures, epilepsy).
—it is prescribed for an infant under 3 months of age.

INFORM YOUR PHYSICIAN BEFORE TAKING THIS DRUG IF
—you have a history of liver disease, or impaired liver function.
—you have a history of kidney disease, or impaired kidney function.
—you have impaired circulation within the brain.
—you have any form of parkinsonism.

Time Required for Apparent Benefit
From 1 to 2 weeks. Periodic urine examinations are required to evaluate response.

Possible Side-Effects *(natural, expected, and unavoidable drug actions)*
None reported.

Possible Adverse Effects *(unusual, unexpected, and infrequent reactions)*

IF ANY OF THE FOLLOWING DEVELOP, DISCONTINUE DRUG AND NOTIFY YOUR PHYSICIAN AS SOON AS POSSIBLE

Mild Adverse Effects
   Allergic Reactions: Itching, skin rash, hives, localized swellings, joint pain and swelling.
   Other Reactions
      Headache, dizziness, drowsiness, weakness.
      Visual disturbances such as overbrightness of lights, changes in color perception, difficulty in focusing, double vision.
      Nausea, vomiting, abdominal discomfort, diarrhea.
      Numbness and/or tingling.

Serious Adverse Effects
  Allergic Reactions
    Anaphylactic reaction (see Glossary).
    Drug fever (see Glossary).
  Idiosyncratic Reactions
    Hemolytic anemia (see Glossary).
    Behavioral disturbances (toxic psychosis).
    Convulsions, usually brief.
    Hepatitis with jaundice (see Glossary).
    Abnormally low white blood cells and/or blood platelets (see Glossary).

CAUTION

1. Infants, young children, and the elderly are more susceptible to behavioral disturbances and convulsions while taking this drug.
2. Some bacteria can develop resistance to this drug rapidly and render it ineffective. Adhere to dosage schedules closely, and take the full amount prescribed.
3. This drug can cause *false* positive results when any of these reagents are used to test the urine for sugar: Benedict's solution, Fehling's solution, Clinitest tablets. A false positive test result does *not* occur with the use of Clinistix or Tes-Tape.

Precautions for Use by Those over 60 Years of Age

The natural decline in kidney function that occurs after 60 may require reduction in dosage and lengthening of dosage intervals. Dosage must be carefully individualized and based upon measurements of kidney function.

Advisability of Use During Pregnancy

Pregnancy Category: C (tentative). See Pregnancy Code inside back cover. Animal reproduction studies in rats and rabbits reveal significant birth defects due to this drug.
Information from adequate studies in pregnant women is not available.
Avoid completely during first 3 months.
Ask physician for guidance.

Advisability of Use While Nursing Infant

No significant amounts of this drug have been found in the milk of mothers with normal kidney function. It can be present in the milk of mothers with reduced kidney function, and it can affect the nursing infant. Ask physician for guidance.

Habit-Forming Potential

None.

Effects of Overdosage

With Moderate Overdose: Nausea, vomiting, lethargy.
With Large Overdose: Behavioral disturbance (toxic psychosis), convulsions, shift of acid-alkaline balance of body chemistry resulting in acidosis with stupor and deep, exaggerated breathing.

Possible Effects of Extended Use
None reported.

Suggested Periodic Examinations While Taking This Drug (at physician's discretion)
Complete blood cell counts.
Liver function tests.
Kidney function tests.

While Taking This Drug, Observe the Following
Foods: No restrictions. Absorption is best when drug is taken 1 hour before eating. However, it may be taken with food if necessary to prevent stomach distress.

Beverages: No restrictions. May be taken with milk.

Alcohol: Use caution until combined effect has been determined. This drug in combination with alcohol may impair alertness, judgment, and physical coordination.

Tobacco Smoking: No interactions expected.

Marijuana Smoking: No interactions expected.

Other Drugs

Nalidixic acid may *increase* the effects of
- dicumarol.
- warfarin (Coumadin, etc.).

The following drugs may *increase* the effects of nalidixic acid
- Vitamin C (in large doses)

The following drugs may *decrease* the effects of nalidixic acid
- antacids may reduce its absorption.
- nitrofurantoin (Furadantin, Macrodantin, etc.)

Driving a Vehicle, Operating Machinery, Engaging in Hazardous Activities: Use caution until full effects of drug have been determined. Drowsiness, dizziness, or visual disturbance can impair ability to engage safely in hazardous activities.

Aviation Note: The use of this drug *may be a disqualification* for the piloting of aircraft. Consultation with a designated Aviation Medical Examiner is advised.

Exposure to Sun: Use caution until sensitivity has been determined. This drug can cause severe and prolonged photosensitivity (see Glossary).

Special Storage Instructions
Keep in a tightly closed container. Protect from light.

NAPROXEN

Year Introduced: 1975

Brand Names

USA	Canada
Anaprox (Syntex)	Apo-Naproxen (Apotex)
Naprosyn (Syntex)	Anaprox (Syntex)
	Naprosyn (Syntex)
	Novonaprox (Novopharm)

Common Synonyms ("Street Names"):   Arthritis medicine, aspirin substitute

Drug Class: Analgesic, Mild; Anti-inflammatory; Fever Reducer (Antipyretic)

Prescription Required: Yes

Available for Purchase by Generic Name: No

Available Dosage Forms and Strengths
Tablets — 250 mg., 275 mg., 375 mg., 500 mg.

Tablet May Be Crushed or Capsule Opened for Administration: Yes

How This Drug Works
Intended Therapeutic Effect(s)
Relief of joint pain, stiffness, inflammation, and swelling associated with arthritis.
Relief of mild to moderate pain from any cause. Relief of menstrual cramping (dysmenorrhea).
Location of Drug Action(s):   Not completely established. It is thought that this drug acts in the brain (at the level of the hypothalamus) and in the inflamed tissues of arthritic joints; also in traumatized tissues and in the menstruating uterus.
Method of Drug Action(s)
Not completely known. It is thought that this drug reduces the tissue concentration of prostaglandins, chemicals involved in the production of inflammation and pain.
By reducing the tissue levels of prostaglandins in the muscular wall of the uterus, this drug relieves menstrual cramping.

Principal Uses of This Drug
As a Single Drug Product: This "aspirin substitute" is used in a variety of conditions to relieve pain and inflammation. While its primary use is to provide symptomatic relief in acute and chronic arthritis, including gout, it is also used to relieve the pain associated with musculo-skeletal injuries, bursitis, tendinitis, menstrual cramping, and minor surgical procedures.

THIS DRUG SHOULD NOT BE TAKEN IF
—you have had an allergic reaction to any dosage form of it previously.
—you are allergic to aspirin (hives, nasal polyps, or asthma caused by aspirin).

—you have an active peptic ulcer, active gastritis, duodenitis, ileitis, or ulcerative colitis.

—it is prescribed for a child under 16 years of age.

INFORM YOUR PHYSICIAN BEFORE TAKING THIS DRUG IF

—you have a history of peptic ulcer or recurrent gastritis, duodenitis, ileitis, or colitis.

—you have diverticulosis.

—you have a history of heart disease.

—you have a tendency to retain water and develop edema.

—you have a history of kidney disease or reduced kidney function.

Time Required for Apparent Benefit

Drug action begins in 1 to 2 hours, reaches a maximum in 2 to 4 hours, and gradually subsides within 24 to 26 hours. Significant improvement may require continuous use on a regular schedule for 1 to 2 weeks.

Possible Side-Effects *(natural, expected, and unavoidable drug actions)*

Prolongation of bleeding time.

Possible Adverse Effects *(unusual, unexpected, and infrequent reactions)*

IF ANY OF THE FOLLOWING DEVELOP, DISCONTINUE DRUG AND NOTIFY YOUR PHYSICIAN AS SOON AS POSSIBLE

Mild Adverse Effects

Allergic Reactions: Itching, rash, hives, localized swellings, spontaneous bruising.

Other Reactions

Headache, lightheadedness, dizziness, ringing in the ears, drowsiness, fatigue, inability to concentrate.

Nausea, vomiting, heartburn, indigestion, abdominal pain, diarrhea, irritation of mouth.

Mild fluid retention (edema) in face or legs.

Serious Adverse Effects

Stomach or intestinal bleeding, mild to severe, with or without the development of ulcer. (Observe for dark-colored stools.)

Hepatitis with jaundice (see Glossary).

Visual disturbances due to corneal changes, lens opacities, retinal changes.

Hearing impairment.

Reduction of white blood cells and/or blood platelets (see Glossary).

Diverticulitis.

CAUTION

This drug's anti-inflammatory and antipyretic effects can make it more difficult to recognize the presence of infection. If you develop any symptoms that suggest an active infection, inform your physician promptly.

Precautions for Use by Those over 60 Years of Age

You may be more sensitive to all of the actions of this drug. Small doses are advisable until your individual response has been determined.

You may be more susceptible to the development of headache, dizziness, confusion, impairment of memory, stomach ulcer, stomach bleeding, and diarrhea.

Advisability of Use During Pregnancy

Pregnancy Category: B (tentative). See Pregnancy Code inside back cover. Animal reproduction studies reveal no birth defects due to this drug. Information from adequate studies in pregnant women is not available. Ask physician for guidance.

Advisability of Use While Nursing Infant

This drug is known to be present in milk in very small amounts. Ask physician for guidance.

Habit-Forming Potential

None.

Effects of Overdosage

With Moderate Overdose: Nausea, vomiting, heartburn.

With Large Overdose: Drowsiness. No other serious or threatening effects reported to date.

Possible Effects of Extended Use

Eye changes such as opacities in the cornea or lens, deterioration of the retina (macular area).

Kidney damage.

Suggested Periodic Examinations While Taking This Drug (at physician's discretion)

Complete blood cell counts to detect development of:
 Anemia, due to silent bleeding from the stomach.
 Reduction of white blood cells.
 Reduction of blood platelets.
Liver function tests.
Kidney function tests.
Complete eye examinations if any change in vision occurs.
Hearing examinations if ringing in the ears or hearing impairment develops.

While Taking This Drug, Observe the Following

Foods: No restrictions. This drug should be taken with food if stomach irritation occurs.

Beverages: No restrictions. May be taken with milk.

Alcohol: Use with caution. The irritant action of alcohol on the stomach lining added to the irritant action of naproxen in sensitive individuals can increase the risk of stomach bleeding or ulceration.

Tobacco Smoking: No interactions expected.

Marijuana Smoking
 Occasional (once or twice weekly):   No effect to mild increase in pain relief from this drug.
 Daily: Moderate increase in pain relief from this drug.

Other Drugs

Naproxen may *increase* the effects of
- anticoagulants of the coumarin family (see Drug Class, Section Three).
- anti-diabetic drugs of the sulfonylurea family (see Drug Class, Section Three).
- phenytoin (Dantoin, Dilantin, etc.).
- sulfonamides (see Drug Class, Section Three).

The following drug may *decrease* the effects of naproxen
- aspirin may hasten its elimination from the body.

Driving a Vehicle, Operating Machinery, Engaging in Hazardous Activities: Use caution until full effect has been determined. This drug can cause drowsiness and dizziness and can impair the ability to engage safely in hazardous activities.

Aviation Note: The use of this drug *may be a disqualification* for the piloting of aircraft. Consultation with a designated Aviation Medical Examiner is advised.

Exposure to Sun: No restrictions.

Special Storage Instructions

Keep in a dry, tightly closed container.

NICOTINIC ACID
(Niacin)

Year Introduced: 1937

Brand Names

USA		Canada
Niacin (Various Manufacturers)	Nico-Span (Key) Nicotinex (Fleming)	Niacin (Various Manufacturers)
Nicalex (Merrell-National)	(Numerous other brand and	Novoniacin (Novopharm)
Nicobid (Armour)	combination brand	
Nicolar (Armour)	names)	

Common Synonyms ("Street Names"): None

Drug Class: Vasodilator; Cholesterol Reducer (Antihyperlipemic)

Prescription Required: For tablets and elixir—No
For capsules—Yes

Available for Purchase by Generic Name: Yes

Available Dosage Forms and Strengths

Tablets — 50 mg., 100 mg., 250 mg., 500 mg.

Prolonged-action tablets — 150 mg.

Capsules — 125 mg., 250 mg., 500 mg.

Prolonged-action capsules — 125 mg., 200 mg., 250 mg., 300 mg., 400 mg., 500 mg.

Elixir — 50 mg. per teaspoonful (5 ml.)

Tablet May Be Crushed or Capsule Opened for Administration

Regular tablets and capsules — Yes

Prolonged-action capsules — No

Nicobid Tempule — Yes, but do not crush or chew contents

How This Drug Works

Intended Therapeutic Effect(s)

Prevention and treatment of pellagra, a disease resulting from deficiency of nicotinic acid and characterized by dermatitis, diarrhea, and mental disturbances.

Increased circulation of blood to the head, thought to be of benefit in the treatment of vertigo, ringing in the ears, and premenstrual headache.

Reduction of the blood levels of cholesterol and triglycerides (using doses of 3 grams daily).

Location of Drug Action(s)

Tissues throughout the body that require nicotinic acid as a component of essential enzyme systems.

Blood vessels in the skin of the "blush area" (the face and neck).

Fatty tissues throughout the body; possibly the liver.

Method of Drug Action(s)

By correcting a deficiency of nicotinic acid in the tissues, this drug in adequate dosage can prevent or relieve the manifestations of pellagra.

Dilation of blood vessels is thought to be limited to the skin, an action of questionable therapeutic value. Increased blood flow within the brain has not been demonstrated.

It is thought that this drug (in large dosage) reduces the initial production of cholesterol and prevents the conversion of fatty tissue to cholesterol and triglycerides.

Principal Uses of This Drug

As a Single Drug Product: This drug is used to treat three unrelated conditions: (1) Pellagra, a deficiency disorder due to inadequate intake of nicotinic acid (niacin, Vitamin B-3). (2) Certain patterns of high blood fats—cholesterol and triglycerides—in individuals considered to be at high risk for the development of coronary artery disease. (3) Vertigo and ringing in the ears thought to be due to impaired blood flow to the inner ear.

THIS DRUG SHOULD NOT BE TAKEN IF

—you have had an allergic reaction to any dosage form of it previously. A combination drug [CD] should not be taken if you are allergic to *any* of its ingredients.

—you have impaired liver function.
—you have an active peptic ulcer (stomach or duodenum).

INFORM YOUR PHYSICIAN BEFORE TAKING THIS DRUG IF
—you have a history of peptic ulcer, liver disease, jaundice, or gall bladder
  disease.
—you have diabetes.
—you have gout.

Time Required for Apparent Benefit
Drug action begins in approximately 15 to 20 minutes and persists for 1 hour.

Possible Side-Effects *(natural, expected, and unavoidable drug actions)*
Flushing, itching, or tingling sensations, and feeling of warmth. Sensitive
individuals may experience orthostatic hypotension (see Glossary).

Possible Adverse Effects *(unusual, unexpected, and infrequent reactions)*
**IF ANY OF THE FOLLOWING DEVELOP, DISCONTINUE DRUG AND NOTIFY
YOUR PHYSICIAN AS SOON AS POSSIBLE**

Mild Adverse Effects
  Allergic Reactions: Skin rash, itching, hives.
  Other Reactions
    Headache, dimness of vision.
    Nausea, indigestion, vomiting, diarrhea.
    Dryness of skin, grayish-black pigmentation of skin folds.
Serious Adverse Effects
  Activation of peptic ulcer.
  Hepatitis with jaundice (see Glossary)—yellow eyes and skin, dark-colored
    urine, light-colored stools.
  Worsening of diabetes and gout.

CAUTION
Small doses (as used for vasodilation) are usually well tolerated and free of
serious adverse effects. Large doses used for prolonged periods of time may
be more hazardous.

Precautions for Use by Those over 60 Years of Age
It is not possible to predict in advance the nature of your response to this
drug. It may relieve your symptoms, have no significant effect, or make
your symptoms worse. Dosage must be carefully individualized.

Advisability of Use During Pregnancy
Pregnancy Category: C (tentative). See Pregnancy Code inside back cover.
  Animal reproduction studies in chicks reveal significant birth defects due
    to this drug.
  Information from adequate studies in pregnant women is not available.
  Ask physician for guidance.

Advisability of Use While Nursing Infant
Presence of drug in milk is not known. Safety for infant not established. Ask
physician for guidance.

Habit-Forming Potential
None.

Effects of Overdosage
With Moderate Overdose: Severe generalized flushing, nausea, vomiting, abdominal cramping, diarrhea.

With Large Overdose: Weakness, lightheadedness, fainting, sweating.

Possible Effects of Extended Use
Disturbance of liver function.

Suggested Periodic Examinations While Taking This Drug (at physician's discretion)
Liver function tests.
Measurement of blood sugar (glucose) levels.
Measurement of blood uric acid levels.

While Taking This Drug, Observe the Following
Foods: No interactions. Advisable to take drug with or following food to reduce stomach irritation.

Beverages: No restrictions.

Alcohol: Use caution until combined effects have been determined. Alcohol used with large doses of this drug may cause excessive lowering of the blood pressure.

Tobacco Smoking: The nicotine in tobacco can cause blood vessel constriction, the opposite of the dilation produced by nicotinic acid. Smoking may reduce the effectiveness of this drug.

Marijuana Smoking: No interactions expected.

Other Drugs

Nicotinic acid may *increase* the effects of

• some anti-hypertensive drugs, and cause excessive lowering of the blood pressure. Dosage adjustments may be necessary for guanethidine (Ismelin, Esimil), mecamylamine (Inversine), methyldopa (Aldomet), pargyline (Eutonyl), and propranolol (Inderal).

Nicotinic acid may *decrease* the effects of

• anti-diabetic drugs, by raising the level of blood sugar. Doses of insulin or oral anti-diabetic drugs may have to be raised or the diet may have to be modified.

Driving a Vehicle, Operating Machinery, Engaging in Hazardous Activities: Usually no restrictions. Determine first that this drug does not cause orthostatic hypotension.

Aviation Note: The use of this drug *may be a disqualification* for the piloting of aircraft. Consultation with a designated Aviation Medical Examiner is advised.

Exposure to Sun: No restrictions.

Special Storage Instructions
Keep in a dry, tightly closed container.

NIFEDIPINE

Year Introduced: 1972

Brand Names

USA	Canada
Procardia (Pfizer)	Adalat (Miles)

Common Synonyms ("Street Names"):   Angina pills, heart pills

Drug Class: Anti-anginal, Calcium channel blocker

Prescription Required: USA: Yes   Canada: Yes

Available for Purchase by Generic Name: USA: No   Canada: No

Available Dosage Forms and Strengths
Capsules — 10 mg.

Tablet May Be Crushed or Capsule Opened for Administration: No

How This Drug Works
   Intended Therapeutic Effect(s):   Reduction in the frequency and severity of pain associated with angina pectoris.
   Location of Drug Action(s):   Specific sites (the calcium channels) in the walls of cells that comprise the heart muscle and the muscular layers of small arteries.
   Method of Drug Action(s):   By blocking the flow of calcium through certain cell walls, this drug impairs the ability of the heart muscle to contract and the ability of the muscular walls of small arteries to constrict. The consequences are (1) the relaxation and prevention of coronary artery constriction, and (2) the reduction of the work load on the heart muscle. The net effects of improved coronary artery blood flow and reduced oxygen demand by the heart muscle are resposible for the reduction in the frequency and severity of angina pain.

Principal Uses of This Drug
   As a Single Drug Product: Used primarily to treat both types of angina, the classical effort-induced angina associated with coronary artery disease (atherosclerosis), and the variant type of angina due to spasm of the coronary artery (Prinzmetal's angina).

THIS DRUG SHOULD NOT BE TAKEN IF
—you have had an allergic reaction to it previously.
—you have active liver disease.

INFORM YOUR PHYSICIAN BEFORE TAKING THIS DRUG IF
—you are taking *any* other drugs at this time.
—you have had a recent stroke or heart attack.
—you have a history of heart disease, especially heart rhythm disturbances.
—you have impaired liver or kidney function.
—you have diabetes.

Time Required for Apparent Benefit
Drug action usually begins in 20 minutes and reaches its peak in 1 to 2 hours. Continuous use on a regular schedule for 1 to 2 weeks is usually necessary to determine this drug's effectiveness in preventing angina.

Possible Side-Effects *(natural, expected, and unavoidable drug actions)*
Flushing and sensation of warmth (25%), sweating, fluid retention (7%), low blood pressure, rapid heart rate.

Possible Adverse Effects *(unusual, unexpected, and infrequent reactions)*

IF ANY OF THE FOLLOWING DEVELOP, DISCONTINUE DRUG AND NOTIFY YOUR PHYSICIAN AS SOON AS POSSIBLE

Mild Adverse Effects
Allergic Reactions: Skin eruptions, itching, hives, drug fever (see Glossary).
Other Reactions: Headache (23%), dizziness (27%), weakness (12%), nervousness (7%), blurred vision.
Palpitation (7%), shortness of breath, cough, wheezing (6%).
Nausea, heartburn (11%), cramps, diarrhea (2%).
Tremors, muscle cramps (8%).

Serious Adverse Effects
Allergic Reactions: Drug-induced hepatitis (very rare).
Idiosyncratic Reactions: Joint stiffness and inflammation.
Other Reactions: *Increased* frequency, duration, or severity of angina on initiation of treatment or following an increase in dosage. (This is thought to be due to an excessive drop in blood pressure with resultant increase in heart rate—a rare reaction.)
Marked drop in blood pressure with fainting.
Impaired sexual function.

Adverse Effects That May Mimic Natural Diseases or Disorders
An allergic skin eruption and swelling of the legs can resemble erysipelas. An allergic reaction within the liver may suggest the development of viral hepatitis.

CAUTION
1. If this drug is used concurrently with a "beta-blocker" drug, you may develop excessively low blood pressure. Consult your physician regarding this possibility.
2. This drug may cause swelling of the feet and ankles. This is not indicative of heart or kidney trouble.
3. If you notice any increase in the frequency, duration or severity of angina pain, inform your physician promptly.

Precautions for Use by Those over 60 Years of Age
It is advisable to begin treatment with small doses and to increase the dosage gradually if needed.
Observe carefully for any tendency to lightheadedness or dizziness that could cause falling and injury.

Advisability of Use During Pregnancy

Pregnancy Category: C (tentative). See Pregnancy Code inside back cover.
Animal reproductive studies reveal toxic effects on the embryo in mice,
rats, and rabbits, and birth defects in rats.
Information from adequate studies in pregnant women is not available.
Avoid this drug during the first 3 months. Use it during the last 6 months
only if clearly needed.

Advisability of Use While Nursing Infant

The presence of this drug in human milk is not known.
If this drug is used, monitor the nursing infant for
poor feeding and possible low blood pressure.

Habit-Forming Potential

None.

Effects of Overdosage

With Moderate Overdose: Flushed and warm skin, sweating, lightheadedness, irritability, tremors, rapid heart rate, low blood pressure.
With Large Overdose: Marked low blood pressure, loss of consciousness.

Possible Effects of Extended Use

None identified.

Suggested Periodic Examinations While Taking This Drug (at physician's discretion)

Measurements of blood pressure in lying, sitting, and standing positions.

While Taking This Drug, Observe the Following

Foods: No specific restrictions. Avoid excessive salt. May be taken with or
following food to reduce stomach irritation.
Beverages: No restrictions. May be taken with milk.
Alcohol: Use caution until the combined effects have been determined.
Alcohol can enhance the blood pressure-lowering effects of this drug.
Tobacco Smoking: To be avoided. Nicotine can inhibit the potential bene-
fits of this drug significantly.

Marijuana Smoking

Occasional (once or twice weekly): No effect to mild and transient additional lowering of the blood pressure.
Daily: Possible increase in heart rate and further lowering of the blood
pressure.

Other Drugs

Nifedipine may *increase* the effects of
- nitroglycerin and the long-acting nitrates in the treatment of angina
(improved anti-anginal effects).

Nifedipine *taken concurrently* with
- beta-blocking drugs (see Drug Class, Section Three) may increase the risk
of worsening angina, inducing low blood pressure, or initiating congestive
heart failure.

Driving a Vehicle, Operating Machinery, Engaging in Hazardous Activities: Usually no restrictions. However, it is advisable to observe for the possible occurrence of excessively low blood pressure with dizziness and weakness; restrict activities accordingly.

Aviation Note: Angina pectoris *is a disqualification* for the piloting of aircraft. Consultation with a designated Aviation Medical Examiner is advised.

Exposure to Sun: No restrictions.

Exposure to Heat: Use caution. Hot environments can enhance the blood pressure-lowering effects of this drug.

Exposure to Cold: Use caution. Cold environments can induce angina and reduce the effectiveness of this drug.

Heavy Exercise or Exertion: Use caution. This drug can increase your tolerance for exercise. Avoid exertion that causes angina or shortness of breath.

Occurrence of Unrelated Illness: The fever associated with serious infections can lower the blood pressure. Observe carefully for the combined effects while taking this drug.

Discontinuation: No withdrawal effects have been reported when this drug is stopped abruptly. However, it is advisable to reduce the dose gradually over a period of 7 to 10 days, and to monitor for the possible development of rebound angina.

Special Storage Instructions

Keep in original container at room temperature. Protect from light, moisture, and excessive heat.

NITROFURANTOIN

Year Introduced: 1953

Brand Names

USA		Canada
Furadantin (Norwich-Eaton)	Macrodantin (Norwich-Eaton)	Apo-Nitrofurantoin (Apotex)
Furalan (Lannett)	Nitrex (Star)	Furatine (ICN)
Furaloid (Edwards)	Nitrodan (Century)	Macrodantin (Norwich-Eaton)
Furantoin (North Amer. Pharm.)	Sarodant (Saron)	Nephronex (Cortunon)
	Urotoin (Scruggs)	Nifuran (Technilab)
		Novofuran (Novopharm)

Common Synonyms ("Street Names"):   None

Drug Class: Antimicrobial (Anti-infective) [Nitrofurans]

Prescription Required: Yes

Available for Purchase by Generic Name: Yes

Available Dosage Forms and Strengths
    Tablets — 50 mg., 100 mg.
    Capsules — 25 mg., 50 mg., 100 mg.
Oral suspension — 25 mg. per teaspoonful (5 ml.)

Tablet May Be Crushed or Capsule Opened for Administration: Yes

How This Drug Works
    Intended Therapeutic Effect(s):   The elimination of infections responsive to
    the action of this drug.
    Location of Drug Action(s):   Any body tissue or fluid in which sufficient
    concentration of the drug can be achieved.
    Method of Drug Action(s):   Not completely established. It is thought that
    this drug prevents growth and multiplication of susceptible bacteria by
    interfering with the function of essential enzyme systems.

Principal Uses of This Drug
    As a Single Drug Product: Because this drug is concentrated in the urine
    and attains only low levels in the blood, its use is limited to the prevention
    or treatment of infections in the urinary tract.

THIS DRUG SHOULD NOT BE TAKEN IF
—you have had an allergic reaction to any dosage form of it previously.
—you have serious impairment of kidney function.
—you are in the last month of pregnancy.
—you cannot abstain from drinking alcohol.
—it is prescribed for an infant under 1 month of age.

INFORM YOUR PHYSICIAN BEFORE TAKING THIS DRUG IF
—you are allergic to any nitrofuran drug.
—you have a history of kidney disease.

Time Required for Apparent Benefit
    From 1 to 2 weeks. Periodic urine examinations required to evaluate re-
    sponse.

Possible Side-Effects *(natural, expected, and unavoidable drug actions)*
    Brown discoloration of the urine, of no significance.

Possible Adverse Effects *(unusual, unexpected, and infrequent reactions)*
    **IF ANY OF THE FOLLOWING DEVELOP, DISCONTINUE DRUG AND NOTIFY
    YOUR PHYSICIAN AS SOON AS POSSIBLE**

    Mild Adverse Effects
        Allergic Reactions: Skin rashes (various kinds), hives, itching, swelling of
        face or extremities, fever, chills.
        Other Reactions
        Nausea, vomiting, diarrhea, abdominal cramps.

Headache, dizziness, drowsiness, muscle aching, temporary loss of hair, impaired color vision, burning and tearing of eyes.

Serious Adverse Effects

Allergic Reactions: Anaphylactic reaction (see Glossary), severe allergic reaction in lungs (giving the appearance of pneumonia), asthma, jaundice, drop in blood pressure, joint pain.

Idiosyncratic Reaction: Hemolytic anemia (see Glossary).

Other Reactions

Peripheral neuritis (see Glossary).

Liver damage with jaundice (see Glossary).

Superinfections (see Glossary).

CAUTION

Troublesome and persistent diarrhea can develop in sensitive individuals. If diarrhea persists more than 24 hours, discontinue this drug and consult your physician for guidance.

Precautions for Use by Those over 60 Years of Age

The natural decline in kidney function that occurs after 60 may require reduction in dosage and lengthening of dosage intervals. Dosage must be carefully individualized and based upon measurements of kidney function.

Advisability of Use During Pregnancy

Pregnancy Category: C (tentative). See Pregnancy Code inside back cover.

Animal reproduction studies: No data available.

Information from adequate studies in pregnant women is not available.

The manufacturers state that this drug is contraindicated just prior to termination of pregnancy.

Ask physician for guidance.

Advisability of Use While Nursing Infant

Drug can be present in milk. Safety for infant not established. Ask physician for guidance.

Habit-Forming Potential

None.

Effects of Overdosage

Nausea, vomiting, abdominal pain, diarrhea.

Possible Effects of Extended Use

Varying degrees of allergic reaction within the lungs, from mild to severe. (Physician should be informed of chest pain, shortness of breath, or cough.)

Superinfections (see Glossary) within the urinary system.

Suggested Periodic Examinations While Taking This Drug (at physician's discretion)

Complete blood cell counts.

Liver function tests.

X-ray examination of lungs (during extended use of drug).

While Taking This Drug, Observe the Following

Foods: No restrictions of food selection. Drug should be taken with meals, or with food or milk if taken at bedtime.

Beverages: No restrictions.

Alcohol: Use with extreme caution until combined effects have been determined. This drug, in combination with alcohol, may cause a disulfiram-like reaction in sensitive individuals (see Glossary).

Tobacco Smoking: No interactions expected.

Marijuana Smoking: No interactions expected.

Other Drugs

The following drug may *increase* the effects of nitrofurantoin
- probenecid (Benemid) may delay its elimination from the body.

The following drugs may *decrease* the effects of nitrofurantoin
- phenobarbital may reduce its absorption and hasten its elimination from the body.
- nalidixic acid (NegGram) may reduce its antimicrobial action and impair its effectiveness in treatment.

Driving a Vehicle, Operating Machinery, Engaging in Hazardous Activities: No restrictions unless dizziness occurs.

Aviation Note: The use of this drug *may be a disqualification* for the piloting of aircraft. Consultation with a designated Aviation Medical Examiner is advised.

Exposure to Sun: No restrictions.

Special Storage Instructions

Keep in a tightly closed, light-resistant container.

NITROGLYCERIN

Year Introduced: 1890

Brand Names

USA		Canada
Nitro-Bid (Marion)	Nitrostat	Nitro-Bid (Roussel)
Nitrodisc (Searle)	(Parke-Davis)	Nitrol (K-U)
Nitro-Dur (Key)	Susadrin (Merrell	Nitrong
Nitroglyn (Key	Dow)	(Rhone-Poulenc)
Pharmaceuticals)	Transderm-Nitro	Nitrostabilin (A & H)
Nitrospan (USV)	(CIBA)	Nitrostat (P.D. & Co.)
		Tridil (AHS)

Common Synonyms ("Street Names"):   Angina pills, heart pills

Drug Class: Anti-anginal, Nitrates

Prescription Required: USA: Yes   Canada: No

Available for Purchase by Generic Name: Yes

Available Dosage Forms and Strengths
Sublingual tablets — 0.15 mg., 0.3 mg., 0.4 mg., 0.6 mg.
Prolonged-action tablets — 1.3 mg., 2.6 mg., 6.5 mg., 9 mg.
Prolonged-action capsules — 2.5 mg., 6.5 mg., 9 mg.
Ointment — 2%
Transmucosal Tablets — 1 mg., 2 mg.
Transdermal System — 2.5 mg., 5 mg., 7.5 mg., 10 mg., 15 mg., all per 24 hours

Tablet May Be Crushed or Capsule Opened for Administration: No; Nitro-Bid Plateau capsules and Nitrospan capsules—Yes, but do not crush or chew contents

How This Drug Works
Intended Therapeutic Effect(s):   Reduction in the frequency and severity of pain associated with angina pectoris (coronary insufficiency).
Location of Drug Action(s):   The muscular tissue in the walls of the blood vessels. The principal site of therapeutic action is the system of coronary arteries in the heart.
Method of Drug Action(s):   This drug acts directly on the muscle cell to produce relaxation. This permits expansion of blood vessels and increases the supply of blood and oxygen to meet the needs of the working heart muscle.

Principal Uses of This Drug
As a Single Drug Product: Used primarily in the treatment of symptomatic coronary artery disease. The rapid-action forms are used to relieve acute attacks of anginal pain at their onset. The sustained-action forms are used to prevent the development of angina.

THIS DRUG SHOULD NOT BE TAKEN IF
—you have had an allergic reaction to any dosage form of it previously.

INFORM YOUR PHYSICIAN BEFORE TAKING THIS DRUG IF
—you have glaucoma.
—you have had an unfavorable response to any vasodilator drug in the past.

Time Required for Apparent Benefit
The action of the sublingual tablet (dissolved under the tongue) begins in 1 to 3 minutes and persists for approximately 20 minutes. The action of the prolonged action preparations begins in approximately 30 minutes and persists for 8 to 12 hours.

Possible Side-Effects *(natural, expected, and unavoidable drug actions)*
Flushing of the face, throbbing in the head, increased heart rate (faster pulse), lightheadedness in upright position (see orthostatic hypotension in Glossary).

Possible Adverse Effects *(unusual, unexpected, and infrequent reactions)*

IF ANY OF THE FOLLOWING DEVELOP, DISCONTINUE DRUG AND NOTIFY YOUR PHYSICIAN AS SOON AS POSSIBLE

Mild Adverse Effects
 Allergic Reactions: Skin rash.
 Other Reactions
  Headache (may be persistent), dizziness, fainting.
  Nausea, vomiting.
Serious Adverse Effects
 Allergic Reactions: Severe dermatitis with peeling of skin.

CAUTION
Many over-the-counter (OTC) medications (see Glossary) for allergies, colds, and coughs contain drugs that may counteract the desired effects of this drug. Ask your physician or pharmacist for guidance before using any such medications.

Precautions for Use by Those over 60 Years of Age
You may be more sensitive to the actions of this drug. Small doses are advisable until your individual response has been determined.
You may be more susceptible to the development of low blood pressure with associated lightheadedness, dizziness, unsteadiness, and falling.

Advisability of Use During Pregnancy
Pregnancy Category: "C" (Tentative). See Pregnancy Code inside back cover.
Animal reproduction studies: No data available.
Information from adequate studies in pregnant women is not available. Ask physician for guidance.

Advisability of Use While Nursing Infant
Presence of drug in milk is not known. Safety for infant not established. Ask physician for guidance.

Habit-Forming Potential
None.

Effects of Overdosage
With Moderate Overdose: Headache, dizziness, marked flushing of the skin.
With Large Overdose: Vomiting, weakness, sweating, fainting, shortness of breath, coma.

Possible Effects of Extended Use
The development of tolerance (see Glossary), which may reduce the drug's effectiveness at recommended doses.
The development of abnormal hemoglobin (red blood cell pigment).

Suggested Periodic Examinations While Taking This Drug (at physician's discretion)

Measurement of internal eye pressure in those individuals with glaucoma or a tendency to glaucoma.

Red blood cell counts and hemoglobin measurements.

While Taking This Drug, Observe the Following

Foods: No restrictions.

Beverages: No restrictions.

Alcohol: Use extreme caution until combined effects have been determined. Avoid alcohol completely in the presence of any side-effects or adverse effects from nitroglycerin. Never use alcohol in the presence of a nitroglycerin headache.

Tobacco Smoking: Nicotine may reduce the effectiveness of this drug. Follow physician's advice regarding smoking, based upon its effect on the condition under treatment and its possible interaction with this drug.

Marijuana Smoking

Occasional (once or twice weekly):   No interactions expected.

Daily: Possible reduced effectiveness of this drug; mild to moderate increase in angina; possible changes in electrocardiogram, confusing interpretation.

Other Drugs

Nitroglycerin may *increase* the effects of

• atropine-like drugs (see Drug Class, Section Three), and cause an increase in internal eye pressure.

• tricyclic antidepressants (see Drug Class, Section Three), and cause excessive lowering of the blood pressure.

Nitroglycerin may *decrease* the effects of

• all choline-like drugs, such as Mestinon, Mytelase, pilocarpine, Prostigmin, and Urecholine.

Nitroglycerin *taken concurrently* with

• anti-hypertensive drugs, may cause severe drop in blood pressure. Careful monitoring of drug response and appropriate dosage adjustments are necessary.

The following drug may *increase* the effects of nitroglycerin

• propranolol (Inderal) may cause additional lowering of the blood pressure. Dosage adjustments may be necessary.

Driving a Vehicle, Operating Machinery, Engaging in Hazardous Activities: Usually no restrictions. Before engaging in hazardous activities, determine that this drug will not cause you to have orthostatic hypotension.

Aviation Note: Coronary artery disease *is a disqualification* for the piloting of aircraft. Consultation with a designated Aviation Medical Examiner is advised.

Exposure to Sun: No restrictions.

Exposure to Cold: Cold environment may reduce the effectiveness of this drug.

Heavy Exercise or Exertion: This drug may improve your ability to be more active without resulting anginal pain. Use caution and avoid excessive exertion that could cause heart injury if warning pain is delayed.

Special Storage Instructions
To prevent loss of strength
- keep tablets in the original glass container.
- do not transfer tablets to a plastic or metallic container (such as a pill box).
- do not place absorbent cotton, paper (such as the prescription label), or other material inside the container.
- do not store other drugs in the same container.
- close the container tightly immediately after each use.
- store at room temperature (59° to 86° F, 15° to 30° C).

Observe the Following Expiration Times
Do not use the sublingual tablet of this drug if older than 60 days from the date of opening the original container. With repeated exposure to air, nitroglycerin gradually loses its strength and becomes ineffective.

NORTRIPTYLINE

Year Introduced: 1964

Brand Names

USA	Canada
Aventyl (Lilly)	Aventyl (Lilly)
Pamelor (Sandoz)	

Common Synonyms ("Street Names"):   None

Drug Class: Antidepressant, Tricyclic

Prescription Required: Yes

Available for Purchase by Generic Name: No

Available Dosage Forms and Strengths
Capsules — 10 mg., 25 mg., 75 mg.
Oral liquid — 10 mg. per teaspoonful (5 ml.)

Tablet May Be Crushed or Capsule Opened for Administration: Yes

How This Drug Works
Intended Therapeutic Effect(s):   Gradual improvement of mood and relief of emotional depression.
Location of Drug Action(s):   Those areas of the brain that determine mood and emotional stability.

Method of Drug Action(s):   Not established. Present thinking is that this drug slowly restores to normal levels certain constitutents of brain tissue (such as norepinephrine) that transmit nerve impulses.

Principal Uses of This Drug
As a Single Drug Product: To relieve the symptoms associated with spontaneous (endogenous) depression, and to initiate the restoration of normal mood. This drug should be used only when a diagnosis of a true, primary depression of significant degree has been established. It should not be used to treat the symptoms of mild and transient (reactive) depression that may be associated with many life situations in the absence of a bona fide affective illness.

THIS DRUG SHOULD NOT BE TAKEN IF
—you have had an allergic reaction to any dosage form of it previously.
—you are taking or have taken within the past 14 days any mono-amine oxidase (MAO) inhibitor drug (see Drug Class, Section Three).
—you are recovering from a recent heart attack.
—you have glaucoma (narrow-angle type).
—it is prescribed for a child under 12 years of age.

INFORM YOUR PHYSICIAN BEFORE TAKING THIS DRUG IF
—you are allergic or sensitive to any other tricyclic antidepressant (see Drug Class, Section Three).
—you have a history of any of the following: diabetes, epilepsy, glaucoma, heart disease, prostate gland enlargement, or overactive thyroid function.
—you plan to have surgery under general anesthesia in the near future.

Time Required for Apparent Benefit
Some benefit may be apparent within the first 1 to 2 weeks. Adequate response may require continuous treatment for 4 to 6 weeks.

Possible Side-Effects *(natural, expected, and unavoidable drug actions)*
Drowsiness, blurring of vision, dryness of mouth, constipation, impaired urination.

Possible Adverse Effects *(unusual, unexpected, and infrequent reactions)*
IF ANY OF THE FOLLOWING DEVELOP, DISCONTINUE DRUG AND NOTIFY YOUR PHYSICIAN AS SOON AS POSSIBLE
Mild Adverse Effects
Allergic Reactions: Skin rash, hives, swelling of face or tongue, drug fever.
Other Reactions
   Nausea, indigestion, irritation of tongue or mouth, peculiar taste.
   Headache, dizziness, weakness, fainting, unsteady gait, tremors.
   Swelling of testicles, breast enlargement, milk formation.
   Fluctuation of blood sugar levels.
Serious Adverse Effects
Allergic Reactions: Hepatitis with jaundice (see Glossary).
Other Reactions
   Confusion (especially in the elderly), hallucinations, agitation, restlessness, nightmares.

Heart palpitation and irregular rhythm.

Bone marrow depression (see Glossary)—fatigue, weakness, fever, sore throat, unusual bleeding or bruising.

Peripheral neuritis (see Glossary)—numbness, tingling, pain, loss of strength in arms and legs.

Parkinson-like disorders (see Glossary)—usually mild and infrequent; more likely to occur in the elderly (over 60 years of age).

Precautions for Use by Those over 60 Years of Age

During the first 2 weeks of treatment observe for the development of confusional reactions—restlessness, agitation, forgetfulness, disorientation, delusions, and hallucinations. Reduction of dosage or discontinuation may be necessary.

Observe for incoordination and instability in stance and gait which may predispose to falling and injury.

This drug can increase the degree of impaired urination associated with prostate gland enlargement (prostatism).

Advisability of Use During Pregnancy

Pregnancy Category: C (tentative). See Pregnancy Code inside back cover. Animal reproduction studies are inconclusive.

Information from adequate studies in pregnant women is not available. Ask physician for guidance.

Advisability of Use While Nursing Infant

This drug may be present in milk in small quantities. Ask physician for guidance.

Habit-Forming Potential

Psychological or physical dependence is rare and unexpected.

Effects of Overdosage

With Moderate Overdose: Confusion, hallucinations, extreme drowsiness, drop in body temperature, heart palpitation, dilated pupils, tremors.

With Large Overdose: Stupor, deep sleep, coma, convulsions.

Possible Effects of Extended Use

None reported.

Suggested Periodic Examinations While Taking This Drug (at physician's discretion)

Complete blood cell counts.

Liver function tests.

Serial blood pressure readings and electrocardiograms.

While Taking This Drug, Observe the Following

Foods: No restrictions.

Beverages: No restrictions.

Alcohol: Avoid completely. This drug can increase markedly the intoxicating effects of alcohol and accentuate its depressant action on brain function.

Tobacco Smoking: No interactions expected.

Marijuana Smoking

Occasional (once or twice weekly):   Transient increase in drowsiness and dryness of mouth.

Daily: Persistent drowsiness, increased dryness of mouth; possible reduced effectiveness of this drug.

Other Drugs

Nortriptyline may *increase* the effects of

- atropine and drugs with atropine-like actions (see Drug Class, Section Three).
- sedatives, sleep-inducing drugs, tranquilizers, antihistamines, and narcotic drugs, and cause oversedation. Dosage adjustments may be necessary.
- levodopa (Dopar, Larodopa, etc.), in its control of Parkinson's disease.

Nortriptyline may *decrease* the effects of

- guanethidine, and reduce its effectiveness in lowering blood pressure.
- other commonly used anti-hypertensive drugs. Ask physician for guidance regarding the need to monitor blood pressure readings and to adjust dosage of antihypertensive medications. (The action of Aldomet is not decreased by tricyclic antidepressants.)

Nortriptyline *taken concurrently* with

- thyroid preparations, may cause impairment of heart rhythm and function. Ask physician for guidance regarding thyroid dosage adjustment.
- ethchlorvynol (Placidyl), may cause delirium.
- quinidine, may cause impairment of heart rhythm and function. Avoid the combined use of these two drugs.
- mono-amine oxidase (MAO) inhibitor drugs (see Drug Class, Section Three), may cause high fever, delirium, and convulsions.

The following drugs may *increase* the effects of nortriptyline

- thiazide diuretics (see Drug Family, Section Three) may slow its elimination from the body. Overdosage may occur.

Driving a Vehicle, Operating Machinery, Engaging in Hazardous Activities: This drug may impair mental alertness, judgment, physical coordination, and reaction time. Avoid hazardous activities.

Aviation Note: The use of this drug *is a disqualification* for the piloting of aircraft. Consultation with a designated Aviation Medical Examiner is advised.

Exposure to Sun: Use caution until sensitivity to sun has been determined. This drug may cause photosensitivity (see Glossary).

Discontinuation: If it has been necessary to use this drug for an extended period of time, do not discontinue it abruptly. Ask physician for guidance regarding dosage reduction and withdrawal. It may be necessary to adjust the dosage of other drugs taken concurrently.

Special Storage Instructions

Keep in a dry, tightly closed container.

NYLIDRIN
(Buphenine)

Year Introduced: 1953

Brand Names

USA	Canada
Arlidin (USV)	Arlidin (USV)
Rolidrin (Robinson)	Arlidin Forte (USV)
	Pervadil (Pharmascience)

Common Synonyms ("Street Names"):   None

Drug Class: Vasodilator

Prescription Required: USA: Yes   Canada: No

Available for Purchase by Generic Name: USA: Yes   Canada: No

Available Dosage Forms and Strengths
    Tablets — 6 mg., 12 mg.

Tablet May Be Crushed or Capsule Opened for Administration: Yes

How This Drug Works
    Intended Therapeutic Effect(s)
        Relief of symptoms associated with impaired circulation of blood in the extremities.
        Relief of vertigo associated with impaired circulation of blood in the inner ear.
    Location of Drug Action(s):   Those sympathetic nerve terminals in the muscles of blood vessel walls that are responsible for vessel dilation. Principal sites are the small arteries of muscles in the extremities, and the small arteries of the labyrinth system in the inner ear.
    Method of Drug Action(s):   By stimulating the action of those nerve terminals responsible for blood vessel dilation, this drug produces expansion of vessel walls. The resulting dilation increases the volume of blood flowing through the vessels. The increase in oxygen and nutrients relieves the symptoms attributable to deficient circulation.

Principal Uses of This Drug
    As a Single Drug Product: Used in a variety of conditions associated with impaired circulation due to spasm of blood vessels. It is used most frequently to treat circulatory disorders of the extremities: arteriosclerosis, night leg cramps, Raynaud's disease, thrombophlebitis, and cold hands, legs, and feet. It is used less frequently to treat circulatory deficiency of the inner ear that is thought to be responsible for vertigo and disturbances of hearing.

THIS DRUG SHOULD NOT BE TAKEN IF
—you have had an allergic reaction to any dosage form of it previously.
—you have just experienced an acute heart attack.

—you have just experienced a stroke.
—you have an active peptic ulcer.

INFORM YOUR PHYSICIAN BEFORE TAKING THIS DRUG IF
—you have a history of coronary heart disease, with or without angina.
—you have a history of heart rhythm disorders, especially attacks of rapid heart action (tachycardia).
—you have a history of stroke or impaired circulation to the brain.
—you have glaucoma.
—you have overactive thyroid function (hyperthyroidism).

Time Required for Apparent Benefit
Drug action begins in approximately 10 minutes and reaches a maximum in 30 minutes. Continuous use on a regular schedule for several weeks may be necessary to determine this drug's effectiveness.

Possible Side-Effects *(natural, expected, and unavoidable drug actions)*
Orthostatic hypotension in sensitive individuals (see Glossary).

Possible Adverse Effects *(unusual, unexpected, and infrequent reactions)*

IF ANY OF THE FOLLOWING DEVELOP, DISCONTINUE DRUG AND NOTIFY YOUR PHYSICIAN AS SOON AS POSSIBLE

Mild Adverse Effects
Nervousness, tremor, weakness, dizziness.
Acid indigestion, nausea, vomiting.
Rapid heart action, palpitation.

Serious Adverse Effects
Increase in internal eye pressure, of importance in glaucoma.

CAUTION
Individuals with extensive or severe impairment of circulation to the brain or heart may respond unfavorably to this drug. Observe closely until the true nature of the response has been determined. Discontinue drug if condition worsens.

Precautions for Use by Those over 60 Years of Age
Only arteries that are temporarily in spasm, and which have walls that are elastic and capable of expanding, can respond to the actions of this drug. Arteries with walls that are hardened and rigid (arteriosclerosis) cannot be dilated by any drug. If symptoms of impaired circulation worsen with the use of this drug, it indicates that blood is being diverted *away* from areas supplied by hardened arteries that are unable to dilate in response to the actions of the drug.
Avoid high doses that could cause a drop in blood pressure—hazardous for anyone with impaired circulation to the brain or heart muscle (coronary artery disease).

Advisability of Use During Pregnancy
Pregnancy Category: C (tentative). See Pregnancy Code inside back cover.
Animal reproduction studies: No data available.
Information from adequate studies in pregnant women is not available.
Ask physician for guidance.

Advisability of Use While Nursing Infant
The presence of this drug in milk is not known. Ask physician for guidance.

Habit-Forming Potential
None.

Effects of Overdosage
With Moderate Overdose: Sudden drop in blood pressure resulting in sense of weakness, dizziness, heart palpitation.

With Large Overdose: Restlessness, tremor, nausea, vomiting, rapid and irregular heart action.

Possible Effects of Extended Use
None reported.

Suggested Periodic Examinations While Taking This Drug (at physician's discretion)
Measurement of internal eye pressure, especially in presence of glaucoma. Heart examinations to detect any significant alteration of heart rhythm.

While Taking This Drug, Observe the Following
Foods: No restrictions of food selection. Drug may be taken with or immediately following food to minimize stomach irritation or nausea.

Beverages: No restrictions. May be taken with milk.

Alcohol: Use with caution until combined effects have been determined. Both alcohol and nylidrin can increase the secretion of stomach acid— potentially harmful to anyone prone to peptic ulcer disease.

Tobacco Smoking: Avoid completely. Nicotine is often a major contributing factor to the disorder under treatment. Also, nicotine can reduce this drug's ability to dilate blood vessels and to improve circulation.

Marijuana Smoking: No interactions expected.

Other Drugs

Nylidrin may *increase* the effects of

- phenothiazines (see Drug Class, Section Three), by increasing their level in the blood.

The following drugs may *decrease* the effects of nylidrin

- metoprolol (Lopressor).
- propranolol (Inderal). It is theoretically possible that metoprolol and propranolol may inhibit the primary actions of nylidrin. If these drugs are taken concurrently, observe for this possible effect.

Driving a Vehicle, Operating Machinery, Engaging in Hazardous Activities: This drug can cause nervousness, weakness, and/or dizziness in sensitive individuals. Use caution until the full effects are determined.

Aviation Note: Serious circulatory disorders *are a disqualification* for the piloting of aircraft. Consultation with a designated Aviation Medical Examiner is advised.

Exposure to Sun: No restrictions.

Exposure to Cold: Avoid as much as possible. This drug may be less effective in cold environments or with the handling of cold objects.

Heavy Exercise or Exertion: No restrictions.

Discontinuation: If this drug has not proved to be significantly beneficial after 1 month of continuous use on a regular schedule, consult your physician regarding the advisability of discontinuing it.

Special Storage Instructions
Keep in a dry, tightly closed container.

NYSTATIN

Year Introduced: 1954

Brand Names

USA	Canada
Mycostatin (Squibb)	Mycostatin (Squibb)
Nilstat (Lederle)	Nadostine (Nadeau)
O-V Statin (Squibb)	Nilstat (Lederle)
Mycolog [CD] (Squibb)	Nyaderm (K-Line)
(Others)	

Common Synonyms ("Street Names"):   None

Drug Class: Antibiotic, Antifungal (Antimycotic)

Prescription Required: USA: Yes   Canada: No

Available for Purchase by Generic Name: USA: Yes   Canada: No

Available Dosage Forms and Strengths

            Tablets — 100,000 units, 500,000 units
    Vaginal tablets — 100,000 units
         Suspension — 100,000 units per ml.
Ointment and cream — 100,000 units per gram
             Lotion — 100,000 units per ml.
             Powder — 100,000 units per gram.

Tablet May Be Crushed or Capsule Opened for Administration: Yes

How This Drug Works
Intended Therapeutic Effect(s):   The elimination of fungus infections responsive to the action of this drug.

Location of Drug Action(s):   Those body tissues and fluids infected by certain strains of fungus, and in which an adequate concentration of the drug can be achieved.

Method of Drug Action(s):   This drug prevents the growth and multiplication of susceptible strains of fungus by attacking the walls of the infecting organism and causing the leakage of essential internal components.

Principal Uses of This Drug
As a Single Drug Product: This drug is used exclusively to treat yeast infections of the skin, mouth, throat, gastro-intestinal tract, and vagina. It is only effective locally since it is not absorbed into the blood stream.

As a Combination Drug Product [CD]:   This drug is available in creams and ointments combined with neomycin, gramicidin, and triamcinolone for the treatment of certain skin infections. It is also available in capsules combined with tetracycline antibiotics for internal use. It is added to these products to prevent the development of a secondary yeast infection in the colon and rectum (see Superinfection in Glossary).

THIS DRUG SHOULD NOT BE TAKEN IF
—you have had an allergic reaction to any dosage form of it previously.

Time Required for Apparent Benefit
Drug action begins immediately on contact with the infecting yeast organisms. Complete cure may require continuous use on a regular schedule for 1 to 3 weeks depending upon the location and extent of the infection.

Possible Side-Effects *(natural, expected, and unavoidable drug actions)*
None reported.

Possible Adverse Effects *(unusual, unexpected, and infrequent reactions)*
IF ANY OF THE FOLLOWING DEVELOP, DISCONTINUE DRUG AND NOTIFY YOUR PHYSICIAN AS SOON AS POSSIBLE

Mild Adverse Effects
Allergic Reactions: Irritation and itching of tissues on local application.
Serious Adverse Effects
None reported.

CAUTION
To accomplish complete cure of infection, it is advisable to continue treatment several days after all symptoms (indications of infection) have disappeared.

Precautions for Use by Those over 60 Years of Age
None.

Advisability of Use During Pregnancy
Pregnancy Category: B (tentative). See Pregnancy Code inside back cover. Animal reproduction studies reveal no birth defects due to this drug. Information from adequate studies in pregnant women is not available. Ask physician for guidance.

Advisability of Use While Nursing Infant
This drug does not appear in the milk. It is considered safe to use while nursing infant.

Habit-Forming Potential
None.

Effects of Overdosage
With Moderate Overdose: Nausea, vomiting, diarrhea.
With Large Overdose: No significant or threatening effects.

Possible Effects of Extended Use
None known.

Suggested Periodic Examinations While Taking This Drug (at physician's discretion)
Laboratory examination at end of treatment course to determine degree of response.

While Taking This Drug, Observe the Following
Foods: No restrictions.
Beverages: No restrictions.
Alcohol: No interactions expected.
Tobacco Smoking: No interactions expected.
Marijuana Smoking: No interactions expected.
Other Drugs: No interactions reported.
Driving a Vehicle, Operating Machinery, Engaging in Hazardous Activities: No restrictions or precautions.
Aviation Note: The use of this drug *may be a disqualification* for the piloting of aircraft. Consultation with a designated Aviation Medical Examiner is advised.
Exposure to Sun: No restrictions.

Special Storage Instructions
Keep tablets in a dry, tightly closed container, at room temperature.
Keep liquid preparations in a cool place. Protect from light and high temperatures. Use within one week after preparation.

ORAL CONTRACEPTIVES

Year Introduced: 1960

Brand Names

USA

Combination Type*
Brevicon (Syntex)
Demulen (Searle)
Demulen 1/35
(Searle)
Enovid-E (Searle)
Enovid 5 mg.
(Searle)
Enovid 10 mg.
(Searle)
Loestrin 1/20
(Parke-Davis)
Loestrin 1.5/30
(Parke-Davis)
Loestrin Fe 1/20
(Parke-Davis)
Loestrin Fe 1.5/30
(Parke-Davis)
Lo/Ovral (Wyeth)
Modicon (Ortho)

Norinyl 1+35
(Syntex)
Norinyl 1+50
(Syntex)
Norinyl 1+80
(Syntex)
Norinyl 2 mg.
(Syntex)
Norlestrin 1/50
(Parke-Davis)
Norlestrin 2.5/50
(Parke-Davis)
Norlestrin Fe 1/50
(Parke-Davis)
Norlestrin Fe
2.5/50
(Parke-Davis)
Ortho-Novum 1/35
(Ortho)
Ortho-Novum 1/50
(Ortho)

Ortho-Novum 1/80
(Ortho)
Ortho-Novum 2
mg. (Ortho)
Ovcon-35 (Mead
Johnson)
Ovcon-50 (Mead
Johnson)
Ovral (Wyeth)
Ovulen (Searle)

"Mini-Pill" Type**
Micronor 0.35 mg.
(Ortho)
Nor-Q.D. (Syntex)
Ovrette (Wyeth)

Canada

Combination Type*
Demulen (Searle)
Enovid (Searle)
Enovid-E (Searle)
Loestrin 1.5/30
(P.D. & Co.)
Min-Ovral (Wyeth)
Norinyl 1+50
(Syntex)
Norinyl 1+80
(Syntex)
Norinyl-2 (Syntex)
Norlestrin 1/50
(P.D. & Co.)

Norlestrin 2.5/50
(P.D. & Co.)
Ortho 0.5/35
(Ortho)
Ortho 10/11
(Ortho)
Ortho 1/35 (Ortho)
Ortho-Novum 0.5
mg. (Ortho)
Ortho-Novum 1/50
(Ortho)
Ortho-Novum 1/80
(Ortho)

Ortho-Novum 2
mg. (Ortho)
Ortho-Novum 5
mg. (Ortho)
Ovral (Wyeth)
Ovulen 0.5 mg.
(Searle)
Ovulen 1 mg.
(Searle)

"Mini-Pill" Type**
Micronor (Ortho)

Common Synonyms ("Street Names"):   O.C.'s, "The Pill"

Drug Class: Oral Contraceptives (Estrogen+Progestin)

*Contains estrogen and progestin.
**Contains progestin only.

Prescription Required: Yes

Available for Purchase by Generic Name: No

Available Dosage Forms and Strengths
Tablets — Numerous combinations of varying strengths (examine package label of drug prescribed)

Tablet May Be Crushed or Capsule Opened for Administration: Yes

How This Drug Works
Intended Therapeutic Effect(s):   The prevention of pregnancy by suppression of ovulation.
Location of Drug Action(s):   Principal actions occur in
• a major control center in the brain known as the hypothalamus.
• the pituitary gland.
Method of Drug Action(s):   When the combination of an estrogen and a progestin are taken in sufficient dosage and on a regular basis, their blood and tissue levels increase to resemble those that occur during pregnancy. This results in suppression of the two pituitary gland hormones that normally produce ovulation (the formation and release of an egg by the ovary). In addition, these drugs may (1) alter the cervical mucus so that it resists the passage of sperm, and (2) alter the lining of the uterus so that it resists implantation of the egg (if ovulation occurs).

Principal Uses of This Drug
As a Single Drug Product: The "Mini-Pill" contains only one component— a progestin. This has been shown to be slightly less effective than the combination of estrogen and progestin in preventing pregnancy.
As a Combination Drug Product [CD]:   Most oral contraceptives consist of a combination of a type of estrogen and a type of progestin. These products are the most effective form of contraception available. While used most commonly to prevent pregnancy, they are sometimes used to treat menstrual irregularity.

THIS DRUG SHOULD NOT BE TAKEN IF
—you are allergic to either of the drugs contained in the brand prescribed (see package label).
—you have now, or have had in the past, any form of phlebitis, embolism, stroke, angina, or heart attack (coronary thrombosis).
—you have active liver disease or impaired liver function.
—you have a history of cancer of the breast or reproductive organs.
—you have abnormal and unexplained vaginal bleeding.

INFORM YOUR PHYSICIAN BEFORE TAKING THIS DRUG IF
—you have had an unfavorable reaction of any kind to any oral contraceptive in the past.
—you have cystic disease of the breasts (cystic mastitis).
—you have fibroid tumors of the uterus.
—you have a history of migraine headaches.
—you have epilepsy.

—you have a history of asthma or heart disease.
—you have diabetes or a tendency to diabetes.
—you have high blood pressure.
—you have sickle cell disease.
—you have a history of endometriosis.
—you plan to have surgery within 1 month.
—you smoke 15 or more cigarettes daily.

Time Required for Apparent Benefit

When the dosage schedule is followed exactly (one pill every scheduled day at the same time), the effectiveness of these drugs approaches 100%. Missed doses are the main reason for treatment failure and the occurrence of pregnancy. However, during the first 10 days of the first month of treatment, another method of birth control is advisable since early ovulation (and possible pregnancy) may occur before these drugs have become fully effective.

Possible Side-Effects *(natural, expected, and unavoidable drug actions)*

Retention of fluid, gain in weight, "breakthrough" bleeding (spotting in middle of menstrual cycle), change in menstrual flow, absence of menstrual flow (during regular use and after permanent withdrawal). There may be an increased tendency to acquire a yeast infection of the genital tissues.

Possible Adverse Effects *(unusual, unexpected, and infrequent reactions)*

IF ANY OF THE FOLLOWING DEVELOP, DISCONTINUE DRUG AND NOTIFY YOUR PHYSICIAN AS SOON AS POSSIBLE

Mild Adverse Effects
Allergic Reactions: Skin rashes, itching, hives.
Other Reactions
  Headache, nervous tension, and irritability.
  Accentuation of migraine headaches.
  Nausea, vomiting, bloating.
  Breast enlargement, tenderness, and secretion.
  Tannish pigmentation of the face.
  Reduced tolerance to contact lenses.
  Impaired color vision: blue tinge to objects, blue halo around lights.

Serious Adverse Effects
Idiosyncratic Reactions: Muscle and joint pains.
Other Reactions
  Thrombophlebitis (inflammation of a vein with the formation of blood clot)—pain or tenderness in thigh or leg, with or without swelling of the foot, ankle, or leg.
  Pulmonary embolism (movement of blood clot to the lung)—sudden shortness of breath and/or pain in the chest, coughing, bloody sputum.
  Stroke (blood clot in the brain)—headaches, blackouts, sudden weakness or paralysis of any part of the body, severe dizziness, drooping of eyelid, double vision, slurred speech, inability to speak.
  Rise in blood pressure—increasing headaches.
  Coronary thrombosis (heart attack)—sudden pain in heart area, weakness.

Retinal thrombosis (blood clot in eye vessels)—sudden impairment or loss of vision.

Hepatitis with jaundice (see Glossary)—yellow eyes and skin, dark-colored urine, light-colored stools.

Emotional depression (may be severe).

Formation of benign liver tumors—discomfort in the right upper abdomen, acute pain in the abdomen due to internal bleeding (from liver tumor).

Gall bladder disease—indigestion and discomfort in the right upper abdomen after eating fatty foods. (Recent studies suggest an increased risk of gall bladder disease in oral contraceptive users.)

CAUTION
1. The incidence of serious adverse effects due to the use of these drugs is very low.* However, you should report any unusual development to your physician promptly for evaluation.
2. Recent studies indicate that women over 30 years of age who smoke and use oral contraceptives are at significantly greater risk of having a serious cardiovascular event than nonusers.*
3. Certain commonly used drugs may reduce the effectiveness of oral contraceptives (some of these are listed in the section Other Drugs, below).

Advisability of Use During Pregnancy
Pregnancy Category: X (tentative). See Pregnancy Code inside back cover.
Animal reproduction studies reveal significant birth defects due to these drugs.

Information from studies in pregnant women indicates that female hormones can masculinize the female fetus. In addition, it is known that estrogenic drugs can predispose the female child to development of cancer of the vagina or cervix following puberty.

Avoid completely during entire pregnancy.

There is a possibility that this drug could be taken during the early weeks of an unrecognized pregnancy. If you have 2 consecutive cycles without menstruation (following the 7-day withdrawal of the drug), notify your physician so an examination for pregnancy can be made.

Advisability of Use While Nursing Infant
The components of this drug are known to be present in milk. Safety for the infant has not been established. Ask physician for guidance. It is generally felt that this drug should not be taken while nursing.

Habit-Forming Potential
None.

Effects of Overdosage
With Moderate Overdose: Headache, nausea, vomiting, fluid retention, abnormal vaginal bleeding, breast enlargement and discomfort.

With Large Overdose: Drowsiness (in some individuals). No serious or dangerous effects reported.

*See table at the end of this Profile.

Possible Effects of Extended Use

Increased growth of fibroid tumors of the uterus.

Gradual rise in blood pressure.

Delayed resumption of normal menstruation after discontinuation of drug, with associated difficulty in establishing pregnancy (impaired fertility).

Gall bladder disease with formation of gallstones.

Suggested Periodic Examinations While Taking This Drug (at physician's discretion)

Regular examinations of the breasts and reproductive organs (pelvic examination of uterus and ovaries, including "Pap" smear).

Liver function tests.

While Taking This Drug, Observe the Following

Foods: No restrictions. Ask physician for guidance regarding salt intake if you experience fluid retention. Ask physician regarding the need for supplemental folic acid (Vitamin Bc).

Beverages: No restrictions.

Alcohol: No interactions expected.

Tobacco Smoking: Recent studies indicate that heavy smoking (15 or more cigarettes daily) in association with the use of oral contraceptives significantly increases the risk of heart attack (coronary thrombosis). Heavy smoking should be considered a contraindication to the use of oral contraceptives.

Marijuana Smoking

Occasional (once or twice weekly): No interactions expected.

Daily: Possible menstrual irregularities; increased "breakthrough" bleeding.

Other Drugs

Oral contraceptives may *increase* the effects of

- meperidine (Demerol, pethidine).
- promazine (Sparine).

Oral contraceptives may *decrease* the effects of

- anticoagulants of the coumarin family. Dosage adjustment may be necessary to protect against clotting.
- anti-diabetic drugs (oral tablets and insulin). Dosage adjustment may be necessary to control diabetes.
- clofibrate (Atromid-S), and prevent the lowering of blood cholesterol or triglycerides.
- guanethidine (Ismelin), and reduce its ability to lower the blood pressure.

The following drugs may *decrease* the effects of oral contraceptives

- ampicillin (Amcill, etc.)
- antihistamines (some)
- chloramphenicol (Chloromycetin, etc.)
- meprobamate (Equanil, Miltown, etc.)
- mineral oil
- phenobarbital (possibly other barbiturates)
- phenylbutazone (Azolid, Butazolidin, etc.)

- phenytoin (Dantoin, Dilantin, etc.)
- rifampin (Rifadin, Rifomycin, Rimactane)
- tetracycline (Achromycin, etc.)

Driving a Vehicle, Operating Machinery, Engaging in Hazardous Activities: Usually no restrictions or precautions. Consult your physician for assessment of individual risk and for guidance regarding specific restrictions.

Aviation Note: Usually no restrictions. However, it is advisable to observe for the rare occurrence of acute disturbance of vision and to restrict activities accordingly.

Exposure to Sun: Use caution until full effect is known. These drugs may cause photosensitivity (see Glossary).

Occurrence of Unrelated Illness: Notify your physician of any illness that causes vomiting or diarrhea; these can interfere with absorption of the drug and reduce its effectiveness.

Discontinuation

If spotting or "breakthrough" bleeding occurs, do not discontinue the drug. If bleeding does not subside, notify your physician.

Remember: failure to take the drug for even 1 day of the dosage schedule may allow pregnancy to occur; use another contraceptive method for the remaining part of the cycle.

It is considered advisable to avoid pregnancy for 6 months after discontinuing these drugs. (This recommendation is based upon the finding of significantly increased chromosome abnormalities in aborted fetuses from women who became pregnant within 6 months of discontinuing oral contraceptives.)

Consult your physician regarding the advisability of continuing or discontinuing this drug prior to any surgery.

Special Storage Instructions

Keep in a dry, tightly closed container. Use of the original container will reduce dosage error.

Comparison of estimated deaths associated with pregnancy and childbirth and with use of oral contraceptives

Age group	Deaths from pregnancy and childbirth*	Deaths from use of oral contraceptives**	
		Non-smokers	Smokers
15–19	10.4	0.6	2.1
20–24	9.5	1.1	4.2
25–29	12.1	1.6	6.1
30–34	22.8	3.0	11.8
35–39	43.7	9.1	31.3
40–44	68.2	17.7	60.9

*Per 100,000 live births.
**Per 100,000 users per year.

ORPHENADRINE

Year Introduced: 1957

Brand Names

USA	Canada
Disipal (Riker)	Disipal (Riker)
Norflex (Riker)	Norflex (Riker)
Norgesic [CD] (Riker)	Norgesic [CD] (Riker)
Norgesic Forte [CD] (Riker)	Norgesic Forte [CD] (Riker)

Common Synonyms ("Street Names"):   None

Drug Class: Muscle Relaxant, Antihistamines, Anti-parkinsonism, Atropine-like Drug

Prescription Required: USA: Yes   Canada: No

Available for Purchase by Generic Name: USA: Yes   Canada: No

Available Dosage Forms and Strengths
Tablets — 50 mg., 100 mg.
Prolonged-action tablets — 100 mg.

Tablet May Be Crushed or Capsule Opened for Administration: Yes

How This Drug Works
Intended Therapeutic Effect(s)
Relief of discomfort associated with acutely painful muscle strain.
Relief of the rigidity, tremor, sluggish movement, and impaired gait associated with Parkinson's disease.

Location of Drug Action(s)
The site of drug action within the brain responsible for the relief of pain due to muscle spasm is unknown.
The site of drug action beneficial in the management of Parkinson's disease is the regulating center in the brain (the basal ganglia) that governs the coordination and efficiency of bodily movements.

Method of Drug Action(s)
The action responsible for the relief of pain associated with muscle strain is not fully established. It may be related to sedative and analgesic effects. This drug does not directly relax muscle in spasm due to strain.
The improvement in Parkinson's disease results from the restoration of a more normal balance of the chemical activities responsible for the transmission of nerve impulses within the basal ganglia.

Principal Uses of This Drug
As a Single Drug Product: Used primarily to relieve the symptoms associated with muscle spasm in two conditions: (1) acute musculo-skeletal injuries such as strains and sprains and (2) all forms of parkinsonism.

As a Combination Drug Product [CD]:   This drug is available in combination with aspirin and caffeine. Aspirin is added to enhance its ability to relieve pain. Caffeine is added to counteract the sedative effects of orphenadrine.

THIS DRUG SHOULD NOT BE TAKEN IF
—you have had an allergic reaction to any dosage form of it previously.

INFORM YOUR PHYSICIAN BEFORE TAKING THIS DRUG IF
—you have glaucoma.
—you have myasthenia gravis.
—you have difficulty emptying the urinary bladder.
—you have a history of heart disease or disturbance of heart rhythm.
—you have a history of peptic ulcer disease.

Time Required for Apparent Benefit
Drug action usually begins in 1 to 2 hours and persists for 8 to 12 hours.

Possible Side-Effects *(natural, expected, and unavoidable drug actions)*
Dryness of the mouth, blurred vision, constipation, slowed urination, drowsiness.

Possible Adverse Effects *(unusual, unexpected, and infrequent reactions)*

IF ANY OF THE FOLLOWING DEVELOP, DISCONTINUE DRUG AND NOTIFY YOUR PHYSICIAN AS SOON AS POSSIBLE

Mild Adverse Effects
  Allergic Reactions: Skin rash, hives, itching.
  Other Reactions
    Headache, lightheadedness, dizziness, weakness, fainting.
    Nausea, vomiting.
    Palpitation, rapid heart action.
Serious Adverse Effects
  Idiosyncratic Reactions: Agitation, hallucinations, tremor.

CAUTION
Many over-the-counter (OTC) medications (see Glossary) for allergies, colds, and coughs contain drugs that can interact unfavorably with this drug. Ask your physician or pharmacist for guidance before using any such medications.

Precautions for Use by Those over 60 Years of Age
You may be more sensitive to all of the actions of this drug. Small doses are advisable until your individual response has been determined.

This drug can increase the degree of impaired urination associated with prostate gland enlargement (prostatism).

You may be more susceptible to the development of impaired thinking, confusion, nightmares, and hallucinations. Careful dosage adjustments are mandatory.

Advisability of Use During Pregnancy
Pregnancy Category: C (tentative). See Pregnancy Code inside back cover. Animal reproduction studies. No data available.
Information from adequate studies in pregnant women is not available. Ask physician for guidance.

Advisability of Use While Nursing Infant
Presence of drug in milk is not known. Safety for infant not established. Ask physician for guidance.

Habit-Forming Potential
None.

Effects of Overdosage
With Moderate Overdose: Marked dryness of mouth and throat, drowsiness, muscle tremors, fainting.
With Large Overdose: Confusion, convulsions, coma, widely dilated pupils, rapid pulse.

Possible Effects of Extended Use
Increased internal eye pressure, possibly glaucoma.
Safety for continuous long-term use has not been established.

Suggested Periodic Examinations While Taking This Drug (at physician's discretion)
Measurement of internal eye pressure (glaucoma detection) on a regular basis.
Complete blood cell counts.

While Taking This Drug, Observe the Following
Foods: No restrictions. May be taken with or after food to prevent stomach irritation.
Beverages: No restrictions.
Alcohol: Use with caution until combined effect has been determined. Alcohol may increase the drowsiness produced by this drug in sensitive individuals.
Tobacco Smoking: No interactions expected.
Marijuana Smoking
Occasional (once or twice weekly):   No effect to mild and transient increase in drowsiness, dryness of mouth, muscle weakness and orthostatic hypotension (see Glossary).
Daily: Moderate to marked drowsiness, dryness of mouth, muscle weakness and incoordination, and significant accentuation of orthostatic hypotension.
Other Drugs
Orphenadrine may *increase* the effects of
• other atropine-like drugs, and intensify their side effects. Dosage adjustments may be necessary.
• levodopa (Dopar, Larodopa, etc.), and improve its effectiveness in the treatment of parkinsonism.

Orphenadrine may *decrease* the effects of
- griseofulvin (Fulvicin, Grifulvin, etc.), and reduce its effectiveness in treating fungus infections.
- phenylbutazone (Azolid, Butazolidin, etc.), and reduce its effectiveness in relieving inflammation and pain.

Orphenadrine *taken concurrently* with
- propoxyphene (Darvon), may cause confusion, nervousness, and tremors in sensitive individuals (probably very rare).
- chlorpromazine (Thorazine), may cause hypoglycemia (see Glossary) in sensitive individuals.

Driving a Vehicle, Operating Machinery, Engaging in Hazardous Activities: This drug may impair mental alertness, physical control, coordination, and reaction time. Determine tolerance before undertaking hazardous activities.

Aviation Note: The use of this drug *is a disqualification* for the piloting of aircraft. Consultation with a designated Aviation Medical Examiner is advised.

Exposure to Sun: No restrictions.

Special Storage Instructions
Keep in a dry, tightly closed container. Protect from light.

OXACILLIN

Year Introduced: 1961

Brand Names

USA	Canada
Bactocill (Beecham)	Prostaphlin (Bristol)
Prostaphlin (Bristol)	

Common Synonyms ("Street Names"):   None

Drug Class: Antibiotic (Anti-infective), Penicillins

Prescription Required: Yes

Available for Purchase by Generic Name: No

Available Dosage Forms and Strengths
Capsules — 250 mg., 500 mg.
Oral suspension — 250 mg. per teaspoonful (5 ml.)

Tablet May Be Crushed or Capsule Opened for Administration: Yes

How This Drug Works

Intended Therapeutic Effect(s):   The elimination of infections responsive to the action of this drug.

Location of Drug Action(s):   Any body tissue or fluid in which sufficient concentration of the drug can be achieved.

Method of Drug Action(s):   This drug destroys susceptible infecting bacteria by interfering with their ability to produce new protective cell walls as they multiply and grow.

Principal Uses of This Drug

As a Single Drug Product: This type of penicillin is used specifically to treat infections caused by strains of staphylococcus bacteria that are resistant to other penicillins.

THIS DRUG SHOULD NOT BE TAKEN IF

—you have had an allergic reaction to any dosage form of it previously.

—you are certain you are allergic to any form of penicillin.

INFORM YOUR PHYSICIAN BEFORE TAKING THIS DRUG IF

—you suspect you may be allergic to penicillin, or you have a history of a previous "reaction" to penicillin.

—you are allergic to cephalopsporin antibiotics (Ancef, Ceporan, Ceporex, Kafocin, Keflex, Keflin, Kefzol, Loridine).

—you are allergic by nature (hayfever, asthma, hives, eczema).

Time Required for Apparent Benefit

Varies with the nature of the infection under treatment; usually from 2 to 5 days.

Possible Side-Effects *(natural, expected, and unavoidable drug actions)*

Superinfections (see Glossary).

Possible Adverse Effects *(unusual, unexpected, and infrequent reactions)*

IF ANY OF THE FOLLOWING DEVELOP, DISCONTINUE DRUG AND NOTIFY YOUR PHYSICIAN AS SOON AS POSSIBLE

Mild Adverse Effects

Allergic Reactions: Skin rashes (various kinds).

Other Reactions: Irritation of mouth or tongue, "black tongue," nausea, vomiting, diarrhea, gaseous indigestion.

Serious Adverse Effects

Allergic Reactions: †Anaphylactic reaction (see Glossary), severe skin reactions, high fever, swollen painful joints, sore throat, unusual bleeding or bruising.

Other Reactions: Abnormally low white blood cell count.

Precautions for Use by Those over 60 Years of Age

It is advisable to evaluate kidney function before and during use of this drug to determine the need for dosage adjustment.

---

†A rare but potentially dangerous reaction characteristic of penicillins.

Natural changes in the skin after 60 may predispose to severe and prolonged itching reactions in the genital and anal regions. This reaction should be reported promptly.

Advisability of Use During Pregnancy
Pregnancy Category: C (tentative). See Pregnancy Code inside back cover. Animal reproduction studies: No data available.

Information from studies in pregnant women indicates no increased risk of defects in 3546 pregnancies exposed to penicillin derivatives.

Ask physician for guidance.

Advisability of Use While Nursing Infant
Drug may be present in milk and may sensitize infant to penicillin. Ask physician for guidance.

Habit-Forming Potential
None.

Effects of Overdosage
Possible nausea, vomiting, and/or diarrhea.

Possible Effects of Extended Use
Superinfections.

Suggested Periodic Examinations While Taking This Drug (at physician's discretion)
Complete blood cell counts.
Liver and kidney function tests.

While Taking This Drug, Observe the Following
Foods: No restrictions of food selection. Drug is most effective when taken on an empty stomach, 1 hour before or 2 hours after eating.
Beverages: No restrictions.
Alcohol: No interactions expected.
Tobacco Smoking: No interactions expected.
Marijuana Smoking: No interactions expected.
Other Drugs

The following drugs may *decrease* the effects of oxacillin
• antacids can reduce absorption of oxacillin.
• chloramphenicol (Chloromycetin)
• erythromycin (Erythrocin, E-Mycin, etc.)
• paromomycin (Humatin)
• tetracyclines (see Drug Class, Section Three)
• troleandomycin (Cyclamycin, TAO)

Driving a Vehicle, Operating Machinery, Engaging in Hazardous Activities: Usually no restrictions. Be alert to the rare occurrence of nausea and/or diarrhea; restrict activities accordingly.

Aviation Note: The use of this drug *may be a disqualification* for the piloting of aircraft. Consultation with a designated Aviation Medical Examiner is advised.

Exposure to Sun: No restrictions.

Special Storage Instructions
Keep capsules in a tightly closed container, at room temperature. Keep oral suspension refrigerated.

Observe the Following Expiration Times
Do not take the oral suspension of this drug if it is older than 3 days when kept at room temperature; 14 days when kept refrigerated.

OXAZEPAM

Year Introduced: 1965

Brand Names

USA	Canada
Serax (Wyeth)	Apo-Oxazepam (Apotex)
	Oxpam (ICN)
	Serax (Wyeth)

Common Synonyms ("Street Names"):   Downs, nerve pills, tranks

Drug Class: Tranquilizer, Mild (Anti-anxiety), Benzodiazepines

Prescription Required: Yes (Controlled Drug, U.S. Schedule IV)*

Available for Purchase by Generic Name: USA: No   Canada: Yes

Available Dosage Forms and Strengths
Tablets — 15 mg.
Capsules — 10 mg., 15 mg., 30 mg.

Tablet May Be Crushed or Capsule Opened for Administration: Yes

How This Drug Works
Intended Therapeutic Effect(s):   Relief of mild to moderate anxiety and nervous tension, without significant sedation.
Location of Drug Action(s):   Thought to be the limbic system of the brain, one of the centers that influence emotional stability.
Method of Drug Action(s):   Not established. Present thinking is that this drug may reduce the activity of certain parts of the limbic system.

Principal Uses of This Drug
As a Single Drug Product: Used primarily as a mild tranquilizer to relieve mild to moderate anxiety and nervous tension. It is useful in relieving the anxiety that accompanies depression, and in managing the agitation associated with alcohol withdrawal.

THIS DRUG SHOULD NOT BE TAKEN IF
—you have had an allergic reaction to any dosage form of it previously.
—it is prescribed for a child under 6 years of age.

*See Schedules of Controlled Drugs inside back cover.

INFORM YOUR PHYSICIAN BEFORE TAKING THIS DRUG IF

—you are allergic to any drugs chemically related to oxazepam: chlordiaz-epoxide, clorazepate, diazepam, flurazepam (see Drug Profiles for brand names).

—you have epilepsy.

—you are taking sedative, sleep-inducing, tranquilizer, antidepressant, or anti-convulsant drugs of any kind.

—you plan to have surgery under general anesthesia in the near future.

Time Required for Apparent Benefit

Approximately 1 to 2 hours. For severe symptoms of some duration, relief may require regular medication for several days.

Possible Side-Effects (natural, expected, and unavoidable drug actions)

Drowsiness, lethargy, unsteadiness in stance and gait.

Possible Adverse Effects (unusual, unexpected, and infrequent reactions)

IF ANY OF THE FOLLOWING DEVELOP, DISCONTINUE DRUG AND NOTIFY YOUR PHYSICIAN AS SOON AS POSSIBLE

Mild Adverse Effects

Allergic Reactions: Skin rashes (various kinds), swelling of face.

Other Reactions: Dizziness, fainting, blurred vision, double vision, slurred speech, headache, nausea.

Serious Adverse Effects

Allergic Reactions: Jaundice (yellow skin coloration; see Glossary), impaired resistance to infection manifested by fever and/or sore throat.

Paradoxical Reactions: Acute excitement, overactivity.

Other Reactions: Prolonged drop in blood pressure; may be hazardous in the elderly.

Precautions for Use by Infants and Children

Safety and effectiveness in children below the age of 6 years have not been established.

Precautions for Use by Those over 60 Years of Age

Natural changes in body functions increase the duration of this drug's actions. It is necessary to use smaller doses with longer intervals between doses to avoid excessive accumulation of the drug in body tissues. Dosage must be carefully individualized and limited to the smallest effective amount.

You may be more susceptible to the development of lightheadedness, impaired thinking and memory, confusion, lethargy, drowsiness, incoordination, unsteady gait and balance, impaired bladder control, and constipation.

Be alert to the possibility of paradoxical responses consisting of excitement, agitation, anger, hostility, and rage.

Advisability of Use During Pregnancy

Pregnancy Category: B (tentative). See Pregnancy Code inside back cover.

Animal reproduction studies reveal no birth defects due to this drug.

Information from adequate studies in pregnant women is not available. Ask physician for guidance.

The findings of some recent studies suggest a possible association between the use of a drug closely related to oxazepam during early pregnancy and the occurrence of birth defects, such as cleft lip. It is advisable to avoid this drug completely during the first 3 months of pregnancy.

Advisability of Use While Nursing Infant

With recommended dosage, drug is probably present in milk. Avoid use if possible. Ask physician for guidance.

Habit-Forming Potential

This drug can cause psychological and/or physical dependence (see Glossary) if used in large doses for an extended period of time.

Effects of Overdosage

With Moderate Overdose: Marked drowsiness, weakness, drunkenness, impairment of stance and gait.

With Large Overdose: Stupor progressing to deep sleep or coma.

Possible Effects of Extended Use

Psychological and/or physical dependence.
Impairment of blood cell production.
Impairment of liver function.

Suggested Periodic Examinations While Taking This Drug (at physician's discretion)

Blood cell counts and liver function tests during long-term use.

While Taking This Drug, Observe the Following

Foods: No restrictions.

Beverages: Large intake of coffee, tea, or cola drinks (because of their caffeine content) may reduce the calming action of this drug.

Alcohol: Use with extreme caution until the combined effect is determined. Alcohol may increase the sedative effects of oxazepam. Oxazepam may increase the intoxicating effects of alcohol.

Tobacco Smoking: Heavy smoking may reduce the calming action of oxazepam.

Marijuana Smoking

Occasional (once or twice weekly):   Mild increase in sedative effect of this drug.

Daily: Marked increase in sedative effect of this drug.

Other Drugs

Oxazepam may *increase* the effects of

- other sedatives, sleep-inducing drugs, tranquilizers, anti-convulsants, and narcotic drugs. Use these only under supervision of a physician. Careful dosage adjustment is necessary.
- oral anticoagulants of the coumarin drug family; ask physician for guidance regarding need for dosage adjustment to prevent bleeding.
- anti-hypertensives, producing excessive lowering of the blood pressure.

Oxazepam *taken concurrently* with

- anti-convulsants, may cause an increase in the frequence or severity of seizures; an increase in the dose of the anti-convulsant may be necessary.
- monoamine oxidase (MAO) inhibitor drugs (see Drug Class, Section Three) may cause extreme sedation, convulsions, or paradoxical excitement or rage.

The following drugs may *increase* the effects of oxazepam

- tricyclic anti-depressants (see Drug Class, Section Three) may increase the sedative effects of oxazepam.

Driving a Vehicle, Operating Machinery, Engaging in Hazardous Activities: This drug can impair mental alertness, judgment, physical coordination, and reaction time. Avoid hazardous activities.

Aviation Note: The use of this drug *is a disqualification* for the piloting of aircraft. Consultation with a designated Aviation Medical Examiner is advised.

Exposure to Sun: No restrictions.

Exposure to Heat: Use caution until effect of excessive perspiration is determined. Because of reduced urine volume, oxazepam may accumulate in the body and produce effects of overdosage.

Heavy Exercise or Exertion: No restrictions in cool or temperate weather.

Discontinuation: If it has been necessary to use this drug for an extended period of time do not discontinue it abruptly. Ask physician for guidance regarding dosage reduction and withdrawal. The dosage of other drugs taken concurrently with oxazepam may also require adjustment.

Special Storage Instructions
Keep in a dry, tightly closed, light-resistant container.

OXYCODONE

Year Introduced: 1950

Brand Names

USA	Canada
Percocet-5 [CD] (Endo)	Supeudol (Sabex)
Percodan [CD] (Endo)	Percocet [CD] (Endo)
Percodan-Demi [CD] (Endo)	Percocet-Demi [CD] (Endo)
Tylox [CD] (McNeil)	Percodan [CD] (Endo)
	Percodan-Demi [CD] (Endo)

Common Synonyms ("Street Names"):   Painkiller, pain reliever, perkies

Drug Class: Analgesic, Mild (Narcotic)

Prescription Required: Yes (Controlled Drug, U.S. Schedule II)*

Available for Purchase by Generic Name: Yes

Available Dosage Forms and Strengths
Tablets — 2.44 mg., 4.88 mg. (in combination with other drugs)

Tablet May Be Crushed or Capsule Opened for Administration: Yes

How This Drug Works
Intended Therapeutic Effect(s)
    Relief of moderate pain.
    Control of coughing.
Location of Drug Action(s)
    Those areas of the brain and spinal cord involved in the perception of pain.
    Those areas of the brain and spinal cord involved in the cough reflex.
Method of Drug Action(s):   Not completely established. It is thought that this drug affects tissue sites that react specifically with opium and its derivatives to relieve pain and cough.

Principal Uses of This Drug
As a Single Drug Product: Used primarily to relieve moderate to severe pain. Although effective in controlling cough, it is seldom used for this purpose.
As a Combination Drug Product [CD]:   This drug is available in combinations with acetaminophen and with aspirin. These milder pain-relievers are added to enhance the analgesic effect and to reduce fever if appropriate.

THIS DRUG SHOULD NOT BE TAKEN IF
—you have had an allergic reaction to any dosage form of it previously.
—it is prescribed for a child under 6 years of age.

INFORM YOUR PHYSICIAN BEFORE TAKING THIS DRUG IF
—you have had an unfavorable reaction to any narcotic drug in the past.
—you are taking any sedatives, sleep-inducing drugs, tranquilizers, other pain-relieving drugs, or antihistamines.
—you have difficulty emptying the urinary bladder.

Time Required for Apparent Benefit
Drug action begins within the first hour and persists for 4 to 5 hours.

Possible Side-Effects *(natural, expected, and unavoidable drug actions)*
Drowsiness, unsteadiness in stance and gait, constipation.

Possible Adverse Effects *(unusual, unexpected, and infrequent reactions)*
IF ANY OF THE FOLLOWING DEVELOP, DISCONTINUE DRUG AND NOTIFY YOUR PHYSICIAN AS SOON AS POSSIBLE

Mild Adverse Effects
    Allergic Reactions: Itching.
    Other Reactions

*See Schedules of Controlled Drugs inside back cover.

Lightheadedness, dizziness, euphoria.
Nausea, vomiting.
Serious Adverse Effects
None reported.

Precautions for Use by Those over 60 Years of Age
The aim of treatment should be to provide the maximal relief of pain consistent with minimal risk and the preservation of ability to function. Dosage should be low at the beginning with adjustment upward according to individual response.
The use of this drug should be limited to short-term treatment only.
You may be more susceptible to the development of dizziness, drowsiness, and constipation.

Advisability of Use During Pregnancy
Pregnancy Category: C (tentative). See Pregnancy Code inside back cover.
Animal reproduction studies: No data available.
Information from adequate studies in pregnant women is not available. Ask physician for guidance.

Advisability of Use While Nursing Infant
Safety not established. Avoid use or avoid nursing. Ask physician for guidance.

Habit-Forming Potential
This drug can produce both psychological and physical dependence (see Glossary). Avoid use over an extended period of time.

Effects of Overdosage
With Moderate Overdose: Marked drowsiness, staggering gait, incoordination.
With Large Overdose: Stupor progressing to coma, slow and shallow breathing, cold and clammy skin, weak and slow pulse.

Possible Effects of Extended Use
Psychological and physical dependence.

Suggested Periodic Examinations While Taking This Drug (at physician's discretion)
None required.

While Taking This Drug, Observe The Following
Foods: No restrictions.
Beverages: No restrictions.
Alcohol: Use with extreme caution. Alcohol can increase this drug's sedative and depressant action on brain function. This drug can increase the intoxicating action of alcohol.
Tobacco Smoking: No interactions expected.

Marijuana Smoking

Occasional (once or twice weekly):   Mild and transient increase in drowsiness and relief of pain.

Daily: Significant increase in drowsiness, relief of pain, and impairment of mental and physical performance.

Other Drugs

Oxycodone may *increase* the effects of

- sedatives, sleep-inducing drugs, tranquilizers, pain-relieving drugs, narcotic drugs, and antihistamines. Dosage adjustments are necessary to prevent excessive sedation.

Oxycodone *taken concurrently* with

- phenytoin (Dantoin, Dilantin, etc.), may cause excessive depression of brain function. Ask physician for guidance regarding dosage adjustment for proper control of seizures.

The following drugs may *increase* the effects of oxycodone

- all drugs with a sedative action: calming drugs, sleep-inducing drugs, tranquilizers, pain relievers, other narcotic drugs, antihistamines. Dosage adjustments are usually necessary to prevent excessive sedation.

The following drugs may *decrease* the effects of oxycodone

- cyproheptadine (Periactin) may reduce its ability to relieve pain.
- methysergide (Sansert) may reduce its ability to relieve pain.

Driving a Vehicle, Operating Machinery, Engaging in Hazardous Activities:
This drug can impair mental alertness, judgment, physical coordination, and reaction time. Avoid hazardous activities.

Aviation Note: The use of this drug *is a disqualification* for the piloting of aircraft. Consultation with a designated Aviation Medical Examiner is advised.

Exposure to Sun: No restrictions.

Discontinuation: If it has been necessary to use this drug for an extended period of time, ask physician for guidance regarding gradual reduction and withdrawal.

Special Storage Instructions

Keep in a dry, tightly closed container. Protect from light.

OXYMETAZOLINE

Year Introduced: 1964

Brand Names

USA	Canada
Afrin (Schering)	Nafrine (Schering)
Neo-Synephrine (Winthrop)	Ocuclear (Schering)
Sinex Long Lasting (Vicks)	

Common Synonyms ("Street Names"):   None

Drug Class: Decongestant

Prescription Required: No

Available for Purchase by Generic Name: USA: Yes   Canada: No

Available Dosage Forms and Strengths
Nasal solution — 0.05%
Nasal spray — 0.05%
Pediatric Nose Drops — 0.025%

How This Drug Works
Intended Therapeutic Effect(s):   Relief of congestion of the nose, sinuses, and throat associated with allergic disorders and infections.

Location of Drug Action(s):   The small blood vessels (arterioles) in the tissues lining the nasal passages, the sinuses, and the throat.

Method of Drug Action(s):   By contracting the walls and thus reducing the size of the arterioles, this drug decreases the volume of blood in the tissues, resulting in shrinkage of tissue mass (decongestion). This expands the nasal airway and enlarges the openings into the sinuses and eustachian tubes.

Principal Uses of This Drug
As a Single Drug Product: Used primarily as a decongestant nose drop or spray to treat swelling and congestion of the nasal membranes due to colds or allergy. It is also used as an eye drop to relieve inflammation and swelling of the conjunctival membranes ("red eyes") due to allergy or chemical irritation.

THIS DRUG SHOULD NOT BE TAKEN IF
—you have had an allergic reaction to any dosage form of it previously.
—it is prescribed for a child under 6 years of age.

INFORM YOUR PHYSICIAN BEFORE TAKING THIS DRUG IF
—you have high blood pressure or heart disease.
—you have diabetes or an overactive thyroid gland (hyperthyroidism).
—you are taking, or have taken within the past 2 weeks, any mono-amine oxidase (MAO) inhibitor drug (see Drug Class, Section Three).

Time Required for Apparent Benefit
Drug action is usually felt within 5 to 30 minutes after application to nasal membranes and may persist for periods of 4 to 12 hours.

Possible Side-Effects *(natural, expected, and unavoidable drug actions)*
Dryness of nose, nervousness, insomnia.

Possible Adverse Effects *(unusual, unexpected, and infrequent reactions)*

IF ANY OF THE FOLLOWING DEVELOP, DISCONTINUE DRUG AND NOTIFY YOUR PHYSICIAN AS SOON AS POSSIBLE

Mild Adverse Effects
Burning and stinging of nose, headache, lightheadedness, heart palpitation, tremor.
Serious Adverse Effects
None reported.

CAUTION
1. Too frequent application of nose drops and sprays containing this drug may cause a secondary "rebound" congestion resulting in a form of dependence (see Glossary).
2. Many over-the-counter (OTC) medications (see Glossary) for allergies, colds, and coughs contain drugs that may interact unfavorably with this drug. Ask your physician or pharmacist for guidance before using any such medications.

Precautions for Use by Those over 60 Years of Age
You may be more sensitive to the stimulant effects of this drug. Small doses are advisable until your individual response has been determined.
You may be more susceptible to the development of high blood pressure, disturbance of heart rhythm, angina, nervousness, or insomnia.

Advisability of Use During Pregnancy
Pregnancy Category: C (tentative). See Pregnancy Code inside back cover. Animal reproduction studies. No data available.
Information from adequate studies in pregnant women is not available. Ask physician for guidance.

Advisability of Use While Nursing Infant
Safety not established. Ask physician for guidance regarding time and frequency of use with relationship to nursing.

Habit-Forming Potential
Frequent or excessive use may cause functional dependence.

Effects of Overdosage
With Moderate Overdose: Headache, restlessness, sweating, heart palpitation.
With Large Overdose: Anxiety, agitation, rapid and irregular pulse.

Possible Effects of Extended Use
Secondary "rebound" congestion and chemical irritation of nasal membranes.

Suggested Periodic Examinations While Taking This Drug (at physician's discretion)
None required.

While Taking This Drug, Observe the Following
Foods: No restrictions.

Beverages: Heavy use of coffee or tea may add to the nervousness or insomnia experienced by sensitive individuals.

Alcohol: No interactions expected.

Tobacco Smoking: No interactions expected. No restrictions (unless directed otherwise by the physician).

Marijuana Smoking: No interactions expected.

Other Drugs

Oxymetazoline *used concurrently* with

• mono-amine oxidase (MAO) inhibitor drugs, may cause dangerous elevation of the blood pressure.

Driving a Vehicle, Operating Machinery, Engaging in Hazardous Activities: No restrictions.

Aviation Note: The use of this drug and the disorder for which this drug is prescribed *may be disqualifications* for the piloting of aircraft. Consultation with a designated Aviation Medical Examiner is advised.

Exposure to Sun: No restrictions.

Special Storage Instructions
Keep in a tightly closed container.

PAPAVERINE

Year Introduced: 1937

Brand Names

USA		Canada
Cerespan (USV)	Pavakey (Key)	None
Pavabid (Marion)	Vasospan (Ulmer)	
Pavacap (Reid-Provident)	(Numerous other brand names)	

Common Synonyms ("Street Names"):   Circulation medicine

Drug Class: Vasodilator

Prescription Required: Yes

Available for Purchase by Generic Name: Yes

Available Dosage Forms and Strengths
                      Tablets — 30 mg., 60 mg., 100 mg., 200 mg., 300 mg.
          Prolonged-action tablets — 200 mg.
      Prolonged-action capsules — 150 mg., 300 mg.
          Capsules, liquid filled — 75 mg., 150 mg.
                        Elixir — 33.3 mg. per teaspoonful (5 ml.)

Tablet May Be Crushed or Capsule Opened for Administration
                      Tablets — Yes
        Prolonged-action capsules — No
    Cerespan and Pavabid capsules — Yes, but do not crush or chew contents

How This Drug Works
  Intended Therapeutic Effect(s):   Relief of symptoms associated with
    • impaired circulation of blood in the extremities.
    • impaired circulation of blood within the brain (in carefully selected
      cases).
  Location of Drug Action(s):   The muscles in the walls of blood vessels. The
    principal therapeutic action is on the small arteries (arterioles).
  Method of Drug Action(s):   By causing direct relaxation and expansion of
    blood vessel walls, this drug increases the volume of blood flowing through
    the vessels. The resulting increase in oxygen and nutrients relieves the
    symptoms attributable to deficient circulation. The mechanism responsible
    for the direct relaxation of muscle is not known.

Principal Uses of This Drug
  As a Single Drug Product: Used in a variety of conditions associated with
    impaired circulation due to spasm of blood vessels. It is used to treat circula-
    tory deficiency of the brain (selected cases) and the major circulatory dis-
    orders of the extremities: Raynaud's disease, thrombophlebitis, night leg
    cramps, and cold hands, legs, and feet.

THIS DRUG SHOULD NOT BE TAKEN IF
—you have had an allergic reaction to any dosage form of it previously.

INFORM YOUR PHYSICIAN BEFORE TAKING THIS DRUG IF
—you have glaucoma.
—you have had a heart attack or a stroke.
—you suffer from poor circulation to the brain or heart (angina).

Time Required for Apparent Benefit
  Drug action begins in 30 to 60 minutes and persists for 4 to 6 hours.

Possible Side-Effects *(natural, expected, and unavoidable drug actions)*
  Lightheadedness and lethargy (lowered blood pressure), flushing of the face,
  sweating, mild constipation.

Possible Adverse Effects *(unusual, unexpected, and infrequent reactions)*

IF ANY OF THE FOLLOWING DEVELOP, DISCONTINUE DRUG AND NOTIFY YOUR PHYSICIAN AS SOON AS POSSIBLE

Mild Adverse Effects
Allergic Reactions: Itching, skin rash.
Other Reactions
Stomach irritation, indigestion, nausea, dryness of mouth and throat. Drowsiness, dizziness, headache.
Serious Adverse Effects
Allergic Reactions: Hepatitis with jaundice (see Glossary).

CAUTION
Individuals with extensive or severe impairment of circulation to the brain or heart may respond unfavorably or not at all to this drug. Observe closely to determine if drug effects are beneficial. Discontinue drug if the condition worsens.

Precautions for Use by Those over 60 Years of Age
It is not possible to predict in advance the nature of your response to this drug. It may relieve your symptoms, have no significant effect, or make your symptoms worse. Dosage must be carefully individualized.

Advisability of Use During Pregnancy
Pregnancy Category: C (tentative). See Pregnancy Code inside back cover.
Animal reproduction studies: No data available.
Information from adequate studies in pregnant women is not available. Ask physician for guidance.

Advisability of Use While Nursing Infant
Drug is known to be present in milk. Safety for infant not established. Ask physician for guidance.

Habit-Forming Potential
None.

Effects of Overdosage
With Moderate Overdose: Nausea, vomiting, marked drowsiness, severe constipation.
With Large Overdose: Weakness, faintness in upright position, flushed and warm face, excessive sweating, stupor, irregular pulse.

Possible Effects of Extended Use
None reported.

Suggested Periodic Examinations While Taking This Drug (at physician's discretion)
Liver function tests.
Measurement of internal eye pressure (if glaucoma is present).

While Taking This Drug, Observe the Following

Foods: No restrictions of food selection. Drug may be taken with or immediately following meals to reduce stomach irritation or nausea.

Beverages: No restrictions.

Alcohol: No interactions expected.

Tobacco Smoking: Nicotine can reduce drug's ability to dilate blood vessels and improve circulation. Follow physician's advice regarding smoking.

Marijuana Smoking: No interactions expected.

Other Drugs

The following drugs may *increase* the effects of papaverine

- sedatives, sleep-inducing drugs, tranquilizers, pain relievers, and narcotic drugs. Observe for excessive sedation.

Driving a Vehicle, Operating Machinery, Engaging in Hazardous Activities: Determine if drug causes drowsiness or dizziness before undertaking hazardous activities.

Aviation Note: Serious circulatory disorders *are a disqualification* for the piloting of aircraft. Consultation with a designated Aviation Medical Examiner is advised.

Exposure to Sun: No restrictions.

Exposure to Heat: Use caution. This drug may cause excessive sweating in hot environments.

Exposure to Cold: Avoid as much as possible. This drug may be less effective in cold environments or with the handling of cold objects.

Heavy Exercise or Exertion: No restrictions.

Special Storage Instructions

Keep in a dry, tightly closed container. Protect from light and excessive heat.

PARA-AMINOSALICYLIC ACID

Year Introduced: 1946

Brand Names

USA		Canada
Parasal (Panray)	Pasna (Barnes-Hind)	Nemasol (ICN)
P.A.S. (Various)	Teebacin (CMC)	
P.A.S. Acid (Kasar)		

Common Synonyms ("Street Names"): TB pills

Drug Class: Antimicrobial, Anti-tuberculosis (Anti-infective)

Prescription Required: USA: Yes   Canada: No

Available for Purchase by Generic Name: USA: Yes   Canada: No

Available Dosage Forms and Strengths
Tablets — 0.5 Gm., 1 Gm.
Powder — 4.18 Gm., 1 pound packets

Tablet May Be Crushed or Capsule Opened for Administration
Regular tablets — Yes
Enteric-coated tablets — No

How This Drug Works
Intended Therapeutic Effect(s):   To increase the effectiveness of other drugs used in the treatment of active tuberculosis.

Location of Drug Action(s):   Those body tissues and fluids in which adequate concentration of the drug can be achieved.

Method of Drug Action(s):   This drug prevents the growth and multiplication of susceptible tuberculosis organisms and renders them more vulnerable to the destructive action of more potent drugs.

Principal Uses of This Drug
As a Single Drug Product: Used primarily to treat active tuberculosis in conjunction with other anti-tuberculosis drugs. This drug is used because of its ability to delay the development of resistance of the tuberculosis bacteria to other more effective drugs.

THIS DRUG SHOULD NOT BE TAKEN IF
—you are allergic to any of the drugs bearing the brand names listed above or to any form of aminosalicylic acid.

INFORM YOUR PHYSICIAN BEFORE TAKING THIS DRUG IF
—you have a history of liver or kidney disease.
—you have a history of peptic ulcer (stomach or duodenum).
—you are taking anticoagulant drugs.
—you have epilepsy.

Time Required for Apparent Benefit
From 3 to 6 months.

Possible Side-Effects *(natural, expected, and unavoidable drug actions)*
Interference with the absorption of Vitamin B–12. (This may result in the development of anemia.)

Possible Adverse Effects *(unusual, unexpected, and infrequent reactions)*

IF ANY OF THE FOLLOWING DEVELOP, DISCONTINUE DRUG AND NOTIFY YOUR PHYSICIAN AS SOON AS POSSIBLE

Mild Adverse Effects
Allergic Reactions: Skin rashes (various kinds), fever, swollen glands.
Other Reactions
Loss of appetite, nausea, vomiting, diarrhea, stomach pain and burning (all common).
Headaches, pains in the arms and/or legs.

Serious Adverse Effects
Allergic Reactions: Hepatitis, with or without jaundice (see Glossary).
Other Reactions
  Bone marrow depression (see Glossary)—fatigue, weakness, fever, sore
    throat, unusual bleeding or bruising.
  Mental and behavioral disturbances.
  Peptic ulceration of stomach.

Precautions for Use by Those over 60 Years of Age
Natural changes in body composition and function that occur after 60 may
  make you more susceptible to the adverse effects of this drug. Small doses
  are advisable until your individual response has been determined.
You may be more prone to develop anemia. Consult your physician regarding
  the need for supplemental iron and vitamin B–12.

Advisability of Use During Pregnancy
Pregnancy Category: C (tentative). See Pregnancy Code inside back cover.
  Animal reproduction studies in rats reveal no birth defects due to this drug.
  Information from limited studies in pregnant women indicates that the risk
    of defects may be doubled.
  Avoid completely during first 3 months.
  Ask physician for guidance.

Advisability of Use While Nursing Infant
Safety for infant not established. Avoid use if possible. Ask physician for
  guidance.

Habit-Forming Potential
None.

Effects of Overdosage
Severe nausea, vomiting, abdominal pain, diarrhea.

Possible Effects of Extended Use
Impaired thyroid function with enlargement of thyroid gland (goiter).

Suggested Periodic Examinations While Taking This Drug (at physician's discretion)
Complete blood cell counts.
Serial determination of blood potassium levels.
Liver, kidney, and thyroid function tests.

While Taking This Drug, Observe the Following
Foods: No restrictions of food selection. Take PAS with meals to reduce
  stomach irritation.
Beverages: No restrictions.
Alcohol: Avoid completely if you have a history of liver disease.
Tobacco Smoking: No interactions expected with PAS. Ask physician for
  guidance regarding smoking.
Marijuana Smoking: No interactions expected.

Other Drugs

PAS may *increase* the effects of
- oral anticoagulants, and cause bleeding. Monitor prothrombin time and adjust dosage of anticoagulant as necessary.
- phenytoin (Dantoin, Dilantin, etc.), to an excessive degree. Dosage reduction of phenytoin may be necessary to prevent toxicity.
- barbiturates, and cause oversedation.

PAS may *decrease* the effects of
- rifampin, by reducing its absorption. Separate doses of each drug by 8 to 12 hours.
- "sulfa" drugs (see Drug Class, Section Three).

PAS *taken concurrently* with
- aspirin, may cause excessive irritation of the stomach, increasing the possibility of stomach ulceration or bleeding.

Driving a Vehicle, Operating Machinery, Engaging in Hazardous Activities: Usually no restrictions. Be alert to the possible occurrence of nausea; restrict activities accordingly.

Aviation Note: The use of this drug *may be a disqualification* for the piloting of aircraft. Consultation with a designated Aviation Medical Examiner is advised.

Exposure to Sun: No restrictions.

Discontinuation: Long-term treatment is required for cure. If you cannot tolerate PAS because of severe stomach irritation, consult your physician so your treatment program can be modified.

Special Storage Instructions
Keep in a tightly closed, light-resistant container. PAS solutions must be refrigerated and kept in a dark place.

Observe the Following Expiration Times
Do not take the liquid form of this drug if it is older than 24 hours.

PAREGORIC
(Camphorated Tincture of Opium)

Year Introduced: 1885

Brand Names

USA		Canada
Opium Tincture (Lilly)	Parepectolin [CD] (Rorer)	Diban [CD] (Robins)
Brown Mixture [CD] (Various)	(Others)	Donnagel-PG [CD] (Robins)
Donnagel-PG [CD] (Robins)		

Common Synonyms ("Street Names"):   PG, PO

Drug Class: Anti-diarrheal (Narcotic)

Prescription Required: Yes (Controlled Drug, U.S. Schedule III)*

Available for Purchase by Generic Name: USA: Yes   Canada: No

Available Dosage Forms and Strengths
Oral liquid mixtures — Opium content 15 to 24 mg. per ounce

How This Drug Works
Intended Therapeutic Effect(s)
Relief of mild to moderate pain.
Relief of intestinal cramping and diarrhea.

Location of Drug Action(s)
Those areas of the brain and spinal cord involved in the perception of pain.
The membranes lining the intestine and the nerve fibers in the wall of the
intestine.

Method of Drug Action(s):   Not completely established. It is thought that
this drug affects tissue sites that react specifically with opium and its derivatives to relieve pain. Morphine, the active ingredient in paregoric, acts in
two ways to relieve cramping and diarrhea: It acts as a local anesthetic on
surface membranes and it blocks the release of acetylcholine, the chemical
that transmits stimulating nerve impulses to the muscular walls of the
intestine.

Principal Uses of This Drug
As a Single Drug Product: Used primarily to relieve intestinal cramping
and diarrhea. Less frequently used as an analgesic.
As a Combination Drug Product [CD]:   This drug is available in combination with kaolin, pectin, and derivatives of atropine. Kaolin and pectin are
added to provide adsorbents that combine with toxins in the intestinal tract
and thereby prevent their absorption. Atropine enhances the antispasmodic effect of paregoric.

*See Schedules of Controlled Drugs inside back cover.

THIS DRUG SHOULD NOT BE TAKEN IF
—you are allergic to any opium derivative (morphine, codeine, papaverine).

INFORM YOUR PHYSICIAN BEFORE TAKING THIS DRUG IF
—you are taking any other sedative, sleep-inducing, tranquilizing, or narcotic drugs at this time.
—you have impaired liver or kidney function.

Time Required for Apparent Benefit
Control of cramping and diarrhea may require several doses over a period of 2 to 6 hours.

Possible Side-Effects *(natural, expected, and unavoidable drug actions)*
Mild drowsiness, lightheadedness, sweating, constipation.

Possible Adverse Effects *(unusual, unexpected, and infrequent reactions)*
IF ANY OF THE FOLLOWING DEVELOP, DISCONTINUE DRUG AND NOTIFY YOUR PHYSICIAN AS SOON AS POSSIBLE

Mild Adverse Effects
Allergic Reactions: Skin rash, hives, itching.
Other Reactions
Nausea, vomiting (in sensitive individuals).
Dizziness, unsteadiness (more common in the elderly, over 60 years of age).
Serious Adverse Effects
None reported.

Precautions for Use by Those over 60 Years of Age
You may be more susceptible to the development of drowsiness, dizziness, unsteadiness, and constipation. Avoid prolonged use.

Advisability of Use During Pregnancy
Pregnancy Category: C (tentative). See Pregnancy Code inside back cover.
Animal reproduction studies: No data available.
Information from studies in pregnant women indicates no increase in defects in 562 exposures to this drug.
Ask physician for guidance.

Advisability of Use While Nursing Infant
The active drug (morphine) is known to be present in milk and may have a depressant effect on the infant. Ask physician for guidance.

Habit-Forming Potential
This drug may produce both psychological and physical dependence (see Glossary) if used in large doses for an extended period of time.

Effects of Overdosage
With Moderate Overdose: Increased drowsiness, nausea, vomiting, constipation.
With Large Overdose: Stupor progressing to deep sleep, slow breathing, slow pulse, flushed and warm skin, small (constricted) pupils.

Possible Effects of Extended Use
Psychological and physical dependence.

Suggested Periodic Examinations While Taking This Drug (at physician's discretion)
None required.

While Taking This Drug, Observe the Following
Foods: Follow diet prescribed to combat diarrhea.

Beverages: No interactions.

Alcohol: Best avoided until diarrhea is controlled. Use with caution if taken concurrently with this drug. Opium (morphine) can intensify the intoxicating effects of alcohol. Alcohol can intensify the depressant action of opium on brain function.

Tobacco Smoking: No interactions expected.

Marijuana Smoking
Occasional (once or twice weekly): Mild and transient increase in drowsiness and relief of pain.
Daily: Significant increase in drowsiness, relief of pain, and impairment of mental and physical performance.

Other Drugs
Paregoric may *increase* the effects of
• all sedatives, sleep-inducing drugs, analgesics,tranquilizers, and narcotic drugs, causing excessive sedation.

The following drugs may *increase* the effects of paregoric
• phenothiazines may enhance its sedative effect.
• tricyclic antidepressants may enhance its sedative effect.

Driving a Vehicle, Operating Machinery, Engaging in Hazardous Activities: Usually no restrictions. However, if used in large doses this drug may impair mental alertness, judgment, reaction time, or coordination. If so, avoid hazardous activities.

Aviation Note: The use of this drug *may be a disqualification* for the piloting of aircraft. Consultation with a designated Aviation Medical Examiner is advised.

Exposure to Sun: No restrictions.

Special Storage Instructions
Keep in a tightly closed, light-resistant container. Avoid exposure to direct sunlight and to excessive heat.

PENICILLIN V

Year Introduced: 1953

Brand Names

USA		Canada
Betapen VK (Bristol)	Repen-VK	Ledercillin VK
Ledercillin VK	(Reid-Provident)	(Lederle)
(Lederle)	Robicillin-VK (Robins)	Nadopen-V (Nadeau)
Penapar VK	SK-Penicillin VK	Novopen-VK
(Parke-Davis)	(Smith Kline &	(Novopharm)
Penicillin VK	French)	Pen-Vee (Wyeth)
(Comer)	Uticillin VK (Upjohn)	Pen-Vee K (Wyeth)
Pen-Vee K (Wyeth)	V-Cillin K (Lilly)	PVF (Frosst)
Pfizerpen VK	Veetids (Squibb)	PVF K (Frosst)
(Pfipharmecs)		V-Cillin K (Lilly)
		VC-K 500 (Lilly)

Common Synonyms ("Street Names"):   None

Drug Class: Antibiotic (Anti-infective), Penicillins

Prescription Required: Yes

Available for Purchase by Generic Name: Yes

Available Dosage Forms and Strengths
       Tablets — 125 mg., 250 mg., 500 mg.
    Oral solutions — 125 mg., 250 mg. per teaspoonful (5 ml.)

Tablet May Be Crushed or Capsule Opened for Administration: Yes

How This Drug Works
  Intended Therapeutic Effect(s):   The elimination of infections responsive to
    the action of this drug.
  Location of Drug Action(s):   Any body tissue or fluid in which sufficient
    concentration of the drug can be achieved.
  Method of Drug Action(s):   This drug destroys susceptible infecting bacteria
    by interfering with their ability to produce new protective cell walls as they
    multiply and grow.

Principal Uses of This Drug
  As a Single Drug Product: This type of penicillin is used primarily to treat
    responsive infections of the upper and lower respiratory tract, the middle
    ear, and the skin. Equally important uses are the prevention of rheumatic
    fever recurrence and the prevention of bacterial endocarditis in individu-
    als with rheumatic heart disease.

THIS DRUG SHOULD NOT BE TAKEN IF
—you have had an allergic reaction to any dosage form of it previously
—you are certain you are allergic to any form of penicillin.

INFORM YOUR PHYSICIAN BEFORE TAKING THIS DRUG IF
—you suspect you may be allergic to penicillin or you have a history of a previous "reaction" to penicillin.
—you are allergic to cephalosporin antibiotics (Ancef, Ceporan, Ceporex, Kafocin, Keflex, Keflin, Kefzol, Loridine).
—you are allergic by nature (hayfever, asthma, hives, eczema).

Time Required for Apparent Benefit
Varies with the nature of the infection under treatment; usually from 2 to 5 days.

Possible Side-Effects *(natural, expected, and unavoidable drug actions)*
Superinfections (see Glossary).

Possible Adverse Effects *(unusual, unexpected, and infrequent reactions)*

IF ANY OF THE FOLLOWING DEVELOP, DISCONTINUE DRUG AND NOTIFY YOUR PHYSICIAN AS SOON AS POSSIBLE

Mild Adverse Effects
Allergic Reactions: Skin rashes (various kinds).
Other Reactions: Irritations of mouth or tongue, "black tongue," nausea, vomiting, diarrhea.
Serious Adverse Effects
Allergic Reactions: †Anaphylactic reaction (see Glossary), severe skin reactions, high fever, swollen painful joints, sore throat, unusual bleeding or bruising.
Other Reactions: Colitis

Precautions for Use by Those over 60 Years of Age
It is advisable to evaluate kidney function before and during use of this drug to determine the need for dosage adjustment.
Natural changes in the skin after 60 may predispose to severe and prolonged itching reactions in the genital and anal regions. This reaction should be reported promptly.

Advisability of Use During Pregnancy
Pregnancy Category: B (tentative). See Pregnancy Code inside back cover.
Animal reproduction studies in mice reveal significant birth defects due to this drug.
Information from studies in pregnant women indicates no increase in defects in 3546 exposures to penicillin derivatives.
Ask physician for guidance.

Advisability of Use While Nursing Infant
Drug may be present in milk and may sensitize infant to penicillin. Ask physician for guidance.

†A rare but potentially dangerous reaction characteristic of penicillins.

Habit-Forming Potential
None.

Effects of Overdosage
Possible nausea, vomiting, and/or diarrhea.

Possible Effects of Extended Use
Superinfections.

Suggested Periodic Examinations While Taking This Drug (at physician's discretion)
Complete blood cell counts.
Liver and kidney function tests.

While Taking This Drug, Observe the Following
Foods: No restrictions of food selection. May be taken at any time (before, during, or after eating, or between meals).

Beverages: No restrictions.

Alcohol: No interactions expected.

Tobacco Smoking: No interactions expected.

Marijuana Smoking: No interactions expected.

Other Drugs
The following drugs may *decrease* the effectiveness of penicillin V
- chloramphenicol (Chloromycetin)
- erythromycin (Erythrocin, E-Mycin, etc.)
- paromomycin (Humatin)
- tetracyclines (see Drug Class, Section Three)
- troleandomycin (Cyclamycin, TAO)

Driving a Vehicle, Operating Machinery, Engaging in Hazardous Activities: Usually no restrictions. Be alert to the rare occurrence of dizziness, nausea, and/or diarrhea; restrict activities accordingly.

Aviation Note: The use of this drug *may be a disqualification* for the piloting of aircraft. Consultation with a designated Aviation Medical Examiner is advised.

Exposure to Sun: No restrictions.

Discontinuation: Certain infections require that this drug be taken for 10 days to prevent the development of rheumatic fever. Ask your physician for guidance regarding the recommended duration of treatment.

Special Storage Instructions
Keep tablets and capsules in a tightly closed, light-resistant container, preferably below 85°F. (30°C). Keep liquid preparations refrigerated.

Observe the Following Expiration Times
Do not take a liquid form of this drug if it is older than 7 days when kept at room temperature; 14 days when kept refrigerated.

PENTAERYTHRITOL TETRANITRATE

Year Introduced: 1951

Brand Names

USA		Canada
Duotrate (Marion)	(Numerous other	Peritrate (P.D.)
Pentritol (Armour)	brand and	Peritrate Forte (P.D.)
Peritrate	combination brand	
(Warner/Chilcott)	names)	
Vaso-80 Unicelles		
(Reid-Provident)		
Miltrate [CD]		
(Wallace)		

Common Synonyms ("Street Names"):   Angina pills, heart pills

Drug Class: Anti-anginal, Nitrates

Prescription Required: USA: Yes   Canada: No

Available for Purchase by Generic Name: USA: Yes   Canada: No

Available Dosage Forms and Strengths
Tablets — 10 mg., 20 mg., 40 mg.
Prolonged-action tablets — 80 mg.
Prolonged-action capsules — 30 mg., 45 mg., 60 mg., 80 mg.

Tablet May Be Crushed or Capsule Opened for Administration
Regular tablets — Yes
Prolonged-action tablets and capsules — No
Duotrate capsules — Yes, but do not crush or chew
contents

How This Drug Works
Intended Therapeutic Effect(s):   Reduction in the frequency and severity of pain associated with angina pectoris (coronary insufficiency).
Location of Drug Action(s):   The muscular tissue in the walls of the blood vessels. The principal site of the therapeutic action is the system of coronary arteries in the heart.
Method of Drug Action(s):   This drug acts directly on the muscle cell to produce relaxation. This permits expansion of blood vessels and increases the supply of blood and oxygen to meet the needs of the working heart muscle.

Principal Uses of This Drug
As a Single Drug Product: Used in the treatment of symptomatic coronary artery disease to prevent the development of effort-induced anginal pain.

As a Combination Drug Product [CD]:   This drug is available in combination with hydroxyzine and with meprobamate. These mild tranquilizers are added to relieve anxiety and nervous tension that are both cause and effect in angina pectoris.

THIS DRUG SHOULD NOT BE TAKEN IF
—you have had an allergic reaction to any dosage form of it previously. A combination drug [CD] should not be taken if you are allergic to *any* of its ingredients.

INFORM YOUR PHYSICIAN BEFORE TAKING THIS DRUG IF
—you have glaucoma.
—you have had an unfavorable response to any vasodilator drug in the past.

Time Required for Apparent Benefit
Drug action begins in 30 to 60 minutes and persists for 4 to 5 hours.

Possible Side-Effects *(natural, expected, and unavoidable drug actions)*
Flushing, lightheadedness in upright position (see orthostatic hypotension in Glossary).

Possible Adverse Effects *(unusual, unexpected, and infrequent reactions)*

IF ANY OF THE FOLLOWING DEVELOP, DISCONTINUE DRUG AND NOTIFY YOUR PHYSICIAN AS SOON AS POSSIBLE

Mild Adverse Effects
  Allergic Reactions: Skin rash.
  Other Reactions
    Headache (may be persistent), dizziness, fainting.
    Nausea, vomiting.
Serious Adverse Effects
  Allergic Reactions: Severe dermatitis with peeling of skin.

CAUTION
Many over-the-counter (OTC) medications (see Glossary) for allergies, colds, and coughs contain drugs that may counteract the desired effects of this drug. Ask your physician or pharmacist for guidance before using any such medications.

Precautions for Use by Those over 60 Years of Age
You may be more sensitive to the actions of this drug. Small doses are advisable until your individual response has been determined.
You may be more susceptible to the development of low blood pressure with associated lightheadedness, dizziness, unsteadiness, and falling.

Advisability of Use During Pregnancy
Pregnancy Category: C (tentative). See Pregnancy Code inside back cover.
Animal reproduction studies: No data available.
Information from adequate studies in pregnant women is not available. Ask physician for guidance.

Advisability of Use While Nursing Infant
Presence of drug in milk is not known. Safety for infant not established. Avoid use if possible. Ask physician for guidance.

Habit-Forming Potential
None.

Effects of Overdosage
With Moderate Overdose: Headache, dizziness, marked flushing of the skin.

With Large Overdose: Vomiting, weakness, sweating, fainting, shortness of breath, coma.

Possible Effects of Extended Use
Development of tolerance (see Glossary), which may reduce the drug's effectiveness at recommended doses.

Development of abnormal hemoglobin (red blood cell pigment).

Suggested Periodic Examinations While Taking This Drug (at physician's discretion)
Measurement of internal eye pressure in those individuals with glaucoma or a tendency to glaucoma.

Red blood cell counts and hemoglobin measurements.

While Taking This Drug, Observe the Following
Foods: No restrictions. This drug is likely to be more effective if taken one-half to 1 hour before eating.

Beverages: No restrictions.

Alcohol: Use with extreme caution until combined effects have been determined. Alcohol may exaggerate the drop in blood pressure experienced by some sensitive individuals. This could be dangerous.

Tobacco Smoking: Nicotine may reduce the effectiveness of this drug. Follow physician's advice regarding smoking, based upon its effect on the condition under treatment and its possible interaction with this drug.

Marijuana Smoking

Occasional (once or twice weekly):   No interactions expected.

Daily: Possible reduced effectiveness of this drug; mild to moderate increase in angina; possible changes in electrocardiogram, confusing interpretation.

Other Drugs

Pentaerythritol may *increase* the effects of

- atropine-like drugs (see Drug Class, Section Three), and cause an increase in internal eye pressure.
- tricyclic antidepressants (see Drug Class, Section Three), and cause excessive lowering of the blood pressure.

Pentaerythritol may *decrease* the effects of

- all choline-like drugs, such as Mestinon, Mytelase, pilocarpine, Prostigmin, and Urecholine.

Pentaerythritol *taken concurrently* with

- anti-hypertensive drugs, may cause severe drop in blood pressure. Careful monitoring of drug response and appropriate dosage adjustments are necessary.

The following drugs may *increase* the effects of pentaerythritol

- propranolol (Inderal) may cause additional lowering of the blood pressure. Dosage adjustments may be necessary.

Driving a Vehicle, Operating Machinery, Engaging in Hazardous Activities: Usually no restrictions. Before engaging in hazardous activities, determine that this drug will not cause orthostatic hypotension.

Aviation Note: Coronary artery disease *is a disqualification* for the piloting of aircraft. Consultation with a designated Aviation Medical Examiner is advised.

Exposure to Sun: No restrictions.

Exposure to Cold: Cold environment may reduce the effectiveness of this drug.

Heavy Exercise or Exertion: This drug may improve your ability to be more active without resulting angina pain. Use caution and avoid excessive exertion that could cause heart injury if warning pain is delayed.

Special Storage Instructions

Keep in a dry, tightly closed container and in a cool place. Protect from heat and light.

PENTAZOCINE

Year Introduced: 1967

Brand Names

USA	Canada
Talwin Compound [CD] (Winthrop)	Talwin (Winthrop)
Talwin Nx [CD] (Winthrop)	Talwin Compound-50 [CD] (Winthrop)

Common Synonyms ("Street Names"):   Painkiller, pain reliever, TS

Drug Class: Analgesic, Mild (Non-narcotic)

Prescription Required: Yes (Controlled Drug, U.S. Schedule IV)*

Available for Purchase by Generic Name: No

Available Dosage Forms and Strengths

Tablets — 50 mg. of pentazocine and 0.5 mg. of naloxone.
Injection — 30 mg. per ml.

*See Schedules of Controlled Drugs inside back cover.

Tablet May Be Crushed or Capsule Opened for Administration: Yes

How This Drug Works

Intended Therapeutic Effect(s):   Relief of mild to moderate pain.

Location of Drug Action(s):   Those areas of the brain and spinal cord involved in the perception of pain.

Method of Drug Action(s):   Not completely established. It has been suggested that the resulting increase in chemicals that transmit nerve impulses somehow contributes to the analgesic effect of this drug.

Principal Uses of This Drug

As a Single Drug Product: Used exclusively to relieve acute or chronic pain of mild to moderate degree from any cause.

As a Combination Drug Product [CD]:   This drug is combined with aspirin to enhance the product's analgesic effect and to utilize aspirin's ability to reduce fever and inflammation if desired.

THIS DRUG SHOULD NOT BE TAKEN IF

—you have had an allergic reaction to any dosage form of it previously.

—it is prescribed for a child under 12 years of age.

INFORM YOUR PHYSICIAN BEFORE TAKING THIS DRUG IF

—you are taking sedatives, sleep-inducing drugs, tranquilizers, antidepressants, or narcotic drugs of any kind.

—you have a history of impaired liver or kidney function.

—you have epilepsy.

—you plan to have surgery under general anesthesia in the near future.

Time Required for Apparent Benefit

Usually 15 minutes to 1 hour when taken orally.

Possible Side-Effects *(natural, expected, and unavoidable drug actions)*

Drowsiness, lightheadedness, weakness, constipation.

Possible Adverse Effects *(unusual, unexpected, and infrequent reactions)*

IF ANY OF THE FOLLOWING DEVELOP, DISCONTINUE DRUG AND NOTIFY YOUR PHYSICIAN AS SOON AS POSSIBLE

Mild Adverse Effects

Allergic Reactions: Skin rash, hives, swelling of face.

Other Reactions

Nausea, vomiting, indigestion, diarrhea.

Headache, dizziness, blurring of vision, flushing and sweating.

Serious Adverse Effects

Marked drop in blood pressure, which may produce fainting.

Mental and behavioral disturbances, hallucinations, tremor.

Bone marrow depression (see Glossary) of a mild and reversible nature (rare).

Interference with urination.

Precautions for Use by Those over 60 Years of Age

You may be more sensitive to all of the actions of this drug. Small doses are advisable until your individual response has been determined.

You may be more susceptible to the development of confusion, disorientation, and drop in blood pressure with resultant weakness, fainting, and falling.

Advisability of Use During Pregnancy

Pregnancy Category: C (tentative). See Pregnancy Code inside back cover. Animal reproduction studies in hamsters reveal significant birth defects due to this drug.

Information from adequate studies in pregnant women is not available. It is advisable to avoid this drug during first 3 months.

Ask physician for guidance.

Advisability of Use While Nursing Infant

Safety not established. Avoid use if possible. Ask physician for guidance.

Habit-Forming Potential

This drug can produce psychological and physical dependence (see Glossary) if used in large doses for an extended period of time.

Effects of Overdosage

With Moderate Overdose: Anxiety, disturbed thoughts, hallucinations, nightmares, progressive drowsiness.

With Large Overdose: Stupor, depressed respiration.

Possible Effects of Extended Use

Psychological and physical dependence.

Suggested Periodic Examinations While Taking This Drug (at physician's discretion)

Complete blood cell counts, if used for an extended period of time.

While Taking This Drug, Observe the Following

Foods: No restrictions.

Beverages: No restrictions.

Alcohol: Use with caution until combined effect is determined. Pentazocine may increase the intoxicating effects of alcohol.

Tobacco Smoking: Heavy smoking may reduce the effectiveness of pentazocine. Consult physician regarding need for dosage adjustment.

Marijuana Smoking

Occasional (once or twice weekly):   No effect to mild increase in pain relief from this drug.

Daily: Moderate increase in pain relief from this drug.

Other Drugs

Pentazocine may *increase* the effects of

• all sedatives, sleep-inducing drugs, tranquilizers, antidepressants. Ask physician for guidance regarding need for dosage adjustment.

Pentazocine may *decrease* the effects of
• narcotic drugs (to a slight degree).

Driving a Vehicle, Operating Machinery, Engaging in Hazardous Activities:
This drug can impair mental alertness, judgment, reaction time, and physical coordination. Use caution until the occurrence of drowsiness, dizziness, and weakness is determined. Avoid hazardous activities.

Aviation Note: The use of this drug *is a disqualification* for the piloting of aircraft. Consultation with a designated Aviation Medical Examiner is advised.

Exposure to Sun: No restrictions.

Discontinuation: If this drug has been taken for an extended period of time, do not discontinue it abruptly. Ask physician for guidance.

Special Storage Instructions
Keep in a dry, tightly closed container.

PENTOBARBITAL

Year Introduced: 1930

Brand Names

USA	Canada
Nembutal (Abbott)	Nembutal (Abbott)
	Novopentobarb
	(Novopharm)
	Pentogen (Technilab)

Common Synonyms ("Street Names"):   Barbs, candy, downers, goofballs, nebbies, nembies, nimby, nemish, nemmies, peanuts, sleepers, stoppers, stumblers, yellow birds, yellow jackets, yellows, yellow submarines

Drug Class: Sedative, Mild; Sleep Inducer (Hypnotic), Barbiturates

Prescription Required: Yes (Controlled Drug, U.S. Schedule II)*

Available for Purchase by Generic Name: Yes

Available Dosage Forms and Strengths
Capsules — 30 mg., 50 mg., 100 mg.
Elixir — 20 mg. per teaspoonful (5 ml.)
Suppositories — 30 mg., 60 mg., 120 mg., 200 mg.

Tablet May Be Crushed or Capsule Opened for Administration
Regular tablets and capsules — Yes
Prolonged-action tablets — No

*See Schedules of Controlled Drugs inside back cover.

How This Drug Works
Intended Therapeutic Effect(s)
With low dosage, relief of mild to moderate anxiety or tension (sedative effect).

With higher dosage taken at bedtime, sedation sufficient to induce sleep (hypnotic effect).

Location of Drug Action(s):   The connecting points (synapses) in the nerve pathways that transmit impulses between the wake-sleep centers of the brain.

Method of Drug Action(s):   Not completely established. Present thinking is that this drug selectively blocks the transmission of nerve impulses by reducing the amount of available norepinephrine, one of the chemicals responsible for impulse transmission.

Principal Uses of This Drug
As a Single Drug Product: This member of the barbiturate class is used in small doses to relieve anxiety and nervous tension, and in larger doses at bedtime to prevent insomnia. It has been largely replaced by the non-barbiturate benzodiazepines for both uses.

As a Combination Drug Product [CD]:   This drug is available in combination with carbromal, another sedative that enhances its effectiveness for inducing sleep.

THIS DRUG SHOULD NOT BE TAKEN IF
—you have had an allergic reaction to any dosage form of it previously.
—you have a history of porphyria.

INFORM YOUR PHYSICIAN BEFORE TAKING THIS DRUG IF
—you are allergic or sensitive to any barbiturate drug.
—you are taking any sedative, sleep-inducing drugs, tranquilizers, antihistamines, pain relievers, or narcotic drugs of any kind.
—you have epilepsy.
—you have a history of liver or kidney disease.
—you plan to have surgery under general anesthesia in the near future.

Time Required for Apparent Benefit
Approximately 30 minutes.

Possible Side-Effects (natural, expected, and unavoidable drug actions)
Drowsiness, lethargy, a sense of mental and physical sluggishness.

Possible Adverse Effects (unusual, unexpected, and infrequent reactions)
IF ANY OF THE FOLLOWING DEVELOP, DISCONTINUE DRUG AND NOTIFY YOUR PHYSICIAN AS SOON AS POSSIBLE

Mild Adverse Effects
Allergic Reactions: Skin rash (various kinds), hives, localized swellings of eyelids, face, or lips, drug fever.

Other Reactions
"Hangover" effect, dizziness, unsteadiness.
Nausea, vomiting, diarrhea.
Joint and muscle pains, most often in the neck, shoulders, and arms.

Serious Adverse Effects
Allergic Reactions
Hepatitis with jaundice (see Glossary).
Severe skin reactions.
Idiosyncratic Reactions: Paradoxical excitement and delirium (rather than sedation).
Other Reactions
Anemia, manifested by weakness and fatigue.
Reduction of blood platelets (see Glossary), resulting in unusual bleeding or bruising.

Precautions for Use by Infants and Children
This drug should not be given to the hyperkinetic child.
Observe for possible paradoxical hyperactivity.

Precautions for Use by Those over 60 Years of Age
Small doses are advisable until tolerance has been determined. The elderly or debilitated may experience agitation, excitement, confusion, and delerium with standard doses (paradoxical reaction).
This drug may cause excessive lowering of body temperature (hypothermia). Keep dosage to a minimum during winter, and dress warmly.
The natural decline in liver function that may occur after 60 can slow the elimination of this drug. Longer intervals between doses may be necessary to avoid overdosage and toxicity.
Note: A barbiturate is not the drug of choice as a sedative or sleep inducer in this age group.

Advisability of Use During Pregnancy
Pregnancy Category: D (tentative). See Pregnancy Code inside back cover.
Animal reproduction studies in mice (but not in rats, rabbits, guinea pigs, or monkeys) reveal significant birth defects due to this drug.
Information from studies in pregnant women indicates no significant increase in defects in 1523 exposures to this drug.
It is advisable to avoid this drug during entire pregnancy.

Advisability of Use While Nursing Infant
Drug is known to be present in milk. Avoid use if possible. Ask physician for guidance.

Habit-Forming Potential
This drug can cause both psychological and physical dependence (see Glossary).

Effects of Overdosage
With Moderate Overdose: Behavior similar to alcoholic intoxication: confusion, slurred speech, physical incoordination, staggering gait, drowsiness.
With Large Overdose: Deepening sleep, coma, slow and shallow breathing, weak and rapid pulse, cold and sweaty skin.

Possible Effects of Extended Use
Psychological and/or physical dependence.
Anemia.

If dose is excessive, a form of chronic drug intoxication can occur—headache, impaired vision, slurred speech, and depression.

Suggested Periodic Examinations While Taking This Drug (at physician's discretion)

Complete blood cell counts.
Liver function tests.

While Taking This Drug, Observe the Following

Foods: No restrictions.

Beverages: No restrictions.

Alcohol: Avoid completely. Alcohol can increase greatly the sedative and depressant actions of this drug on brain function.

Tobacco Smoking: No interactions expected.

Marijuana Smoking

Occasional (once or twice weekly):   Mild, transient increase in drowsiness, unsteadiness, and impairment of mental and physical performance.

Daily: Marked, prolonged drowsiness, unsteadiness, and significantly impaired mental and physical performance.

Other Drugs

Pentobarbital may *increase* the effects of

- other sedatives, sleep-inducing drugs, tranquilizers, antihistamines, pain relievers, and narcotic drugs, and cause oversedation. Ask your physician for guidance regarding dosage adjustment.

Pentobarbital may *decrease* the effects of

- oral anticoagulants of the coumarin family (see Drug Class, Section Three). Ask physician for guidance regarding prothrombin time testing and adjustment of the anticoagulant dosage.
- aspirin, and reduce its pain-relieving action.
- cortisone and related drugs, by hastening their elimination from the body.
- oral contraceptives, by hastening their elimination from the body.
- griseofulvin (Fulvicin, Grisactin, etc.), and reduce its effectiveness in treating fungus infections.
- phenylbutazone (Azolid, Butazolidin, etc.), and reduce its effectiveness in treating inflammation and pain.

Pentobarbital *taken concurrently* with

- anti-convulsants, may cause a change in the pattern of epileptic seizures. Careful dosage adjustments are necessary to achieve a balance of actions that will give the best protection from seizures.

The following drugs may *increase* the effects of pentobarbital

- both mild and strong tranquilizers may increase the sedative and sleep-inducing actions of barbiturate drugs and cause oversedation.
- isoniazid (INH, Isozide, etc.) may prolong the action of barbiturate drugs.
- antihistamines may increase the sedative effects of barbiturate drugs.
- oral anti-diabetic drugs of the sulfonylurea type may prolong the sedative effects of barbiturate drugs.

- mono-amine oxidase (MAO) inhibitor drugs (see Drug Class, Section Three) may prolong the sedative effects of barbiturate drugs.

Driving a Vehicle, Operating Machinery, Engaging in Hazardous Activities: This drug can produce drowsiness and impair mental alertness, judgment, physical coordination, and reaction time. Avoid hazardous activities.

Aviation Note: The use of this drug *is a disqualification* for the piloting of aircraft. Consultation with a designated Aviation Medical Examiner is advised.

Exposure to Sun: Use caution until sensitivity has been determined. Some barbiturates can cause photosensitivity (see Glossary).

Exposure to Cold: The elderly may experience excessive lowering of body temperature while taking this drug. Keep dosage to a minimum during winter and dress warmly.

Discontinuation: If it has been necessary to use this drug for an extended period of time, do not discontinue it abruptly. Ask physician for guidance regarding dosage adjustment and withdrawal. It may also be necessary to adjust the dose of other drugs taken concurrently with it.

Special Storage Instructions

Keep tablets and capsules in a dry, tightly closed container. Keep elixir in a tightly closed, amber glass container.

PERPHENAZINE

Year Introduced: 1963

Brand Names

USA	Canada
Trilafon (Schering)	Apo-Perphenazine (Apotex)
Etrafon [CD] (Schering)	Phenazine (ICN)
Triavil [CD] (Merck Sharp & Dohme)	Trilafon (Schering)
	Etrafon [CD] (Schering)
	Triavil [CD] (MSD)

Common Synonyms ("Street Names"): None

Drug Class: Tranquilizer, Strong (Anti-psychotic) [Phenothiazines]

Prescription Required: Yes

Available for Purchase by Generic Name: USA: No   Canada: Yes

Available Dosage Forms and Strengths

Tablets — 2 mg., 4 mg., 8 mg., 16 mg.
Prolonged-action tablets — 8 mg.
Concentrate — 16 mg. per teaspoonful (5 ml.)
Injection — 5 mg. per ml.

Tablet May Be Crushed or Capsule Opened for Administration
Tablets — Yes

Prolonged-action tablets — No

How This Drug Works
Intended Therapeutic Effect(s):   Restoration of emotional calm. Relief of severe anxiety, agitation, and psychotic behavior.

Location of Drug Action(s):   Those nerve pathways in the brain that utilize the tissue chemical dopamine for the transmission of nerve impulses.

Method of Drug Action(s):   Not completely established. Present theory is that by inhibiting the action of dopamine, this drug acts to correct an imbalance of nerve impulse transmissions that is thought to be responsible for certain mental disorders.

Principal Uses of This Drug
As a Single Drug Product: This member of the phenothiazine class is used primarily to treat acute and chronic psychotic disorders such as agitated depression, schizophrenia, and similar states of mental dysfunction. It is used less frequently to relieve severe nausea or vomiting.

As a Combination Drug Product [CD]:   This drug is available in combination with amitriptyline, an effective antidepressant. In some cases of severe agitated depression, the combination of a specific antipsychotic drug and a specific antidepressant drug will be more effective than either drug used alone.

THIS DRUG SHOULD NOT BE TAKEN IF
—you have had an allergic reaction to any dosage form of it previously.

—you have a blood or bone marrow disorder.

—you have impaired liver function.

—it is prescribed for a child under 12 years of age.

INFORM YOUR PHYSICIAN BEFORE TAKING THIS DRUG IF
—you are allergic or sensitive to any phenothiazine drug (see Drug Class, Section Three).

—you are taking sedatives, sleep-inducing drugs, other tranquilizers, antidepressants, antihistamines, or narcotic drugs of any kind.

—you have epilepsy.

—you plan to have surgery under general or spinal anesthesia in the near future.

Time Required for Apparent Benefit
Some benefit may be apparent during first week. Maximal benefit may require continuous use for several weeks.

Possible Side-Effects *(natural, expected, and unavoidable drug actions)*
Drowsiness (usually mild), blurring of vision, nasal congestion, dryness of mouth, constipation, impaired urination.

Possible Adverse Effects *(unusual, unexpected, and infrequent reactions)*

IF ANY OF THE FOLLOWING DEVELOP, DISCONTINUE DRUG AND NOTIFY YOUR PHYSICIAN AS SOON AS POSSIBLE

Mild Adverse Effects

Allergic Reactions: Skin rashes (various kinds), hives, itching, local or generalized swelling.

Other Reactions: Headaches, mild insomnia.

Serious Adverse Effects

Allergic Reactions: Anaphylactic reaction (see Glossary), severe skin reactions, asthma.

Idiosyncratic Reactions: High fever.

Other Reactions

Parkinson-like disorders (see Glossary).

Hepatitis with jaundice (see Glossary).

Bone marrow depression (see Glossary)—usually mild and very rare.

Muscle spasms involving the face and neck—rolling eyes, grimacing, clamping jaws, difficult speech and swallowing, twisting and bending of the neck, rounding and protrusion of the tongue.

Generalized convulsions.

CAUTION

1. Many over-the-counter (OTC) medications (see Glossary) for allergies, colds, and coughs contain drugs that can interact unfavorably with this drug. Ask your physician or pharmacist for guidance before using any such medications.
2. Antacids that contain aluminum and/or magnesium can prevent the absorption of this drug and reduce its effectiveness.
3. Obtain prompt evaluation of any disturbance or change in vision.

Precautions for Use by Those over 60 Years of Age

You may be more sensitive to all of the actions of this drug. Small doses are advisable until your individual response has been determined.

You may be more susceptible to the development of drowsiness, lethargy, constipation, lowering of body temperature (hypothermia), and excessive drop in blood pressure on arising from lying or sitting position (see orthostatic hypotension in Glossary).

This drug can increase the degree of impaired urination associated with prostate gland enlargement (prostatism).

You may also be more susceptible to the development of Parkinson-like disorders and/or tardive dyskinesia (see discussion of these terms in Glossary). These conditions must be recognized early since they may become unresponsive to treatment and irreversible. Consult your physician promptly if suggestive symptoms develop.

Advisability of Use During Pregnancy

Pregnancy Category: C (tentative). See Pregnancy Code inside back cover. Animal reproduction studies in mice and rats reveal significant birth defects due to this drug.

Information from adequate studies in pregnant women is not available. It is advisable to avoid this drug during first 3 months.
Ask physician for guidance.

Advisability of Use While Nursing Infant
Safety not established. Avoid use if possible. Ask physician for guidance.

Habit-Forming Potential
None.

Effects of Overdosage
With Moderate Overdose: Marked drowsiness, weakness, slurred speech, staggering gait, muscle spasms of face, neck, arms, and legs, convulsions.
With Large Overdose: Stupor progressing to deep sleep and coma.

Possible Effects of Extended Use
Tardive dyskinesia (see Glossary).

Suggested Periodic Examinations While Taking This Drug (at physician's discretion)
Complete blood cell counts, especially during first 3 months.
Liver function tests.
Periodic electrocardiograms.
Periodic examinations of tongue for development of fine, wave-like, rippling movements (involuntary) that could indicate the beginning of tardive dyskinesia.

While Taking This Drug, Observe the Following
Foods: No restrictions.
Beverages: No restrictions.
Alcohol: Use extreme caution until combined effects have been determined. Alcohol may increase the sedative action of perphenazine and accentuate its depressant effects on brain function. Perphenazine may increase the intoxicating action of alcohol.
Tobacco Smoking: No interactions expected.
Marijuana Smoking
Occasional (once or twice weekly):   No effect to mild and transient increase in drowsiness and accentuation of orthostatic hypotension (see Glossary); some risk of precipitating latent psychoses (in predisposed individuals).
Daily: Moderate increase in drowsiness, significant accentuation of orthostatic hypotension; increased risk of precipitating latent psychoses, confusing interpretation of mental status and of drug responses.
Other Drugs
Perphenazine may *increase* the effects of
- all sedatives, sleep-inducing drugs, other tranquilizers, antidepressants, antihistamines, and narcotic drugs, and cause oversedation. Ask physician for guidance regarding dosage adjustment.
- mono-amine oxidase (MAO) inhibitor drugs (see Drug Class, Section Three), and cause excessive lowering of the blood pressure.

- reserpine (and related drugs), and cause excessive lowering of the blood pressure.
- atropine and atropine-like drugs (see Drug Class, Section Three).

Perphenazine may *decrease* the effects of
- appetite suppressant drugs (Pre-Sate, Preludin, Dexedrine, etc.).
- levodopa (Dopar, Larodopa, Parda, etc.), and reduce its effectiveness in the treatment of Parkinson's disease (shaking palsy).

Perphenazine *taken concurrently* with
- anti-convulsants, may cause a change in the pattern of epileptic seizures. Ask physician for guidance regarding dosage adjustment of the anti-convulsant.
- anti-hypertensive drugs (see Drug Class, Section Three), may cause excessive lowering of the blood pressure. Use this combination very cautiously and ask physician for guidance regarding dosage adjustment.
- quinidine, may impair heart function. Avoid this combination of drugs.

The following drugs may *increase* the effects of perphenazine
- tricyclic antidepressants (see Drug Class, Section Three)
- all sedatives, sleep-inducing drugs, and other tranquilizers, both mild and strong

Driving a Vehicle, Operating Machinery, Engaging in Hazardous Activities: This drug may impair mental alertness, judgment, physical coordination, and reaction time. Avoid hazardous activities.

Aviation Note: The use of this drug *is a disqualification* for the piloting of aircraft. Consultation with a designated Aviation Medical Examiner is advised.

Exposure to Sun: Use caution until sensitivity has been determined. This drug may cause photosensitivity (see Glossary).

Exposure to Heat: Use caution until combined effect has been determined. This drug may impair regulation of body temperature and produce increased risk of heat stroke.

Heavy Exercise or Exertion: No restriction in moderate temperatures.

Discontinuation: If it has been necessary to use this drug for an extended period of time, do not discontinue it suddenly. Ask physician for guidance regarding dosage reduction and withdrawal. It may also be necessary to adjust the dosage of other drugs taken concurrently with it.

Special Storage Instructions
Keep liquid concentrate in a tightly closed, amber glass container. Protect all liquid forms from light.

PHENAZOPYRIDINE

Year Introduced: 1927

Brand Names

USA

Pyridium
 (Parke-Davis)
Azo Gantanol [CD]
 (Roche)
Azo Gantrisin [CD]
 (Roche)
Pyridium Plus [CD]
 (Parke-Davis)

Thiosulfil-A [CD]
 (Ayerst)
Urobiotic [CD]
 (Roerig)
(Numerous other
 brand and
 combination brand
 names)

Canada

Phenazo (ICN)
Pyridium (P.D.)
Pyronium (Pro Doc)
Azo Gantrisin [CD]
 (Roche)
Azotrex [CD] (Bristol)

Common Synonyms ("Street Names"):   Bladder pills, cystitis pills

Drug Class: Urinary Analgesic

Prescription Required: USA: Yes   Canada: No

Available for Purchase by Generic Name: USA: Yes   Canada: No

Available Dosage Forms and Strengths
 Tablets — 100 mg., 200 mg.

Tablet May Be Crushed or Capsule Opened for Administration: No

How This Drug Works
 Intended Therapeutic Effect(s):   Relief of pain and discomfort associated
  with acute irritation of the lower urinary tract, as in cystitis, urethritis, and
  prostatitis.
 Location of Drug Action(s):   The sensory nerve endings in the lining of the
  lower urinary tract (bladder and urethra).
 Method of Drug Action(s):   By its local anesthetic effect on the tissues lining
  the lower urinary tract, this drug provides symptomatic relief of pain,
  burning, pressure, and sense of urgency to void.

Principal Uses of This Drug
 As a Single Drug Product: Used exclusively in the treatment of lower urinary tract infections to relieve the urgency to urinate and the discomfort
  that accompanies the passage of urine.
 As a Combination Drug Product [CD]:   This drug is available in combinations with several anti-infective drugs that are commonly used to treat
  urinary tract infections. Each combination product provides a drug to
  eradicate the infection and a drug to relieve discomfort during the early
  period of treatment.

THIS DRUG SHOULD NOT BE TAKEN IF
—you have had an allergic reaction to any dosage form of it previously.
—you have active hepatitis.

INFORM YOUR PHYSICIAN BEFORE TAKING THIS DRUG IF
—you have a history of serious liver or kidney disease.

Time Required for Apparent Benefit
Drug action usually begins in 1 to 2 hours and persists for 3 to 5 hours.

Possible Side-Effects *(natural, expected, and unavoidable drug actions)*
Reddish-orange discoloration of the urine, of no significance.

Possible Adverse Effects *(unusual, unexpected, and infrequent reactions)*

IF ANY OF THE FOLLOWING DEVELOP, DISCONTINUE DRUG AND NOTIFY YOUR PHYSICIAN AS SOON AS POSSIBLE

Mild Adverse Effects
Allergic Reactions: Skin rash.
Other Reactions
Headache, dizziness.
Indigestion, abdominal cramping.
Serious Adverse Effects
Allergic Reactions: Hepatitis with or without jaundice (see Glossary).
Idiosyncratic Reactions: Hemolytic anemia (see Glossary) in sensitive individuals (may occur in the presence of impaired kidney function).

CAUTION
It is important to understand that this drug is only an analgesic, and that its action is limited to the relief of symptoms. It has no curative effect on the underlying condition responsible for the symptoms. Consult your physician regarding the need for specific anti-infective therapy.

Precautions for Use by Those over 60 Years of Age
The natural decline in kidney function that occurs after 60 may require that you use smaller doses.
Observe for the development of a yellowish coloration of the eyes or skin—an indication of excessive drug accumulation. Report this to your physician.

Advisability of Use During Pregnancy
Pregnancy Category: C (tentative). See Pregnancy Code inside back cover.
Animal reproduction studies: No data available.
Information from studies in pregnant women indicates no increase in defects in 1109 exposures to this drug.
Ask physician for guidance.

Advisability of Use While Nursing Infant
Presence of drug in milk is not known. Ask physician for guidance.

Habit-Forming Potential
None.

Effects of Overdosage
With Moderate Overdose: Nausea, indigestion, abdominal distress, vomiting.

With Large Overdose: Hemolytic anemia (in sensitive individuals), skin discoloration, altered hemoglobin resulting in shortness of breath and weakness.

Possible Effects of Extended Use
Orange-yellow discoloration of the skin.
Hemolytic anemia.

Suggested Periodic Examinations While Taking This Drug (at physician's discretion)
If used on a long-term basis, red blood cell counts and liver function tests.

While Taking This Drug, Observe the Following
Foods: No restrictions.
Beverages: No restrictions.
Alcohol: No interactions expected.
Tobacco Smoking: No interactions expected.
Marijuana Smoking: No interactions expected.
Other Drugs: No significant interaction with other drugs has been reported.
Driving a Vehicle, Operating Machinery, Engaging in Hazardous Activities: No restrictions.
Aviation Note: The use of this drug *may be a disqualification* for the piloting of aircraft. Consultation with a designated Aviation Medical Examiner is advised.
Exposure to Sun: No restrictions.

Special Storage Instructions
Keep in a dry, tightly closed container.

PHENIRAMINE

Year Introduced: 1951

Brand Names

USA		Canada
Triaminic [CD] (Dorsey)	Ursinus [CD] (Dorsey)	Triaminic [CD] (Anca)
Triaminic Juvelets [CD] (Dorsey)	(Numerous other brand and combination brand names)	Triaminic AC [CD] (Anca)
Triaminic Oral Infant Drops [CD] (Dorsey)		Triaminic Expectorant [CD] (Anca)
Tussagesic [CD] (Dorsey)		Triaminicin [CD] (Anca)
		Triaminicol DM [CD] (Anca)

Common Synonyms ("Street Names"):   Allergy pills, cold tablets

Drug Class: Antihistamines

Prescription Required: For low-strength formulations—No
For high-strength formulations—Yes

Available for Purchase by Generic Name: USA: Yes   Canada: No

Available Dosage Forms and Strengths
Tablets — 12.5 mg., 25 mg. (in combination with other drugs)
Syrup — 6.25 mg. per teaspoonful (5 ml.) (in combination with other drugs)
Pediatric drops — 10 mg. per ml. (in combination with other drugs)

Tablet May Be Crushed or Capsule Opened for Administration: Yes

How This Drug Works
Intended Therapeutic Effect(s):   Relief of symptoms associated with hayfever (allergic rhinitis) and with allergic reactions in the skin, such as itching, swelling, hives, and rash.
Location of Drug Action(s):   Those hypersensitive tissues that release excessive histamine as part of an allergic reaction. The principal tissue sites are the eyes, the nose, and the skin.
Method of Drug Action(s):   This drug reduces the intensity of the allergic response by blocking the action of histamine after it has been released from sensitized tissue cells.

Principal Uses of This Drug
As a Single Drug Product: Used primarily to provide symptomatic relief in allergic and related disorders: seasonal and perennial allergic rhinitis (hayfever), allergic conjunctivitis, and vasomotor rhinitis.
As a Combination Drug Product [CD]:   Often combined with other antithistamines and decongestants to enhance their ability to reduce tissue swelling and secretions in allergic and infectious disorders of the upper respiratory tract. It is a common ingredient in cold and cough remedies.

THIS DRUG SHOULD NOT BE TAKEN IF
—you have had an allergic reaction to any dosage form of it previously.
—you are taking, or have taken during the past 2 weeks, any mono-amine oxidase (MAO) inhibitor drug (see Drug Class, Section Three).
—it has been prescribed for a newborn infant.

INFORM YOUR PHYSICIAN BEFORE TAKING THIS DRUG IF
—you have had an unfavorable reaction to any antihistamine drug in the past.
—you have glaucoma.
—you have a history of asthma, peptic ulcer disease, or impairment of urinary bladder function.
—you plan to have surgery under general anesthesia in the near future.

Time Required for Apparent Benefit
Drug action begins in approximately 30 minutes, reaches a maximum in 1 hour, and subsides in 4 to 6 hours.

Possible Side-Effects *(natural, expected, and unavoidable drug actions)*
Drowsiness, sense of weakness, dryness of nose, mouth, and throat, constipation.

Possible Adverse Effects *(unusual, unexpected, and infrequent reactions)*

IF ANY OF THE FOLLOWING DEVELOP, DISCONTINUE DRUG AND NOTIFY YOUR PHYSICIAN AS SOON AS POSSIBLE

Mild Adverse Effects
Allergic Reactions: Skin rash, hives.
Other Reactions
  Headache, dizziness, inability to concentrate, nervousness, blurring of vision, double vision, difficulty in urination.
  Nausea, vomiting, diarrhea.

Serious Adverse Effects
Idiosyncratic Reactions: Emotional and behavioral disturbances: confusion, agitation, inappropriate actions.

Precautions for Use by Those over 60 Years of Age
You may be more susceptible to the development of drowsiness, dizziness, and lethargy and to impairment of thinking, judgment, and memory.
This drug can increase the degree of impaired urination associated with prostate gland enlargement (prostatism).

Advisability of Use During Pregnancy
Pregnancy Category: C (tentative). See Pregnancy Code inside back cover.
Animal reproduction studies: No data available.
Information from studies in pregnant women indicates no significant increase in defects in 2442 exposures to this drug.
Ask physician for guidance.

Advisability of Use While Nursing Infant
This drug may impair milk formation and make nursing difficult. It is known to be present in milk. Avoid use or stop nursing. Ask physician for guidance.

Habit-Forming Potential
None.

Effects of Overdosage
With Moderate Overdose: Marked drowsiness, confusion, incoordination, unsteady gait, muscle tremors. In children: excitement, hallucinations, overactivity, convulsions.
With Large Overdose: Stupor progressing to coma, fever, flushed face, dilated pupils, weak pulse, shallow breathing.

Possible Effects of Extended Use
None reported.

Suggested Periodic Examinations While Taking This Drug (at physician's discretion)

Complete blood cell counts.

While Taking This Drug, Observe the Following

Foods: No restrictions. Stomach irritation can be reduced if drug is taken after eating.

Beverages: Coffee and tea may help to reduce the drowsiness caused by most antihistamines.

Alcohol: Use with extreme caution until combined effect has been determined. The combination of alcohol and antihistamines can cause rapid and marked sedation.

Tobacco Smoking: No interactions expected.

Marijuana Smoking

Occasional (once or twice weekly): Mild increase in drowsiness and dryness of mouth.

Daily: Moderate to marked increase in drowsiness and dryness of mouth; possible accentuation of impaired thinking.

Other Drugs

Pheniramine may *increase* the effects of

- sedatives, sleep-inducing drugs, tranquilizers, antidepressants, pain relievers, and narcotic drugs, and result in oversedation. Careful dosage adjustments are necessary.
- atropine and drugs with atropine-like action (see Drug Class, Section Three).

The following drugs may *increase* the effects of pheniramine

- all sedatives, sleep-inducing drugs, tranquilizers, pain relievers, and narcotic drugs may exaggerate its sedative action and cause oversedation.
- mono-amine oxidase (MAO) inhibitor drugs (see Drug Class, Section Three) may delay its elimination from the body, thus exaggerating and prolonging its action.

The following drugs may *decrease* the effects of pheniramine

- amphetamines (Benzedrine, Dexedrine, Desoxyn, etc.) may reduce the drowsiness caused by most antihistamines.

Driving a Vehicle, Operating Machinery, Engaging in Hazardous Activities: This drug may impair mental alertness, judgment, physical coordination, and reaction time. Avoid hazardous activities until full sedative effect has been determined.

Aviation Note: The use of this drug *may be a disqualification* for the piloting of aircraft. Consultation with a designated Aviation Medical Examiner is advised.

Exposure to Sun: No restrictions.

Special Storage Instructions

Keep in a dry, tightly closed, light-resistant container.

PHENOBARBITAL
(Phenobarbitone)

Year Introduced: 1912

Brand Names

USA		Canada
Barbita (Vortech)	Solfoton (Poythress)	Gardenal (Poulenc)
Luminal (Winthrop)	Solu-barb (Fellows)	Luminal (Winthrop)
Sedadrops (Merrell Dow)	(Numerous other combination brand names)	
SK-Phenobarbital (Smith Kline & French)		

Common Synonyms ("Street Names"):   Barbs, candy, downers, goofballs, peanuts, phennies, phenos, sleepers, stoppers, stumblers

Drug Class: Sedative, Mild, Sleep Inducer (Hypnotic), Barbiturates

Prescription Required: Yes (Controlled Drug, U.S. Schedule IV)*

Available for Purchase by Generic Name: Yes

Available Dosage Forms and Strengths

Tablets — 8 mg., 15 mg., 16 mg., 30 mg., 32 mg., 50 mg., 65 mg., 100 mg.
Capsules — 16 mg.
Prolonged-action capsules — 65 mg.
Elixir — 20 mg. per teaspoonful (5 ml.)
Liquid — 15 mg. per teaspoonful (5 ml.)
Drops — 16 mg. per ml.

Tablet May Be Crushed or Capsule Opened for Administration
Regular tablets and capsules — Yes
Prolonged-action capsules — No

How This Drug Works
Intended Therapeutic Effect(s)
With low dosage, relief of mild to moderate anxiety or tension (sedative effect).
With higher dosage taken at bedtime, sedation sufficient to induce sleep (hypnotic effect).
With continuous dosage on a regular schedule, prevention of epileptic seizures (anti-convulsant effect).
Location of Drug Action(s):   The connecting points (synapses) in the nerve pathways that transmit impulses between the wake-sleep centers of the brain.

*See Schedules of Controlled Drugs inside back cover.

Method of Drug Action(s):   Not completely established. Present thinking is that this drug selectively blocks the transmission of nerve impulses by reducing the amount of available norepinephrine, one of the chemicals responsible for impulse transmission.

Principal Uses of This Drug
As a Single Drug Product: This barbiturate drug has two primary uses: (1) as a mild sedative to relieve anxiety, nervous tension, and insomnia; and (2) as an anti-convulsant to control grand mal epilepsy and all types of partial seizures. It is also used to control febrile seizures of childhood.

As a Combination Drug Product [CD]:   This drug is available in many combinations with derivatives of belladonna, an antispasmodic commonly used to treat functional disorders of the gastro-intestinal tract. It is also available in combination with bronchodilators for the treatment of asthma.

THIS DRUG SHOULD NOT BE TAKEN IF
—you have had an allergic reaction to any dosage form of it previously.
—you have a history of porphyria.

INFORM YOUR PHYSICIAN BEFORE TAKING THIS DRUG IF
—you are allergic or sensitive to any barbiturate drug.
—you are taking any sedative, sleep-inducing drugs, tranquilizers, antihistamines, pain relievers, or narcotic drugs of any kind.
—you have epilepsy.
—you have a history of liver or kidney disease.
—you plan to have surgery under general anesthesia in the near future.

Time Required for Apparent Benefit
Approximately 1 hour.

Possible Side-Effects *(natural, expected, and unavoidable drug actions)*
Drowsiness, lethargy, a sense of mental and physical sluggishness.

Possible Adverse Effects *(unusual, unexpected, and infrequent reactions)*

IF ANY OF THE FOLLOWING DEVELOP, DISCONTINUE DRUG AND NOTIFY YOUR PHYSICIAN AS SOON AS POSSIBLE

Mild Adverse Effects
Allergic Reactions: Skin rashes (various kinds), hives, localized swellings of eyelids, face, or lips, drug fever (see Glossary).
Other Reactions
"Hangover" effect, dizziness, unsteadiness.
Nausea, vomiting, diarrhea.
Joint and muscle pains, most often in the neck, shoulders, and arms.
Serious Adverse Effects
Allergic Reactions
Hepatitis with jaundice (see Glossary).
Severe skin reactions.
Idiosyncratic Reactions: Paradoxical excitement and delirium (rather than sedation).

Other Reactions
Anemia, manifested by weakness and fatigue.
Reduction of blood platelets (see Glossary), resulting in unusual bleeding
or bruising.

Precautions for Use by Infants and Children
This drug should not be given to the hyperkinetic child.
Observe for possible paradoxical hyperactivity.
Children under 11 years of age metabolize this drug rapidly and may require
higher maintenance doses than adults to achieve optimal drug levels.
Changes associated with puberty characteristically slow the metabolism of
this drug and permit its gradual accumulation. Monitor the blood levels of
young adolescents every 3 months to detect rising concentrations and
subtle toxicity. Reduce dosage as indicated.

Precautions for Use by Those over 60 Years of Age
Small doses are advisable until tolerance has been determined. The elderly
or debilitated may experience agitation, excitement, confusion, and delirium with standard doses (paradoxical reaction).
This drug may cause excessive lowering of body temperature (hypothermia).
Keep dosage to a minimum during winter, and dress warmly.
The natural decline in liver function that may occur after 60 can slow the
elimination of this drug. Longer intervals between doses may be necessary
to avoid overdosage and toxicity.
Note: A barbiturate is not the drug of choice as a sedative or sleep inducer
in this age group.

Advisability of Use During Pregnancy
Pregnancy Category: B (tentative). See Pregnancy Code inside back
cover.
Animal reproduction studies are conflicting.
Information from studies in pregnant women indicates no increase in de-
fects in 8037 exposures to this drug.
It is advisable to avoid this drug during first 3 months.
Ask physician for guidance.

Advisability of Use While Nursing Infant
Drug is known to be present in milk. Avoid use if possible. Ask physician for
guidance.

Habit-Forming Potential
This drug can cause both psychological and physical dependence (see Glossary).

Effects of Overdosage
With Moderate Overdose: Behavior similar to alcoholic intoxication: confusion, slurred speech, physical incoordination, staggering gait, drowsiness.
With Large Overdose: Deepening sleep, coma, slow and shallow breathing,
weak and rapid pulse, cold and sweaty skin.

Possible Effects of Extended Use
Psychological and/or physical dependence.

Anemia.

If dose is excessive, a form of chronic drug intoxication can occur: headache, impaired vision, slurred speech, and depression.

Suggested Periodic Examinations While Taking This Drug (at physician's discretion)
Complete blood cell counts.

Liver function tests.

While Taking This Drug, Observe the Following
Foods: No restrictions.

Beverages: No restrictions.

Alcohol: Avoid completely. Alcohol can increase greatly the sedative and depressant actions of this drug on brain function.

Tobacco Smoking: No interactions expected.

Marijuana Smoking

Occasional (once or twice weekly):   Mild, transient increase in drowsiness, unsteadiness, and impairment of mental and physical performance.

Daily: Marked, prolonged drowsiness, unsteadiness, and significantly impaired mental and physical performance.

Other Drugs

Phenobarbital may *increase* the effects of

- other sedatives, sleep-inducing drugs, tranquilizers, antihistamines, pain relievers, and narcotic drugs, and cause oversedation. Ask your physician for guidance regarding dosage adjustments.

Phenobarbital may *decrease* the effects of

- oral anticoagulants of the coumarin family. Ask physician for guidance regarding prothrombin time testing and adjustment of the anticoagulant dosage.
- aspirin, and reduce its pain relieving action.
- cortisone and related drugs, by hastening their elimination from the body.
- oral contraceptives, by hastening their elimination from the body.
- griseofulvin (Fulvicin, Grisactin, etc.), and reduce its effectiveness in treating fungus infections.
- phenylbutazone (Azolid, Butazolidin, etc.), and reduce its effectiveness in treating inflammation and pain.

Phenobarbital *taken concurrently* with

- anti-convulsants, may cause a change in the pattern of epileptic seizures. Careful dosage adjustments are necessary to achieve a balance of actions that will give the best protection from seizures.

The following drugs may *increase* the effects of phenobarbital

- both mild and strong tranquilizers may increase the sedative and sleep-inducing actions of barbiturate drugs and cause oversedation.
- isoniazid (INH, Isozide, etc.) may prolong the action of barbiturate drugs.

- antihistamines may increase the sedative effects of barbiturate drugs.
- oral anti-diabetic drugs of the sulfonylurea type may prolong the sedative effect of barbiturate drugs.
- mono-amine oxidase (MAO) inhibitor drugs may prolong the sedative effects of barbiturate drugs.

Driving a Vehicle, Operating Machinery, Engaging in Hazardous Activities: This drug can produce drowsiness and can impair mental alertness, judgment, physical coordination, and reaction time. Avoid hazardous activities.

Aviation Note: The use of this drug *is a disqualification* for the piloting of aircraft. Consultation with a designated Aviation Medical Examiner is advised.

Exposure to Sun: Use caution until sensitivity has been determined. Some barbiturates can cause photosensitivity (see Glossary).

Exposure to Cold: The elderly may experience excessive lowering of body temperature while taking this drug. Keep dosage to a minimum during winter and dress warmly.

Discontinuation: If it has been necessary to use this drug for an extended period of time, do not discontinue it abruptly. Ask physician for guidance regarding dosage adjustment and withdrawal. It may also be necessary to adjust the doses of other drugs taken concurrently with it.

Special Storage Instructions

Keep tablets and capsules in a dry, tightly closed container. Keep elixir in a tightly closed, amber glass bottle.

PHENTERMINE

Year Introduced: 1952

Brand Names

USA	Canada
Fastin (Beecham)	Fastin (Beecham)
Ionamin (Pennwalt)	Ionamin (Pennwalt)
Tora (Tutag)	
Unifast Unicelles (Reid-Provident)	

Common Synonyms ("Street Names"):   Diet pills

Drug Class: Appetite Suppressant (Anorexiant), Amphetamine-like Drug

Prescription Required: Yes (Controlled Drug, U.S. Schedule IV)*

*See Schedules of Controlled Drugs inside back cover.

Available for Purchase by Generic Name: USA: Yes   Canada: No

Available Dosage Forms and Strengths
    Tablets — 8 mg., 37.5 mg.
    Capsules — 15 mg., 30 mg., 37.5 mg.
Prolonged-action capsules — 15 mg., 30 mg.

Tablet May Be Crushed or Capsule Opened for Administration
Regular tablets and capsules — Yes
    Prolonged-action capsules — No

How This Drug Works
    Intended Therapeutic Effect(s)   The suppression of appetite in the management of weight reduction using low-calorie diets.
    Location of Drug Action(s):   Not completely established. The site of therapeutic action is thought to be the appetite-regulating center located in the hypothalamus of the brain.
    Method of Drug Action(s):   Not established. This drug is thought to resemble the amphetamines in its action, diminishing hunger by altering the chemical control of nerve impulse transmission in the brain center which regulates appetite.

Principal Uses of This Drug
    As a Single Drug Product: Used exclusively for the short-term control of appetite in conjunction with other treatment measures designed to reduce body weight. Its effectiveness in suppressing the appetite is usually limited to 6 to 12 weeks.

THIS DRUG SHOULD NOT BE TAKEN IF
—you have had an allergic reaction to any dosage form of it previously.
—you have glaucoma.
—you are taking, or have taken during the past 2 weeks, any mono-amine oxidase (MAO) inhibitor drug (see Drug Class, Section Three).
—it is prescribed for a child under 12 years of age.

INFORM YOUR PHYSICIAN BEFORE TAKING THIS DRUG IF
—you have had an unfavorable reaction to any amphetamine-like drug in the past.
—you have high blood pressure or any form of heart disease.
—you have an overactive thyroid gland (hyperthyroidism).
—you have a history of serious anxiety or nervous tension.

Time Required for Apparent Benefit
Drug action begins in approximately 1 hour and persists for 10 to 14 hours (if the prolonged-action capsule is used).

Possible Side-Effects *(natural, expected, and unavoidable drug actions)*
Nervousness, insomnia.

Possible Adverse Effects *(unusual, unexpected, and infrequent reactions)*

IF ANY OF THE FOLLOWING DEVELOP, DISCONTINUE DRUG AND NOTIFY YOUR PHYSICIAN AS SOON AS POSSIBLE

Mild Adverse Effects
  Allergic Reactions: Skin rash, hives.
  Other Reactions
    Dryness of the mouth, nausea, diarrhea.
    Headache, dizziness, restlessness, tremor.
    Fast and forceful heart action (heart palpitation).
Serious Adverse Effects
  None reported.

CAUTION
The appetite-suppressing action of this drug may disappear after several weeks of continuous use, regardless of the size of the dose. *Do not increase the dose* beyond that prescribed.

Precautions for Use by Those over 60 Years of Age
You may be more sensitive to the stimulant effects of this drug. Small doses are advisable until your individual response has been determined.
You may be more susceptible to the development of nervousness, agitation, insomnia, high blood pressure, disturbance of heart rhythm, or angina.

Advisability of Use During Pregnancy
Pregnancy Category: C (tentative). See Pregnancy Code inside back cover.
  Animal reproduction studies: No data available.
  Information from adequate studies in pregnant women is not available.
  Ask physician for guidance.

Advisability of Use While Nursing Infant
Drug is present in milk. Safety for infant not established. Ask physician for guidance.

Habit-Forming Potential
This drug is related to amphetamine and can cause severe psychological dependence (see Glossary). Avoid large doses and prolonged use.

Effects of Overdosage
With Moderate Overdose: Nervous irritability, overactivity, insomnia, personality change, tremor.
With Large Overdose: Initial excitement, dilated pupils, rapid pulse, confusion, disorientation, bizarre behavior, hallucinations, convulsions, and coma.

Possible Effects of Extended Use
Severe psychological dependence.
Skin eruptions.

Suggested Periodic Examinations While Taking This Drug (at physician's discretion)
None required.

While Taking This Drug, Observe the Following
Foods: Avoid foods rich in tyramine (see Glossary). This drug in combination with tyramine may cause excessive rise in blood pressure.
Beverages: Avoid beverages prepared from meat or yeast extracts. Avoid chocolate drinks.
Alcohol: Avoid beer, Chianti wines, and vermouth.
Tobacco Smoking: No interactions expected.
Marijuana Smoking
Occasional (once or twice weekly):   Mild and transient increased heart rate; mild reduction of stimulant effect and appetite suppressant effect of this drug.
Daily: Persistent rapid heart rate; possible heart rhythm disturbance (in sensitive individuals); significant reduction of stimulant effect of this drug.
Other Drugs
Phentermine may *decrease* the effects of
• the major anti-hypertensive drugs, impairing their ability to lower blood pressure. The drugs most affected are guanethidine (Ismelin), hydralazine (Apresoline), methyldopa (Aldomet), reserpine (Serpasil, etc.).

Phentermine *taken concurrently* with
• mono-amine oxidase (MAO) inhibitor drugs (see Drug Class, Section Three), may cause a dangerous rise in blood pressure. Withhold the use of phentermine for a minimum of 2 weeks after discontinuing any MAO inhibitor drug.

Driving a Vehicle, Operating Machinery, Engaging in Hazardous Activities: This drug may impair the ability to safely engage in hazardous activities. Use caution until full effect has been determined.
Aviation Note: The use of this drug *is a disqualification* for the piloting of aircraft. Consultation with a designated Aviation Medical Examiner is advised.
Exposure to Sun: No restrictions.
Discontinuation: If this drug has been used for an extended period of time, do not discontinue it suddenly. Ask physician for guidance regarding gradual reduction and withdrawal.

Special Storage Instructions
Keep in a dry, tightly closed container.

PHENYLBUTAZONE

Year Introduced: 1949

Brand Names

USA	Canada	
Azolid (USV)	Algoverine (Rougier)	Neo-Zoline (Neolab)
Butazolidin (Geigy)	Butazolidin (Geigy)	Novobutazone
Apo-Phenylbutazone	Intrabutazone	(Novopharm)
(Apotex)	(Organon)	Phenbuff (Sands)
	Nadozone (Nadeau)	

Common Synonyms ("Street Names"):   None

Drug Class: Analgesic, Mild; Anti-inflammatory; Fever Reducer (Antipyretic)

Prescription Required: Yes

Available for Purchase by Generic Name: Yes

Available Dosage Forms and Strengths
Tablets — 100 mg.
Capsules — 100 mg.

Tablet May Be Crushed or Capsule Opened for Administration: Yes

How This Drug Works
Intended Therapeutic Effect(s):   Symptomatic relief of inflammation, swelling, pain, and tenderness associated with arthritis, tendinitis, bursitis, and superficial phlebitis. (This drug does not correct the underlying disease process.)
Location of Drug Action(s):   Areas of inflammation in
• the soft tissue structures of joints (tendons, ligaments, bursas, etc.).
• the superficial veins.
Method of Drug Action(s):   Not completely established. Present thinking is that this drug acts somewhat like aspirin, by suppressing the formation of prostaglandins (chemicals involved in the production of inflammation).

Principal Uses of This Drug
As a Single Drug Product: This potent anti-inflammatory drug is used primarily for the short-term relief of pain associated with moderately severe arthritis, gout, bursitis, tendinitis, and superficial thrombophlebitis. Because of its potential for serious toxicity, it is not considered to be an "aspirin substitute." Its use should be limited to those conditions that do not respond to less toxic drugs.

THIS DRUG SHOULD NOT BE TAKEN IF
—you are allergic to any of the drugs bearing the brand names listed above or to oxyphenbutazone (Oxalid, Tandearil).
—you have had a severe reaction to any drug in the past (ask physician for guidance).
—you have a history of blood or bone marrow disease.

—you have a history of stomach or intestinal ulceration, or recurrent indigestion of a serious nature.

—you have a history of disease or impaired function of the thyroid, heart, liver, or kidneys.

—you have high blood pressure.

—it is prescribed for a mild or trivial condition.

—it is prescribed for a child under 15 years of age.

—it is prescribed for anyone in a state of senility.

INFORM YOUR PHYSICIAN BEFORE TAKING THIS DRUG IF

—you are taking any other drugs at this time, either prescription drugs or over-the-counter drugs (see OTC drugs in Glossary).

—you are on long-term anticoagulant drugs.

—you have glaucoma.

Time Required for Apparent Benefit

Usually 2 to 7 days.

Possible Side-Effects *(natural, expected, and unavoidable drug actions)*

Retention of salt and water in the body with decreased formation of urine.

Possible Adverse Effects *(unusual, unexpected, and infrequent reactions)*

IF ANY OF THE FOLLOWING DEVELOP, DISCONTINUE DRUG AND NOTIFY YOUR PHYSICIAN AS SOON AS POSSIBLE

Mild Adverse Effects

Allergic Reactions: Skin rashes (various kinds), hives, itching, fever.

Other Reactions

Indigestion, stomach pain, nausea, vomiting, diarrhea.

Progressive gain in weight and rise in blood pressure due to water retention; these are indications to discontinue this drug.

Serious Adverse Effects

Allergic Reactions: Severe skin reactions, high fever, swollen and painful joints, salivary gland enlargement, anaphylactic reaction (see Glossary).

Other Reactions

Bone marrow depression (see Glossary)—fatigue, weakness, fever, sore throat, mouth irritation, unusual bleeding or bruising.

Hepatitis with or without jaundice (see Glossary).

Kidney damage with impaired function.

Stomach and intestinal ulceration and/or bleeding, with dark red to black discoloration of stools.

Blood pressure elevation, heart damage.

Eye damage: injury to optic nerve and retina, with impaired vision.

Ear damage: hearing loss.

Lethargy, confusion, nervousness.

Precautions for Use by Those over 60 Years of Age

The natural changes in body composition and function that occur after 60 may cause greater susceptibility to the more serious adverse effects of this drug. Many authorities advise that this drug not be used by this age group.

Advisability of Use During Pregnancy

Pregnancy Category: C (tentative). See Pregnancy Code inside back cover. Animal reproduction studies reveal evidence of embryo toxicity. Information from adequate studies in pregnant women is not available. It is advisable to avoid use of this drug during entire pregnancy if possible. Ask physician for guidance.

Advisability of Use While Nursing Infant

Drug is known to be present in milk. Safety for infant not established. Ask physician for guidance.

Habit-Forming Potential

None.

Effects of Overdosage

With Moderate Overdose: Headache, insomnia, dizziness, mental and behavioral disturbance.

With Large Overdose: Hallucinations, convulsions, coma.

Possible Effects of Extended Use

Bone marrow depression (see Glossary).

Development of thyroid gland enlargement (goiter), with or without impaired function.

Suggested Periodic Examinations While Taking This Drug (at physician's discretion)

Complete blood cell counts and urine analysis should be made before drug is taken and during course of treatment at intervals of 1 to 2 weeks. Evaluation of thyroid gland size and functional status.

While Taking This Drug, Observe the Following

Foods: Avoid heavily salted foods. Drug should be taken with or following food to minimize stomach irritation.

Beverages: No restrictions of beverage selection. May be taken with milk to minimize stomach irritation.

Alcohol: Best avoided because of its irritant effect on stomach, with increased risk of ulceration and bleeding.

Tobacco Smoking: No interactions expected.

Marijuana Smoking

Occasional (once or twice weekly):   No effect to mild increase in pain relief from this drug.

Daily: Moderate increase in pain relief from this drug.

Other Drugs

Phenylbutazone may *increase* the effects of

- oral anticoagulants of the coumarin type (see Drug Class, Section Three); consult physician regarding need for dosage adjustment to prevent bleeding.
- anti-diabetic drugs of the sulfonylurea family (see Drug Class, Section Three). Consult physician regarding dosage adjustment to prevent hypoglycemia.

- insulin preparations; consult physician regarding dosage adjustment to prevent "insulin reaction" (hypoglycemia).
- lithium (Lithane, Eskalith, Lithotabs, etc.), and increase the risk of lithium toxicity.
- the penicillins (see Drug Class, Section Three).
- sulfonamide ("sulfa") drugs (see Drug Class, Section Three).

Phenylbutazone may *decrease* the effects of
- antihistamines (see Drug Class, Section Three).
- barbiturates (see Drug Class, Section Three).
- digitoxin; consult physician regarding need for dosage adjustment.
- griseofulvin, by hastening its destruction.
- oral contraceptives, by hastening their destruction.
- zoxazolamine (Flexin), by hastening its destruction.

Phenylbutazone *taken concurrently* with
- indomethacin, may increase the risk of stomach ulceration.
- phenytoin (Dantoin, Dilantin, etc.), may cause excessive levels of phenytoin, resulting in toxic effects on the brain. Dosage reduction may be necessary.

The following drugs may *decrease* the effects of phenylbutazone
- aspirin and related drugs
- barbiturates (see Drug Class, Section Three)
- tricyclic antidepressants (Elavil, Tofranil, etc.)

Driving a Vehicle, Operating Machinery, Engaging in Hazardous Activities: Use caution until occurrence of lethargy, confusion, and impairment of vision or hearing is determined.

Aviation Note: The use of this drug *may be a disqualification* for the piloting of aircraft. Consultation with a designated Aviation Medical Examiner is advised.

Exposure to Sun: Use caution until sensitivity is determined. Phenylbutazone can cause photosensitivity (see Glossary).

Discontinuation: This drug should be discontinued after 7 days if a favorable response has not occurred. If drug has been used for a longer period of time, consult physician regarding dosage adjustment for any of the following drugs taken concurrently with phenylbutazone: oral anticoagulant drugs, oral anti-diabetic medications, insulin preparations, barbiturates, digitoxin, phenytoin.

Special Storage Instructions
Keep in a dry, tightly closed container.

PHENYLEPHRINE

Year Introduced: 1949

Brand Names

USA		Canada
Alconefrin (Webcon)	Clistin-D [CD]	Neo-Synephrine
Anti-B Nasal Spray	(McNeil)	(Sterling)
(DePree)	Demazin [CD]	Prefrin (Allergan)
Coricidin Nasal Mist	(Schering)	Duo-Medihaler [CD]
(Schering)	Duo-Medihaler [CD]	(Riker)
Isophrin (Riker)	(Riker)	
Neo-Synephrine	4-Way Nasal Spray	
(Winthrop)	[CD]	
Nostril (Boehringer-	(Bristol-Myers)	
Ingleheim)	Naldecon [CD]	
Sinarest Nasal Spray	(Bristol)	
(Pharmacraft)	(Numerous other	
Sinex (Vicks)	combination brand	
Synasal Spray (Texas	names)	
Pharm.)		
Chlor-Trimeton		
Expectorant [CD]		
(Schering)		

Common Synonyms ("Street Names"):   None

Drug Class: Decongestant

Prescription Required: No

Available for Purchase by Generic Name: USA: Yes   Canada: No

Available Dosage Forms and Strengths

Tablets — 5 mg., 10 mg. (in combination with other drugs)
Solution — 0.125%, 0.16%, 0.2%, 0.25%, 0.5%, 1%
Ophthalmic solutions — 0.08%, 0.12%, 2.5%, 10%
Nasal jelly — 0.5%
(Examine drug label of combination products.)

Tablet May Be Crushed or Capsule Opened for Administration

Dimetapp — No
Demazin — No
Naldecon — No

How This Drug Works

Intended Therapeutic Effect(s):   Relief of congestion of the nose, sinuses, and throat associated with allergic disorders and infections.

Location of Drug Action(s):   The small blood vessels (arterioles) in the tissues lining the nasal passages, the sinuses, and the throat.

Method of Drug Action(s): By contracting the walls and thus reducing the size of the arterioles, this drug decreases the volume of blood in the tissues, resulting in shrinkage of tissue mass (decongestion). This expands the nasal airway and enlarges the openings into the sinuses and eustachian tubes.

Principal Uses of This Drug

As a Single Drug Product: Used primarily in nose drops and sprays to relieve swelling and congestion in the nose and sinuses.

As a Combination Drug Product [CD]: This drug is available in a variety of combinations. Combined with another decongestant and two antihistamines, the product is widely used to treat infections and allergic conditions of the upper respiratory tract. Combined with isoproterenol as an inhalant for the treatment of acute asthma, this drug improves breathing by reducing the swelling and congestion of the bronchial passages.

THIS DRUG SHOULD NOT BE TAKEN IF

—you have had an allergic reaction to any dosage form of it previously.

INFORM YOUR PHYSICIAN BEFORE TAKING THIS DRUG IF

—you have high blood pressure or heart disease.
—you have diabetes or an overactive thyroid gland (hyperthyroidism).
—you are taking, or have taken within the past 2 weeks, any mono-amine oxidase (MAO) inhibitor drug (see Drug Class, Section Three).

Time Required for Apparent Benefit

Drug action is usually felt within 5 to 30 minutes after application to nasal membranes and may persist for 4 hours.

Possible Side-Effects *(natural, expected, and unavoidable drug actions)*

Dryness of the nose and throat.

Possible Adverse Effects *(unusual, unexpected, and infrequent reactions)*

IF ANY OF THE FOLLOWING DEVELOP, DISCONTINUE DRUG AND NOTIFY YOUR PHYSICIAN AS SOON AS POSSIBLE

Mild Adverse Effects
Allergic Reactions: None reported.
Other Reactions: Burning and stinging of nose, headache, lightheadedness, heart palpitation, tremor.
Serious Adverse Effects
None reported.

CAUTION

1. Too frequent application of nose drops and sprays containing this drug may cause a secondary "rebound" congestion resulting in functional dependence (see Glossary).
2. Many over-the-counter (OTC) medications (see Glossary) for allergies, colds, and coughs contain drugs that may interact unfavorably with this drug. Ask your physician or pharmacist for guidance before using any such medications.

Precautions for Use by Those over 60 Years of Age

You may be more sensitive to the stimulant effects of this drug. Small doses are advisable until your individual response has been determined.

You may be more susceptible to the development of high blood pressure, disturbance of heart rhythm, angina, nervousness, or insomnia.

Advisability of Use During Pregnancy

Pregnancy Category: C (tentative). See Pregnancy Code inside back cover.

Animal reproduction studies in rabbits reveal significant birth defects due to this drug.

Information from studies in pregnant women is conflicting. Limited studies indicate possible increased risk for defects during first 3 months. Larger studies indicate no increase in defects in 4194 exposures during entire pregnancy.

Avoid completely during first 3 months.

Ask physician for guidance.

Advisability of Use While Nursing Infant

Safety not established. Ask physician for guidance regarding time and frequency of use with relationship to nursing.

Habit-Forming Potential

Frequent or excessive use may cause functional dependence.

Effects of Overdosage

With Moderate Overdose: Headache, heart palpitation, vomiting.

With Large Overdose: Elevation of blood pressure, slow and forceful pulse.

Possible Effects of Extended Use

Secondary "rebound" congestion and chemical irritation of nasal membranes.

Suggested Periodic Examinations While Taking This Drug (at physician's discretion)

None required.

While Taking This Drug, Observe the Following

Foods: No restrictions. Oral dosage forms should be taken after eating to reduce stomach irritation.

Beverages: No restrictions.

Alcohol: No interactions expected.

Tobacco Smoking: No interactions expected. No restrictions (unless directed otherwise by physician).

Marijuana Smoking: No interactions expected.

Other Drugs

Phenylephrine *taken concurrently* with

• mono-amine oxidase (MAO) inhibitor drugs (see Drug Class, Section Three), may cause dangerous elevation of the blood pressure.

Driving a Vehicle, Operating Machinery, Engaging in Hazardous Activities: No restrictions.

Aviation Note: The use of this drug *may be a disqualification* for the piloting of aircraft. Consultation with a designated Aviation Medical Examiner is advised.

Exposure to Sun: No restrictions.

Special Storage Instructions
Keep in a tightly closed container. Protect from light.

PHENYLPROPANOLAMINE

Year Introduced: 1948

Brand Names

USA		Canada
Dexatrim (Thompson)	Sinubid [CD]	Naldecol [CD]
Propadrine (Merck	(Parke-Davis)	(Bristol)
Sharp & Dohme)	Sinutab [CD]	Ornade [CD] (SK&F)
Propagest (Carnrick)	(Warner/Chilcott)	Sinutab [CD] (P.D.)
Allerest [CD]	Triaminic [CD]	Tuss-Ornade [CD]
(Pharmacraft)	(Dorsey)	(SK&F)
Contac [CD] (Menley	Triaminicin [CD]	
& James)	(Dorsey)	
Dietac [CD] (Menley	Triaminicol [CD]	
& James)	(Dorsey)	
Dimetapp [CD]	Tussagesic [CD]	
(Robins)	(Dorsey)	
Naldecon [CD]	Tuss-Ornade [CD]	
(Bristol)	(Smith Kline &	
Ornade [CD] (Smith	French)	
Kline & French)	Voxin-PG [CD]	
Ornex [CD] (Menley	(Norwich-Eaton)	
& James)	(Numerous other	
Sine-Off [CD]	combination brand	
(Menley & James)	names)	

Common Synonyms ("Street Names"):   None

Drug Class: Decongestant

Prescription Required: For low-strength formulations—No
For high-strength formulations—Yes

Available for Purchase by Generic Name: USA: Yes   Canada: No

Available Dosage Forms and Strengths

Tablets — 25 mg., 50 mg.

Capsules — 25 mg., 50 mg.

Prolonged-action capsules — 75 mg.

Elixir — 20 mg. per teaspoonful (5 ml.)

Syrup — 12.5 mg. per ml.

(Also marketed in a variety of tablets, capsules, syrups, solutions, and sprays in combination with other drugs. Strength varies according to drug product; examine drug label.)

Tablet May Be Crushed or Capsule Opened for Administration

Regular tablets and capsules — Yes

Prolonged-action capsules — No

Dimetapp — No

Allerest, Contac, Ornade, and

Tuss-Ornade capsules — Yes, but do not crush or chew contents

How This Drug Works

Intended Therapeutic Effect(s)

Relief of congestion of the nose, sinuses, and throat associated with allergic disorders and infections.

Suppression of appetite in the management of weight reduction using low-calorie diets.

Location of Drug Action(s)

The small blood vessels (arterioles) in the tissues lining the nasal passages, the sinuses, and the throat.

The appetite-regulating center within the hypothalamus of the brain.

Method of Drug Action(s)

By contracting the walls and thus reducing the size of the arterioles, this drug decreases the volume of blood in the tissues, resulting in shrinkage of tissue mass (decongestion). This expands the nasal airway and enlarges the openings into the sinuses and eustachian tubes.

By altering the chemical control of nerve impulse transmission within the appetite-regulating center, this drug can temporarily reduce hunger in some individuals.

Principal Uses of This Drug

As a Single Drug Product: This drug is currently used for two purposes: (1) As a nasal decongestant and (2) as an appetite suppressant for weight control.

As a Combination Drug Product [CD]:   This drug is available in numerous combinations. It is often combined with other decongestants and antihistamines in preparations used to treat nasal allergies, headcolds, and sinusitis. Similar formulations are combined with aspirin or acetaminophen for treatment of sinus headache. This drug is also combined with expectorants and cough suppressants, such as dextromethorphan, in the formulation of cough syrups.

THIS DRUG SHOULD NOT BE TAKEN IF

—you have had an allergic reaction to any dosage form of it previously.

INFORM YOUR PHYSICIAN BEFORE TAKING THIS DRUG IF
—you have high blood pressure or heart disease.
—you have an overactive thyroid gland (hyperthyroidism) or diabetes.
—you have difficulty emptying the urinary bladder.
—you are taking, or have taken during the past 2 weeks, any mono-amine oxidase (MAO) inhibitor drug (see Drug Class, Section Three).
—you are taking any form of digitalis (Digitoxin, Digoxin, etc.).
—you plan to have surgery under general anesthesia in the near future.

Time Required for Apparent Benefit
Drug action begins in 30 to 60 minutes and persists for 3 to 4 hours.

Possible Side-Effects *(natural, expected, and unavoidable drug actions)*
Nervousness, insomnia, increase in blood pressure in sensitive individuals.

Possible Adverse Effects *(unusual, unexpected, and infrequent reactions)*

IF ANY OF THE FOLLOWING DEVELOP, DISCONTINUE DRUG AND NOTIFY YOUR PHYSICIAN AS SOON AS POSSIBLE

Mild Adverse Effects
Allergic Reactions: None reported when drug is taken orally.
Other Reactions
Headache, dizziness, rapid and forceful heart action.
Nausea, vomiting.
Serious Adverse Effects
Idiosyncratic Reactions: Acute temporary mental derangement (psychotic episodes).

CAUTION
1. Do not exceed recommended dose. Large doses can cause dangerous increase in blood pressure. Too frequent application of nose drops and sprays containing this drug may cause a secondary "rebound" congestion resulting in functional dependence (see Glossary).
2. Many over-the-counter (OTC) medications (see Glossary) for allergies, colds, and coughs contain drugs that may interact unfavorably with this drug. Ask your physician or pharmacist for guidance before using any such medications.

Precautions for Use by Those over 60 Years of Age
You may be more sensitive to the stimulant effects of this drug. Small doses are advisable until your individual response has been determined.
You may be more susceptible to the development of high blood pressure, disturbance of heart rhythm, angina, nervousness, or insomnia.

Advisability of Use During Pregnancy
Pregnancy Category: D (tentative). See Pregnancy Code inside back cover.
Animal reproduction studies: No data available.
Information from studies in pregnant women is conflicting. Limited studies indicate significantly increased risk for defects during first 3 months. Larger studies indicate no increase in defects in 2489 exposures during entire pregnancy.

Avoid completely during first 3 months.
Ask physician for guidance.

Advisability of Use While Nursing Infant
Drug is known to be present in milk and to have adverse effects on the infant. Avoid drug or stop nursing. Ask physician for guidance.

Habit-Forming Potential
Frequent or excessive use of nasal solutions containing this drug may lead to functional dependence.

Effects of Overdosage
With Moderate Overdose: Marked nervousness, restlessness, headache, heart palpitation, sweating, nausea, vomiting.

With Large Overdose: Anxiety, confusion, delirium, muscular tremors, rapid and irregular pulse.

Possible Effects of Extended Use
Secondary "rebound" congestion of nasal membranes.

Suggested Periodic Examinations While Taking This Drug (at physician's discretion)
None required.

While Taking This Drug, Observe the Following
Foods: No restrictions.

Beverages: Excessive coffee or tea may add to the nervousness or insomnia caused by this drug in sensitive individuals.

Alcohol: No interactions expected.

Tobacco Smoking: No interactions expected. No restrictions (unless advised otherwise by your physician).

Marijuana Smoking

Occasional (once or twice weekly): Mild and transient increased heart rate; mild reduction of appetite suppressant effect of this drug.

Daily: Persistent rapid heart rate; possible heart rhythm disturbance (in sensitive individuals).

Other Drugs

Phenylpropanolamine may *increase* the effects of

• epinephrine (Adrenalin, Bronkaid Mist, Vaponefrin, etc.), and cause excessive stimulation of the heart and an increase in blood pressure. Use caution and avoid excessive dosage.

Phenylpropanolamine may *decrease* the effects of

• the anti-hypertensive drugs, and reduce their effectiveness in lowering blood pressure. Ask physician if any dosage adjustment is necessary to maintain proper blood pressure control.

Phenylpropanolamine *taken concurrently* with

• digitalis preparations (Digitoxin, Digoxin, etc.), may cause serious disturbances of heart rhythm.

- ergot-related preparations (Cafergot, Ergotrate, Migral, Wigraine, etc.), may cause serious increase in blood pressure.
- guanethidine, may result in reduced effectiveness of both drugs.

The following drugs may *increase* the effects of phenylpropanolamine

- mono-amine oxidase (MAO) inhibitor drugs (see Drug Class, Section Three). The combined effects may cause a dangerous increase in blood pressure.
- tricyclic antidepressants (see Drug Class, Section Three). The combined effects may cause excessive stimulation of the heart and blood pressure.

Driving a Vehicle, Operating Machinery, Engaging in Hazardous Activities: No restrictions unless dizziness occurs.

Aviation Note: The use of this drug *may be a disqualification* for the piloting of aircraft. Consultation with a designated Aviation Medical Examiner is advised.

Exposure to Sun: No restrictions.

Special Storage Instructions
Keep in a tightly closed, light-resistant container. Avoid excessive heat.

PHENYLTOLOXAMINE

Year Introduced: 1959

Brand Names

USA	Canada
Naldecon [CD] (Bristol)	Naldecol [CD] (Bristol)
Percogesic [CD] (Rho Mu)	Sinutab [CD] (P.D. & Co.)
Sinubid [CD] (Parke-Davis)	Tussionex [CD] (Pennwalt)
Tussionex [CD] (Pennwalt)	

Common Synonyms ("Street Names"): None

Drug Class: Antihistamines

Prescription Required: USA: Yes for some (Controlled Drug Schedule C-III [Tussionex])*
Canada: Yes for some (Controlled Drug Schedule N [Tussionex])

Available for Purchase by Generic Name: No

*See Schedules of Controlled Drugs inside back cover.

Available Dosage Forms and Strengths

Several combination drugs containing phenyltoloxamine are available as capsules, tablets, prolonged-action tablets, syrups, and pediatric drops. Read the product label carefully to learn the contents and the strength of each ingredient.

Tablet May Be Crushed or Capsule Opened for Administration

Regular tablets — Yes
Naldecon tablets — No
Ask your pharmacist for guidance

How This Drug Works

Intended Therapeutic Effect(s):   Relief of symptoms associated with hayfever (allergic rhinitis) and with allergic reactions and infections of the nose, sinuses and throat.

Location of Drug Action (s):   Those hypersensitive tissues that release excessive histamine as part of an allergic reaction. The principal tissue sites are the mucous membranes of the upper respiratory passages.

Method of Drug Action(s):   This drug reduces the intensity of the allergic response by blocking the action of histamine after it has been released from sensitized tissue cells.

Principal Uses of This Drug

As a Single Drug Product: This drug is not available in a single entity preparation.

As a Combination Drug Product [CD]:   This drug is available in combination with another antihistamine and two decongestants for use in treating nasal allergies, headcolds, and sinusitis. It is also combined with acetaminophen for the treatment of sinus headache. A combination of this drug and hydrocodone is a widely used cough remedy.

THIS DRUG SHOULD NOT BE TAKEN IF

—you have had an allergic reaction to any dosage form of it previously.
—you are subject to acute attacks of asthma.
—you have glaucoma (narrow-angle type).
—you have difficulty emptying the urinary bladder.
—it has been prescribed for a newborn infant.

INFORM YOUR PHYSICIAN BEFORE TAKING THIS DRUG IF

—you have had an unfavorable reaction to any antihistamine drug in the past.
—you have a history of peptic ulcer disease.
—you plan to have surgery under general anesthesia in the near future.

Time Required for Apparent Benefit

Drug action usually begins in 30 minutes, reaches its peak in 1 to 2 hours, and subsides in 4 to 6 hours.

Continuous use on a regular schedule for 2 to 4 days is usually necessary to determine this drug's effectiveness in relieving the symptoms of allergic and/or infectious disorders of the upper respiratory tract.

Possible Side-Effects *(natural, expected, and unavoidable drug actions)*
Drowsiness, sense of weakness, dryness of nose, mouth, and throat, constipation.

Possible Adverse Effects *(unusual, unexpected, and infrequent reactions)*

IF ANY OF THE FOLLOWING DEVELOP, DISCONTINUE DRUG AND NOTIFY YOUR PHYSICIAN AS SOON AS POSSIBLE

Mild Adverse Effects
  Allergic Reactions: Skin rash, hives.
  Other Reactions
    Headache, dizziness, inability to concentrate, impaired coordination, nervousness, blurring of vision, double vision, difficulty in urination, insomnia, tremors.
    Nausea, vomiting, diarrhea, stomach distress.
    Reduced tolerance for contact lenses (possible).
Serious Adverse Effects
  Drop in blood pressure, palpitation, convulsions.

Precautions for Use by Infants and Children
Adhere strictly to prescribed doses and dosage schedules. Do not exceed recommended amounts.

Precautions for Use by Those over 60 Years of Age
You may be more susceptible to the development of drowsiness, dizziness, and lethargy and to impairment of thinking, judgment, and memory.
This drug can increase the degree of impaired urination associated with prostate gland enlargement (prostatism).

Advisability of Use During Pregnancy
Pregnancy Category: C (tentative). See Pregnancy Code inside back cover.
  Animal reproduction studies: No data available.
  Information from adequate studies in pregnant women is not available.
  Ask physician for guidance.

Advisability of Use While Nursing Infant
This drug is probably present in the mother's milk. It is advisable to avoid use of this drug or to refrain from breast-feeding.

Habit-Forming Potential
None.

Effects of Overdosage
With Moderate Overdose: Marked drowsiness, confusion, incoordination, unsteady gait, muscle tremors. In children, excitement, hallucinations, overactivity, convulsions.
With Large Overdose: Stupor progressing to coma, fever, flushed face, dilated pupils, weak pulse, shallow breathing.

Possible Effects of Extended Use
None reported.

Suggested Periodic Examinations While Taking This Drug (at physician's discretion)

None.

While Taking This Drug, Observe the Following

Foods: No restrictions. Timing of Drug and Food: May be taken after eating to reduce stomach irritation.

Beverages: No restrictions. This drug may be taken with milk.

Alcohol: Use with extreme caution until combined effect has been determined. The combination of alcohol and antihistamines can cause rapid and marked sedation.

Tobacco Smoking: No interactions expected.

Marijuana Smoking

Occasional (once or twice weekly):   No effect to mild increase in sedation. Daily: Possibly a significant increase in sedation.

Other Drugs

Phenyltoloxamine may *increase* the effects of

- sedatives, sleep-inducing drugs, tranquilizers, antidepressants, pain relievers, and narcotic drugs, and result in oversedation. Careful dosage adjustments are necessary.
- atropine and drugs with atropine-like action (see Drug Class, Section Three).

Phenyltoloxamine may *decrease* the effects of

- oral anticoagulants, and reduce their protective action. Consult physician regarding prothrombin time testing and dosage adjustment.
- cortisone and related drugs (See Drug Class, Section Three).

Phenyltoloxamine *taken concurrently* with

- phenytoin (Dantoin, Dilantin, etc.), may change the pattern of epileptic seizures. Dosage adjustments may be necessary for proper control of epilepsy.

The following drugs may *increase* the effects of phenyltoloxamine:

- all sedatives, sleep-inducing drugs, tranquilizers, pain relievers, and narcotic drugs may exaggerate its sedative action and cause oversedation.

The following drugs may *decrease* the effects of phenyltoloxamine:

- the amphetamines (Benzedrine, Dexedrine, Desoxyn, etc.) may reduce the drowsiness caused by most antihistamines.

Driving a Vehicle, Operating Machinery, Engaging in Hazardous Activities: This drug may impair mental alertness, judgment, physical coordination, and reaction time. Avoid hazardous activities until full sedative effect has been determined.

Aviation Note: The use of this drug *is a disqualification* for the piloting of aircraft. Consultation with a designated Aviation Medical Examiner is advised.

Exposure to Sun: Use caution until sensitivity has been determined. This type of drug may cause photosensitivity (see Glossary).

Exposure to Cold: The elderly should dress warmly and use caution to prevent hypothermia.

Special Storage Instructions
Keep in a dry, tightly closed, light-resistant container.

PHENYTOIN
(formerly Diphenylhydantoin)

Year Introduced: 1938

Brand Names

USA		Canada
Dihycon (Consol. Midland)	Diphenylan (Lannett)	Dilantin (P.D.)
Dilantin (Parke-Davis)	Dilantin w/Phenobarbital [CD] (Parke-Davis)	Novophenytoin (Novopharm)

Common Synonyms ("Street Names"): Epilepsy medicine

Drug Class: Anti-convulsant, Hydantoins

Prescription Required: Yes

Available for Purchase by Generic Name: USA: Yes   Canada: No

Available Dosage Forms and Strengths
Tablets — 50 mg.
Capsules (prompt) — 30 mg., 100 mg.
Capsules (extended) — 30 mg., 100 mg.
Oral suspension — 30 mg., 125 mg. per 5 ml. teaspoonful
Injection — 50 mg. per ml.

Tablet May Be Crushed or Capsule Opened for Administration: Yes

How This Drug Works
Intended Therapeutic Effect(s): Prevention of epileptic seizures (anti-convulsant effect).
Location of Drug Action(s): Those areas of the brain that initiate and sustain episodes of excessive electrical discharges responsible for epileptic seizures.
Method of Drug Action(s): Not completely established. It is thought that by promoting the loss of sodium from nerve fibers, this drug lowers and stabilizes their excitability and inhibits the repetitious spread of electrical impulses along nerve pathways. This action may prevent seizures altogether, or it may reduce their frequency and severity.

Principal Uses of This Drug

As a Single Drug Product: Used primarily as an anti-epileptic drug to control grand mal, psychomotor, myoclonic, and focal seizures. Though not officially approved, this drug is also used to initiate treatment of trigeminal neuralgia; it is sometimes effective in relieving the severe facial pain of this disorder.

As a Combination Drug Product [CD]:   This drug is available in combination with phenobarbital, another effective anticonvulsant. Some seizure disorders require the combined effects of these two drugs for effective control.

THIS DRUG SHOULD NOT BE TAKEN IF

—you are allergic to any of the drugs bearing the brand names listed above or you have had an allergic reaction or an unfavorable response to any hydantoin drug.

INFORM YOUR PHYSICIAN BEFORE TAKING THIS DRUG IF

—you have a history of liver disease or impaired liver function.
—you plan to have surgery under general anesthesia in the near future.

Time Required for Apparent Benefit

Dosage must be individualized. Continuous use on a regular schedule for 7 to 10 days is needed to achieve satisfactory response.

Possible Side-Effects *(natural, expected, and unavoidable drug actions)*

Sluggishness or drowsiness (in sensitive individuals).
Pink to red to brown coloration of the urine.

Possible Adverse Effects *(unusual, unexpected, and infrequent reactions)*

IF ANY OF THE FOLLOWING DEVELOP, DISCONTINUE DRUG AND NOTIFY YOUR PHYSICIAN AS SOON AS POSSIBLE

Mild Adverse Effects
  Allergic Reactions: Skin rash, drug fever (see Glossary).
  Other Reactions
    Headache, dizziness, staggering, slurred speech, confusion, muscle twitching.
    Nausea, vomiting, constipation.
    Joint aches and pains.
    Excessive growth of hair (more common in young girls).
Serious Adverse Effects
  Allergic Reactions: Severe skin reactions—peeling, bruising, blistering. Enlargement of lymph glands.
  Idiosyncratic Reactions: Hemolytic anemia (see Glossary).
  Other Reactions
    Bone marrow depression (see Glossary)—weakness, fever, sore throat, abnormal bruising or bleeding.
    Swelling and tenderness of the gums (more common in children).
    Hepatitis with jaundice (see Glossary)—yellow eyes and skin, dark-colored urine, light-colored stools.

CAUTION

1. Some brand name capsules of this drug have a significantly longer duration of action than generic name capsules of the same strength. To assure a correct dosing schedule, it is necessary to distinguish between "prompt" action and "extended" action capsules. Do not substitute one for the other without your physician's knowledge and guidance.
2. When used for the treatment of epilepsy, this drug must not be stopped abruptly.
3. The wide variation of this drug's action from person to person requires careful individualization of dosage schedules.
4. Total daily dosage should not exceed 600 mg. for adults (proportionately less for children).
5. Regularity of drug use is essential for the successful management of seizure disorders.
6. Shake the suspension form of this drug to mix it thoroughly before measuring the dose. Use a standard measuring device to assure that the dose is based upon a 5 ml. teaspoon.
7. Side-effects and mild adverse effects are usually most apparent during the first several days of treatment, and often subside with continued use.
8. It may be necessary to take Vitamin Bc (folic acid) to prevent anemia while taking this drug. Consult your physician.
9. It is advisable to carry a card of personal identification with a notation that you are taking this drug (see Table 19 and Section Six).

Precautions for Use by Infants and Children

In mild epilepsy satisfactory control may be achieved with blood levels below the therapeutic range of 7 to 22 mcg/ml.

Monitor for hypocalcemia, incipient rickets, and need for supplemental vitamin D.

The elimination half-time in some children is comparatively short, requiring more than 1 dose per 24 hours.

Precautions for Use by Those over 60 Years of Age

The natural changes in body composition and function that occur after 60 may make you more sensitive to all of the actions of this drug. Smaller doses will probably be necessary to prevent symptoms of overdosage or toxicity.

The primary intent of this drug is to prevent seizures. Any dosage adjustment must be made under the close supervision of your physician.

Advisability of Use During Pregnancy

Pregnancy Category: D (tentative). See Pregnancy Code inside back cover.

Animal reproduction studies in mice and rats reveal significant birth defects due to this drug.

Information from studies in pregnant women is conflicting. Limited studies suggest a significant increase in defects due to this drug. Avoid completely during first 3 months if possible.

Discuss with your physician the advantages and possible disadvantages of using this drug during pregnancy. It is advisable to use the smallest maintenance dose that will prevent seizures.

The newborn infants of mothers who take this drug during pregnancy may develop abnormal bleeding or serious hemorrhage due to a deficiency of certain clotting factors in the blood. Consult your physician regarding the advisability of taking Vitamin K during the last month of pregnancy.

Advisability of Use While Nursing Infant
This drug is known to be present in milk. Ask physician for guidance with regard to nursing.

Habit-Forming Potential
None.

Effects of Overdosage
With Moderate Overdose: Jerky eye movements, staggering gait, imbalance, slurred speech, drowsiness.
With Large Overdose: Deep sleep progressing to coma, drop in blood pressure, slow and shallow breathing.

Possible Effects of Extended Use
Development of lymph gland enlargement and toxic change.
Development of peripheral neuritis (see Glossary).

Suggested Periodic Examinations While Taking This Drug (at physician's discretion)
Measurements of drug level in blood.
Complete blood cell counts.
Liver function tests.
Evaluation of lymph glands.

While Taking This Drug, Observe the Following
Foods: No interactions. The drug may be taken with or following food to reduce the possibility of nausea. Consult physician regarding the need for additional Vitamin D.
Beverages: No restrictions.
Alcohol: Use with extreme caution until combined effects have been determined. Alcohol (in large quantities or with continuous use) may reduce this drug's effectiveness in preventing seizures.
Tobacco Smoking: No interactions expected.
Marijuana Smoking
Occasional (once or twice weekly):   No effect to mild increase in drowsiness and unsteadiness; little influence on anticonvulsant effect of drug.
Daily: Moderate increase in drowsiness, unsteadiness, and impaired thinking; possible decrease of anticonvulsant effect of drug.
Other Drugs
Phenytoin may *increase* the effects of
• anticoagulants of the coumarin family (see Drug Class, Section Three), and cause abnormal bleeding or hemorrhage.
• anti-hypertensive drugs, and cause excessive lowering of the blood pressure.
• sedatives and sleep-inducing drugs, and cause oversedation.

- griseofulvin (Fulvicin, Grifulvin, etc.).
- methotrexate.
- propranolol (Inderal).
- quinidine.

Phenytoin may *decrease* the effects of
- cortisone and related drugs (see Drug Class, Section Three).
- methadone (Dolophine), by hastening its elimination. (Withdrawal symptoms may result.)
- oral contraceptives

Phenytoin *taken concurrently* with
- barbiturates, may cause an initial change in the pattern of seizures. Dosage adjustments may be necessary.
- tricyclic antidepressants, may require adjustment of the phenytoin dosage to control seizures produced by the antidepressants (when they are used in high doses).
- digitalis preparations, may cause unpredictable toxic effects by either drug. Careful observation and dosage adjustments are essential.

The following drugs may *increase* the effects of phenytoin
- anticoagulants of the coumarin family (see Drug Class, Section Three)
- disulfiram (Antabuse)
- isoniazid (INH, Niconyl, Isozide, Rimifon)
- phenylbutazone (Azolid, Butazolidin, etc.)
- para-aminosalicylic acid (PAS)
- aspirin (in large doses)
- mild tranquilizers (Librium, Valium, Serax, Dalmane)
- chloramphenicol (Chloromycetin)
- estrogens (Premarin, etc.)
- methylphenidate (Ritalin)
- phenothiazines (Compazine, Thorazine)
- certain "sulfa" drugs (Gantrisin, Orisul)

    Reduced doses of phenytoin may be necessary to prevent phenytoin toxicity.

The following drugs may *decrease* the effects of phenytoin
- alcohol
- antihistamines (some)
- glutethimide (Doriden)

Driving a Vehicle, Operating Machinery, Engaging in Hazardous Activities: Use caution until the full effects of this drug have been determined. Rarely, it can cause drowsiness, and impair mental alertness, vision, and physical coordination. Avoid hazardous activities if such symptoms occur. It is essential that you adhere to a schedule of drug dosage that will prevent seizures.

Aviation Note: The use of this drug and the disorder for which this drug is prescribed *are disqualifications* for the piloting of aircraft. Consultation with a designated Aviation Medical Examiner is advised.

Exposure to Sun: Use caution until full effect has been determined. This drug may cause photosensitivity (see Glossary).

Occurrence of Unrelated Illness: Notify your physician of any illness or injury that causes you to make any alterations in your regular dosage schedule.

Discontinuation: Do not discontinue this drug abruptly if you are taking it for epilepsy or seizure disorders. Sudden withdrawal of any anti-convulsant drug can cause severe and repeated seizures.

Special Storage Instructions
Keep in a dry, tightly closed container.

PILOCARPINE

Year Introduced: 1875

Brand Names

USA		Canada
Almocarpine (Ayerst)	Pilocar (Cooper Vision)	Isopto-Carpine (Alcon)
Isopto-Carpine (Alcon)	Pilocel (Bio Products)	Minims (Smith & Nephew)
Ocusert Pilo-20 and -40 (CIBA)	Pilomiotin (Cooper Vision)	Miocarpine (Cooper Vision)
		Ocusert Pilo-20 and -40 (Alza)
		P.V. Carpine (Allergan)

Common Synonyms ("Street Names"):   Glaucoma drops.

Drug Class: Anti-glaucoma (Miotic)

Prescription Required: USA: Yes   Canada: No

Available for Purchase by Generic Name: USA: Yes   Canada: No

Available Dosage Forms and Strengths
Eye drop solution — 0.25%, 0.5%, 1%, 1.5%, 2%, 3%, 4%, 5%, 6%, 8%, 10%
    Ocuserts — 20 mcg., 40 mcg.

How This Drug Works
Intended Therapeutic Effect(s):   Reduction of elevated internal eye pressure, of benefit in the management of glaucoma.

Location of Drug Action(s):   The parasympathetic nerve terminals in the muscles of the eye that constrict the pupil.

Method of Drug Action(s):   By directly stimulating constriction of the pupil, this drug enlarges the canal in the anterior chamber of the eye and promotes the drainage of excess fluid (aqueous humor), thus lowering the internal eye pressure.

Principal Uses of This Drug

As a Single Drug Product: This drug is used exclusively in the form of eye drops and plastic inserts for the management of glaucoma. Selection of the appropriate dosage strength must be carefully individualized.

THIS DRUG SHOULD NOT BE TAKEN IF

—you have had an allergic reaction to any dosage form of it previously.
—you are subject to attacks of bronchial asthma.

INFORM YOUR PHYSICIAN BEFORE TAKING THIS DRUG IF

—you have a history of bronchial asthma.

Time Required for Apparent Benefit

Drug action begins in 15 to 30 minutes, reaches a maximal effect in 60 to 75 minutes, and gradually subsides in 4 to 8 hours. Continuous use on a regular schedule is necessary to control internal eye pressure (as in the treatment of glaucoma).

Possible Side-Effects *(natural, expected, and unavoidable drug actions)*

Temporary impairment of vision, usually lasting 2 to 3 hours after installation of drops.

Possible Adverse Effects *(unusual, unexpected, and infrequent reactions)*

IF ANY OF THE FOLLOWING DEVELOP, DISCONTINUE DRUG AND NOTIFY YOUR PHYSICIAN AS SOON AS POSSIBLE

Mild Adverse Effects
  Allergic Reactions: Itching of the eyes, itching and/or swelling of the eyelids.
  Other Reactions: Headache, heart palpitation, trembling.
Serious Adverse Effects
  Provocation of acute asthma in susceptible individuals.

Precautions for Use by Those over 60 Years of Age

Maintain personal cleanliness to prevent eye infections. Report promptly any indication of possible infection involving the eyes.

Advisability of Use During Pregnancy

Pregnancy Category: C (tentative). See Pregnancy Code inside back cover.
  Animal reproduction studies in rats reveal significant birth defects due to this drug.
  Information from adequate studies in pregnant women is not available.
  Limit use to the smallest effective dose.
  Ask physician for guidance.

Advisability of Use While Nursing Infant
Drug may be present in milk in small quantities. Ask physician for guidance.

Habit-Forming Potential
None.

Effects of Overdosage
With Moderate Overdose: Flushing of the face, increased flow of saliva, and sweating may result from absorption with excessive use of pilocarpine eye drops.

With Large Overdose: If solution is swallowed: nausea, vomiting, diarrhea, profuse sweating, rapid pulse, difficult breathing, loss of consciousness.

Possible Effects of Extended Use
Continuous use may lead to the development of tolerance and the loss of effectiveness in reducing internal eye pressure. Ask physician how this may be avoided.

Suggested Periodic Examinations While Taking This Drug (at physician's discretion)
Measurements of internal eye pressure on a regular basis.
Examination of the eyes for the development of cataracts.

While Taking This Drug, Observe the Following
Foods: No restrictions.

Beverages: No restrictions.

Alcohol: Use caution until combined effect has been determined. This drug may prolong the action of alcohol on the brain.

Tobacco Smoking: No interactions expected.

Marijuana Smoking
Occasional (once or twice weekly):   No effect to mild and transient additional decrease in internal eye pressure.
Daily: Sustained additional decrease in internal eye pressure.

Other Drugs
The following drugs may *decrease* the effects of pilocarpine
- atropine and atropine-like drugs (see Drug Class, Section Three)
- amphetamine and related drugs (see Drug Class, Section Three)
- cortisone and related drugs (see Drug Class, Section Three)
- members of the phenothiazine family (see Drug Class, Section Three). Consult physician regarding the need for dosage adjustments.

Driving a Vehicle, Operating Machinery, Engaging in Hazardous Activities: Use caution until full effect on vision (ability to focus properly) has been determined.

Aviation Note: The use of this drug *may be a disqualification* for the piloting of aircraft. Consultation with a designated Aviation Medical Examiner is advised.

Exposure to Sun: No restrictions.

Discontinuation: Periodic discontinuation of this drug and temporary substitution of another drug may be necessary to preserve its effectiveness in treating glaucoma.

Special Storage Instructions
Keep in a tightly closed, light-resistant bottle.

Do Not Use This Drug if It Is Older Than
the expiration date stated on the label.

PIROXICAM

Year Introduced: 1978

Brand Names

USA	Canada
Feldene (Pfizer)	Feldene (Pfizer)

Common Synonyms ("Street Names"):   Arthritis pill

Drug Class: Anti-arthritics, Aspirin Substitute

Prescription Required: USA: Yes   Canada: Yes

Available for Purchase by Generic Name: No

Available Dosage Forms and Strengths
Capsules — 10 mg., 20 mg.

Tablet May Be Crushed or Capsule Opened for Administration: Yes

How This Drug Works
Intended Therapeutic Effect(s):   Relief of joint pain, stiffness, inflammation, and swelling associated with the major types of arthritis.
Location of Drug Action(s):   Primarily in the inflamed tissues of arthritic joints.
Method of Drug Action(s):   Not completely known. It is thought that this drug reduces the tissue concentration of prostaglandins, chemicals involved in the production of inflammation and pain.

Principal Uses of This Drug
As a Single Drug Product: To provide symptomatic relief in the management of rheumatoid arthritis (and related conditions), osteoarthritis, and gout. This drug does not alter the basic disease process, and should not be considered as curative.

THIS DRUG SHOULD NOT BE TAKEN IF
—you have had a significant allergic reaction to it previously.
—you are allergic to aspirin.
—you have active peptic ulcer disease, regional enteritis, or ulcerative colitis.

INFORM YOUR PHYSICIAN BEFORE TAKING THIS DRUG IF
—you are allergic to any other aspirin substitute.
—you have a history of peptic ulcer disease, regional enteritis, ulcerative colitis, or gastro-intestinal bleeding.

—you have impaired liver or kidney function.
—you are currently taking any anticoagulant drug ("blood thinner").
—you plan to have surgery of any type in the near future.

Time Required for Apparent Benefit
Drug action usually begins in 1 hour and reaches its peak in 4 hours. Continuous use on a regular schedule for 2 weeks is usually necessary to determine this drug's effectiveness in relieving the symptoms of arthritis.

Possible Side-Effects *(natural, expected, and unavoidable drug actions)*
Prolongation of the bleeding time.

Possible Adverse Effects *(unusual, unexpected, and infrequent reactions)*

IF ANY OF THE FOLLOWING DEVELOP, DISCONTINUE DRUG AND NOTIFY YOUR PHYSICIAN AS SOON AS POSSIBLE

Mild Adverse Effects
Allergic Reactions: Skin rash, itching.
Other Reactions: Headache, dizziness, drowsiness, nervousness, insomnia, blurred vision, ringing in the ears.
Loss of appetite, indigestion, abdominal discomfort, nausea, vomiting, constipation, diarrhea.
Mild urinary disturbances: urinary frequency or discomfort.

Serious Adverse Effects
Development of peptic ulcer, with or without bleeding.
Mild anemia due to "silent" blood loss from the stomach (less than that caused by aspirin).
Fluid retention (of importance with heart disease or high blood pressure).

CAUTION
1. If possible, limit dose to 20 mg. daily. Do not exceed 40 mg. daily, and then for no more than 5 days.
2. This drug's anti-inflammatory and antipyretic effects can make it more difficult to recognize the presence of infection. If you develop any symptoms that suggest an active infection, notify your physician promptly.

Precautions for Use by Infants and Children
Safety and effectiveness in children under 12 years of age have not been established.

Precautions for Use by Those over 60 Years of Age
You may be more sensitive to all of the actions of this drug. Small doses are advisable until your individual response has been determined.
You may be more susceptible to the development of headache, dizziness, stomach ulcer, stomach bleeding, and diarrhea.

Advisability of Use During Pregnancy
Pregnancy Category: B (tentative). See Pregnancy Code inside back cover.
Animal reproduction studies reveal no birth defects due to this drug. However, some impairment and delay in the birth process was noted.
Information from adequate studies in pregnant women is not available.
Use this drug only if necessary. Avoid it during the last month of pregnancy.

Advisability of Use While Nursing Infant
The presence of this drug in breast milk is not known.
Ask physician for guidance.

Habit-Forming Potential
None noted to date.

Effects of Overdosage
With Moderate Overdose: Possible stomach irritation with nausea and vomiting.
With Large Overdose: Increased risk of gastro-intestinal bleeding. No serious or threatening effects reported to date.

Possible Effects of Extended Use
Development of anemia due to "silent" bleeding from the stomach.

Suggested Periodic Examinations While Taking This Drug (at physician's discretion)
Complete blood cell counts.
Liver and kidney function tests.

While Taking This Drug, Observe the Following
Foods: No restrictions. Ask physician regarding the use of salt. May be taken with or following food to reduce stomach irritation.
Beverages: No restrictions. May be taken with milk.
Alcohol: Use with caution. The irritant action of alcohol on the stomach lining, added to the irritant action of piroxicam in sensitive individuals, can increase the risk of stomach bleeding or ulceration.
Tobacco Smoking: No interactions expected.
Marijuana Smoking
Occasional (once or twice weekly): No effect to mild increase in pain relief from this drug.
Daily: Moderate increase in pain relief from this drug.
Other Drugs
Piroxicam may *increase* the effects of
• lithium by delaying its elimination and raising its blood levels; monitor carefully for lithium toxicity.

Piroxicam *taken concurrently* with
• oral anticoagulants requires careful monitoring of combined effects until more experience establishes a predictable pattern. Piroxicam can prolong the bleeding time.
Driving a Vehicle, Operating Machinery, Engaging in Hazardous Activities: This drug infrequently causes drowsiness and/or dizziness. If these drug effects occur, avoid all hazardous activities.
Aviation Note: The use of this drug *may be a disqualification* for the piloting of aircraft. Consultation with a designated Aviation Medical Examiner is advised.
Exposure to Sun: No restrictions.

Special Storage Instructions
Keep capsules in a dry, tightly closed container at room temperature.

POTASSIUM

Year Introduced: 1939

Brand Names

USA

Kaochlor (Adria)
Kaon (Adria)
Kay Ciel (Berlex)
K-Lor (Abbott)
Klorvess (Dorsey)

Klotrix
   (Mead Johnson)
K-Lyte
   (Mead Johnson)

Slow-K (CIBA)
Twin-K-Cl (Boots)
Trikates (Lilly)
Kelyum (Pennwalt)

Canada

Kalium Durules
   (Astra)
Kaochlor (Adria)
Kaon (Adria)
Kay Ciel (Pentagone)
K-10 (Beecham)

K Cl 5% and 20%
   (Rougier)
K-Long (Adria)
K-Lor (Abbott)
K-Lyte (Bristol)
K-Sol (ICN)

Micro-K Extencaps
   (Robins)
Neo-K (Neolab)
Slo-Pot (ICN)
Slow-K (CIBA)

Common Synonyms ("Street Names"):   None

Drug Class: Potassium Preparations

Prescription Required: USA: Yes   Canada: No

Available for Purchase by Generic Name: Yes

Available Dosage Forms and Strengths:

Tablets — 2 mEq., 2.5 mEq., 5 mEq.*
Slow-release capsules — 8 mEq.
Effervescent tablets — 20 mEq., 25 mEq., 50 mEq.
Enteric coated tablets — 4 mEq., 13.4 mEq.
Wax matrix tablets — 6.7 mEq., 8 mEq., 10 mEq.
Powder — 15 mEq., 20 mEq., 25 mEq. per packet
Elixir — 20 mEq. per tablespoonful (15 ml.)
Oral liquid — 10 mEq. per tablespoonful (15 ml.)
— 15 mEq. per teaspoonful (5 ml.)
— 20 mEq. per tablespoonful (15 ml.)
— 30 mEq. per tablespoonful (15 ml.)
— 40 mEq. per tablespoonful (15 ml.)
— 45 mEq. per tablespoonful (15 ml.)

*Milliequivalent—the number of grams of potassium contained in one milliliter of a normal solution.

Tablet May Be Crushed or Capsule Opened for Administration
   Regular tablets — Yes
Slow-release tablets — No

How This Drug Works
Intended Therapeutic Effect(s):   The prevention or treatment of potassium deficiency.

Location of Drug Action(s):   Within the cells of most body tissues.

Method of Drug Action(s):   By maintaining or replenishing the normal potassium content of cells, this drug preserves or restores such normal cellular functions as the transmission of nerve impulses, the contraction of muscle fibers, the regulation of kidney function, and the secretion of stomach juices.

Principal Uses of This Drug
As a Single Drug Product: This drug is used primarily in conjunction with those diuretics that cause excessive loss of potassium from the body. Potassium preparations are usually given to stabilize the blood level within the normal range. Dosage adjustments may be necessary.

THIS DRUG SHOULD NOT BE TAKEN IF
—you have had an allergic reaction to any of the drugs bearing the brand names listed above or to any potassium preparation previously.
—you have severe impairment of kidney function.
—you are taking any drug that contains either spironolactone or triamterene.

INFORM YOUR PHYSICIAN BEFORE TAKING THIS DRUG IF
—you are taking any cortisone-like drug (see Drug Class, Section Three).
—you are taking any digitalis preparation.
—you are taking any diuretic drug (see Drug Class, Section Three).
—you have Addison's disease (adrenal gland deficiency).
—you have diabetes.
—you have any form of heart disease.
—you have a history of kidney disease or impaired kidney function.
—you have a history of intestinal obstruction.
—you have a history of familial periodic paralysis.

Time Required for Apparent Benefit
When used to correct potassium deficiency, these preparations are usually beneficial within 12 to 24 hours.

Possible Side-Effects *(natural, expected, and unavoidable drug actions)*
A mild laxative effect for some individuals.

Possible Adverse Effects *(unusual, unexpected, and infrequent reactions)*
IF ANY OF THE FOLLOWING DEVELOP, DISCONTINUE DRUG AND NOTIFY YOUR PHYSICIAN AS SOON AS POSSIBLE

Mild Adverse Effects
Nausea, vomiting, abdominal discomfort, diarrhea. (These usually occur if potassium is taken undiluted or on an empty stomach.)

Serious Adverse Effects

Potassium accumulation, resulting in abnormally high blood levels (see Effects of Overdosage, below). Immediate treatment is mandatory.

Potassium in enteric-coated tablets can cause ulceration, perforation, narrowing, and obstruction of the small intestine. Report promptly the development of abdominal pain, vomiting, or evidence of intestinal bleeding.

Potassium in slow-release (wax matrix) tablets can cause ulceration of the stomach. Report the development of persistent indigestion or stomach discomfort.

CAUTION

1. Dosage must be individualized. Periodic evaluation of overall condition and blood potassium levels is essential to safe and effective management. Excessively high blood levels of potassium can occur without warning. Do not exceed the prescribed dose.
2. Inform your physician promptly if you are taking a tablet form of this drug and you become aware of any difficulty in swallowing.
3. If you have chronic constipation, it is advisable that you avoid potassium in tablet form.
4. Some salt substitutes contain a large amount of potassium. If you are using a salt substitute, consult your physician regarding its continued use or any necessary adjustment in the dosage of your potassium preparation.

Precautions for Use by Those over 60 Years of Age

Your potassium balance must be maintained within strict limitations. Serious adverse effects can occur when the potassium level is either above or below the normal range. Adhere to your dosage schedule exactly.

Advisability of Use During Pregnancy

Pregnancy Category: C (tentative). See Pregnancy Code inside back cover.
Animal reproduction studies: No data available.
Information from adequate studies in pregnant women is not available. Ask physician for guidance.
Potassium preparations can be used safely during pregnancy. Adhere strictly to prescribed dosage. Inform your physician promptly if symptoms suggestive of overdosage develop.

Advisability of Use While Nursing Infant

The presence of these drugs in milk is not known. Ask your physician for guidance.

Habit-Forming Potential

None.

Effects of Overdosage

With Moderate Overdose: Lethargy, weakness and heaviness of legs, numbness and tingling in the extremities, confusion.

With Large Overdose: Paralysis of the extremities, irregular heart rhythm, drop in blood pressure, convulsions, coma, heart arrest.

Possible Effects of Extended Use
Reduced absorption of Vitamin B-12, resulting in anemia (in some individuals).

Suggested Periodic Examinations While Taking This Drug (at physician's discretion)
Measurement of blood potassium levels.

Electrocardiograms, to monitor changes that reflect the potassium content of blood and body tissues.

Measurement of red blood cell counts and hemoglobin levels to detect development of anemia during extended use of drug.

While Taking This Drug, Observe the Following
Foods: Consult your physician regarding the advisability of eating potassium-rich foods. Potassium preparations should be taken with or following food to reduce the possibility of stomach irritation.

Beverages: The effervescent tablets, powder, elixir, and oral liquid preparations of potassium should be well diluted in cold water or juice and taken after meals. If you are on a low-sodium diet, consult your physician regarding the selection of beverage to use for dissolving potassium powder or diluting potassium liquids. Beverages with a high sodium content include Clamato juice, Gatorade, tomato juice, and V-8 juice.

Alcohol: No interactions expected. However, alcoholic beverages can intensify any stomach irritation due to potassium preparations.

Tobacco Smoking: No interactions expected.

Marijuana Smoking: No interactions expected.

Other Drugs

Potassium *taken concurrently* with

- spironolactone or triameterene, may cause an excessive rise in the blood potassium level. This can be extremely dangerous; avoid the concurrent use of these diuretics and any form of potassium.
- digitalis preparations, requires very careful monitoring of the dosage and effects of both drugs.

The following drugs may *decrease* the effects of potassium

- thiazide diuretics (see Drug Class, Section Three) may promote the loss of potassium from the body (hence the need for potassium preparations to maintain normal blood and tissue levels).

Driving a Vehicle, Operating Machinery, Engaging in Hazardous Activities: No restrictions in the absence of symptoms indicative of overdosage.

Aviation Note: Serious cardiovascular disorders *are a disqualification* for the piloting of aircraft. Consultation with a designated Aviation Medical Examiner is advised.

Exposure to Sun: No restrictions.

Occurrence of Unrelated Illness: Inform your physician of any illness that causes vomiting or diarrhea.

Discontinuation: Do not discontinue any potassium preparation suddenly if you are taking digitalis. Ask your physician for guidance if you find it necessary to reduce or discontinue potassium medication for any reason.

Special Storage Instructions
Keep all tablets in a dry, tightly closed container.
Keep elixir and oral liquid in tightly closed, light-resistant containers.

PRAZEPAM

Year Introduced: 1969

Brand Names

USA	Canada
Centrax (Parke-Davis)	None

Common Synonyms ("Street Names"):   Downs, nerve pills, tranks, tranquilizers

Drug Class: Tranquilizer, Mild (Anti-anxiety), Benzodiazepines

Prescription Required: Yes (Controlled Drug, U.S. Schedule IV)*

Available for Purchase by Generic Name: No

Available Dosage Forms and Strengths
Capsules — 5 mg., 10 mg., 20 mg.
Tablets — 10 mg.

Tablet May Be Crushed or Capsule Opened for Administration: Yes

How This Drug Works
Intended Therapeutic Effect(s):   Relief of mild to moderate anxiety and nervous tension, and relief of symptoms during alcohol withdrawal.

Location of Drug Action(s):   Thought to be the limbic system of the brain, one of the centers that influence emotional stability.

Method of Drug Action(s):   It is thought that by enhancing the effects of the nerve transmitter gamma-aminobutyric acid (GABA), this drug reduces the hyperexcitability of certain nerve pathways in the limbic system and thereby produces a calming effect.

Principal Uses of This Drug
As a Single Drug Product: Used primarily for the short-term management of anxiety and nervous tension states, and to control the acute agitation, tremors, delirium, and hallucinations often associated with detoxification of the alcoholic patient.

THIS DRUG SHOULD NOT BE TAKEN IF
—you have had an allergic reaction to it previously.
—you have acute narrow-angle glaucoma.

*See Schedules of Controlled Drugs inside back cover.

INFORM YOUR PHYSICIAN BEFORE TAKING THIS DRUG IF
—you are allergic to any benzodiazepine drug (see Drug Class, Section Three).
—you have a history of alcoholism or drug abuse.
—you are pregnant or planning pregnancy.
—you have impaired liver or kidney function.
—you are currently taking any sedative, sleep-inducing, tranquilizer, or anti-convulsant drug.
—you have a history of a psychotic disorder or severe emotional depression.
—you have asthma, emphysema, or myasthenia gravis.
—you plan to have surgery under general anesthesia in the near future.

Time Required for Apparent Benefit
Drug action usually begins in 1 hour and reaches its peak in 6 hours. Continuous use on a regular schedule for 5 to 7 days is usually necessary to determine this drug's effectiveness in relieving anxiety and nervous tension.

Possible Side-Effects *(natural, expected, and unavoidable drug actions)*
Lethargy (11%), drowsiness (6%), unsteadiness (5%).
"Hangover" effects on the day following bedtime use.

Possible Adverse Effects *(unusual, unexpected, and infrequent reactions)*
IF ANY OF THE FOLLOWING DEVELOP, DISCONTINUE DRUG AND NOTIFY YOUR PHYSICIAN AS SOON AS POSSIBLE

Mild Adverse Effects
Allergic Reactions: Skin rash, hives, itching.
Other Reactions: Dizziness (8%), weakness (7%), fainting, confusion, blurred vision, double vision, slurred speech, sweating, nausea.

Serious Adverse Effects
Paradoxical responses of excitement, agitation, anger, rage, and aggressive behavior.

Natural Diseases or Disorders That May Be Activated By This Drug
Acute intermittent porphyria can be activated by other drugs of this chemical class.

CAUTION
1. This drug should not be discontinued abruptly if it has been taken continuously for more than 4 weeks.
2. The concurrent use of over-the-counter drug products that contain antihistamines (allergy and cold preparations, sleep aids) can cause excessive sedation in sensitive individuals.
3. If this drug is taken at bedtime to induce sleep, significant impairment of intellectual and motor function may persist into the following day. Under these circumstances, it is advisable to avoid hazardous activities and the use of alcohol.

Precautions for Use by Those over 60 Years of Age
It is advisable to use smaller doses at longer intervals to avoid overdosage.
Increased lethargy and indifference are common adverse effects and may result in reduced intake of food and beverages, causing debility, dehydration, and progressive inactivity.

Increased fatigue, muscle weakness, and low blood pressure may predispose
to falls and possible injury.

The development of disturbing dreams and nightmares may require the use
of another class of sedatives.

Be alert to the possible occurrence of "paradoxical" reactions consisting of
agitation, combativeness, anger, and rage.

Advisability of Use During Pregnancy

Pregnancy Category: C (tentative). See Pregnancy Code inside back cover.
No information is available from animal reproduction studies.

Some human studies suggest a possible association between the use of
other drugs of this chemical class and birth defects such as cleft lip and
heart malformations. A cause-and-effect relationship has not been established. Information from adequate studies in pregnant women is not
available.

The consistent use of this drug during pregnancy may cause the development of the "floppy infant" syndrome—a newborn infant with weakness,
lethargy, unresponsiveness, poor muscle tone, depressed breathing, and
low body temperature. Another possible result is the "infant withdrawal"
syndrome—irritability due to the development of dependence upon the
drug during fetal life.

Avoid use of this drug during entire pregnancy if possible.

Advisability of Use While Nursing Infant

The presence of this drug in human milk is not known. However, other drugs
of this chemical class are present in significant amounts. If this drug is used,
observe infant for drowsiness, lethargy, and poor feeding.

Habit-Forming Potential

This drug is liable to abuse. Psychological and/or physical dependence can
occur with long-term use.

Effects of Overdosage

With Moderate Overdose: Increased drowsiness and lethargy, impaired
concentration and memory, confusion, unsteadiness, tremor, hallucinations.

With Large Overdose: Stupor progressing to deep sleep and coma, depressed breathing, low blood pressure.

Possible Effects of Extended Use

Psychological and/or physical dependence.

Suggested Periodic Examinations While Taking This Drug (at physician's discretion)

Complete blood cell counts. Liver function tests.

While Taking This Drug, Observe the Following

Foods: No restrictions. Food increases the absorption of this drug. It may
be taken with food or on an empty stomach.

Beverages: Avoid excessive intake of caffeine-containing drinks: coffee, tea,
cola. May be taken with milk.

Alcohol: Use with extreme caution until the combined effects have been determined. Alcohol may increase the depressant effects of this drug on brain function. It is advisable to avoid alcohol completely—throughout the day and night—if it is necessary to drive or to engage in any hazardous activity.

Tobacco Smoking: Heavy smoking may reduce the calming action of this drug.

Marijuana Smoking

Occasional (once or twice weekly): Transient increase in drowsiness lasting 2 to 6 hours.

Daily: Marked increase in drowsiness and significant impairment of intellectual and psychomotor performance. Avoid all hazardous activities.

Other Drugs

Prazepam may *increase* the effects of

- all other drugs that depress brain function: sedatives, sleep-inducing drugs, tranquilizers, pain relievers, anticonvulsants, antihistamines, narcotics. These drugs will also increase the effects of prazepam and cause oversedation.

The following drugs may *decrease* the effects of prazepam

- all drugs containing caffeine: Cafergot, Cope, Nodoz, etc.

Driving a Vehicle, Operating Machinery, Engaging in Hazardous Activities: This drug can impair intellectual function, judgment, motor performance, and coordination, can slow reaction time, and can impair vision. Should these drug effects occur, restrict your activities accordingly.

Aviation Note: The use of this drug *is a disqualification* for the piloting of aircraft. Consultation with a designated Aviation Medical Examiner is advised.

Exposure to Sun: No restrictions.

Exposure to Heat: Use caution until the effects of excessive perspiration are determined. If urine volume is reduced, drug excretion may be delayed, resulting in drug accumulation and excessive sedation.

Exposure to Cold: The elderly should dress warmly and avoid situations that could induce hypothermia (excessively low body temperature).

Discontinuation: Avoid sudden discontinuation if this drug has been taken continuously over 4 to 6 weeks. The dose should be tapered gradually to prevent a withdrawal reaction. Ask your physician for guidance.

Special Storage Instructions

Keep in a dry, tightly closed container at room temperature.

PRAZOSIN

Year Introduced: 1975

Brand Names

USA	**Canada**
Minipress (Pfizer)	Minipress (Pfizer)
Minizide [CD] (Pfizer)	

Common Synonyms ("Street Names"):   Blood pressure pills

Drug Class: Anti-hypertensive (Hypotensive)

Prescription Required: Yes

Available for Purchase by Generic Name: No

Available Dosage Forms and Strengths
   Capsules — 0.5 mg. (in Canada only), 1.0 mg., 2.0 mg., 5.0 mg.

Tablet May Be Crushed or Capsule Opened for Administration: Yes

How This Drug Works
   Intended Therapeutic Effect(s):   Reduction of high blood pressure.
   Location of Drug Action(s):   The muscles in the walls of blood vessels. The
      principal therapeutic action occurs in the small arteries (arterioles).
   Method of Drug Action(s):   By causing direct relaxation and expansion of
      blood vessel walls, this drug lowers the pressure of the blood within. The
      mechanism of this direct action is not known.

Principal Uses of This Drug
   As a Single Drug Product: This anti-hypertensive drug is used as a "step 2"
      medication in conjunction with other anti-hypertensive drugs in the treat-
      ment of moderate to severe high blood pressure.
   As a Combination Drug Product [CD]:   This drug is available in combina-
      tion with polythiazide, a diuretic of the thiazide class of drugs that are
      usually used as "step 1" medications to initiate treatment for hypertension.
      By utilizing two different methods of drug action, this combination product
      is more effective and more convenient for long-term use.

THIS DRUG SHOULD NOT BE TAKEN IF
—you have had an allergic reaction to it previously.
—you are experiencing mental depression.

INFORM YOUR PHYSICIAN BEFORE TAKING THIS DRUG IF
—you have experienced lightheadedness and/or fainting with use of other
   anti-hypertensive drugs (see Drug Class, Section Three).
—you have a history of mental depression.
—you have impaired circulation to the brain, or a history of stroke.
—you have coronary heart disease, with or without angina.
—you have active liver disease or impaired liver function.
—you plan to have surgery under general anesthesia in the near future.

Time Required for Apparent Benefit

Drug action begins in 30 minutes and reaches a peak in 2 to 3 hours.
Continuous use on a regular schedule for 4 to 6 weeks (with appropriate dosage adjustments) may be necessary to determine this drug's full effectiveness in lowering your blood pressure.

Possible Side-Effects *(natural, expected, and unavoidable drug actions)*

Lightheadedness or feeling of impending faint on arising from a sitting or lying position (see orthostatic hypotension in Glossary).

Possible Adverse Effects *(unusual, unexpected, and infrequent reactions)*

IF ANY OF THE FOLLOWING DEVELOP, DISCONTINUE DRUG AND NOTIFY YOUR PHYSICIAN AS SOON AS POSSIBLE

Mild Adverse Effects

Allergic Reactions: Skin rash, itching.
Other Reactions
  Headache (7.8%),* dizziness (10.3%), drowsiness (7.6%), lack of energy (6.9%), weakness (6.5%).
  Restlessness, agitation, disturbed sleep, depression.
  Blurred vision, ringing in ears, nasal congestion, dryness of mouth.
  Palpitation (5.3%), rapid heart action, shortness of breath.
  Nausea (4.9%), vomiting, abdominal discomfort, diarrhea, urinary frequency.

Serious Adverse Effects

Episodes of very rapid heart rate (120 to 160 beats per minute) followed by fainting.
Sudden drop in blood pressure—with or without fainting—can occur within 30 to 90 minutes after the *first dose.* Be alert to this possibility, so accidental fall and injury can be prevented.
Precipitation of angina in presence of coronary heart disease.
Fluid retention (edema) resulting in weight gain.
Reduced sexual potency (less than 1%).

CAUTION

1. Do not begin treatment with doses greater than 1 mg. daily. Dosage increases must be carefully adjusted according to individual response.
2. Do not exceed a total dose of 20 mg. per 24 hours.
3. Impaired kidney function may increase some individuals' sensitivity to the actions of this drug.

Precautions for Use by Those over 60 Years of Age

Begin treatment with no more than 1 mg. per day for the first 3 days. Subsequent increases in dosage must be very gradual and carefully supervised by your physician.
Use extreme caution when adding other anti-hypertensive drugs to be taken concurrently.

*The percentage figures represent the frequency of occurrence of the respective adverse reaction in patients using this drug to date.

The occurrence of orthostatic hypotension can cause unexpected falls and injury. Sit or lie down promptly if you feel lightheaded or dizzy.

If you have impaired circulation to the brain, or coronary heart disease, excessive lowering of the blood pressure should be avoided. Report any occurrence of lightheadedness, dizziness, or chest pain to your physician promptly.

Advisability of Use During Pregnancy
Pregnancy Category: B (tentative). See Pregnancy Code inside back cover. Animal reproduction studies reveal no birth defects due to this drug. Information from adequate studies in pregnant women is not available. Ask physician for guidance.

Advisability of Use While Nursing Infant
The presence of this drug in milk is not known. Ask physician for guidance.

Habit-Forming Potential
None.

Effects of Overdosage
With Moderate Overdose: Marked lightheadedness or dizziness in upright position (orthostatic hypotension), headache, rapid heart action, generalized flushing of skin.

With Large Overdose: Collapse of circulation—extreme weakness, loss of consciousness, cold and sweaty skin, weak and rapid pulse.

Possible Effects of Extended Use
None reported.

Suggested Periodic Examinations While Taking This Drug (at physician's discretion)
Measurements of blood pressure in lying, sitting, and standing positions.

While Taking This Drug, Observe the Following
Foods: No restrictions.

Beverages: No restrictions.

Alcohol: Use with extreme caution until combined effect has been determined. Alcohol can exaggerate the blood pressure-lowering action of this drug and cause excessive reduction.

Tobacco Smoking: The nicotine in tobacco can contribute significantly to this drug's ability to intensify coronary insufficiency (angina) in susceptible individuals. Follow your physician's advice regarding the use of tobacco.

Marijuana Smoking
Occasional (once or twice weekly):   No effect to mild and transient accentuation of orthostatic hypotension (see Glossary).

Daily: Significant accentuation of orthostatic hypotension, requiring dosage adjustment in sensitive individuals.

Other Drugs

Prazosin may *increase* the effects of
- other anti-hypertensive drugs (see Drug Class, Section Three), and cause excessive lowering of the blood pressure. Careful dosage adjustments are necessary.

Prazosin *taken concurrently with*
- amitriptyline (Elavil) or chlorpromazine (Thorazine, etc.), may cause acute agitation.

The following drugs may *increase* the effects of prazosin
- all other anti-hypertensive drugs (see Drug Class, Section Three). Careful dosage adjustments are necessary.
- nitroglycerin can prolong the effects of prazosin.

The following drugs may *decrease* the effects of prazosin
- amphetamines (Benzedrine, Dexedrine, Synatan, etc.) can impair its blood pressure-lowering action.

Driving a Vehicle, Operating Machinery, Engaging in Hazardous Activities: Avoid hazardous activities until the possibility of orthostatic hypotension has been determined.

Aviation Note: Hypertension (high blood pressure) *is a disqualification* for the piloting of aircraft. Consultation with a designated Aviation Medical Examiner is advised.

Exposure to Sun: No restrictions.

Exposure to Cold: Use caution until combined effect has been determined. Cold may increase this drug's ability to cause coronary insufficiency (angina) in susceptible individuals.

Heavy Exercise or Exertion: Use caution until combined effect has been determined. Excessive exertion can increase this drug's ability to cause coronary insufficiency (angina) in susceptible individuals. Isometric exercises—the "overload" technique for strengthening individual muscles—can raise the blood pressure significantly. Ask your physician for guidance regarding participation in this form of exercise.

Discontinuation: If you find it necessary to discontinue this drug for any reason, inform your physician so proper adjustments can be made in the doses of other drugs you may be taking.

Special Storage Instructions
Keep in a dry, tightly closed container.

PREDNISOLONE

Year Introduced: 1955

Brand Names

USA	Canada
Delta-Cortef (Upjohn)	Inflamase (Cooper Vision)
Fernisolone (Ferndale)	Meticortelone (Schering)
Sterane (Pfipharmecs)	Nova-Pred (Nova)
(Others)	Novoprednisolone
	(Novopharm)

Common Synonyms ("Street Names"):   Cortisone medicine

Drug Class: Cortisone-like Drug, Adrenocortical Steroids

Prescription Required: Yes

Available for Purchase by Generic Name: Yes

Available Dosage Forms and Strengths
   Tablets — 1 mg., 5 mg.

Tablet May Be Crushed or Capsule Opened for Administration: Yes

How This Drug Works
   Intended Therapeutic Effect(s):   The symptomatic relief of inflammation
   (swelling, redness, heat and pain) in any tissue, and from many causes.
   (Cortisone-like drugs do not correct the underlying disease process.)
   Location of Drug Action(s):   Significant biological effects occur in most tissues throughout the body. The principal actions of therapeutic doses occur
   at sites of inflammation and/or allergic reaction, regardless of the nature
   of the causative injury or illness.
   Method of Drug Action(s):   Not completely established. Present thinking is
   that cortisone-like drugs probably inhibit several mechanisms within the
   tissues that induce inflammation. Well-regulated dosage aids the body in
   restoring normal stability. However, prolonged use or excessive dosage can
   impair the body's defense mechanisms against infectious disease.

Principal Uses of This Drug
   As a Single Drug Product: This member of the cortisone class of drugs is
   used to treat a wide variety of allergic and inflammatory conditions. It is
   used primarily in the management of serious skin disorders, bronchial
   asthma, regional enteritis, ulcerative colitis, and all types of major rheumatic disorders including most forms of arthritis, bursitis, tendinitis, and
   related conditions.

THIS DRUG SHOULD NOT BE TAKEN IF
—you have had an allergic reaction to any dosage form of it previously.
—you have an active peptic ulcer (stomach or duodenum).
—you have an active infection of the eye caused by the herpes simplex virus
   (ask your eye doctor for guidance).
—you have active tuberculosis.

INFORM YOUR PHYSICIAN BEFORE TAKING THIS DRUG IF
—you have had an unfavorable reaction to any cortisone-like drug in the past.
—you have a history of tuberculosis.
—you have diabetes or a tendency to diabetes.
—you have a history of peptic ulcer disease.
—you have glaucoma or a tendency to glaucoma.
—you have a deficiency of thyroid function (hypothyroidism).
—you have high blood pressure.
—you have myasthenia gravis.
—you have a history of thrombophlebitis.
—you plan to have surgery of any kind in the near future, especially if under general anesthesia.

Time Required for Apparent Benefit
Evidence of beneficial drug action is usually apparent in 24 to 48 hours. Dosage must be individualized to give reasonable improvement. This is usually accomplished in 4 to 10 days. It is unwise to demand complete relief of all symptoms. The effective dose varies with the nature of the disease and with the patient. During long-term use it is essential that the smallest effective dose be determined and maintained.

Possible Side-Effects *(natural, expected, and unavoidable drug actions)*
Retention of salt and water, gain in weight, increased sweating, increased appetite, increased susceptibility to infection.

Possible Adverse Effects *(unusual, unexpected, and infrequent reactions)*

IF ANY OF THE FOLLOWING DEVELOP, DISCONTINUE DRUG AND NOTIFY YOUR PHYSICIAN AS SOON AS POSSIBLE

Mild Adverse Effects
    Allergic Reactions: Skin rash.
    Other Reactions
        Headache, dizziness, insomnia.
        Acid indigestion, abdominal distention.
        Muscle cramping and weakness.
        Irregular menstrual periods.
        Acne, excessive growth of facial hair.
Serious Adverse Effects
    Mental and emotional disturbances of serious magnitude.
    Reactivation of latent tuberculosis.
    Development of peptic ulcer.
    Increased blood pressure.
    Development of inflammation of the pancreas.
    Thrombophlebitis (inflammation of a vein with the formation of blood clot)
        —pain or tenderness in thigh or leg, with or without swelling of the foot, ankle, or leg.
    Pulmonary embolism (movement of blood clot to the lung)—sudden shortness of breath, pain in the chest, coughing, bloody sputum.

CAUTION
1. It is advisable to carry a card of personal identification with a notation that you are taking this drug if your course of treatment is to exceed 1 week (see Table 19 and Section Six).
2. Do not discontinue this drug abruptly.
3. While taking this drug, immunization procedures should be given with caution. If vaccination against measles, smallpox, rabies, or yellow fever is required, discontinue this drug 72 hours before vaccination and do not resume for at least 14 days after vaccination.

Precautions for Use by Those over 60 Years of Age
The "cortisone-related" drugs should be used very sparingly after 60, and only when the disorder under treatment is unresponsive to adequate trials of non-cortisone drugs. Prolonged use should be avoided.

The continuous use of this drug (even in small doses) can increase the severity of diabetes, enhance fluid retention, raise the blood pressure, weaken resistance to infection, induce stomach ulcer, and accelerate the development of cataract and softening of the bones (osteoporosis).

In sensitive individuals, cortisone-related drugs can cause serious emotional disturbance and disruptive behavior.

Advisability of Use During Pregnancy
Pregnancy Category: C (tentative). See Pregnancy Code inside back cover.

Animal reproduction studies in mice, rats, and rabbits reveal significant birth defects due to this drug.

Information from adequate studies in pregnant women is not available. Ask physician for guidance.

If use of this drug is considered necessary, limit dosage and duration of use as much as possible. Following birth, the infant should be examined for possible defective function of the adrenal glands (deficiency of adrenal cortical hormones).

Advisability of Use While Nursing Infant
Drug is known to be present in milk. Ask physician for guidance.

Habit-Forming Potential
Use of this drug to suppress symptoms over an extended period of time may produce a state of functional dependence (see Glossary). In the treatment of conditions like rheumatoid arthritis and asthma, it is advisable to try alternate-day drug administration to keep the daily dose as small as possible and to attempt drug withdrawal after periods of reasonable improvement. Such procedures may reduce the degree of "steroid rebound"—the return of symptoms as the drug is withdrawn.

Effects of Overdosage
With Moderate Overdose: Excessive fluid retention, swelling of extremities, flushing of the face, nervousness, stomach irritation, weakness.

With Large Overdose: Severe headache, convulsions, heart failure in susceptible individuals, emotional and behavioral disturbances.

Possible Effects of Extended Use

Development of increased blood sugar, possibly diabetes.

Increased fat deposits on the trunk of the body ("buffalo hump"), rounding of the face ("moon face"), and thinning of the arms and legs.

Thinning and fragility of the skin, easy bruising.

Loss of texture and strength of the bones, resulting in spontaneous fractures.

Development of increased internal eye pressure, possibly glaucoma.

Development of cataracts.

Retarded growth and development in children.

Suggested Periodic Examinations While Taking This Drug (at physician's discretion)

Measurement of blood potassium levels.

Measurement of blood sugar levels 2 hours after eating.

Measurement of blood pressure at regular intervals.

Eye examination at regular intervals.

Chest X-ray if history of previous tuberculosis.

Determination of the rate of development of the growing child to detect retardation of normal growth.

While Taking This Drug, Observe the Following

Foods: No interactions. Ask physician regarding need to restrict salt intake or to eat potassium-rich foods. During long-term use of this drug it is advisable to have a high protein diet.

Beverages: No restrictions.

Alcohol: No interactions expected.

Tobacco Smoking: Nicotine increases the blood levels of naturally produced cortisone and related hormones. Heavy smoking may add to the expected actions of this drug and requires close observation for excessive effects.

Marijuana Smoking

Occasional (once or twice weekly):   No interactions expected.

Daily: Additional impairment of immunity due to this drug.

Other Drugs

Prednisolone may *increase* the effects of

- barbiturates and other sedatives and sleep-inducing drugs, causing oversedation.

Prednisolone may *decrease* the effects of

- insulin and oral anti-diabetic drugs, by raising the level of blood sugar. Doses of anti-diabetic drugs may have to be raised.
- anticoagulants of the coumarin family. Monitor prothrombin times closely and adjust dosage accordingly.
- choline-like drugs (Mestinon, pilocarpine, Prostigmin), and reduce their effectiveness in treating glaucoma and myasthenia gravis.

Prednisolone *taken concurrently* with

- thiazide diuretics, may cause excessive loss of potassium. Monitor blood levels of potassium on physician's advice.

- atropine-like drugs, (see Drug Class, Section Three) may cause increased internal eye pressure and initiate or aggravate glaucoma.
- digitalis preparations, requires close monitoring of body potassium stores to prevent digitalis toxicity.
- stimulant drugs (Adrenalin, amphetamines, ephedrine, etc.), may increase internal eye pressure and initiate or aggravate glaucoma.

The following drugs may *increase* the effects of prednisolone
- indomethacin (Indocin, Indocid)
- aspirin

The following drugs may *decrease* the effects of prednisolone
- barbiturates
- phenytoin (Dantoin, Dilantin, etc.)
- antihistamines (some)
- chloral hydrate (Noctec, Somnos)
- glutethimide (Doriden)
- phenylbutazone (Azolid, Butazolidin, etc.) may reduce its effectiveness following a brief initial increase in effectiveness.
- propranolol (Inderal)

Driving a Vehicle, Operating Machinery, Engaging in Hazardous Activities: Usually no restrictions or precautions. Be alert to the rare occurrence of dizziness; restrict activities accordingly.

Aviation Note: The use of this drug *is a disqualification* for the piloting of aircraft. Consultation with a designated Aviation Medical Examiner is advised.

Exposure to Sun: No restrictions.

Occurrence of Unrelated Illness

This drug may decrease natural resistance to infection. Notify your physician if you develop an infection of any kind.

This drug may reduce your body's ability to respond appropriately to the stress of acute illness, injury, or surgery. Keep your physician fully informed of any significant changes in your state of health.

Discontinuation

If you have been taking this drug for an extended period of time, do not discontinue it abruptly. Ask physician for guidance regarding gradual withdrawal.

For a period of 2 years after discontinuing this drug, it is essential in the event of illness, injury, or surgery that you inform attending medical personnel that you used this drug in the past. The period of inadequate response to stress following the use of cortisone-like drugs may last for 1 to 2 years.

Special Storage Instructions

Keep in a tightly closed container. Protect from light.

PREDNISONE

Year Introduced: 1955

Brand Names

USA	Canada
Deltasone (Upjohn)	Apo-Prednisone (Apotex)
Meticorten (Schering)	Colisone (Frosst)
Orasone (Rowell)	Deltasone (Upjohn)
SK-Prednisone (Smith Kline & French)	Novoprednisone (Novopharm)
	Paracort (P.D. & Co.)
	Winpred (ICN)

Common Synonyms ("Street Names"):   Cortisone medicine

Drug Class: Cortisone-like Drug, Adrenocortical Steroids

Prescription Required: Yes

Available for Purchase by Generic Name: Yes

Available Dosage Forms and Strengths
Tablets — 1 mg., 2.5 mg., 5 mg., 10 mg., 20 mg., 25 mg., 50 mg.
Syrup — 5 mg. per teaspoonful (5 ml.)

Tablet May Be Crushed or Capsule Opened for Administration: Yes

How This Drug Works
Intended Therapeutic Effect(s):   The symptomatic relief of inflammation (swelling, redness, heat and pain) in any tissue, and from many causes. (Cortisone-like drugs do not correct the underlying disease process.)
Location of Drug Action(s):   Significant biological effects occur in most tissues throughout the body. The principal actions of therapeutic doses occur at sites of inflammation and/or allergic reaction, regardless of the nature of the causative injury or illness
Method of Drug Action(s):   Not completely established. Present thinking is that cortisone-like drugs probably inhibit several mechanisms within the tissues that induce inflammation. Well-regulated dosage aids the body in restoring normal stability. However, prolonged use or excessive dosage can impair the body's defense mechanisms against infectious disease.

Principal Uses of This Drug
As a Single Drug Product: This member of the cortisone class of drugs is used to treat a wide variety of allergic and inflammatory conditions. It is used primarily in the management of serious skin disorders, bronchial asthma, regional enteritis, ulcerative colitis, and all types of major rheumatic disorders including most forms of arthritis, bursitis, tendinitis, and related conditions.

THIS DRUG SHOULD NOT BE TAKEN IF
—you are allergic to any of the drugs bearing the brand names listed above.
—you have an active peptic ulcer (stomach or duodenum).

—you have an active infection of the eye caused by the herpes simplex virus (ask your eye doctor for guidance).
—you have active tuberculosis.

INFORM YOUR PHYSICIAN BEFORE TAKING THIS DRUG IF
—you have had an unfavorable reaction to any cortisone-like drug in the past.
—you have a history of tuberculosis.
—you have diabetes or a tendency to diabetes.
—you have a history of peptic ulcer disease.
—you have glaucoma or a tendency to glaucoma.
—you have a deficiency of thyroid function (hypothyroidism).
—you have high blood pressure.
—you have myasthenia gravis.
—you have a history of thrombophlebitis.
—you plan to have surgery of any kind in the near future, especially if under general anesthesia.

Time Required for Apparent Benefit
Evidence of beneficial action is usually apparent in 24 to 48 hours. Dosage must be individualized to give reasonable improvement; this is usually accomplished in 4 to 10 days. It is unwise to demand complete relief of all symptoms. The effective dose varies with the nature of the disease and with the patient. During long-term use it is essential that the smallest effective dose be determined and maintained.

Possible Side-Effects *(natural, expected, and unavoidable drug actions)*
Retention of salt and water, gain in weight, increased sweating, increased appetite, increased susceptibility to infection.

Possible Adverse Effects *(unusual, unexpected, and infrequent reactions)*

IF ANY OF THE FOLLOWING DEVELOP, DISCONTINUE DRUG AND NOTIFY YOUR PHYSICIAN AS SOON AS POSSIBLE

Mild Adverse Effects
Allergic Reactions: Skin rash.
Other Reactions
Headache, dizziness, insomnia.
Acid indigestion, abdominal distention.
Muscle cramping and weakness.
Irregular menstrual periods.
Acne, excessive growth of facial hair.
Serious Adverse Effects
Mental and emotional disturbances of serious magnitude.
Reactivation of latent tuberculosis.
Development of peptic ulcer.
Increased blood pressure.
Development of inflammation of the pancreas.
Thrombophlebitis (inflammation of a vein with the formation of blood clot)
—pain or tenderness in thigh or leg, with or without swelling of the foot, ankle, or leg.

Pulmonary embolism (movement of blood clot to the lung)—sudden shortness of breath, pain in the chest, coughing, bloody sputum.

CAUTION

1. It is advisable to carry a card of personal identification with a notation that you are taking this drug if your course of treatment is to exceed 1 week (see Table 19 and Section Six).
2. Do not discontinue this drug abruptly.
3. While taking this drug, all immunization procedures should be used with caution. If vaccination against measles, smallpox, rabies, or yellow fever is required, discontinue this drug 72 hours before vaccination and do not resume it for at least 14 days after vaccination.

Precautions for Use by Those over 60 Years of Age

The "cortisone-related" drugs should be used very sparingly after 60, and only when the disorder under treatment is unresponsive to adequate trials of non-cortisone drugs. Prolonged use should be avoided.

The continuous use of this drug (even in small doses) can increase the severity of diabetes, enhance fluid retention, raise the blood pressure, weaken resistance to infection, induce stomach ulcer, and accelerate the development of cataract and softening of the bones (osteoporosis).

In sensitive individuals, cortisone-related drugs can cause serious emotional disturbance and disruptive behavior.

Advisability of Use During Pregnancy

Pregnancy Category: C (tentative). See Pregnancy Code inside back cover.
Animal reproduction studies in rats reveal significant birth defects due to this drug.

Information from adequate studies in pregnant women is not available. Ask physician for guidance.

If use of this drug is considered necessary, limit dosage and duration of use as much as possible. Following birth, the infant should be examined for possible defective function of the adrenal glands (deficiency of adrenal cortical hormones).

Advisability of Use While Nursing Infant

Drug is known to be present in milk. Ask physician for guidance.

Habit-Forming Potential

Use of this drug to suppress symptoms over an extended period of time may produce a state of functional dependence (see Glossary). In the treatment of conditions like rheumatoid arthritis and asthma, it is advisable to try alternate-day drug administration to keep the daily dose as small as possible and to attempt drug withdrawal after periods of reasonable improvement. Such procedures may reduce the degree of "steroid rebound"—the return of symptoms as the drug is withdrawn.

Effects of Overdosage

With Moderate Overdose: Excessive fluid retention, swelling of extremities, flushing of the face, nervousness, stomach irritation, weakness.

With Large Overdose: Severe headache, convulsions, heart failure in susceptible individuals, emotional and behavioral disturbances.

Possible Effects of Extended Use
Development of increased blood sugar, possibly diabetes.

Increased fat deposits on the trunk of the body ("buffalo hump"), rounding of the face ("moon face"), and thinning of the arms and legs.

Thinning and fragility of the skin, easy bruising.

Loss of strength and texture of the bones, resulting in spontaneous fractures.

Development of increased internal eye pressure, possibly glaucoma.

Development of cataracts.

Retarded growth and development in children.

Suggested Periodic Examinations While Taking This Drug (at physician's discretion)
Measurement of blood potassium levels.

Measurement of blood sugar levels 2 hours after eating.

Measurement of blood pressure at regular intervals.

Chest X-ray if history of previous tuberculosis.

Determination of the rate of development of the growing child to detect retardation of normal growth.

While Taking This Drug, Observe the Following
Foods: No interactions. Ask physician regarding need to restrict salt intake or to eat potassium-rich foods. During long-term use of this drug it is advisable to have a high protein diet.

Beverages: No restrictions.

Alcohol: No interactions expected.

Tobacco Smoking: Nicotine increases the blood levels of naturally produced cortisone and related hormones. Heavy smoking may add to the expected actions of this drug and requires close observation for excessive effects.

Marijuana Smoking

Occasional (once or twice weekly): No interactions expected.

Daily: Additional impairment of immunity due to this drug.

Other Drugs

Prednisone may *increase* the effects of

• barbiturates and other sedatives and sleep-inducing drugs, and cause oversedation.

Prednisone may *decrease* the effects of

• anticoagulants of the coumarin family. Monitor prothrombin times closely and adjust dosage accordingly.

• choline-like drugs (Mestinon, pilocarpine, Prostigmin), and reduce their effectiveness in treating glaucoma and myasthenia gravis.

• insulin and oral anti-diabetic drugs, by raising the level of blood sugar. Doses of anti-diabetic drugs may have to be raised.

Prednisone *taken concurrently* with
- atropine-like drugs, (see Drug Class, Section Three) may cause increased internal eye pressure and initiate or aggravate glaucoma.
- digitalis preparations, requires close monitoring of body potassium stores to prevent digitalis toxicity.
- stimulant drugs (Adrenalin, amphetamines, ephedrine, etc.), may increase internal eye pressure and initiate or aggravate glaucoma.
- thiazide diuretics, may cause excessive loss of potassium. Monitor blood levels of potassium on physician's advice.

The following drugs may *increase* the effects of prednisone
- aspirin
- indomethacin (Indocin, Indocid)

The following drugs may *decrease* the effects of prednisone
- antihistamines (some)
- barbiturates
- chloral hydrate (Noctec, Somnos)
- glutethimide (Doriden)
- phenylbutazone (Azolid, Butazolidin, etc.) may reduce its effectiveness following a brief, initial increase in effectiveness.
- phenytoin (Dantoin, Dilantin, etc.)
- propranolol (Inderal)

Driving a Vehicle, Operating Machinery, Engaging in Hazardous Activities: Usually no restrictions or precautions. Be alert to the rare occurrence of dizziness; restrict activities accordingly.

Aviation Note: The use of this drug *is a disqualification* for the piloting of aircraft. Consultation with a designated Aviation Medical Examiner is advised.

Exposure to Sun: No restrictions.

Occurrence of Unrelated Illness

This drug may decrease natural resistance to infection. Notify your physician if you develop an infection of any kind.

This drug may reduce your body's ability to respond appropriately to the stress of acute illness, injury, or surgery. Keep your physician fully informed of any significant changes in your state of health.

Discontinuation

If you have been taking this drug for an extended period of time, do not discontinue it abruptly. Ask physician for guidance regarding gradual withdrawal.

For a period of 2 years after discontinuing this drug, it is essential in the event of illness, injury, or surgery that you inform attending medical personnel that you used this drug in the past. The period of inadequate response to stress following the use of cortisone-like drugs may last 1 to 2 years.

Special Storage Instructions
Keep in a tightly closed container. Protect from light.

PRIMIDONE

Year Introduced: 1954

Brand Names

USA	Canada
Mysoline (Ayerst)	Apo-Primidone (Apotex)
	Mysoline (Ayerst)
	Sertan (Pharmascience)

Common Synonyms ("Street Names"):   Epilepsy medicine

Drug Class: Anti-convulsant

Prescription Required: Yes

Available for Purchase by Generic Name: Yes

Available Dosage Forms and Strengths
    Tablets — 50 mg., 250 mg.
    Suspension — 250 mg. per teaspoonful (5 ml.)

Tablet May Be Crushed or Capsule Opened for Administration: Yes

How This Drug Works
   Intended Therapeutic Effect(s):   Prevention of epileptic seizures (anti-convulsant effect).
   Location of Drug Action(s):   Those areas of the brain that initiate and sustain episodes of excessive electrical discharges responsible for epileptic seizures.
   Method of Drug Action(s):   Not completely established. This drug reduces and stabilizes the excitability of nerve fibers and inhibits the repetitious spread of electrical impulses along nerve pathways. This action may prevent seizures altogether, or it may reduce their frequency and severity. (Part of this drug's action is attributable to phenobarbital, one of its conversion products in the body.)

Principal Uses of This Drug
   As a Single Drug Product: This drug is used exclusively as an anti-epileptic medication to control generalized grand mal seizures and all types of partial seizures. It can be used to supplement the anticonvulsant action of phenytoin.

THIS DRUG SHOULD NOT BE TAKEN IF
—you have had an allergic reaction to any dosage form of it previously.
—you are allergic to phenobarbital.
—you have a history of porphyria.

INFORM YOUR PHYSICIAN BEFORE TAKING THIS DRUG IF
—you have had an allergic reaction to any barbiturate drug (see Drug Class, Section Three).

—you have a history of liver or kidney disease.
—you have a history of systemic lupus erythematosus.
—you plan to have surgery under general anesthesia in the near future.

Time Required for Apparent Benefit

Dosage must be individualized. Continuous use on a regular schedule for 2 to 3 weeks is needed to evaluate response. Dosage adjustments may be necessary from time to time.

Possible Side-Effects *(natural, expected, and unavoidable drug actions)*

Drowsiness, lethargy, a sense of mental and physical sluggishness.

Possible Adverse Effects *(unusual, unexpected, and infrequent reactions)*

IF ANY OF THE FOLLOWING DEVELOP, DISCONTINUE DRUG AND NOTIFY YOUR PHYSICIAN AS SOON AS POSSIBLE

Mild Adverse Effects

Allergic Reactions: Skin rash.
Other Reactions
Dizziness, vertigo, unsteadiness, impaired coordination.
Reduced appetite, nausea, vomiting.
Nervous irritability, emotional disturbances.

Serious Adverse Effects

Allergic Reactions
Enlargement of lymph glands.
Severe skin reactions.
Idiosyncratic Reactions: Anemia due to deficiency of Vitamin Bc (folic acid).
Other Reactions
Visual disturbances, double vision.
Sexual impotence.
Personality changes, abnormal behavior.
Symptoms suggesting systemic lupus erythematosus (see Glossary).
Bone marrow depression (see Glossary)—fatigue, weakness, fever, sore throat, abnormal bruising or bleeding.

CAUTION

1. This drug must not be stopped abruptly.
2. The wide variation of this drug's action from person to person requires careful individualization of dosage schedules.
3. Total daily dosage should not exceed 2000 mg.
4. Regularity of drug use is essential for the successful management of seizure disorders.
5. Shake the suspension form of this drug to mix it thoroughly before measuring the dose. Use a standard measuring device to assure that the dose is based upon a 5 ml. teaspoon.
6. Side-effects and mild adverse effects are usually most apparent during the first several days of treatment and often subside with continued use.
7. It may be necessary to take Vitamin Bc (folic acid) to prevent anemia while taking this drug. Consult your physician.

8. It is advisable that you carry a card of personal identification with a notation that you are taking this drug (see Table 19 and Section Six).

Precautions for Use by Infants and Children
This drug should be used with caution in the hyperkinetic child.

Observe for possible paradoxical hyperactivity.

Children under 11 years of age may metabolize the derived phenobarbital rapidly and may require higher maintenance doses than adults to achieve optimal drug levels.

Changes associated with puberty characteristically slow the metabolism of phenobarbital and permit its gradual accumulation. Monitor the blood levels of young adolescents every 3 months to detect rising concentrations and subtle toxicity. Reduce dosage as indicated.

Precautions for Use by Those over 60 Years of Age
The natural changes in body composition and function that occur after 60 may make you more sensitive to all of the actions of this drug. Smaller doses will probably be necessary to prevent symptoms of overdosage or toxicity.

The primary intent of this drug is to prevent seizures. Any dosage adjustment must be under the close supervision of your physician.

Advisability of Use During Pregnancy
Pregnancy Category: C (tentative). See Pregnancy Code inside back cover.

Animal reproduction studies in mice reveal significant birth defects due to this drug.

Information from adequate studies in pregnant women is not available.

However, recent reports suggest a possible association between the use of this drug during the first 3 months of pregnancy and the development of birth defects in the fetus. Discuss with your physician the advantages and possible disadvantages of using this drug during pregnancy. It is advisable to use the smallest maintenance dose that will prevent seizures.

The newborn infants of mothers who take this drug during pregnancy may develop abnormal bleeding or serious hemorrhage due to a deficiency of certain clotting factors in the blood. Consult your physician regarding the advisability of taking Vitamin K during the last month of pregnancy.

Advisability of Use While Nursing Infant
This drug is known to be present in milk in substantial amounts. Observe the nursing infant for drowsiness. Ask physician for guidance.

Habit-Forming Potential
None.

Effects of Overdosage
With Moderate Overdose: Drowsiness, jerky eye movements, blurred vision, staggering gait, incoordination, slurred speech.

With Large Overdose: Deep sleep progressing to coma, slow and shallow breathing, weak and rapid pulse.

Possible Effects of Extended Use

Lymph gland enlargement.

Thyroid gland enlargement.

Anemia.

Reduced blood levels of calcium and phosphorus, leading to rickets in children and loss of bone texture (osteomalacia) in adults.

Suggested Periodic Examinations While Taking This Drug (at physician's discretion)

Complete blood cell counts.

Evaluation of lymph glands.

Measurements of blood levels of calcium and phosphorus.

While Taking This Drug, Observe the Following

Foods: No restrictions. This drug may be taken with or following food to reduce the possibility of nausea. Consult your physician regarding the need for additional Vitamin D.

Beverages: No restrictions.

Alcohol: Use with extreme caution until combined effects have been determined. Alcohol can increase the sedative action of this drug and (in large quantities or with continuous use) may reduce its effectiveness in preventing seizures.

Tobacco Smoking: No interactions expected.

Marijuana Smoking

Occasional (once or twice weekly):   No effect to mild increase in drowsiness and unsteadiness; little influence on anticonvulsant effect of drug.

Daily: Moderate increase in drowsiness, unsteadiness, and impaired thinking; possible decrease of anticonvulsant effect of drug.

Other Drugs: This drug is closely related to the barbiturates and yields phenobarbital as a conversion product in the body. See PHENOBARBITAL Drug Profile for possible interactions with other drugs.

Driving a Vehicle, Operating Machinery, Engaging in Hazardous Activities: Use caution until the full effects of this drug have been determined. It can cause drowsiness and impair mental alertness, vision, and physical coordination. Avoid hazardous activities if such symptoms occur.

Aviation Note: The use of this drug and the disorder for which this drug is prescribed *are disqualifications* for the piloting of aircraft. Consultation with a designated Aviation Medical Examiner is advised.

Exposure to Sun: No restrictions.

Occurrence of Unrelated Illness: Notify your physician of any illness or injury that prevents the use of this drug according to your regular dosage schedule.

Discontinuation: Do not discontinue this drug abruptly. Sudden withdrawal of any anti-convulsant drug can cause severe and repeated seizures.

Special Storage Instructions

Keep in a tightly closed container. Protect the liquid suspension from light.

PROBENECID

Year Introduced: 1951

Brand Names

USA		Canada
Benacen (Cenci)	ColBENEMID [CD]	Benemid (MSD)
Benemid (Merck	(Merck Sharp &	Benuryl (ICN)
Sharp & Dohme)	Dohme)	
Probalan (Lannett)		
SK-Probenecid (Smith		
Kline & French)		

Common Synonyms ("Street Names"):   Gout pills

Drug Class: Anti-gout

Prescription Required: USA: Yes   Canada: No

Available for Purchase by Generic Name: USA: Yes   Canada: No

Available Dosage Forms and Strengths
Tablets — 500 mg.

Tablet May Be Crushed or Capsule Opened for Administration: Yes

How This Drug Works
  Intended Therapeutic Effect(s)
    Prevention of acute episodes of gout through maintenance of normal uric
      acid blood levels.
    Maintenance of high blood levels of penicillin.
  Location of Drug Action(s)
    The tubular systems of the kidney that regulate the uric acid content of the
      urine.
    The tubular systems of the kidney that regulate the elimination of penicil-
      lin.
  Method of Drug Action(s)
    By acting on the tubular systems of the kidney to increase the amount of
      uric acid excreted in the urine, this drug reduces the level of uric acid
      in the blood and body tissues.
    By acting on the tubular systems of the kidney to decrease the amount of
      penicillin excreted in the urine, this drug prolongs the presence of peni-
      cillin in the blood.

Principal Uses of This Drug
  As a Single Drug Product: Used primarily in the long-term treatment of
    gout to prevent acute attacks. While effective for prevention, it has no bene-
    ficial effects in relieving the joint inflammation and pain of the acute epi-
    sode. In fact, it may aggravate and prolong the symptoms of acute gout.

As a Combination Drug Product [CD]:   This drug is available in combination with colchicine, the drug of choice for the treatment of acute gout. Each drug has a different mechanism of action; when used in combination they provide both relief of the acute manifestations of gout and some measure of protection from recurrence of acute attacks.

THIS DRUG SHOULD NOT BE TAKEN IF
—you have had an allergic reaction to any dosage form of it previously.
—you are experiencing an attack of acute gout at the present time.
—it is prescribed for a child under 2 years of age.

INFORM YOUR PHYSICIAN BEFORE TAKING THIS DRUG IF
—you have a history of kidney stones or kidney disease.
—you have a history of peptic ulcer disease.
—you have a disease of the bone marrow or blood cells.
—you are taking any drug product that contains aspirin or aspirin-like drugs

Time Required for Apparent Benefit
Drug action begins in 2 hours, reaches a peak in 4 hours, and subsides in 12 to 24 hours. Continuous use on a regular schedule for several months is needed to prevent acute attacks of gout.

Possible Side-Effects *(natural, expected, and unavoidable drug actions)*
Development of kidney stones (composed of uric acid). Ask physician for guidance regarding their prevention.

Possible Adverse Effects *(unusual, unexpected, and infrequent reactions)*

IF ANY OF THE FOLLOWING DEVELOP, DISCONTINUE DRUG AND NOTIFY YOUR PHYSICIAN AS SOON AS POSSIBLE

Mild Adverse Effects
Allergic Reactions: Skin rashes, itching, drug fever (see Glossary).
Other Reactions
Headache, dizziness, flushing.
Reduced appetite, nausea, vomiting, sore gums.
Serious Adverse Effects
Allergic Reactions: Anaphylactic reaction (see Glossary).
Idiosyncratic Reactions: Hemolytic anemia (see Glossary).
Other Reactions
Bone marrow depression (see Glossary)—fatigue, weakness, fever, sore throat, unusual bleeding or bruising.
Liver damage.
Kidney damage.

CAUTION
Acute attacks of gout may occur after this drug is started on a regular dosage schedule. If symptoms suggestive of gout develop, consult your physician for guidance.

Precautions for Use by Those over 60 Years of Age
The natural decline in kidney function that occurs after 60 may require adjustment of your dosage.

You may be more susceptible to the serious adverse effects of this drug. Report promptly the development of *any* of the symptoms listed above.

Advisability of Use During Pregnancy
Pregnancy Category: C (tentative). See Pregnancy Code inside back cover.

Animal reproduction studies: No data available.

Information from adequate studies in pregnant women is not available. Ask physician for guidance.

Advisability of Use While Nursing Infant
Presence of drug in milk is not known. Avoid use if possible.

Habit-Forming Potential
None.

Effects of Overdosage
With Moderate Overdose: Stomach irritation, nausea, vomiting.

With Large Overdose: Severe nervous agitation, delirium, convulsions, coma, difficulty in breathing.

Possible Effects of Extended Use
Development of kidney damage in sensitive individuals.

Suggested Periodic Examinations While Taking This Drug (at physician's discretion)
Complete blood cell counts.

Liver and kidney function tests.

While Taking This Drug, Observe the Following
Foods: Follow physician's advice regarding the need for a low purine diet. Drug may be taken after eating to reduce stomach irritation or nausea.

Beverages: A large intake of coffee, tea, or cola beverages may reduce the effectiveness of treatment. It is advisable to drink no less than 5 to 6 pints of liquids every 24 hours.

Alcohol: No interactions expected with this drug, but alcohol may impair successful management of gout.

Tobacco Smoking: No interactions expected.

Marijuana Smoking

Occasional (once or twice weekly):   No significant interactions expected.

Daily: Possible increase in blood uric acid level.

Other Drugs

Probenecid may *increase* the effects of

- acetohexamide (Dymelor), and cause hypoglycemia. Dosage adjustments may be necessary for smooth control of diabetes.
- allopurinol (Zyloprim), and add to its elimination of uric acid.
- oral anticoagulants (see Drug Class, Section Three), and increase the risk of abnormal bleeding or hemorrhage.

- indomethacin (Indocin, Indocid), and enhance its potential for causing adverse effects. Reduced dosage may be necessary.
- nitrofurantoin (Furadantin).
- sulfinpyrazone (Anturane).

Probenecid may *decrease* the effects of
- ethacrynic acid (Edecrin), and reduce its diuretic action.

Probenecid *taken concurrently* with
- penicillin preparations (see Drug Class, Section Three), may cause a threefold to fivefold increase in penicillin blood levels, greatly increasing the effectiveness of each penicillin dose.
- para-aminosalicylic acid (PAS), may slow its elimination and increase its blood levels by 50%.
- sulfonamide ("sulfa") drugs (see Drug Class, Section Three), may slow their elimination and cause excessive accumulation during long-term use.

The following drugs may *decrease* the effects of probenecid
- aspirin and aspirin-like drugs may reduce its effectiveness in eliminating uric acid from the body.
- ethacrynic acid (Edecrin) may reduce its effectiveness in eliminating uric acid from the body.
- thiazide diuretics (see Drug Class, Section Three) may impair its effectiveness by raising the levels of uric acid in the blood.

Driving a Vehicle, Operating Machinery, Engaging in Hazardous Activities: Usually no restrictions. Be alert to the rare occurrence of dizziness and/or nausea; restrict activities accordingly.

Aviation Note: The use of this drug *may be a disqualification* for the piloting of aircraft. Consultation with a designated Aviation Medical Examiner is advised.

Exposure to Sun: No restrictions.

Discontinuation: Do not discontinue this drug without consulting your physician. At the time of discontinuation, consult the Other Drugs section (above) to see if you are taking any drugs which may require dosage adjustments.

Special Storage Instructions

Keep in a dry, tightly closed container.

PROCAINAMIDE

Year Introduced: 1950

Brand Names

USA	Canada
Procan SR (Parke-Davis)	Pronestyl (Squibb)
Pronestyl (Squibb)	
Pronestyl-SR (Squibb)	
Sub-Quin (Scrip)	

Common Synonyms ("Street Names"):   Heart regulator

Drug Class: Heart Rhythm Regulator (Anti-arrhythmic)

Prescription Required: Yes

Available for Purchase by Generic Name: USA: Yes   Canada: No

Available Dosage Forms and Strengths

Tablets — 250 mg., 375 mg., 500 mg.
Prolonged-action tablets — 250 mg., 500 mg., 750 mg.
Capsules — 250 mg., 375 mg., 500 mg.
Injection — 100 mg. per ml., 500 mg. per ml.

Tablet May Be Crushed or Capsule Opened for Administration: Yes

How This Drug Works

Intended Therapeutic Effect(s):   Correction of certain heart rhythm disorders.

Location of Drug Action(s):   The heart muscle and the tissues that comprise the electrical conduction system of the heart.

Method of Drug Action(s):   By slowing the activity of the pacemaker and delaying the transmission of electrical impulses through the conduction system and muscle of the heart, this drug assists in restoring normal heart rate and rhythm.

Principal Uses of This Drug

As a Single Drug Product: Used exclusively to control the following disturbances of heart rhythm: atrial fibrillation, paroxysmal atrial tachycardia, premature ventricular contractions, and ventricular tachycardia.

THIS DRUG SHOULD NOT BE TAKEN IF

—you have had an allergic reaction to any dosage form of it previously.
—you have myasthenia gravis.

INFORM YOUR PHYSICIAN BEFORE TAKING THIS DRUG IF

—you are allergic to procaine (Novocain) or to other local anesthetics of the "–caine" drug family, such as those commonly used for measuring the internal eye pressure (glaucoma testing) and for dental procedures.
—you have a history of kidney disease or impaired kidney function.
—you have a history of liver disease or impaired liver function.

—you have a history of lupus erythematosus.
—you are taking any form of digitalis.
—you plan to have surgery under general anesthesia in the near future.

Time Required for Apparent Benefit
Drug action begins within 30 to 60 minutes when taken by mouth and within a few minutes when given by intramuscular or intravenous injection.

Possible Side-Effects *(natural, expected, and unavoidable drug actions)*
Drop in blood pressure, mild and infrequent with oral administration but more common and pronounced with intramuscular or intravenous administration.

Possible Adverse Effects *(unusual, unexpected, and infrequent reactions)*
IF ANY OF THE FOLLOWING DEVELOP, DISCONTINUE DRUG AND NOTIFY YOUR PHYSICIAN AS SOON AS POSSIBLE

Mild Adverse Effects
Allergic Reactions: Itching, skin rash, hives, drug fever (see Glossary).
Other Reactions
  Nausea, vomiting, abdominal pain, bitter taste, diarrhea.
  Weakness, lightheadedness.
Serious Adverse Effects
Idiosyncratic Reactions: Hemolytic anemia (see Glossary).
Other Reactions
  Mental depression, hallucinations, abnormal behavior.
  Reduced white blood cell counts—fever, sore throat, respiratory tract infections.
  Reduced blood platelet counts (see Glossary)—abnormal bleeding or bruising.

CAUTION
1. The appearance of symptoms suggestive of arthritis should be reported immediately; they could indicate the development of a lupus erythematosus-like disorder.
2. Dosage schedules must be carefully individualized.

Precautions for Use by Those over 60 Years of Age
You may be more susceptible to the blood pressure-lowering effects of this drug. Report promptly the development of lightheadedness, dizziness, weakness, or sense of impending faint. Use caution to prevent falls.

Advisability of Use During Pregnancy
Pregnancy Category: C (tentative). See Pregnancy Code inside back cover.
Animal reproduction studies: No data available.
Information from adequate studies in pregnant women is not available.
Ask physician for guidance.

Advisability of Use While Nursing Infant
The presence of this drug in milk is not known. Ask physician for guidance.

Habit-Forming Potential
None.

Effects of Overdosage
With Moderate Overdose: Loss of appetite, nausea, drop in blood pressure, lightheadedness, weakness, intensification of abnormal heart rhythm.
With Large Overdose: Stupor, failure of circulation, heart arrest.

Possible Effects of Extended Use
Lupus erythematosus-like disorder (see Glossary; this is a frequent and serious reaction with prolonged use of this drug)—joint pain and swelling (may be several joints), muscle ache, chest pain associated with breathing (pleurisy), fever, skin rash.

Suggested Periodic Examinations While Taking This Drug (at physician's discretion)
Complete blood cell counts.
Blood examinations for the development of lupus erythematosus (LE) cells and anti-nuclear antibodies.
Electrocardiograms to monitor the full effect of the drug on the mechanisms that influence heart rate and rhythm.

While Taking This Drug, Observe the Following
Foods: No restrictions or precautions.
Beverages: Avoid excessive coffee, tea, and cola beverages because of their caffeine content. Avoid iced drinks.
Alcohol: No interactions expected.
Tobacco Smoking: No interactions expected. It is advisable to discontinue all smoking in the presence of serious heart rhythm disorders. Ask physician for guidance.
Marijuana Smoking: No interactions expected.
Other Drugs
Procainamide may *increase* the effects of
• anti-hypertensive drugs, and cause excessive lowering of the blood pressure (see Drug Class, Section Three).
• atropine-like drugs (see Drug Class, Section Three).

Procainamide may *decrease* the effects of
• ambenonium (Mytelase).
• neostigmine (Prostigmin).
• pryridostigmine (Mestinon).
The beneficial effect of these three drugs in the treatment of myasthenia gravis may be reduced.

Procainamide *taken concurrently* with
• propranolol in the presence of recent heart damage (acute myocardial infarction), may increase the depressant action of propranolol on the heart muscle.

• kanamycin, neomycin, or streptomycin, may cause severe muscle weakness and impairment of breathing.

The following drugs may *increase* the effects of procainamide
• acetazolamide (Diamox)
• sodium bicarbonate (see ANTACIDS Drug Profile)

Driving a Vehicle, Operating Machinery, Engaging in Hazardous Activities: Usually no restrictions. Use caution if this drug causes lightheadedness or weakness.

Aviation Note: The use of this drug and the disorder for which this drug is prescribed *may be disqualifications* for the piloting of aircraft. Consultation with a designated Aviation Medical Examiner is advised.

Exposure to Sun: No restrictions.

Discontinuation: This drug should be discontinued if symptoms of lupus erythematosus develop.

Special Storage Instructions

Keep tablets and capsules in tightly closed containers and at room temperature.

Keep injectable form (vials) at room temperature. Protect from light, freezing, and excessive heat.

Do Not Use the Injectable Solution of This Drug if

it is darker than a pale yellow.

PROCHLORPERAZINE

Year Introduced: 1956

Brand Names

USA	Canada
Compazine (Smith Kline & French)	Stemetil (Poulenc)
Combid [CD] (Smith Kline & French)	Combid [CD] (SK & F)

Common Synonyms ("Street Names"):   None

Drug Class: Tranquilizer, Strong (Anti-psychotic), Antinausea (Antiemetic), Phenothiazines

Prescription Required: Yes

Available for Purchase by Generic Name: No

Available Dosage Forms and Strengths
Tablets — 5 mg., 10 mg., 25 mg.
Prolonged-action capsules — 10 mg., 15 mg., 30 mg., 75 mg.
Syrup — 5 mg. per teaspoonful (5 ml.)
Suppositories — 2.5 mg., 5 mg., 25 mg.
Concentrate — 10 mg. per ml.
Injection — 5 mg. per ml.

Tablet May Be Crushed or Capsule Opened for Administration
Regular tablets — Yes
Prolonged-action capsules — No
Combid and Compazine spansule — Yes, but do not crush or chew contents

How This Drug Works
Intended Therapeutic Effect(s)
Relief of severe nausea and vomiting.
Restoration of emotional calm; relief of severe anxiety, agitation, and/or psychotic behavior.

Location of Drug Action(s)
The nerve pathways in the brain that stimulate the vomiting center.
The nerve pathways in the limbic system of the brain that influence emotion and behavior.

Method of Drug Action(s)
By blocking the action of one of the chemicals (acetylcholine) responsible for the transmission of nerve impulses, this drug prevents excessive stimulation of the vomiting center.
By blocking the action of another chemical (dopamine) responsible for the transmission of nerve impulses within certain brain structures, this drug restores a more normal balance of factors controlling emotional state and behavior.

Principal Uses of This Drug
As a Single Drug Product: This member of the phenothiazine class is used primarily to relieve severe nausea and vomiting. Although it has sedative and antipsychotic effects as well, it is seldom used as a major tranquilizer.

As a Combination Drug Product [CD]:   This drug is available in combination with isopropamide, a synthetic antispasmodic. By utilizing the calming action of prochlorperazine and the muscle-relaxing action of isopropamide, the combination drug is effective in relieving the symptoms associated with peptic ulcer disease, functional diarrhea, and irritable bowel syndrome (spastic colon).

THIS DRUG SHOULD NOT BE TAKEN IF
—you have had an allergic reaction to any dosage form of it previously.
—you have a blood or bone marrow disorder.
—it is prescribed for a child under 2 years of age or weighing under 20 pounds.

INFORM YOUR PHYSICIAN BEFORE TAKING THIS DRUG IF
—you are allergic or sensitive to any phenothiazine drug (see Drug Class, Section Three).
—you are taking sedatives, sleep-inducing drugs, tranquilizers, antidepressants, antihistamines, or narcotic drugs of any kind.
—you have glaucoma.
—you have epilepsy.
—you have a liver, heart, or lung disorder, especially asthma or emphysema.
—you have a history of peptic ulcer.
—you plan to have surgery under general or spinal anesthesia in the near future.

Time Required for Apparent Benefit
Approximately 1 to 2 hours. In treating nervous and mental disorders, maximal benefit may require regular use for several weeks.

Possible Side-Effects (natural, expected, and unavoidable drug actions)
Drowsiness, blurring of vision, dryness of the mouth, nasal congestion, constipation, impaired urination.

Possible Adverse Effects (unusual, unexpected, and infrequent reactions)

IF ANY OF THE FOLLOWING DEVELOP, DISCONTINUE DRUG AND NOTIFY YOUR PHYSICIAN AS SOON AS POSSIBLE

Mild Adverse Effects
Allergic Reactions: Skin rashes (various kinds), hives, low-grade fever.
Other Reactions
    Dizziness, lightheadedness in upright position and feeling of impending faint (see orthostatic hypotension in Glossary).
    Menstrual irregularity.
Serious Adverse Effects
Allergic Reactions: Hepatitis with jaundice (see Glossary), usually within the first 4 weeks.
Other Reactions
    Bone marrow depression (see Glossary).
    Parkinson-like disorders (see Glossary).
    Spasms of the muscles of the face, neck, back, and extremities, causing rolling of the eyes, grimacing, clamping of the jaw, protrusion of the tongue, difficulty in swallowing, arching of the back, cramping of the hands and feet.

CAUTION
1. Many over-the-counter (OTC) medications (see Glossary) for allergies, colds, and coughs contain drugs that can interact unfavorably with this drug. Ask your physician or pharmacist for guidance before using any such medications.
2. Antacids that contain aluminum and/or magnesium can prevent the absorption of this drug and reduce its effectiveness.
3. Obtain prompt evaluation of any disturbance or change in vision.

4. Children with acute illness ("flu"-like infections, measles, chickenpox, etc.) are very susceptible to adverse effects involving muscular spasms of the face, neck, back, or extremities when this drug is used to control nausea and vomiting. Observe closely and notify physician if such reactions occur.

Precautions for Use by Those over 60 Years of Age

You may be more sensitive to all of the actions of this drug. Small doses are advisable until your individual response has been determined.

You may be more susceptible to the development of drowsiness, lethargy, constipation, lowering of body temperature (hypothermia), and excessive drop in blood pressure on arising from a lying or sitting position (see orthostatic hypotension in Glossary).

This drug can increase the degree of impaired urination associated with prostate gland enlargement (prostatism)

You may also be more susceptible to the development of Parkinson-like disorders and/or tardive dyskinesia (see discussion of these terms in Glossary). These conditions must be recognized early since they may become unresponsive to treatment and irreversible. Consult your physician promptly if suggestive symptoms develop.

Advisability of Use During Pregnancy

Pregnancy Category: B (tentative). See Pregnancy Code inside back cover.
Animal reproduction studies in mice and rats reveal significant birth defects due to this drug.
Information from studies in pregnant women indicates no increase in defects in 2097 exposures to this drug.
It is advisable to avoid use of this drug during first 3 months.
Ask physician for guidance.

Advisability of Use While Nursing Infant

Drug is known to be present in milk. Avoid use if possible. Ask physician for guidance.

Habit-Forming Potential

None.

Effects of Overdosage

With Moderate Overdose: Marked drowsiness, weakness, tremor, restlessness, agitation.
With Large Overdose: Stupor, deep sleep, coma, convulsions.

Possible Effects of Extended Use

Tardive dyskinesia (see Glossary).

Suggested Periodic Examinations While Taking This Drug (at physician's discretion)

Complete blood cell counts, especially during first 3 months of treatment.
Liver function tests.
Careful inspection of the tongue for early evidence of fine, involuntary, wave-like movements that could indicate the beginning of tardive dyskinesia.

While Taking This Drug, Observe the Following

Foods: No restrictions.

Beverages: No restrictions.

Alcohol: Use with extreme caution until combined effect has been determined. Alcohol can increase the sedative action of prochlorperazine and accentuate its depressant effects on brain function. Prochlorperazine may increase the intoxicating effects of alcohol.

Tobacco Smoking: No interactions expected.

Marijuana Smoking

Occasional (once or twice weekly):   No effect to mild increase in anti-nausea effect of this drug.

Daily: Moderate increase in anti-nausea effect of this drug.

Other Drugs

Prochlorperazine may *increase* the effects of

- all sedatives, sleep-inducing drugs, other tranquilizers, antihistamines, and narcotic drugs, and produce oversedation. Ask physician for guidance regarding dosage adjustment.
- all drugs containing atropine or having an atropine-like action (see Drug Class, Section Three).
- phenytoin (Dantoin, Dilantin, etc.).

Prochlorperazine may *decrease* the effects of

- levodopa (Dopar, Larodopa, etc.), and reduce its effectiveness in the treatment of Parkinson's disease (shaking palsy).
- appetite suppressant drugs (Pre-Sate, Preludin, Benzedrine, Dexedrine, etc.).

Prochlorperazine *taken concurrently* with

- quinidine, may impair heart function. Avoid the combined use of these two drugs.

The following drugs may *increase* the effects of prochlorperazine

- tricyclic antidepressants (see Drug Class, Section Three).

Driving a Vehicle, Operating Machinery, Engaging in Hazardous Activities: This drug can impair mental alertness, judgment, and physical coordination. Avoid hazardous activities.

Aviation Note: The use of this drug *is a disqualification* for the piloting of aircraft. Consultation with a designated Aviation Medical Examiner is advised.

Exposure to Sun: Use caution until sensitization has been determined. This drug can produce photosensitivity (see Glossary).

Exposure to Heat: Use caution and avoid excessive heat. This drug may impair the regulation of body temperature and increase the risk of heat stroke.

Discontinuation: If it has been necessary to use this drug for an extended period of time, do not discontinue it suddenly. Ask physician for guidance regarding dosage reduction and withdrawal. Upon discontinuation of this drug, it may also be necessary to adjust the dosages of other drugs taken concurrently with it.

Special Storage Instructions
Keep in a tightly closed, light-resistant container.

PROMETHAZINE

Year Introduced: 1945

Brand Names

USA		Canada
Fellozine (Fellows)	Prorex (Hyrex)	Histanil
Ganphen (Tutag)	Provigan	(Pharmascience)
K-Phen (Kay)	(Reid-Provident)	Phenergan
Pentazine (Century)	Remsed (Endo)	(Rhône-Poulenc)
Phenergan (Wyeth)	Sigazine (Sig: Pharm.)	
Phenerhist (Rocky	ZiPan (Savage)	
Mtn.)		

Common Synonyms ("Street Names"):   Allergy pills, nausea pills

Drug Class: Antinausea (Anti-emetic), Antihistamines, Phenothiazines

Prescription Required: USA: Yes   Canada: No

Available for Purchase by Generic Name: USA: Yes   Canada: No

Available Dosage Forms and Strengths
Tablets — 12.5 mg., 25 mg., 50 mg.
Syrup — 6.25 mg., 25 mg. per teaspoonful (5 ml.)
Suppositories — 12.5 mg., 25 mg., 50 mg.
Injection — 25 mg. per ml., 50 mg. per ml.
Also available in cough preparations of various compositions (examine product labels)

Tablet May Be Crushed or Capsule Opened for Administration: Yes

How This Drug Works
Intended Therapeutic Effect(s)
Relief of symptoms associated with hayfever (allergic rhinitis) and with allergic reactions in the skin, such as itching, swelling, hives, and rash.
Prevention and management of the nausea, vomiting, and dizziness associated with motion sickness.
The production of mild sedation and light sleep.
Location of Drug Action(s)
Those hypersensitive tissues that release excessive histamine as part of an allergic reaction. Principal tissue sites are the eyes, the nose, and the skin.
The nerve pathways connecting the organ of equilibrium (the labyrinth) in the inner ear with the vomiting center in the brain.
The site in the brain of this drug's action responsible for sedation and sleep is unknown.

Method of Drug Action(s)

This drug reduces the intensity of the allergic response by blocking the action of histamine after it has been released from sensitized tissue cells.

This drug also reduces the sensitivity of the nerve endings in the labyrinth and blocks the transmission of excessive nerve impulses to the vomiting center.

The way in which this drug produces sedation and light sleep is unknown.

Principal Uses of This Drug

As a Single Drug Product: This versatile drug shares the characteristics of two major drug classes, the antihistamines and the phenothiazines. It is used to provide symptomatic relief in allergic disorders (hay fever, hives, etc.), to produce mild sedation, and to control nausea and vomiting.

As a Combination Drug Product [CD]: This drug is often combined with analgesics such as aspirin or codeine to enhance their pain-relieving action by producing mild sedation. It is also used in cough mixtures for its drying (antihistaminic) effect.

THIS DRUG SHOULD NOT BE TAKEN IF

—you have had an allergic reaction to any dosage form of it previously.

—you have a blood or bone marrow disorder.

—you have glaucoma (narrow-angle type).

—it is prescribed for a newborn infant.

INFORM YOUR PHYSICIAN BEFORE TAKING THIS DRUG IF

—you are allergic or sensitive to any phenothiazine drug (see Drug Class, Section Three).

—you are taking any sedatives, sleep-inducing drugs, tranquilizers, other antihistamines, antidepressants, or narcotic drugs of any kind.

—you have a history of recurring peptic ulcer.

—you have a history of prostate gland enlargement.

—you plan to have surgery under general anesthesia in the near future.

Time Required for Apparent Benefit

Usually 1 to 2 hours when taken orally.

Possible Side-Effects *(natural, expected, and unavoidable drug actions)*

Drowsiness, blurred vision, dryness of the mouth, inability to concentrate.

Possible Adverse Effects *(unusual, unexpected, and infrequent reactions)*

IF ANY OF THE FOLLOWING DEVELOP, DISCONTINUE DRUG AND NOTIFY YOUR PHYSICIAN AS SOON AS POSSIBLE

Mild Adverse Effects

Dizziness, weakness.

Serious Adverse Effects

Paradoxical Reactions: hyperexcitability, abnormal movements of arms and legs, nightmares.

Other Reactions

Parkinson-like disorders (see Glossary).

Muscle spasms of the face, neck, back, and extremities, causing rolling of the eyes, twisting of the neck, arching of the back, spasms of the hands and feet.

Bone marrow depression (see Glossary), mild and very rare.

Hepatitis with jaundice (see Glossary), very rare.

CAUTION

Children with acute illness ("flu"-like infections, measles, chickenpox, etc.) are very susceptible to adverse effects involving muscular spasms of the face, neck, back, or extremities when this drug is used to control nausea and vomiting. Observe closely and notify physician if such reactions occur.

Precautions for Use by Those over 60 Years of Age

You may be more susceptible to the development of drowsiness, dizziness, and lethargy and to impairment of thinking, judgment, and memory.

This drug can increase the degree of impaired urination associated with prostate gland enlargement (prostatism).

Advisability of Use During Pregnancy

Pregnancy Category: B (tentative). See Pregnancy Code inside back cover. Animal reproduction studies reveal no birth defects due to this drug. Information from studies in pregnant women indicates no increase in defects in 746 exposures to this drug.

Ask physician for guidance.

Advisability of Use While Nursing Infant

Apparently safe; ask physician for guidance regarding dosage. Observe infant for evidence of sedation.

Habit-Forming Potential

None.

Effects of Overdosage

With Moderate Overdose: Marked drowsiness, weakness, unsteady stance and gait, agitation, delirium.

With Large Overdose: Deep sleep, coma, convulsions.

Possible Effects of Extended Use

Bone marrow depression.

Suggested Periodic Examinations While Taking This Drug (at physician's discretion)

Complete blood cell counts.

While Taking This Drug, Observe the Following

Foods: Take drug with or following food if it causes irritation of stomach.

Beverages: No restrictions.

Alcohol: Use with extreme caution until combined effect has been determined. Alcohol can increase the sedative action of promethazine and accentuate its depressant effects on brain function. Promethazine can increase the intoxicating action of alcohol.

Tobacco Smoking: No interactions expected.

Marijuana Smoking

Occasional (once or twice weekly):   Mild increase in drowsiness and dryness of mouth.

Daily: Moderate to marked increase in drowsiness and dryness of mouth; possible accentuation of impaired thinking.

Other Drugs

Promethazine may *increase* the effects of

- all sedatives, sleep-inducing drugs, pain-relieving drugs, other antihistamines, tranquilizers, and narcotic drugs, and cause oversedation. Ask physician for guidance regarding dosage adjustment.
- atropine and drugs with an atropine-like action (see Drug Class, Section Three).

Driving a Vehicle, Operating Machinery, Engaging in Hazardous Activities: This drug can cause drowsiness and dizziness. Avoid hazardous activities until its effect has been determined.

Aviation Note: The use of this drug *is a disqualification* for the piloting of aircraft. Consultation with a designated Aviation Medical Examiner is advised.

Exposure to Sun: Use caution until sensitivity has been determined. This drug can cause photosensitivity (see Glossary).

Special Storage Instructions

Keep in a tightly closed container. Protect from light.

PROPANTHELINE

Year Introduced: 1953

Brand Names

USA	Canada
Norpanth (Vortech)	Banlin (Technilab)
Pro-Banthine (Searle)	Novopropanthil
SK-Propantheline (Smith	(Novopharm)
Kline & French)	Pro-Banthine (Searle)
	Propanthel (ICN)

Common Synonyms ("Street Names"):   Stomach relaxer

Drug Class: Antispasmodic, Atropine-like Drug

Prescription Required: USA: Yes   Canada: No

Available for Purchase by Generic Name: USA: Yes   Canada: No

Available Dosage Forms and Strengths

Tablets — 7.5 mg., 15 mg.

Tablet May Be Crushed or Capsule Opened for Administration
Regular tablets — Yes
Prolonged-action tablets — No

How This Drug Works
Intended Therapeutic Effect(s):   Relief of discomfort resulting from excessive activity and spasm of the digestive tract (esophagus, stomach, intestine, and colon).

Location of Drug Action(s):   The terminal nerve fibers of the parasympathetic nervous system that control the activity of the gastrointestinal tract.

Method of Drug Action(s):   By blocking the action of the chemical (acetylcholine) that transmits impulses at parasympathetic nerve endings, this drug prevents stimulation of muscular contraction and glandular secretion within the organ involved. This results in reduced overall activity, including the prevention or relief of muscle spasm.

Principal Uses of This Drug
As a Single Drug Product: This synthetic atropine-like drug is used primarily in the management of peptic ulcer disease. It is also used as an antispasmodic to relieve the symptoms associated with "nervous stomach."

THIS DRUG SHOULD NOT BE TAKEN IF
—you have had an allergic reaction to any dosage form of it previously.
—your stomach cannot empty properly into the intestine (pyloric obstruction).
—you are unable to empty the urinary bladder completely.
—you have glaucoma (narrow-angle type).
—you have severe ulcerative colitis.

INFORM YOUR PHYSICIAN BEFORE TAKING THIS DRUG IF
—you have glaucoma (open-angle type).
—you have angina or coronary heart disease.
—you have chronic bronchitis.
—you have a hiatal hernia.
—you have enlargement of the prostate gland.
—you have myasthenia gravis.
—you have a history of peptic ulcer disease.
—you plan to have surgery under general anesthesia in the near future.

Time Required for Apparent Benefit
Drug action begins in 1 to 2 hours and persists for approximately 6 hours.

Possible Side-Effects *(natural, expected, and unavoidable drug actions)*
Blurring of vision (impairment of focus), dryness of the mouth and throat, constipation, hesitancy in urination. (Nature and degree of side-effects depend upon individual susceptibility and drug dosage.)

Possible Adverse Effects *(unusual, unexpected, and infrequent reactions)*

IF ANY OF THE FOLLOWING DEVELOP, DISCONTINUE DRUG AND NOTIFY YOUR PHYSICIAN AS SOON AS POSSIBLE

Mild Adverse Effects
Allergic Reactions: Skin rash, hives.
Other Reactions
Dilation of pupils, causing sensitivity to light.
Flushing and dryness of the skin (reduced sweating).
Rapid heart action.
Lightheadedness, dizziness, unsteady gait.

Serious Adverse Effects
Idiosyncratic Reactions: Acute confusion, delirium, erratic behavior.
Other Reactions: Development of acute glaucoma (in susceptible individuals).

CAUTION
Many over-the-counter (OTC) medications (see Glossary) for allergies, colds, and coughs contain drugs that can interact unfavorably with this drug. Ask your physician or pharmacist for guidance before using any such medication.

Precautions for Use by Those over 60 Years of Age
You may be more sensitive to all of the actions of this drug. Small doses are advisable until your individual response has been determined.
This drug can increase the degree of impaired urination associated with prostate gland enlargement (prostatism).

Advisability of Use During Pregnancy
Pregnancy Category: C (tentative). See Pregnancy Code inside back cover.
Animal reproduction studies: No data available.
Information from adequate studies in pregnant women is not available. Ask physician for guidance.

Advisability of Use While Nursing Infant
This drug may impair the formation of milk and make nursing difficult. It is reported not to be present in milk. Ask physician for guidance regarding nursing.

Habit-Forming Potential
None.

Effects of Overdosage
With Moderate Overdose: Marked dryness of the mouth, dilated pupils, blurring of near vision, rapid pulse, heart palpitation, headache, difficulty in urination.
With Large Overdose: Extremely dilated pupils, rapid pulse and breathing, hot skin, high fever, excitement, confusion, hallucinations, delirium, eventual loss of consciousness, convulsions, coma.

Possible Effects of Extended Use

Chronic constipation, severe enough to result in fecal impaction. (Constipation should be treated promptly with effective laxatives.)

Suggested Periodic Examinations While Taking This Drug (at physician's discretion)

Measurement of internal eye pressure to detect any significant increase that could indicate developing glaucoma.

While Taking This Drug, Observe the Following

Foods: No interaction with drug. Effectiveness is greater if drug is taken one-half to 1 hour before eating. Follow diet prescribed for condition under treatment.

Beverages: No interactions. As allowed by prescribed diet.

Alcohol: No interactions expected with this drug. Follow physician's advice regarding use of alcohol (based upon its effect on the condition under treatment).

Tobacco Smoking: No interactions expected. Follow physician's advice regarding smoking.

Marijuana Smoking

Occasional (once or twice weekly):   Mild increase in drowsiness and dryness of mouth.

Daily: Moderate to marked increase in drowsiness and dryness of mouth.

Other Drugs

Propantheline may *increase* the effects of

• all other drugs having atropine-like actions (see Drug Class, Section Three).

Propantheline may *decrease* the effects of

• pilocarpine eye drops, and reduce their effectiveness in lowering internal eye pressure in the treatment of glaucoma.

Propantheline *taken concurrently* with

• mono-amine oxidase (MAO) inhibitor drugs (see Drug Class, Section Three), may cause an exaggerated response to normal doses of atropine-like drugs. It is best to avoid atropine-like drugs for 2 weeks after the last dose of any MAO inhibitor drug.

• haloperidol (Haldol), may significantly increase internal eye pressure (dangerous in glaucoma).

The following drugs may *increase* the effects of propantheline

• tricyclic antidepressants
• those antihistamines that have an atropine-like action
• meperidine (Demerol, pethidine)
• methylphenidate (Ritalin)
• orphenadrine (Disipal, Norflex)
• those phenothiazines that have an atropine-like action (see Drug Class, Section Three, for brand names)

Driving a Vehicle, Operating Machinery, Engaging in Hazardous Activities: This drug may produce blurred vision, drowsiness, or dizziness. Avoid hazardous activities if these drug effects occur.

Aviation Note: The use of this drug and the disorder for which this drug is prescribed *may be disqualifications* for the piloting of aircraft. Consultation with a designated Aviation Medical Examiner is advised.

Exposure to Sun: No restrictions.

Exposure to Heat: Use extreme caution. The use of this drug in hot environments may significantly increase the risk of heat stroke.

Heavy Exercise or Exertion: Use caution in warm or hot environments. This drug may impair normal perspiration (heat loss) and interfere with the regulation of body temperature.

Special Storage Instructions
Keep in a tightly closed container. Protect from light.

PROPOXYPHENE

Year Introduced: 1955

Brand Names

USA
Darvon (Lilly)
Darvon-N (Lilly)
Dolene (Lederle)
SK-65 (Smith Kline & French)
S-Pain-65 (Saron)
Darvocet-N [CD] (Lilly)
Darvon Compound [CD] (Lilly)
Darvon Compound-65 [CD] (Lilly)
Darvon-N w/ASA [CD] (Lilly)

Darvon w/ASA [CD] (Lilly)
Dolene AP-65 [CD] (Lederle)
Dolene Compound-65 [CD] (Lederle)
SK-65 APAP [CD] (Smith Kline & French)
SK-65 Compound [CD] (Smith Kline & French)
Wygesic [CD] (Wyeth)

Canada
Darvon-N (Lilly)
Novopropoxyn (Novopharm)
642 (Frosst)

Common Synonyms ("Street Names"):   Painkiller, pain reliever

Drug Class: Analgesic, Mild

Prescription Required: Yes (Controlled Drug, U.S. Schedule IV)*

Available for Purchase by Generic Name: Yes

*See Schedules of Controlled Drugs inside back cover.

Available Dosage Forms and Strengths

Tablets — 100 mg.
Capsules — 32 mg., 65 mg.
Oral suspension — 50 mg. per teaspoonful (5 ml.)

Tablet May Be Crushed or Capsule Opened for Administration: Yes

How This Drug Works

Intended Therapeutic Effect(s):   Relief of mild to moderate pain.

Location of Drug Action(s):   Those areas of the brain and spinal cord involved in the perception of pain.

Method of Drug Action(s):   Not completely established. It has been suggested that the resulting increase in chemicals that transmit nerve impulses somehow contributes to the analgesic effect of this drug.

Principal Uses of This Drug

As a Single Drug Product: This drug is used exclusively as an analgesic to relieve mild to moderate pain of any origin.

As a Combination Drug Product [CD]:   It is often combined with aspirin or acetaminophen to enhance its analgesic effects. Some combinations also contain caffeine to counteract the sedative effects of the analgesics.

THIS DRUG SHOULD NOT BE TAKEN IF

—you have had an allergic reaction to any dosage form of it previously. A combination drug [CD] should not be taken if you are allergic to *any* of its ingredients.

—it is prescribed for a child under 12 years of age.

INFORM YOUR PHYSICIAN BEFORE TAKING THIS DRUG IF

—you are taking sedatives, sleep-inducing drugs, tranquilizers, antidepressants, or narcotic drugs of any kind.

Time Required for Apparent Benefit

Usually 1 to 2 hours.

Possible Side-Effects *(natural, expected, and unavoidable drug actions)*

Drowsiness, lightheadedness, constipation.

Possible Adverse Effects *(unusual, unexpected, and infrequent reactions)*

IF ANY OF THE FOLLOWING DEVELOP, DISCONTINUE DRUG AND NOTIFY YOUR PHYSICIAN AS SOON AS POSSIBLE

Mild Adverse Effects

Allergic Reactions: Skin rashes.

Other Reactions

Nausea, vomiting, abdominal discomfort.

Headache, dizziness, weakness, blurred vision, mild behavioral disturbances.

Serious Adverse Effects

Allergic Reactions: Hepatitis with jaundice (very rare).

Other Reactions: Paradoxical excitement, agitation, and insomnia.

Precautions for Use by Those over 60 Years of Age

The aim of treatment should be to provide the maximal relief of pain consistent with minimal risk and the preservation of ability to function. Dosage should be low at the beginning with adjustment upward according to individual response.

The use of this drug should be limited to short-term treatment only.

You may be more susceptible to the development of dizziness, drowsiness, and constipation.

Advisability of Use During Pregnancy

Pregnancy Category: C (tentative). See Pregnancy Code inside back cover.

Animal reproduction studies reveal no birth defects due to this drug.

Information from studies in pregnant women indicates no significant increase in defects in 2914 exposures to this drug.

Ask physician for guidance.

Advisability of Use While Nursing Infant

Drug is known to be present in milk. Safety for infant not established. Ask physician for guidance.

Habit-Forming Potential

Can produce psychological and physical dependence (see Glossary) if used in large doses for an extended period of time.

Effects of Overdosage

With Moderate Overdose: Mental and behavioral disturbance, marked drowsiness progressing to stupor.

With Large Overdose: Coma, convulsions, depression of respiration.

Possible Effects of Extended Use

Psychological and physical dependence.

Suggested Periodic Examinations While Taking This Drug (at physician's discretion)

None.

While Taking This Drug, Observe the Following

Foods: No restrictions.

Beverages: No restrictions.

Alcohol: Use with caution until combined effect is determined. Alcohol can increase this drug's depressant action on the brain. Propoxyphene may increase the intoxicating effects of alcohol.

Tobacco Smoking: Heavy smoking may reduce the effectiveness of propoxyphene.

Marijuana Smoking

Occasional (once or twice weekly): No effect to mild increase in pain relief from this drug.

Daily: Moderate increase in pain relief from this drug.

Other Drugs
Propoxyphene may *increase* the effects of
- sedatives, sleep-inducing drugs, tranquilizers, and narcotic drugs; dosage adjustment may be necessary to avoid excessive sedation.

Propoxyphene *taken concurrently* with
- orphenadrine (Disipal, Norflex, Norgesic), may cause anxiety, confusion, or tremors (probably very rare).

The following drugs may *increase* the effects of propoxyphene
- aspirin and related drugs; combined action increases effectiveness in relieving pain.
- acetaminophen; combined action increases effectiveness in relieving pain.

Driving a Vehicle, Operating Machinery, Engaging in Hazardous Activities: This drug can impair mental alertness, judgment, and physical coordination. Use caution until occurrence of drowsiness and/or dizziness is determined.

Aviation Note: The use of this drug *may be a disqualification* for the piloting of aircraft. Consultation with a designated Aviation Medical Examiner is advised.

Exposure to Sun: No restrictions.

Special Storage Instructions
Keep in a dry, tightly closed container.

PROPRANOLOL

Year Introduced: 1965

Brand Names

USA	Canada
Inderal (Ayerst)	Apo-Propranolol (Apotex)
Inderal LA (Ayerst)	Detensol (Desbergers)
Inderide [CD] (Ayerst)	Inderal (Ayerst)
	Inderal-LA (Ayerst)
	Novopranol (Novopharm)
	Inderide [CD] (Ayerst)

Common Synonyms ("Street Names"):   Blood pressure pills, heart pills

Drug Class: Anti-anginal, Anti-hypertensive (Hypotensive), Heart Rhythm Regulator (Anti-arrhythmic), Migraine Preventive, Beta-Adrenergic Blocker

Prescription Required: Yes

Available for Purchase by Generic Name: USA: No   Canada: Yes

Available Dosage Forms and Strengths
Tablets — 10 mg., 20 mg., 40 mg., 80 mg.

Prolonged-action capsules — 80 mg., 120 mg., 160 mg.

Injection — 1 mg. per ml.

Tablet May Be Crushed or Capsule Opened for Administration: Yes, but
do not chew or crush contents.

How This Drug Works
Intended Therapeutic Effect(s)
Reduction in the frequency and intensity of pain associated with angina pectoris (coronary insufficiency).

Prevention and treatment of heart rhythm disorders (arrhythmias).

Reduction of high blood pressure.

Reduction in the frequency of migraine headaches.

Note: Not effective in relieving the pain of a headache that has already started.

Location of Drug Action(s): Principal sites of therapeutic actions include
- the heart pacemaker and tissues that comprise the electrical conduction system.
- the heart muscle.
- the vasomotor center in the brain that influences the control of the sympathetic nervous system over blood vessels (principally arterioles) throughout the body.
- sympathetic nerve terminals in blood vessel walls.
- possibly the kidneys.

Method of Drug Action(s): Not completely established. By blocking certain actions of the sympathetic nervous system, this drug
- reduces the rate and the contraction force of the heart, thus lowering the oxygen requirement of the heart muscle. This reduces the occurrence of angina.
- prolongs the conduction time of nerve impulses through the heart, of benefit in the management of rhythm disorders.
- reduces the degree of contraction of blood vessel walls, resulting in their relaxation and expansion and lowering of the blood pressure.
- inhibits the release of renin by the kidneys, resulting in further lowering of the blood pressure.
- prevents the spasm of arterioles within the head that is thought to initiate migraine headache.

Principal Uses of This Drug
As a Single Drug Product: This first "beta-blocker" drug is used primarily to treat several serious cardiovascular disorders: classical effort-induced angina, certain types of heart rhythm disturbance, and high blood pressure. It is also beneficial in preventing the reoccurrence of heart attacks (myocardial infarction). In addition, it is used to reduce the frequency and severity of migraine headache. Other uses (not "officially approved" at this time) include the control of physical manifestations of anxiety and nervous tension (as in stage fright), the control of familial tremors, and the control of the symptoms associated with a markedly over-active thyroid gland (thyrotoxicosis).

As a Combination Drug Product [CD]:   This drug is available in combination with hydrochlorothiazide for the treatment of hypertension. This combination product provides a "step 1" antihypertensive (the thiazide diuretic) and a "step 2" antihypertensive (propranolol) for greater effectiveness and convenience.

THIS DRUG SHOULD NOT BE TAKEN IF
—you have had an allergic reaction to any dosage form of it previously.
—you are subject to episodes of asthma.
—you are presently experiencing seasonal hay fever.
—you are taking, or have taken within the past 2 weeks, any mono-amine oxidase (MAO) inhibitor drug (see Drug Class, Section Three).

INFORM YOUR PHYSICIAN BEFORE TAKING THIS DRUG IF
—you have a history of serious heart disease, with or without episodes of heart failure.
—you have a history of hay fever (allergic rhinitis), asthma, chronic bronchitis, or emphysema.
—you have a history of overactive thyroid function (hyperthyroidism).
—you have a history of low blood sugar (hypoglycemia).
—you have a history of impaired liver or kidney function.
—you have diabetes.
—you are taking any form of digitalis or quinidine.
—you are taking any form of reserpine.
—you plan to have surgery under general anesthesia in the near future.

Time Required for Apparent Benefit
Drug action begins in 1 hour, reaches a maximum within 4 hours, and subsides in 6 to 8 hours. Full effectiveness can be determined only by continuous use on a regular schedule for several weeks, during which time dosage is carefully adjusted according to individual response (this can vary widely from person to person).

Possible Side-Effects *(natural, expected, and unavoidable drug actions)*
Lethargy and fatigability, cold hands and feet, lightheadedness in upright position (see orthostatic hypotension in Glossary).

Possible Adverse Effects *(unusual, unexpected, and infrequent reactions)*

IF ANY OF THE FOLLOWING DEVELOP, DISCONTINUE DRUG AND NOTIFY YOUR PHYSICIAN AS SOON AS POSSIBLE

Mild Adverse Effects
Allergic Reactions: Skin rashes, temporary loss of hair, drug fever.
Other Reactions
Reduced appetite, nausea, vomiting, diarrhea.
Insomnia, vivid dreaming.
Serious Adverse Effects
Idiosyncratic Reactions: Acute behavioral disturbances: disorientation, confusion, hallucinations, amnesia.

Other Reactions
Reduced heart muscle strength and reserve.
Increased risk of asthma.
Emotional depression.
Reduction of white blood cells resulting in fever and sore throat.
Reduction of blood platelets (see Glossary), resulting in unusual bleeding
or bruising.

CAUTION
1. *Do not discontinue this drug suddenly if you have angina (coronary heart disease).* Include a notation on your card of personal identification that you are taking this drug (see Table 19 and Section Six).
2. Hot weather and the fever associated with infection can reduce the blood pressure significantly, requiring adjustment of dosage.
3. Report the development of any tendency to emotional depression.

Precautions for Use by Those over 60 Years of Age
The basic rule in treating high blood pressure after 60 is to proceed *cautiously.* The elevated systolic blood pressure often present after 60 is not necessarily a threat to health, and can serve as an adaptive and compensatory change with age that should not be altered drastically. The goals of treatment must be adjusted to the natural changes in body function that occur with aging. Unacceptably high blood pressure should be reduced without creating the risks associated with excessively low blood pressure.
It is advisable to start treatment with small doses and to monitor the blood pressure response frequently. Sudden, rapid, and excessive reduction of blood pressure can predispose to stroke or heart attack.
You may be more susceptible to the development of orthostatic hypotension with resultant lightheadedness, dizziness, unsteadiness, fainting, and falling. Report such symptoms to your physician promptly.

Advisability of Use During Pregnancy
Pregnancy Category: C (tentative). See Pregnancy Code inside back cover.
Animal reproduction studies reveal evidence of embryo toxicity.
Information from adequate studies in pregnant women is not available.
It is advisable to avoid use of this drug during first 3 months if possible.
Ask physician for guidance.

Advisability of Use While Nursing Infant
Drug is present in milk in small amounts. Ask physician for guidance.

Habit-Forming Potential
None

Effects of Overdosage
With Moderate Overdose: General weakness, slow pulse, orthostatic hypotension.
With Large Overdose: Marked drop in blood pressure, fainting, weak and slow pulse, cold and sweaty skin, convulsions.

Possible Effects of Extended Use

Reduced reserve of heart muscle strength, which may result from prolonged use of high doses.

Suggested Periodic Examinations While Taking This Drug (at physician's discretion)

Complete blood cell counts, including platelet counts.
Evaluation of heart function.

While Taking This Drug, Observe the Following

Foods: No interactions with drug. Follow physician's advice regarding salt and total calorie intake. Drug is absorbed best when taken before eating.

Beverages: No restrictions.

Alcohol: Use with caution until combined effect has been determined. Alcohol may exaggerate this drug's ability to lower blood pressure and may increase its mild sedative action.

Tobacco Smoking: Follow physician's advice regarding use of tobacco. Nicotine may reduce this drug's effectiveness in treating angina, heart irregularities, and high blood pressure.

Marijuana Smoking

Occasional (once or twice weekly): No effect to mild and transient cooling of hands and/or feet.

Daily: More marked and persistent coldness of hands and/or feet.

Other Drugs

Propranolol may *increase* the effects of

• oral anti-diabetic drugs and insulin, causing or prolonging hypoglycemia. Careful dosage adjustments are necessary.
• other anti-hypertensive drugs, and cause excessive lowering of the blood pressure. Careful dosage adjustments are necessary.
• barbiturates and narcotic drugs, and cause dangerous oversedation.
• reserpine, and cause excessive sedation and depression.

Propranolol may *decrease* the effects of

• antihistamines, and reduce their effectiveness in treating allergies.
• anti-inflammatory drugs, including aspirin, cortisone, phenylbutazone (Azolid, Butazolidin, etc.), oxyphenbutazone (Oxalid, Tandearil).

Propranolol *taken concurrently* with

• digitalis preparations (digitoxin, digoxin, etc.), may cause adverse interactions—excessive slowing of heart action and reduction of digitalis effectiveness in treating heart failure. Careful dosage adjustments are necessary.
• quinidine, may cause excessive slowing of the heart. Careful dosage adjustments are necessary.

The following drugs may *increase* the effects of propranolol

• phenytoin (Dantoin, Dilantin, etc.) may exaggerate its sedative action on the brain.

Driving a Vehicle, Operating Machinery, Engaging in Hazardous Activities: Avoid hazardous activities until the full extent of drowsiness or lethargy has been determined.

Aviation Note: The use of this drug *may be a disqualification* for the piloting of aircraft. Consultation with a designated Aviation Medical Examiner is advised.

Exposure to Sun: No restrictions.

Exposure to Cold: Use caution until combined effect has been determined. If you are subject to Raynaud's phenomenon, this drug may exaggerate further the impaired circulation in hands and feet.

Heavy Exercise or Exertion: Avoid levels of exertion which produced severe angina prior to the use of this drug. Isometric exercises—the "overload" technique for strengthening individual muscles—can raise the blood pressure significantly. The use of this drug may intensify the hypertensive response to isometric exercises. Ask your physician for guidance.

Occurrence of Unrelated Illness: If an illness causes vomiting and interrupts the regular use of this drug, notify your physician as soon as possible.

Discontinuation: This drug must not be discontinued abruptly. Gradual withdrawal over a period of 2 or more weeks is necessary to prevent serious increase of angina or risk of heart attack. Ask your physician for guidance.

Special Storage Instructions
Keep in a dry, tightly closed container.

PROTRIPTYLINE

Year Introduced: 1967

Brand Names

USA	Canada
Vivactil (Merck Sharp & Dohme)	Triptil (MSD)

Common Synonyms ("Street Names"): None

Drug Class: Antidepressant, Tricyclic

Prescription Required: Yes

Available for Purchase by Generic Name: No

Available Dosage Forms and Strengths
Tablets — 5 mg., 10 mg.

Tablet May Be Crushed or Capsule Opened for Administration: Yes

How This Drug Works

Intended Therapeutic Effect(s):   Gradual improvement of mood and relief of emotional depression.

Location of Drug Action(s):   Those areas of the brain that determine mood and emotional stability.

Method of Drug Action(s):   Not established. Present thinking is that this drug slowly restores to normal levels certain constituents of brain tissue (such as norepinephrine) that transmit nerve impulses.

Principal Uses of This Drug

As a Single Drug Product: To relieve the symptoms associated with spontaneous (endogenous) depression, and to initiate the restoration of normal mood. This drug should be used only when a diagnosis of a true, primary depression of significant degree has been established. It should not be used to treat the symptoms of mild and transient (reactive) depression that may be associated with many life situations in the absence of a bona fide affective illness.

THIS DRUG SHOULD NOT BE TAKEN IF

—you have had an allergic reaction to any dosage form of it previously.

—you are taking or have taken within the past 14 days any mono-amine oxidase (MAO) inhibitor drug (see Drug Class, Section Three).

—you are recovering from a recent heart attack.

—you have glaucoma (narrow-angle type).

—it is prescribed for a child under 12 years of age.

INFORM YOUR PHYSICIAN BEFORE TAKING THIS DRUG IF

—you are allergic or sensitive to any other tricyclic antidepressant (see Drug Class, Section Three).

—you have a history of any of the following: diabetes, epilepsy, glaucoma, heart disease, prostate gland enlargement, or overactive thyroid function.

—you plan to have surgery under general anesthesia in the near future.

Time Required for Apparent Benefit

Some benefit may be apparent within the first 1 to 2 weeks. Adequate response may require continuous treatment for 4 to 6 weeks.

Possible Side-Effects *(natural, expected, and unavoidable drug actions)*

Drowsiness, blurring of vision, dryness of mouth, constipation, impaired urination.

Possible Adverse Effects *(unusual, unexpected, and infrequent reactions)*

IF ANY OF THE FOLLOWING DEVELOP, DISCONTINUE DRUG AND NOTIFY YOUR PHYSICIAN AS SOON AS POSSIBLE

Mild Adverse Effects

Allergic Reactions: Skin rash, hives, swelling of face or tongue, drug fever.

Other Reactions

Nausea, indigestion, irritation of tongue or mouth, peculiar taste.

Headache, dizziness, weakness, fainting, unsteady gait, tremors.

Swelling of testicles, breast enlargement, milk formation.

Fluctuation of blood sugar levels.

Serious Adverse Effects

Allergic Reactions: Hepatitis with jaundice (see Glossary).

Other Reactions

Confusion (especially in the elderly), hallucinations, agitation, restlessness, nightmares.

Heart palpitation and irregular rhythm.

Bone marrow depression (see Glossary)—fatigue, weakness, fever, sore throat, unusual bleeding or bruising.

Peripheral neuritis (see Glossary)—numbness, tingling, pain, loss of strength in arms and legs.

Parkinson-like disorders (see Glossary)—usually mild and infrequent; more likely to occur in the elderly (over 60 years of age).

Precautions for Use by Those over 60 Years of Age

During the first 2 weeks of treatment observe for the development of confusional reactions—restlessness, agitation, forgetfulness, disorientation, delusions, and hallucinations. Reduction of dosage or discontinuation may be necessary.

Observe for incoordination and instability in stance and gait which may predispose to falling and injury.

This drug can increase the degree of impaired urination associated with prostate gland enlargement (prostatism).

Advisability of Use During Pregnancy

Pregnancy Category: B (tentative). See Pregnancy Code inside back cover. Animal reproduction studies reveal no birth defects due to this drug. Information from adequate studies in pregnant women is not available. Ask physician for guidance.

Advisability of Use While Nursing Infant

This drug may be present in milk in small quantities. Ask physician for guidance.

Habit-Forming Potential

Psychological or physical dependence is rare and unexpected.

Effects of Overdosage

With Moderate Overdose: Confusion, hallucinations, extreme drowsiness, drop in body temperature, heart palpitation, dilated pupils, tremors.

With Large Overdose: Stupor, deep sleep, coma, convulsions.

Possible Effects of Extended Use

None reported.

Suggested Periodic Examinations While Taking This Drug (at physician's discretion)

Complete blood cell counts.

Liver function tests.

Serial blood pressure readings and electrocardiograms.

While Taking This Drug, Observe the Following

Foods: No restrictions.

Beverages: No restrictions.

Alcohol: Avoid completely. This drug can increase markedly the intoxicating effects of alcohol and accentuate its depressant action on brain function.

Tobacco Smoking: No interactions expected.

Marijuana Smoking

Occasional (once or twice weekly):   Transient increase in drowsiness and dryness of mouth.

Daily: Persistent drowsiness, increased dryness of mouth; possible reduced effectiveness of this drug.

Other Drugs

Protriptyline may *increase* the effects of

- atropine and drugs with atropine-like actions (see Drug Class, Section Three).
- sedatives, sleep-inducing drugs, tranquilizers, antihistamines, narcotic drugs, and cause oversedation. Dosage adjustments may be necessary.
- levodopa (Dopar, Larodopa, etc.), in its control of Parkinson's disease.

Protriptyline may *decrease* the effects of

- guanethidine, and reduce its effectiveness in lowering blood pressure.
- other commonly used anti-hypertensive drugs. Ask physician for guidance regarding the need to monitor blood pressure readings and to adjust dosage of anti-hypertensive medications. (The action of Aldomet is not decreased by tricyclic antidepressants.)

Protriptyline *taken concurrently* with

- thyroid preparations, may cause impairment of heart rhythm and function. Ask physician for guidance regarding thyroid dosage adjustment.
- ethchlorvynol (Placidyl), may cause delirium.
- quinidine, may impair heart rhythm and function. Avoid the combined use of these two drugs.
- mono-amine oxidase (MAO) inhibitor drugs (see Drug Class, Section Three), may cause high fever, delirium, and convulsions.

The following drugs may *increase* the effects of protriptyline

- thiazide diuretics (see Drug Class, Section Three) may slow its elimination from the body. Overdosage may result.

Driving a Vehicle, Operating Machinery, Engaging in Hazardous Activities: This drug may impair mental alertness, judgment, physical coordination, and reaction time. Avoid hazardous activities.

Aviation Note: The use of this drug *is a disqualification* for the piloting of aircraft. Consultation with a designated Aviation Medical Examiner is advised.

Exposure to Sun: Use caution until sensitivity to sun has been determined. This drug may cause photosensitivity (see Glossary).

Discontinuation: If it has been necessary to use this drug for an extended period of time, do not discontinue it abruptly. Ask physician for guidance regarding dosage reduction and withdrawal. It may be necessary to adjust the dosage of other drugs taken concurrently.

Special Storage Instructions

Keep in a dry, tightly closed container.

PSEUDOEPHEDRINE
(Isoephedrine)

Year Introduced: 1957

Brand Names

USA

Afrinol (Schering)
Cenafed (Century)
Neo-Synephrinol Day
  Relief (Winthrop)
Novafed (Merrell
  Dow)
Ro-Fedrin
  (Robinson)
Sudafed
  (Burroughs
  Wellcome)
Sudafed S.A.
  (Burroughs
  Wellcome)
Actifed [CD]
  (Burroughs
  Wellcome)
Actifed-C
  Expectorant [CD]
  (Burroughs
  Wellcome)
Deconamine [CD]
  (Berlex)

Dimacol [CD]
  (Robins)
Disophrol [CD]
  (Schering)
Drixoral [CD]
  (Schering)
Fedahist [CD] (Rorer)
Fedrazil [CD]
  (Burroughs
  Wellcome)
Isoclor [CD]
  (American Critical
  Care)
Novafed A [CD]
  (Merrell Dow)
Phenergan
  Compound [CD]
  (Wyeth)
(Other combination
  brand names)

Canada

Eltor (Dow)
Profedrine (Pro Doc)
Pseudofrin (Trianon)
Robidrine (Robins)
Sudafed (B.W.)
Actifed [CD] (B.W.)

Common Synonyms ("Street Names"):   None

Drug Class: Decongestant

Prescription Required: USA: No   Canada: No

Available for Purchase by Generic Name: Yes

Available Dosage Forms and Strengths
Tablets — 30 mg., 60 mg.
Prolonged-action tablets — 120 mg.
Prolonged-action capsules — 60 mg., 120 mg.
Syrups — 30 mg. per teaspoonful (5 ml.)

Tablet May Be Crushed or Capsule Opened for Administration
Regular tablets — Yes
Prolonged-action tablets and capsules — No
Afrinol Repetab — No
Disophrol Chronotab — No
Drixoral — No
Isoclor Timesules, Novafed A capsules,
Sudafed SA capsules — Yes, but do not crush or chew contents

How This Drug Works
Intended Therapeutic Effect(s):   Relief of congestion of the nose, sinuses, and throat associated with allergic disorders and infections.

Location of Drug Action(s):   The small blood vessels (arterioles) in the tissues lining the nasal passages, the sinuses, and the throat.

Method of Drug Action(s):   By contracting the walls and thus reducing the size of the arterioles, this drug decreases the volume of blood in the tissues, resulting in shrinkage of tissue mass (decongestion). This expands the nasal airway and enlarges the openings into the sinuses and eustachian tubes.

Principal Uses of This Drug
As a Single Drug Product: Used exclusively as a decongestant in the treatment of allergic and infectious conditions of the nose, sinuses, and eustachian tubes, such as allergic rhinitis (hay fever), headcolds, sinusitis, and the "ear blockage" that occurs with air travel.

As a Combination Drug Product [CD]:   This drug is frequently combined with antihistamines to enhance the drying effect on the membranes of the upper respiratory tract. It may also be present in cough remedies used to treat tracheobronchitis.

THIS DRUG SHOULD NOT BE TAKEN IF
—you have had an allergic reaction to any dosage form of it previously.

INFORM YOUR PHYSICIAN BEFORE TAKING THIS DRUG IF
—you have high blood pressure or heart disease.
—you have an overactive thyroid gland (hyperthyroidism) or diabetes.
—you have difficulty emptying the urinary bladder.
—you are taking, or have taken during the past 2 weeks, any mono-amine oxidase (MAO) inhibitor drug (see Drug Class, Section Three).
—you are taking any form of digitalis (digitoxin, digoxin, etc.).
—you plan to have surgery under general anesthesia in the near future.

Time Required for Apparent Benefit

Drug action begins in 15 to 20 minutes, reaches a maximum in approximately 1 hour, and persists for 3 to 4 hours. (The prolonged action capsules may act for 12 hours.)

Possible Side-Effects *(natural, expected, and unavoidable drug actions)*

Nervousness, insomnia.

Possible Adverse Effects *(unusual, unexpected, and infrequent reactions)*

IF ANY OF THE FOLLOWING DEVELOP, DISCONTINUE DRUG AND NOTIFY YOUR PHYSICIAN AS SOON AS POSSIBLE

Mild Adverse Effects
Allergic Reactions: Skin rash (rare).
Other Reactions: Headache, dizziness, heart palpitation, tremor (in sensitive individuals).
Serious Adverse Effects
None reported.

CAUTION

Many over-the-counter (OTC) medications (see Glossary) for allergies, colds, and coughs contain drugs that may interact unfavorably with this drug. Ask your physician or pharmacist for guidance before using any such medications.

Precautions for Use by Those over 60 Years of Age

You may be more sensitive to the stimulant effects of this drug. Small doses are advisable until your individual response has been determined.
You may be more susceptible to the development of high blood pressure, disturbance of heart rhythm, angina, nervousness, or insomnia.

Advisability of Use During Pregnancy

Pregnancy Category: C (tentative). See Pregnancy Code inside back cover.
Animal reproduction studies: No data available.
Information from adequate studies in pregnant women is not available.
Ask physician for guidance.

Advisability of Use While Nursing Infant

Drug is known to be present in milk and to have adverse effects on the infant. Avoid drug or discontinue nursing. Ask physician for guidance.

Habit-Forming Potential

None.

Effects of Overdosage

With Moderate Overdose: Marked nervousness, restlessness, headache, rapid or irregular heart action, sweating, nausea, vomiting.
With Large Overdose: Anxiety, confusion, delirium, muscle tremors, rapid and irregular pulse.

Possible Effects of Extended Use

None reported.

Suggested Periodic Examinations While Taking This Drug (at physician's discretion)
None required.

While Taking This Drug, Observe the Following
Foods: No restrictions.

Beverages: Excessive coffee or tea may increase the nervousness or insomnia caused by this drug in sensitive individuals.

Alcohol: No interactions expected.

Tobacco Smoking: No interactions expected. No restrictions unless advised otherwise by your physician.

Marijuana Smoking
Occasional (once or twice weekly):   No effect to mild and transient increased heart rate.

Daily: Persistent rapid heart rate; possible heart rhythm disturbance (in sensitive individuals).

Other Drugs
Pseudoephedrine may *increase* the effects of
- epinephrine (Adrenalin, Bronkaid Mist, Vaponefrin, etc.), and cause excessive stimulation of the heart and an increase in blood pressure. Use caution and avoid excessive dosage.

Pseudoephedrine may *decrease* the effects of
- anti-hypertensive drugs, and reduce their effectiveness in lowering blood pressure. Ask physician if any dosage adjustment is necessary to maintain proper blood pressure control.

Pseudoephedrine *taken concurrently* with
- digitalis preparations (digitoxin, digoxin, etc.), may cause serious disturbances of heart rhythm.
- ergot-related preparations (Cafergot, Ergotrate, Migral, Wigraine, etc.), may cause serious increase in blood pressure.
- guanethidine, may result in reduced effectiveness of both drugs.

The following drugs may *increase* the effects of pseudoephedrine
- mono-amine oxidase (MAO) inhibitor drugs (see Drug Class, Section Three). The combined effects may cause a dangerous increase in blood pressure.
- tricyclic antidepressants (see Drug Class, Section Three). The combined effects may cause excessive stimulation of the heart and/or elevation of blood pressure.

Driving a Vehicle, Operating Machinery, Engaging in Hazardous Activities:
No restrictions unless dizziness occurs.

Aviation Note: The use of this drug *may be a disqualification* for the piloting of aircraft. Consultation with a designated Aviation Medical Examiner is advised.

Exposure to Sun: No restrictions.

Special Storage Instructions
Keep in a tightly closed, light-resistant container. Avoid excessive heat.

PYRILAMINE
(Mepyramine)

Year Introduced: 1944

Brand Names

USA		Canada
Nervine Nighttime Sleep-Aid (Miles)	Sominex (Beecham)	Triaminicin [CD] (Anca)
Pyma [CD] (Fellows)	Triaminic [CD] (Dorsey)	Triaminicin w/Codeine [CD]
Pyristan [CD] (Arcum)	Triaminic Juvelets [CD] (Dorsey)	(Anca)
Robitussin Night Relief Cold Formula [CD] (Robins)	Triaminic Oral Infant Drops [CD] (Dorsey)	
Rynatan [CD] (Wallace)		

Common Synonyms ("Street Names"):   Allergy pills

Drug Class: Antihistamines

Prescription Required: No

Available for Purchase by Generic Name: Yes

Available Dosage Forms and Strengths
> Capsules — 25 mg.
> Tablets — 25 mg.
> Tablets — 12.5 mg., 50 mg. (in combination with other drugs)
> Syrup — 6.25 mg. per 5 ml. teaspoonful (in combination with other drugs)
> Pediatric drops — 10 mg. per ml. (in combination with other drugs)

Tablet May Be Crushed or Capsule Opened for Administration: Yes

How This Drug Works
> **Intended Therapeutic Effect(s):**   Relief of symptoms associated with hayfever (allergic rhinitis) and with allergic reactions in the skin, such as itching, swelling, hives, and rash.
> **Location of Drug Action(s):**   Those hypersensitive tissues that release excessive histamine as part of an allergic reaction. The principal tissue sites are the eyes, the nose, and the skin.
> **Method of Drug Action(s):**   This drug reduces the intensity of the allergic response by blocking the action of histamine after it has been released from sensitized tissue cells.

Principal Uses of This Drug
> **As a Single Drug Product:**   Because drowsiness is a prominent side effect of this antihistamine, it is used alone as a nighttime sleep aid.

As a Combination Drug Product [CD]:   It is available in combination with other antihistamines and decongestants in allergy and cold preparations.

THIS DRUG SHOULD NOT BE TAKEN IF
—you have had an allergic reaction to any dosage form of it previously.
—you are taking, or have taken during the past 2 weeks, any mono-amine oxidase (MAO) inhibitor drug (see Drug Class, Section Three).
—it has been prescribed for a newborn infant.

INFORM YOUR PHYSICIAN BEFORE TAKING THIS DRUG IF
—you have had an unfavorable reaction to any antihistamine drug in the past.
—you have glaucoma.
—you have a history of asthma, peptic ulcer disease, or impairment of urinary bladder function.
—you plan to have surgery under general anesthesia in the near future.

Time Required for Apparent Benefit
Drug action begins in approximately 30 minutes, reaches a maximum in 1 hour, and subsides in 4 to 6 hours.

Possible Side-Effects (*natural, expected, and unavoidable drug actions*)
Drowsiness, sense of weakness, dryness of nose, mouth, and throat, constipation.

Possible Adverse Effects (*unusual, unexpected, and infrequent reactions*)

IF ANY OF THE FOLLOWING DEVELOP, DISCONTINUE DRUG AND NOTIFY YOUR PHYSICIAN AS SOON AS POSSIBLE

Mild Adverse Effects
Allergic Reactions: Skin rash, hives.
Other Reactions
Headache, dizziness, inability to concentrate, nervousness, blurring of vision, double vision, difficulty in urination.
Nausea, vomiting, diarrhea.
Serious Adverse Effects
Idiosyncratic Reactions: Emotional and behavioral disturbances—confusion, agitation, inappropriate actions.

Precautions for Use by Those over 60 Years of Age
You may be more susceptible to the development of drowsiness, dizziness, and lethargy and to impairment of thinking, judgment, and memory.
This drug can increase the degree of impaired urination associated with prostate gland enlargement (prostatism).

Advisability of Use During Pregnancy
Pregnancy Category: B (tentative). See Pregnancy Code inside back cover.
Animal reproduction studies reveal no birth defects due to this drug.
Information from studies in pregnant women indicates no significant increase in defects in 392 exposures to this drug.
Ask physician for guidance.

Advisability of Use While Nursing Infant
This drug may impair milk formation and make nursing difficult. It is known to be present in milk. Avoid use or discontinue nursing. Ask physician for guidance.

Habit-Forming Potential
None.

Effects of Overdosage
With Moderate Overdose: Marked drowsiness, confusion, incoordination, unsteady gait, muscle tremors. In children: excitement, hallucinations, overactivity, convulsions.

With Large Overdose: Stupor progressing to coma, fever, flushed face, dilated pupils, weak pulse, shallow breathing.

Possible Effects of Extended Use
None.

Suggested Periodic Examinations While Taking This Drug (at physician's discretion)
Complete blood cell counts.

While Taking This Drug, Observe the Following
Foods: No restrictions. Stomach irritation can be reduced if drug is taken after eating.

Beverages: Coffee and tea may help to reduce the drowsiness caused by most antihistamines.

Alcohol: Use with extreme caution until combined effect has been determined. The combination of alcohol and antihistamines can cause rapid and marked sedation.

Tobacco Smoking: No interactions expected.

Marijuana Smoking

Occasional (once or twice weekly):   Mild increase in drowsiness and dryness of mouth.

Daily: Moderate to marked increase in drowsiness and dryness of mouth; possible accentuation of impaired thinking.

Other Drugs

Pyrilamine may *increase* the effects of

- sedatives, sleep-inducing drugs, tranquilizers, antidepressants, pain relievers, and narcotic drugs, and cause oversedation. Careful dosage adjustments are necessary.
- atropine and drugs with atropine-like action (see Drug Class, Section Three).

The following drugs may *increase* the effects of pyrilamine

- all sedatives, sleep-inducing drugs, tranquilizers, pain relievers, and narcotic drugs may exaggerate its sedative action and cause oversedation.
- mono-amine oxidase (MAO) inhibitor drugs (see Drug Class, Section Three) may delay its elimination from the body, thus exaggerating and prolonging its action.

The following drugs may *decrease* the effects of pyrilamine
- amphetamines (Benzedrine, Dexedrine, Desoxyn, etc.) may reduce the drowsiness caused by most antihistamines.

Driving a Vehicle, Operating Machinery, Engaging in Hazardous Activities: This drug may impair mental alertness, judgment, physical coordination, and reaction time. Avoid hazardous activities until full sedative effect has been determined.

Aviation Note: The use of this drug *may be a disqualification* for the piloting of aircraft. Consultation with a designated Aviation Medical Examiner is advised.

Exposure to Sun: No restrictions.

Special Storage Instructions
Keep in a dry, tightly closed, light-resistant container.

QUINIDINE

Year Introduced: 1918

Brand Names

USA	Canada
Cardioquin (Purdue-Frederick)	Biquin Durules (Astra)
Cin-Quin (Rowell)	Cardioquin (Purdue Frederick)
Duraquin (Parke-Davis)	Quinaglute (Pentagone)
Quinaglute (Berlex)	Quinate (Rougier)
Quinidex Extendtabs (Robins)	Quinidex Extendtabs (Robins)
Quinora (Key)	*Quinobarb [CD] (Welcker-Lyster)
SK-Quinidine (Smith Kline & French)	

Common Synonyms ("Street Names"):   Heart regulator

Drug Class: Heart Rhythm Regulator (Anti-arrhythmic)

Prescription Required: USA: Yes   Canada: No

Available for Purchase by Generic Name: Yes

Available Dosage Forms and Strengths
Tablets — 100 mg., 200 mg., 275 mg., 330 mg.
Prolonged-action tablets — 300 mg., 324 mg., 330 mg.
Capsules — 100 mg., 200 mg., 300 mg.
Injection — 50 mg. per ml., 80 mg. per ml., 200 mg. per ml.

*Quinobarb contains phenylethylbarbiturate, a sedative of the barbiturate drug family.

Tablet May Be Crushed or Capsule Opened for Administration
Regular tablets and capsules — Yes
Prolonged-action tablets, Quinaglute, Quinidex — No

How This Drug Works

Intended Therapeutic Effect(s): Correction of certain heart rhythm disorders.

Location of Drug Action(s): The heart muscle and the tissues that comprise the electrical conduction system of the heart.

Method of Drug Action(s): By slowing the activity of the pacemaker and delaying the transmission of electrical impulses through the conduction system and muscle of the heart, this drug assists in restoring normal heart rate and rhythm.

Principal Uses of This Drug

As a Single Drug Product: Used primarily to control the following types of abnormal heart rhythm: atrial fibrillation and flutter, paroxysmal atrial tachycardia, paroxysmal ventricular tachycardia, premature atrial and ventricular contractions.

As a Combination Drug Product [CD]: This drug is available (in Canada) in combination with a barbiturate, a mild sedative that is added to allay the anxiety and nervous tension that often accompany heart rhythm disorders.

THIS DRUG SHOULD NOT BE TAKEN IF

—you have had an allergic reaction to any dosage form of it previously.
—you presently have an acute infection of any kind.

INFORM YOUR PHYSICIAN BEFORE TAKING THIS DRUG IF

—you are now taking, or have taken within the past 2 weeks, any digitalis preparation.
—you have a history of thyroid gland overactivity (hyperthyroidism).
—you have a history of angina or previous heart attack.
—you plan to have surgery under general anesthesia in the near future.

Time Required for Apparent Benefit

Drug action begins in 1 hour, reaches a maximum in 2 to 4 hours, and gradually subsides within 18 to 24 hours. On regular daily dosage, accumulation persists for 4 to 5 days.

Possible Side-Effects *(natural, expected, and unavoidable drug actions)*

Drop in blood pressure, resulting in lightheadedness in upright position (see orthostatic hypotension in Glossary).

Possible Adverse Effects *(unusual, unexpected, and infrequent reactions)*

IF ANY OF THE FOLLOWING DEVELOP, DISCONTINUE DRUG AND NOTIFY YOUR PHYSICIAN AS SOON AS POSSIBLE

Mild Adverse Effects

Allergic Reactions: Rash, hives, drug fever, skin eruption with peeling.

Other Reactions

Loss of appetite, nausea, vomiting, diarrhea.

Dizziness, ringing in the ears.

Sudden fainting (due to drop in blood pressure).

Serious Adverse Effects
Allergic Reactions: Abnormal bruising due to allergic destruction of blood platelets (see Glossary).
Idiosyncratic Reactions: Confusion, delirium, and agitated behavior.
Other Reactions
Hemolytic anemia (see Glossary).
Worsening of psoriasis (in sensitive individuals).
Bone marrow depression (see Glossary)—fatigue, weakness, fever, sore throat, abnormal bruising or bleeding.

CAUTION
1. The effects of this drug are very unpredictable because of the wide variation in response from person to person. Dosage adjustments must be based upon individual reaction. Notify your physician of any events that you suspect may be drug-related.
2. It is advisable to carry a card of personal identification that includes a notation that you are taking this drug (see Table 19 and Section Six).

Precautions for Use by Those over 60 Years of Age
You may be more sensitive to all of the actions of this drug. Small doses are mandatory until your individual response has been determined.
You may be more susceptible to its blood pressure-lowering effect. Report promptly the development of lightheadedness, dizziness, weakness, or sense of impending faint. Use caution to prevent falls.

Advisability of Use During Pregnancy
Pregnancy Category: C (tentative). See Pregnancy Code inside back cover.
Animal reproduction studies: No data available.
Information from adequate studies in pregnant women is not available. Ask physician for guidance.

Advisability of Use While Nursing Infant
Drug is known to be present in milk. Safety for infant not established. Ask physician for guidance.

Habit-Forming Potential
None.

Effects of Overdosage
With Moderate Overdose: Headache, dizziness, blurred vision, ringing in the ears, nausea, vomiting, diarrhea, confusion.
With Large Overdose: Severe drop in blood pressure, difficulty in breathing, collapse of circulation.

Possible Effects of Extended Use
None reported.

Suggested Periodic Examinations While Taking This Drug (at physician's discretion)
Complete blood cell counts.
Electrocardiograms.

While Taking This Drug, Observe the Following

Foods: No restrictions. Follow prescribed diet.

Beverages: Use caffeine-containing beverages (coffee, tea, cola) sparingly.

Alcohol: No interactions expected.

Tobacco Smoking: No interactions expected. However, nicotine can increase the irritability of the heart and can confuse interpretation of this drug's action. Follow physician's advice regarding smoking.

Marijuana Smoking

Occasional (once or twice weekly):   No effect to mild and transient accentuation of orthostatic hypotension (see Glossary).

Daily: Possible accentuation of orthostatic hypotension, requiring dosage adjustment in sensitive individuals.

Other Drugs

Quinidine may *increase* the effects of

- anticoagulants, and cause abnormal bleeding or hemorrhage. Careful dosage adjustment is necessary.
- anti-hypertensive drugs, and cause excessive lowering of the blood pressure.
- atropine-like drugs (see Drug Class, Section Three).

Quinidine may *decrease* the effects of

- choline-like drugs such as Mestinon, Mytelase, pilocarpine, Prostigmin, and Urecholine, and reduce their effectiveness in the treatment of glaucoma and myasthenia gravis.

Quinidine *taken concurrently* with

- reserpine (and related drugs), may cause serious disturbances of heart rhythm.
- digitalis preparations, may cause excessive slowing of the heart. Dosage adjustment of both drugs is essential. Digoxin may reach toxic levels.
- propranolol (Inderal), may cause excessive slowing of the heart.

The following drugs may *increase* the effects of quinidine

- phenytoin (Dantoin, Dilantin, etc.)
- pyrimethamine (Daraprim)

Driving a Vehicle, Operating Machinery, Engaging in Hazardous Activities: Usually no restrictions. Avoid hazardous activities if dizziness or lightheadedness occurs.

Aviation Note: The use of this drug *may be a disqualification* for the piloting of aircraft. Consultation with a designated Aviation Medical Examiner is advised.

Exposure to Sun: No restrictions.

Special Storage Instructions

Keep in a tightly closed container. Protect from light.

RANITIDINE

Note: This is an Abbreviated Drug Profile of a newly-marketed drug to be used in the treatment of peptic ulcer disease. It has demonstrated significant advantages over similar drugs in current use. As additional information becomes available, it will be provided in subsequent editions of this book.

Year Introduced: 1983

Brand Names

USA	Canada
Zantac (Glaxo)	Zantac (Glaxo)

Common Synonyms ("Street Names"):   Ulcer pills

Drug Class: Anti-peptic ulcer, Histamine H_2 Blocker

Prescription Required: USA: Yes   Canada: Yes

Available Dosage Forms and Strengths
Tablets — 150 mg.

Tablet May Be Crushed or Capsule Opened for Administration: Yes

How This Drug Works
Intended Therapeutic Effect(s): The relief of symptoms associated with active peptic ulcer, and the acceleration of ulcer healing.
Method of Drug Action(s): By blocking the action of histamine, this drug effectively inhibits the secretion of stomach acid and thus creates a more favorable environment for ulcer healing.

Principal Uses of This Drug
As a Single Drug Product: Used primarily for the short-term treatment of active duodenal ulcer and the prevention of ulcer recurrence. Also used for the treatment of excessive stomach acid secretion, such as occurs in the Zollinger-Ellison Syndrome.

INFORM YOUR PHYSICIAN BEFORE TAKING THIS DRUG IF
—you have a history of liver or kidney disease, or impaired liver or kidney function.
—you have glaucoma.

Time Required for Apparent Benefit
Drug action usually begins in 1 hour and reaches its peak in 2 to 3 hours. Continuous use on a regular schedule for 2 to 4 weeks is usually necessary to determine this drug's effectiveness in accelerating the healing of duodenal ulcer.

Possible Adverse Effects *(unusual, unexpected, and infrequent reactions)*

IF ANY OF THE FOLLOWING DEVELOP, DISCONTINUE DRUG AND NOTIFY YOUR PHYSICIAN AS SOON AS POSSIBLE

Mild Adverse Effects
Allergic Reactions: Skin rash.
Other Reactions: Headache, malaise, dizziness.
Nausea, abdominal pain, constipation, diarrhea.

Serious Adverse Effects
Increased internal eye pressure—aggravation of glaucoma.
Drug-induced hepatitis (rare). Reduced white blood cell counts and blood platelet counts (thought to be insignificant).

CAUTION
1. Do not discontinue this drug abruptly. Ask your physician for guidance regarding gradual withdrawal.
2. After discontinuation of this drug, inform your physician promptly if you experience a return of symptoms indicative of ulcer reactivation.

Advisability of Use During Pregnancy
Pregnancy Category: B (tentative). See Pregnancy Code inside back cover.
Animal reproduction studies reveal no birth defects due to this drug.
Information from adequate studies in pregnant women is not available.
Use only if clearly needed. Ask physician for guidance.

Advisability of Use While Nursing Infant
This drug is present in human milk. Ask physician for guidance.

Suggested Periodic Examinations While Taking This Drug (at physician's discretion)
Complete blood cell counts. Liver function tests.

While Taking This Drug, Observe the Following
Foods: Follow your physician's advice regarding diet.
This drug may be taken with or following food.
Beverages: Caffeine-containing beverages (coffee, tea, cola drinks) may increase stomach acidity, reduce the effectiveness of this drug, and delay ulcer healing. This drug may be taken with milk.
Alcohol: No interactions expected. However, alcoholic beverages may increase stomach acidity, reduce the effectiveness of this drug, and delay ulcer healing.
Tobacco Smoking: No interactions expected. However, nicotine may increase stomach acidity, reduce the effectiveness of this drug, and perpetuate peptic ulcer disease.
Other Drugs: No significant drug interactions reported to date.
Driving a Vehicle, Operating Machinery, Engaging in Hazardous Activities:
Use caution until it has been determined that dizziness does not occur.

Aviation Note: The use of this drug *may be a disqualification* for the piloting of aircraft. Consultation with a designated Aviation Medical Examiner is advised.

Special Storage Instructions

Keep in a dry, tightly closed container at room temperature. Protect from light.

RESERPINE
(Deserpidine, Rauwolfia)

Year Introduced: 1953

Brand Names

USA

Arcum R-S (Arcum)
Broserpine (Brothers)
DeSerpa (de Leon)
Elserpine (Canright)
Hyperine (Sutliff & Case)
Lemiserp (Lemmon)
Raudixin (Squibb)
Rauloydin (Tutag)
Rau-Sed (Squibb)
Rauserpin (Ferndale)
Reserpaneed (Hanlon)
Reserpoid (Upjohn)

Sandril (Lilly)
Serp (Scrip)
Serpalan (Lannett)
Serpanray (Panray)
Serpasil (CIBA)
Serpate (Vale)
Serpena (Haag)
Sertabs (Table Rock)
Sertina (Fellows)
SK-Reserpine (Smith
   Kline & French)

Tensin (Standex)
T-Serp (Tennessee)
Demi-Regroton [CD]
   (USV)
Rauzide [CD]
   (Squibb)
Regroton [CD] (USV)
Ser-Ap-Es [CD]
   (CIBA)
(Numerous
   combination brand
   names)

Canada

Reserfia (Medic)
Serpasil (CIBA)
Ser-Ap-Es [CD] (CIBA)

Common Synonyms ("Street Names"):   Blood pressure pills

Drug Class: Anti-hypertensive (Hypotensive)

Prescription Required: Yes

Available for Purchase by Generic Name: Yes

Available Dosage Forms and Strengths
Tablets — 0.1 mg., 0.25 mg., 0.5 mg., 1 mg.
Prolonged-action Capsules — 0.5 mg.
Injection — 2.5 mg. per ml.

Tablet May Be Crushed or Capsule Opened for Administration: Yes

How This Drug Works
Intended Therapeutic Effect(s):   Reduction of high blood pressure.

Location of Drug Action(s):   The storage sites of norepinephrine in the nerve terminals of the sympathetic nervous system.

Method of Drug Action(s):   By displacing the nerve impulse transmitter norepinephrine from nerve terminals, this drug reduces the ability of the sympathetic nervous system to maintain the degree of blood vessel constriction responsible for high blood pressure. The reduced availability of norepinephrine results in relaxation of blood vessel walls and lowering of the blood pressure.

Principal Uses of This Drug
As a Single Drug Product: Used primarily as a "step 2" anti-hypertensive drug in the treatment of high blood pressure. Originally introduced as a tranquilizer for the treatment of psychotic states (schizophrenia), it is no longer used for this purpose.

As a Combination Drug Product [CD]:   This drug is available in combination with most of the thiazide diuretics, the conventional "step 1" antihypertensive medication. One popular product combines reserpine, hydrochlorothiazide, and hydralazine, a "step 2 or 3" anti-hypertensive drug. These combinations are more effective for treating moderate to severe hypertension.

THIS DRUG SHOULD NOT BE TAKEN IF
—you have had an allergic reaction to any dosage form of it previously.
—you are emotionally depressed.
—you have an active peptic ulcer (stomach or duodenal).
—you have active ulcerative colitis.

INFORM YOUR PHYSICIAN BEFORE TAKING THIS DRUG IF
—you have a history of emotional depression.
—you have a history of peptic ulcer, ulcerative colitis, or gall stones.
—you have epilepsy.
—you are taking oral anticoagulants.
—you are taking any form of digitalis, quinidine, or any mono-amine oxidase (MAO) inhibitor drug (see Drug Class, Section Three).
—you plan to have surgery under general anesthesia in the near future.

Time Required for Apparent Benefit
Continuous use on a regular schedule for 3 weeks is usually necessary to determine this drug's full effectiveness in lowering the blood pressure.

Possible Side-Effects *(natural, expected, and unavoidable drug actions)*
Drowsiness and lethargy (especially during first few weeks), reddening of the eyes, nasal stuffiness (frequent), dryness of the mouth, increased hunger contractions, acid indigestion, intestinal cramping, diarrhea, water retention.

Possible Adverse Effects *(unusual, unexpected, and infrequent reactions)*

IF ANY OF THE FOLLOWING DEVELOP, DISCONTINUE DRUG AND NOTIFY
YOUR PHYSICIAN AS SOON AS POSSIBLE

Mild Adverse Effects
Allergic Reactions: Skin rash, itching, spontaneous bruising.
Other Reactions
  Nausea, vomiting, diarrhea.
  Headache, dizziness, nasal congestion, nosebleeds.
  Breast enlargement, milk production, change in menstrual pattern.

Serious Adverse Effects
Idiosyncratic Reactions: Paradoxical nervousness, agitation, nightmares,
  confusion, hallucinations.
Other Reactions
  Parkinson-like disorders (see Glossary).
  Mental depression.
  Activation of stomach or duodenal ulcer.
  Impaired sex drive, potency, and performance.

CAUTION
1. It is advisable to discontinue this drug at the first sign of despondency, loss
   of appetite, early morning awakening (insomnia), or impaired sex drive or
   performance. Notify your physician of this action promptly.
2. Hot weather and the fever associated with infection can reduce the blood
   pressure significantly, requiring adjustment of dosage.

Precautions for Use by Those over 60 Years of Age
The basic rule in treating high blood pressure after 60 is to proceed *cautiously.* The elevated systolic blood pressure often present after 60 is not
necessarily a threat to health, and can serve as an adaptive and compensatory change with age that should not be altered drastically. The goals of
treatment must be adjusted to the natural changes in body function that
occur with aging. Unacceptably high blood pressure should be reduced
without creating the risks associated with excessively low blood pressure.
It is advisable to start treatment with small doses and to monitor the blood
pressure response frequently. Sudden, rapid, and excessive reduction of
blood pressure can predispose to stroke or heart attack.
You may be more susceptible to the development of orthostatic hypotension
with resultant lightheadedness, dizziness, unsteadiness, fainting, and falling. Report such symptoms to your physician promptly.

Advisability of Use During Pregnancy
Pregnancy Category: C (tentative). See Pregnancy Code inside back cover.
  Animal reproduction studies in rats reveal significant birth defects due to
    this drug.
  Information from adequate studies in pregnant women is not available.
  Avoid completely during first 3 months.
  Ask physician for guidance.

Advisability of Use While Nursing Infant

This drug is known to be present in milk. Avoid use or discontinue nursing. Ask physician for guidance.

Habit-Forming Potential

None.

Effects of Overdosage

With Moderate Overdose: Marked drowsiness, slow and weak pulse, slow and shallow breathing, diarrhea.

With Large Overdose: Stupor progressing to deep sleep or coma, flushing of skin, decreased body temperature, severe depression of breathing and heart action.

Possible Effects of Extended Use

Recent reports that reserpine can cause cancer in laboratory test animals are under study by the Food and Drug Administration to assess the significance of this finding with regard to human use. Until a determination is made, it is advisable to avoid the use of this drug if you have a personal history or a strong family history of cancer. Ask your physician for guidance.

Suggested Periodic Examinations While Taking This Drug (at physician's discretion)

Complete blood cell counts.
Eye examinations for impaired vision.

While Taking This Drug, Observe the Following

Foods: Avoid highly spiced foods. Ask physician for guidance if you are subject to acid indigestion or have a history of peptic ulcer.

Beverages: Avoid heavy use of carbonated drinks.

Alcohol: Use with extreme caution until combined effect has been determined. This drug can increase the intoxicating effect of alcohol.

Tobacco Smoking: No interactions expected. Follow physician's advice regarding smoking.

Marijuana Smoking

Occasional (once or twice weekly):   Mild and transient increase in drowsiness.

Daily: Significant increase in drowsiness; possible accentuation of lowered blood pressure due to this drug; possible precipitation of depression due to this drug.

Other Drugs

Reserpine may *increase* the effects of

- other anti-hypertensive drugs, and cause excessive lowering of blood pressure. Careful dosage adjustments are necessary.
- sedatives, sleep-inducing drugs, tranquilizers, antihistamines, pain relievers, and narcotic drugs, and cause oversedation.

Reserpine may *decrease* the effects of

- levodopa (Dopar, Larodopa, etc.), and reduce its effectiveness in the treatment of Parkinson's disease.
- aspirin, and reduce its pain-relieving action.

Reserpine *taken concurrently* with

- oral anticoagulants, may cause unpredictable fluctuations in coagulation control. Ask physician for guidance regarding prothrombin time testing and dosage adjustment.
- anti-convulsants, may cause a serious change in the pattern of epileptic seizures. Some individuals may require an increase in the dose of anti-convulsants.
- digitalis preparations and quinidine, may cause serious disturbances of heart rhythm. Careful dosage adjustments are necessary.
- mono-amine oxidase (MAO) inhibitor drugs, may cause severe emotional depression, cramping, and diarrhea.

The following drugs may *increase* the effects of reserpine

- propranolol (Inderal) may increase its sedative effect and cause oversedation.
- members of the phenothiazine family (see Drug Class, Section Three) may increase both the sedative effect and the blood pressure-lowering action.

Driving a Vehicle, Operating Machinery, Engaging in Hazardous Activities: This drug can impair mental alertness, judgment, physical coordination, and reaction time. Avoid hazardous activities if you experience drowsiness, lethargy, or dizziness.

Aviation Note: The use of this drug and the disorder for which this drug is prescribed *are disqualifications* for the piloting of aircraft. Consultation with a designated Aviation Medical Examiner is advised.

Exposure to Sun: No restrictions.

Heavy Exercise or Exertion: Isometric exercises—the "overload" technique for strengthening individual muscles—can raise the blood pressure significantly. The use of this drug may intensify the hypertensive response to isometric exercises. Ask your physician for guidance.

Discontinuation: Upon stopping this drug, careful readjustments of dosages will be necessary for the following drugs if taken concurrently with reserpine: other anti-hypertensives, oral anticoagulants, anti-convulsants.

Special Storage Instructions
Keep in a dry, tightly closed container.

RIFAMPIN

Year Introduced: 1967 (Europe)
                        1971 (USA)

Brand Names

USA	Canada
Rifadin (Merrell Dow)	Rifadin (Dow)
Rifomycin (Various	Rimactane (CIBA)
Manufacturers)	Rofact (ICN)
Rimactane (CIBA)	
Rifamate [CD] (Merrell	
Dow)	

Common Synonyms ("Street Names"):   TB drug

Drug Class: Antibiotic (Anti-infective), Rifamycins

Prescription Required: Yes

Available for Purchase by Generic Name: No

Available Dosage Forms and Strengths
  Capsules — 150 mg., 300 mg.

Tablet May Be Crushed or Capsule Opened for Administration: Yes

How This Drug Works
  Intended Therapeutic Effect(s):   The treatment of active tuberculosis, in
  conjunction with other drugs.
  Location of Drug Action(s):   Those body tissues and fluids in which adequate
  concentration of the drug can be achieved. The principal site of therapeutic action is the lung.
  Method of Drug Action(s):   This drug prevents the growth and multiplication of susceptible tuberculosis organisms by interfering with enzyme systems involved in the formation of essential proteins.

Principal Uses of This Drug
  As a Single Drug Product: This antibiotic drug is used primarily to treat
  active tuberculosis. It is usually given concurrently with other antitubercular drugs to enhance its effectiveness. It is also used to eliminate the meningitis germ (meningococcus) from the throats of healthy carriers. It is not
  effective in the treatment of active meningitis.
  As a Combination Drug Product [CD]:   This drug is available in combination with isoniazid, another antitubercular drug that delays the development of resistant strains of the tuberculosis germ.

THIS DRUG SHOULD NOT BE TAKEN IF
—you are allergic to any of the drugs bearing the brand names listed above or
  to any rifamycin drug.
—you have active liver disease.
—it is prescribed for a child under 5 years of age.

INFORM YOUR PHYSICIAN BEFORE TAKING THIS DRUG IF
—you are pregnant.
—you have a history of liver disease or impaired liver function.
—you are taking oral contraceptives (any form of "the pill").
—you are taking anticoagulants.

Time Required for Apparent Benefit
Varies with nature of infection under treatment; may be from 4 to 6 weeks.

Possible Side-Effects *(natural, expected, and unavoidable drug actions)*
Red, orange, or brown discoloration of tears, sweat, saliva, sputum, urine, or stool.
Yellow discoloration of skin (not jaundice).
Note: In the absence of symptoms indicating illness, any discoloration is a harmless drug effect and does not indicate toxicity.
Superinfections (see Glossary).

Possible Adverse Effects *(unusual, unexpected, and infrequent reactions)*

IF ANY OF THE FOLLOWING DEVELOP, DISCONTINUE DRUG AND NOTIFY YOUR PHYSICIAN AS SOON AS POSSIBLE

Mild Adverse Effects
Allergic Reactions: Skin rash (various kinds), hives, itching, irritation of mouth or tongue, fever.
Other Reactions
Loss of appetite, heartburn, nausea, vomiting, abdominal cramps, diarrhea.
Headache, drowsiness, dizziness, disturbed vision, impaired hearing, vague numbness or tingling.
Mild menstrual irregularity.
Serious Adverse Effects
Liver damage, causing jaundice (see Glossary).
Abnormally low blood platelets (see Glossary)—unusual bleeding or bruising.

Precautions for Use by Those over 60 Years of Age
The natural changes in body composition and function that occur after 60 may make you more susceptible to the adverse effects of this drug. Report promptly the development of *any* of the symptoms listed above.

Advisability of Use During Pregnancy
Pregnancy Category: C (tentative). See Pregnancy Code inside back cover.
Animal reproduction studies in rodents reveal significant birth defects due to this drug.
Information from adequate studies in pregnant women is not available.
It is advisable to avoid use of this drug during first 3 months if possible.
Ask physician for guidance.

Advisability of Use While Nursing Infant
Safety for infant not established. Ask physician for guidance.

Habit-Forming Potential
None.

Effects of Overdosage
Nausea, vomiting, drowsiness, unconsciousness, severe liver damage, jaundice.

Possible Effects of Extended Use
Superinfections (see Glossary).

Suggested Periodic Examinations While Taking This Drug (at physician's discretion)
Complete blood cell counts.
Liver and kidney function tests.
Hearing acuity tests if hearing loss is suspected.

While Taking This Drug, Observe the Following
Foods: No restrictions of food selection. Most effective when taken 1 hour before or 2 hours after eating.
Beverages: No restrictions.
Alcohol: Avoid while taking this drug if you have a history of liver disease.
Tobacco Smoking: No interactions expected.
Marijuana Smoking: No interactions expected.
Other Drugs
  Rifampin may *decrease* the effects of
  • oral contraceptives, and impair their effectiveness in preventing pregnancy.

  Rifampin *taken concurrently* with
  • oral anticoagulants, may cause unpredictable changes in blood coagulation. Monitor blood prothrombin time closely and adjust dosage accordingly.

  The following drugs may *decrease* the effects of rifampin
  • para-aminosalicylic acid (PAS) may interfere with its absorption. Take each drug separately, 6 to 8 hours apart.
Driving a Vehicle, Operating Machinery, Engaging in Hazardous Activities:
Restricted only if you experience dizziness, impaired balance, or impaired vision.
Aviation Note: The use of this drug *may be a disqualification* for the piloting of aircraft. Consultation with a designated Aviation Medical Examiner is advised.
Exposure to Sun: No restrictions.
Discontinuation: It is advisable not to interrupt or discontinue this drug without consulting your physician. Interrupted or intermittent administration can increase the possibility of allergic reactions.

Special Storage Instructions
Keep in a dry, tightly closed, light-resistant container.

SECOBARBITAL

Year Introduced: 1936

Brand Names

USA	Canada
Seconal (Lilly)	Novosecobarb
Tuinal [CD] (Lilly)	(Novopharm)
	Secogen (Technilab)
	Seconal (Lilly)
	Seral (Medic)
	Tuinal [CD] (Lilly)

Common Synonyms ("Street Names"):   Barbs, bullets, candy, downers, F-40s, goofballs, peanuts, pink ladies, pinks, red birds, red devils, red lilies, reds, seccy, seggy, sleepers, stoppers, stumblers; for Tuinal, a brand of amobarbital with secobarbital: Christmas trees, double trouble, jelly beans, rainbows, tooies, tuies.

Drug Class: Sedative, Mild; Sleep Inducer (Hypnotic), Barbiturates

Prescription Required: Yes (Controlled Drug, U.S. Schedule II)*

Available for Purchase by Generic Name: Yes

Available Dosage Forms and Strengths
Tablets — 100 mg.
Capsules — 50 mg., 100 mg.
Elixir — 22 mg. per teaspoonful (5 ml.)
Suppositories — 30 mg., 60 mg., 120 mg., 200 mg.
Injection — 50 mg. per ml.

Tablet May Be Crushed or Capsule Opened for Administration: Yes

How This Drug Works
Intended Therapeutic Effect(s)
With low dosage, relief of mild to moderate anxiety or tension (sedative effect).
With higher dosage taken at bedtime, sedation sufficient to induce sleep (hypnotic effect).
Location of Drug Action(s):   The connecting points (synapses) in the nerve pathways that transmit impulses between the wake-sleep centers of the brain.
Method of Drug Action(s):   Not completely established. Present thinking is that this drug selectively blocks the transmission of nerve impulses by reducing the amount of available norepinephrine, one of the chemicals responsible for impulse transmission.

*See Schedules of Controlled Drugs inside back cover.

Principal Uses of This Drug

As a Single Drug Product: Used primarily as a bedtime sedative for the short-term treatment of insomnia. It usually loses its effectiveness after 2 weeks of continuous use. Because of their potential for producing dependence (addiction), the barbiturates have been largely replaced by the benzodiazepines.

As a Combination Drug Product [CD]: This short-acting barbiturate (3 to 4 hours) is available in combination with amobarbital, an intermediate-acting barbiturate (6 to 8 hours). This combination is designed to induce sleep quickly and to maintain it for most of the night.

THIS DRUG SHOULD NOT BE TAKEN IF

—you have had an allergic reaction to any dosage form of it previously.

—you have a history of porphyria.

INFORM YOUR PHYSICIAN BEFORE TAKING THIS DRUG IF

—you are allergic or sensitive to any barbiturate drug.

—you are taking any sedative, sleep-inducing drugs, tranquilizers, antihistamines, pain relievers, or narcotic drugs of any kind.

—you have epilepsy.

—you have a history of liver or kidney disease.

—you plan to have surgery under general anesthesia in the near future.

Time Required for Apparent Benefit

Approximately 30 minutes.

Possible Side-Effects *(natural, expected, and unavoidable drug actions)*

Drowsiness, lethargy, and sense of mental or physical sluggishness as "hangover" effects.

Possible Adverse Effects *(unusual, unexpected, and infrequent reactions)*

IF ANY OF THE FOLLOWING DEVELOP, DISCONTINUE DRUG AND NOTIFY YOUR PHYSICIAN AS SOON AS POSSIBLE

Mild Adverse Effects

Allergic Reactions: Skin rashes (various kinds), hives, localized swellings of eyelids, face, or lips, drug fever.

Other Reactions

"Hangover" effect, dizziness, unsteadiness.

Nausea, vomiting, diarrhea.

Joint and muscle pains, most often in the neck, shoulder, and arms.

Serious Adverse Effects

Allergic Reactions: Hepatitis with jaundice (see Glossary), severe skin reactions.

Idiosyncratic Reactions: Paradoxical excitement and delirium (rather than sedation).

Other Reactions

Anemia—weakness and fatigue.

Abnormally low blood platelets (see Glossary)—unusual bleeding or bruising.

Precautions for Use by Infants and Children

Use not sanctioned by the U.S. Food and Drug Administration (FDA). Informed consent advised.

Precautions for Use by Those over 60 Years of Age

Small doses are advisable until tolerance has been determined. The elderly or debilitated may experience agitation, excitement, confusion, and delirium, with standard doses (paradoxical reaction).

This drug may also cause excessive lowering of body temperature (hypothermia). Keep dosage to a minimum during winter, and dress warmly.

The natural decline in liver function that may occur after 60 can slow the elimination of this drug. Longer intervals between doses may be necessary to avoid overdosage and toxicity

Note: A barbiturate is not the drug of choice as a sedative or sleep inducer in this age group.

Advisability of Use During Pregnancy

Pregnancy Category: B (tentative). See Pregnancy Code inside back cover. Animal reproduction studies reveal no birth defects due to this drug. Information from studies in pregnant women indicates no increase in defects in 4248 exposures to this drug.
Ask physician for guidance.

Advisability of Use While Nursing Infant

Drug is known to be present in milk. Ask physician for guidance.

Habit-Forming Potential

This drug can cause both psychological and physical dependence (see Glossary).

Effects of Overdosage

With Moderate Overdose: Behavior similar to alcoholic intoxication: confusion, slurred speech, physical incoordination, staggering gait, drowsiness.

With Large Overdose: Deepening sleep, coma, slow and shallow breathing, weak and rapid pulse, cold and sweaty skin.

Possible Effects of Extended Use

Psychological and/or physical dependence.
Anemia.
If dose is excessive, a form of chronic drug intoxication can occur: headache, impaired vision, slurred speech, and depression.

Suggested Periodic Examinations While Taking This Drug (at physician's discretion)

Complete blood cell counts.
Liver function tests.

While Taking This Drug, Observe the Following

Foods: No restrictions.
Beverages: No restrictions.
Alcohol: Avoid completely. Alcohol can increase greatly the sedative and depressant actions of this drug on brain function.

Tobacco Smoking: No interactions expected.

Marijuana Smoking

Occasional (once or twice weekly):   Mild, transient increase in drowsiness, unsteadiness, and impairment of mental and physical performance.

Daily: Marked, prolonged drowsiness, unsteadiness, and significantly impaired mental and physical performance.

Other Drugs

Secobarbital may *increase* the effects of

- other sedatives, sleep-inducing drugs, tranquilizers, antihistamines, pain relievers, and narcotic drugs, and cause oversedation. Ask your physician for guidance regarding dosage adjustments.

Secobarbital may *decrease* the effects of

- oral anticoagulants of the coumarin drug class. Ask physician for guidance regarding prothrombin time testing and adjustments of the anticoagulant dosage.
- aspirin, and reduce its pain-relieving action.
- cortisone and related drugs, by hastening their elimination from the body.
- oral contraceptives, by hastening their elimination from the body.
- griseofulvin (Fulvicin, Grisactin, etc.), and reduce its effectiveness in treating fungus infections.
- phenylbutazone (Azolid, Butazolidin, etc.), and reduce its effectiveness in treating inflammation and pain.

Secobarbital *taken concurrently* with

- anti-convulsants, may cause a change in the pattern of epileptic seizures. Careful dosage adjustments are necessary to achieve a balance of actions that will give the best protection from seizures.

The following drugs may *increase* the effects of secobarbital

- both mild and strong tranquilizers may increase the sedative and sleep-inducing actions and cause oversedation.
- isoniazid (INH, Isozide, etc.) may prolong the action of barbiturate drugs.
- antihistamines may increase the sedative effects of barbiturate drugs.
- oral anti-diabetic drugs of the sulfonylurea type may prolong the sedative effect of barbiturate drugs.
- mono-amine oxidase (MAO) inhibitor drugs may prolong the sedative effect of barbiturate drugs.

Driving a Vehicle, Operating Machinery, Engaging in Hazardous Activities: This drug can produce drowsiness and can impair mental alertness, judgment, physical coordination, and reaction time. Avoid hazardous activities.

Aviation Note: The use of this drug *is a disqualification* for the piloting of aircraft. Consultation with a designated Aviation Medical Examiner is advised.

Exposure to Sun: Use caution until sensitivity has been determined. Some barbiturates can cause photosensitivity (see Glossary).

Exposure to Cold: The elderly may experience excessive lowering of body temperature while taking this drug. Keep dosage to a minimum during winter and dress warmly.

Discontinuation: If it has been necessary to use this drug for an extended period of time, do not discontinue it abruptly. Ask physician for guidance regarding dosage adjustment and withdrawal. It may also be necessary to adjust the doses of other drugs taken concurrently with it.

Special Storage Instructions

Keep tablets and capsules in a dry, tightly closed container. Keep elixir in a tightly closed, amber glass bottle. Keep suppositories refrigerated.

SPIRONOLACTONE

Year Introduced: 1962

Brand Names

USA	Canada
Aldactone (Searle)	Aldactone (Searle)
Aldactazide [CD] (Searle)	Aldactazide [CD] (Searle)

Common Synonyms ("Street Names"):   Water pills

Drug Class: Anti-hypertensive (Hypotensive), Diuretic

Prescription Required: Yes

Available for Purchase by Generic Name: USA: Yes   Canada: No

Available Dosage Forms and Strengths
Tablets — 25 mg., 100 mg.

Tablet May Be Crushed or Capsule Opened for Administration: Yes

How This Drug Works
Intended Therapeutic Effect(s)
Elimination of excessive fluid retention (edema) without loss of potassium from the body.
Reduction of high blood pressure.
Location of Drug Action(s):   The tubular systems of the kidney that determine the final composition of the urine.
Method of Drug Action(s):   By increasing the elimination of salt and water but not potassium from the body (through increased urine production), this drug reduces the volume of fluid in the blood and body tissues and lowers the sodium content throughout the body. These changes may produce a lowering of the blood pressure.

Principal Uses of This Drug
As a Single Drug Product: This mild diuretic is used as part of the treatment program for the management of congestive heart failure and disorders of the liver and kidney that are accompanied by excessive fluid retention (edema). It is also used in conjunction with other measures to treat high blood pressure. It is used primarily in situations where it is advisable to prevent the loss of potassium from the body.

As a Combination Drug Product [CD]:   This drug is available in combination with hydrochlorothiazide, a different kind of diuretic that promotes
the loss of potassium from the body. Spironolactone is used in this combination to counteract the potassium-wasting effect of the thiazide diuretic.

THIS DRUG SHOULD NOT BE TAKEN IF
—you have had an allergic reaction to any dosage form of it previously.
—you have seriously impaired kidney function.

INFORM YOUR PHYSICIAN BEFORE TAKING THIS DRUG IF
—you have a history of kidney or liver disease.
—you are taking anticoagulant drugs or any form of digitalis.
—you plan to have surgery under general anesthesia in the near future.

Time Required for Apparent Benefit
Maximal diuretic effect requires continuous use for 3 to 5 days. Continuous
use on a regular schedule for 2 or more weeks may be necessary to determine
this drug's effectiveness in lowering your blood pressure.

Possible Side-Effects (*natural, expected, and unavoidable drug actions*)
Usually none, unless there is excessive loss of salt and water from the body
or excessive retention of potassium (see Effects of Overdosage, below).

Possible Adverse Effects (*unusual, unexpected, and infrequent reactions*)

**IF ANY OF THE FOLLOWING DEVELOP, DISCONTINUE DRUG AND NOTIFY
YOUR PHYSICIAN AS SOON AS POSSIBLE**

Mild Adverse Effects
    Allergic Reactions: Skin rashes (various kinds), hives, drug fever.
    Other Reactions
        Headache, drowsiness, lethargy, confusion.
        Indigestion, nausea, vomiting, diarrhea.
        Enlargement and sensitivity of the male breasts.
        Menstrual irregularities, deepening of the female voice.
Serious Adverse Effects
    Stomach ulceration and bleeding.

CAUTION
It is advisable not to use potassium supplements or deliberately to increase
your intake of potassium-rich foods while using this diuretic drug.

Precautions for Use by Those over 60 Years of Age
The natural decline in kidney function that occurs after 60 may predispose
to excessive retention of potassium in the body. It is advisable to limit the
use of this drug to periods of 2 to 3 weeks.
You may be more sensitive to the actions of this drug. Small doses are advisable until your individual response has been determined.
If you are taking this drug to treat high blood pressure, remember that warm
weather and fever can reduce your blood pressure and make it necessary
to adjust your dosage.
Overdosage and extended use of this drug can cause excessive loss of body
water, thickening (increased viscosity) of the blood, and an increased tend-

ency of the blood to clot, predisposing to stroke, heart attack, or thrombophlebitis.

Advisability of Use During Pregnancy

Pregnancy Category: B (tentative). See Pregnancy Code inside back cover.

Animal reproduction studies reveal no birth defects due to this drug. Information from adequate studies in pregnant women is not available.

Ask physician for guidance.

Advisability of Use While Nursing Infant

Presence of this drug in milk is not known. Ask physician for guidance.

Habit-Forming Potential

None.

Effects of Overdosage

With Moderate Overdose: Imbalance of body water, salt, and potassium, causing thirst, drowsiness, fatigue, weakness, nausea, vomiting.

With Large Overdose: Marked lethargy, irregular heart action, excessive drop in blood pressure.

Possible Effects of Extended Use

Retention of potassium in the body, resulting in blood potassium levels above the normal range. This can have an adverse effect on the regulation of heart rhythm and performance.

Suggested Periodic Examinations While Taking This Drug (at physician's discretion)

Kidney function tests.

Measurements of blood sodium, chloride, and potassium levels.

While Taking This Drug, Observe the Following

Foods: Do not restrict the intake of salt (or salted foods) unless directed to do so by your physician.

Beverages: No restrictions.

Alcohol: No interactions expected.

Tobacco Smoking: No interactions expected.

Marijuana Smoking

Occasional (once or twice weekly): No effect to mild increase in thirst and/or urinary frequency.

Daily: Moderate increase in thirst and/or urinary frequency; possible accentuation of orthostatic hypotention (see Glossary).

Other Drugs

Spironolactone may *increase* the effects of

• other anti-hypertensive drugs, and cause excessive lowering of the blood pressure. Dosage adjustments are necessary.

Spironolactone may *decrease* the effects of
- oral anticoagulants, and reduce their protective action. Ask physician for guidance regarding prothrombin time testing and dosage adjustments.
- digitalis preparations, if excessive potassium is retained in the body.

Spironolactone *taken concurrently* with
- triamterene, may cause excessive (dangerous) retention of potassium in the body. Avoid the simultaneous use of these two drugs.

The following drug may *decrease* the effects of spironolactone
- aspirin (in large doses)

Driving a Vehicle, Operating Machinery, Engaging in Hazardous Activities: No restrictions unless drowsiness or confusion occurs.

Aviation Note: Serious cardiovascular disorders *are a disqualification* for the piloting of aircraft. Consultation with a designated Aviation Medical Examiner is advised.

Exposure to Sun: No restrictions.

Heavy Exercise or Exertion: Isometric exercises—the "overload" technique for strengthening individual muscles—can raise the blood pressure significantly. Ask your physician for guidance regarding participation in this form of exercise.

Discontinuation: Consult physician for guidance regarding the need to readjust the dosage schedule of the following drugs taken concurrently with spironolactone: anticoagulants, anti-hypertensives, digitalis.

Special Storage Instructions
Keep in a dry, tightly closed, light-resistant container.

SULFAMETHOXAZOLE

Year Introduced: 1961

Brand Names

USA	Canada
Gantanol (Roche)	Apo-Sulfamethoxazole
Azo Gantanol [CD]	(Apotex)
(Roche)	Gantanol (Roche)
Bactrim [CD] (Roche)	Apo-Sulfatrim [CD]
Bactrim DS [CD] (Roche)	(Apotex)
Septra [CD] (Burroughs	Apo-Sulfatrim-DS [CD]
Wellcome)	(Apotex)
Septra DS [CD]	Novotrimal [CD]
(Burroughs Wellcome)	(Novopharm)
	Novotrimel DS [CD]
	(Novopharm)
	Bactrim [CD] (Roche)
	Bactrim DS [CD] (Roche)
	Septra [CD] (B.W. Ltd.)
	Septra DS [CD] (B.W.
	Ltd.)

Common Synonyms ("Street Names"):   Sulfa drug

Drug Class: Antimicrobial (Anti-infective), Sulfonamides

Prescription Required: Yes

Available for Purchase by Generic Name: Yes

Available Dosage Forms and Strengths
     Tablets — 500 mg., 1 gram
     Oral suspension — 500 mg. per teaspoonful (5 ml.)

Tablet May Be Crushed or Capsule Opened for Administration: Yes

How This Drug Works
Intended Therapeutic Effect(s):   The elimination of infections responsive to
the action of this drug.
Location of Drug Action(s):   Any body tissue or fluid in which sufficient
concentration of the drug can be achieved.
Method of Drug Action(s):   This drug prevents the growth and multiplication of susceptible bacteria by interfering with their formation of folic acid,
an essential nutrient.

Principal Uses of This Drug
As a Single Drug Product: This member of the sulfonamide class ("sulfa"
drugs) is used to treat a variety of bacterial and protozoal infections. It is
used most commonly to treat certain infections of the urinary tract.

As a Combination Drug Product [CD]: This drug is available in combination with phenazopyridine, an analgesic drug that relieves the discomfort associated with acute infections of the urinary bladder and urethra. This combination provides early symptomatic relief while the underlying infection is being eradicated. This drug is also available in combination with another antibacterial drug—trimethoprim. This combination is quite effective in the treatment of certain types of middle ear infection, bronchitis, pneumonia, and certain infections of the intestinal tract and the urinary tract.

THIS DRUG SHOULD NOT BE TAKEN IF
—you are allergic to any sulfonamide ("sulfa") drug (see Drug Class, Section Three).
—you are in the ninth month of pregnancy.
—it is prescribed for an infant under 2 months of age.

INFORM YOUR PHYSICIAN BEFORE TAKING THIS DRUG IF
—you are allergic to any of the drugs chemically related to the sulfonamide ("sulfa") drugs: acetazolamide (Diamox), oral anti-diabetics, and thiazide diuretics (see respective Drug Classes, Section Three).
—you are allergic by nature and have a history of hayfever, asthma, hives or eczema.
—you have a history of serious liver or kidney disease.
—you have a history of acute intermittent porphyria.
—you have ever had anemia caused by a drug.
—you are now taking any of the following drugs:
  methotrexate
  oral anticoagulants
  oral anti-diabetic preparations
  oxyphenbutazone (Oxalid, Tandearil)
  phenylbutazone (Azolid, Butazolidin, etc.)
  phenytoin (Dantoin, Dilantin, etc.)
  probenecid (Benemid)
—you plan to have surgery under pentothal anesthesia while taking this drug.

Time Required for Apparent Benefit
Varies with nature of infection under treatment; usually 2 to 5 days.

Possible Side-Effects *(natural, expected, and unavoidable drug actions)*
Brownish discoloration of urine, of no significance.
Superinfections (see Glossary).

Possible Adverse Effects *(unusual, unexpected, and infrequent reactions)*

IF ANY OF THE FOLLOWING DEVELOP, DISCONTINUE DRUG AND NOTIFY YOUR PHYSICIAN AS SOON AS POSSIBLE

Mild Adverse Effects
Allergic Reactions: Skin rashes (various kinds), hives, itching, swelling of face, redness of eyes.

Other Reactions
Reduced appetite, nausea, vomiting, abdominal pain, diarrhea, irritation of mouth.
Headache, impaired balance, dizziness, ringing in ears, numbness and tingling of extremities, acute mental or behavioral disturbance.

Serious Adverse Effects
Allergic Reactions: Anaphylactic reaction (see Glossary), fever, swollen glands, swollen painful joints.
Idiosyncratic Reactions: Hemolytic anemia (see Glossary).
Other Reactions
Bone marrow depression (see Glossary)—fatigue, weakness, fever, sore throat, unusual bleeding or bruising.
Hepatitis with or without jaundice (see Glossary).
Kidney damage with reduction of urine formation.

CAUTION

1. A large intake of water (up to 2 quarts daily) is mandatory to ensure an adequate volume of dilute urine.
2. Shake liquid dosage forms thoroughly before measuring each dose.

Precautions for Use by Those over 60 Years of Age

The natural changes in body composition and function that occur after 60 may increase your susceptibility to the more serious adverse effects of the sulfonamide drugs.
Small doses taken at longer intervals often achieve adequate blood and tissue drug levels.
Report promptly the development of reduced urine volume, fever, sore throat, unusual bleeding or bruising, or skin irritation with itching, particularly in the genital or anal regions.

Advisability of Use During Pregnancy

Pregnancy Category: C (tentative). See Pregnancy Code inside back cover.
Animal reproduction studies in rats reveal significant birth defects due to this drug.
Information from adequate studies in pregnant women is not available.
It is advisable to avoid use of this drug during first 3 months and just prior to termination of pregnancy.
Ask physician for guidance.

Advisability of Use While Nursing Infant

Drug known to be present in milk and known to have adverse effects on infant. Avoid use. Ask physician for guidance.

Habit-Forming Potential

None.

Effects of Overdosage

With Moderate Overdose: Nausea, vomiting, abdominal pain, possibly diarrhea.
With Large Overdose: Blood in urine, reduced urine formation.

Possible Effects of Extended Use
Development of thyroid gland enlargement (goiter) with or without reduced thyroid function (hypothyroidism).

Superinfections.

Suggested Periodic Examinations While Taking This Drug (at physician's discretion)
Complete blood cell counts, weekly for the first 8 weeks.

Liver and kidney function tests.

While Taking This Drug, Observe the Following
Foods: No restrictions of food selection. Drug may be taken immediately after eating to minimize irritation of stomach.

Beverages: No restriction of beverage selection. However, total liquid intake should be no less than 4 pints every 24 hours while taking a sulfonamide.

Alcohol: Use with caution until combined effect is determined. Sulfonamide drugs can increase the intoxicating effects of alcohol.

Tobacco Smoking: No interactions expected.

Marijuana Smoking: No interactions expected.

Other Drugs

Sulfamethoxazole may *increase* the effects of
- oral anticoagulants (see Drug Class, Section Three). Dosage adjustments may be necessary to prevent abnormal bleeding or hemorrhage.
- oral anti-diabetic preparations (see Drug Class, Section Three). Dosage adjustments may be necessary to prevent hypoglycemia (see Glossary).
- methotrexate.
- phenytoin (Dantoin, Dilantin, etc.). Dosage adjustments may be necessary to prevent toxic effects on the brain.

Sulfamethoxazole may *decrease* the effects of
- penicillin.

Sulfamethoxazole *taken concurrently* with
- methenamine, may cause crystal formation and kidney blockage.
- isoniazid, may cause hemolytic anemia (see Glossary).

The following drugs may *increase* the effects of sulfamethoxazole
- aspirin
- oxyphenbutazone (Oxalid, Tanderaril)
- phenylbutazone (Azolid, Butazolidin, etc.)
- probenecid (Benemid)
- promethazine (Phenergan, etc.)
- sulfinpyrazone (Anturane)
- trimethoprim (Syraprim)

The following drugs may *decrease* the effects of sulfamethoxazole
- paraldehyde (Paral)
- para-aminosalicylic acid (PAS)

Driving a Vehicle, Operating Machinery, Engaging in Hazardous Activities: No restrictions unless dizziness or disturbance of balance occurs.

Aviation Note: The use of this drug *may be a disqualification* for the piloting of aircraft. Consultation with a designated Aviation Medical Examiner is advised.

Exposure to Sun: Use caution until sensitivity is determined. Some sulfonamide drugs can cause photosensitivity (see Glossary).

Discontinuation: Dosage adjustment may be necessary for the following drugs if taken concurrently with sulfamethoxazole: oral anticoagulants, oral anti-diabetic preparations, phenytoin.

After (not during) treatment with a sulfonamide drug, ask physician for guidance regarding the need for supplemental Vitamin C to correct any deficiency due to therapy.

Special Storage Instructions
Keep in a tightly closed, light-resistant container.

SULFASALAZINE

Year Introduced: 1949

Brand Names

USA	Canada
Azulfidine (Pharmacia)	Apo-Sulfasalazine
Azulfidine EN-tabs	(Apotex)
(Pharmacia)	Salazopyrin (Pharmacia)
SAS-500 (Rowell)	SAS-500 (ICN)

Common Synonyms ("Street Names"):   Sulfa drug

Drug Class: Antimicrobial (Anti-infective), Sulfonamides

Prescription Required: Yes

Available for Purchase by Generic Name: USA: Yes   Canada: No

Available Dosage Forms and Strengths
Tablets — 500 mg.
Enteric-coated tablets — 500 mg.
Oral suspension — 250 mg. per teaspoonful (5 ml.)

Tablet May Be Crushed or Capsule Opened for Administration
Regular tablets — Yes
Enteric-coated tablets — No
Azulfidine Entab — No

How This Drug Works

Intended Therapeutic Effect(s)

The reduction of inflammation, ulceration and bleeding associated with the active form of chronic ulcerative colitis.

The prevention of recurrence of active ulcerative colitis.

Location of Drug Action(s):   The inflamed and ulcerated tissues in the diseased areas of the colon.

Method of Drug Action(s):   Not completely established. Possible beneficial effects include

- an anti-infective action which prevents the growth and multiplication of certain bacteria in the colon by interfering with their formation of folic acid, an essential nutrient.
- an anti-inflammatory action which reduces the formation of prostaglandins, tissue chemicals that induce inflammation, tissue destruction and diarrhea.

Principal Uses of This Drug

As a Single Drug Product: This member of the sulfonamide class ("sulfa" drugs) is used exclusively to treat inflammatory diseases of the lower intestinal tract—regional enteritis (Crohn's disease) and ulcerative colitis. It is usually taken by mouth, but may also be used in retention enemas.

THIS DRUG SHOULD NOT BE TAKEN IF

—you are allergic to any sulfonamide ("sulfa") drug (see Drug Class, Section Three).

—you are allergic to salicylates: aspirin, choline salicylate, sodium salicylate.

—you are in the ninth month of pregnancy.

—it is prescribed for an infant under 2 months of age.

INFORM YOUR PHYSICIAN BEFORE TAKING THIS DRUG IF

—you are allergic to any of the drugs chemically related to the sulfonamide ("sulfa") drugs: acetazolamide (Diamox), oral anti-diabetics, and thiazide diuretics (see respective Drug Classes, Section Three).

—you are allergic by nature and have a history of hayfever, asthma, hives or eczema.

—you have a history of serious liver or kidney disease.

—you have a history of acute intermittent porphyria.

—you have ever had anemia caused by a drug.

—you are now taking any of the following drugs:

    methotrexate

    oral anticoagulants

    oral anti-diabetic preparations

    oxyphenbutazone (Oxalid, Tandearil)

    phenylbutazone (Azolid, Butazolidin, etc.)

    phenytoin (Dantoin, Dilantin, etc.)

    probenecid (Benemid)

—you plan to have surgery under pentothal anesthesia while taking this drug.

Time Required for Apparent Benefit
Varies with severity and duration of colitis; usually from 1 to 3 weeks.

Possible Side-Effects *(natural, expected, and unavoidable drug actions)*
Orange-yellow discoloration of urine, of no significance.

Possible Adverse Effects *(unusual, unexpected, and infrequent reactions)*
IF ANY OF THE FOLLOWING DEVELOP, DISCONTINUE DRUG AND NOTIFY YOUR PHYSICIAN AS SOON AS POSSIBLE

Mild Adverse Effects
Allergic Reactions: Skin rashes (various kinds), hives, itching, swelling of face, redness of eyes.

Other Reactions
Reduced appetite, nausea, vomiting, abdominal pain, diarrhea (may be bloody), irritation of mouth.

Headache, impaired balance, dizziness, ringing in ears, numbness and tingling of extremities, acute mental or behavioral disturbance.

Serious Adverse Effects
Allergic Reactions: Anaphylactic reaction (see Glossary), fever, swollen glands, swollen painful joints.

Idiosyncratic Reactions: Hemolytic anemia (see Glossary).

Other Reactions
Bone marrow depression (see Glossary)—fatigue, weakness, fever, sore throat, unusual bleeding or bruising.

Hepatitis with or without jaundice (see Glossary).

Kidney damage with reduction of urine formation.

Peripheral Neuritis (see Glossary).

Pancreatitis—severe abdominal pain, nausea and vomiting.

Pneumonitis—inflammatory reaction within the lung.

Reduced formation of sperm, reversible infertility.

CAUTION
A large intake of water (up to 2 quarts daily) is mandatory to ensure an adequate volume of dilute urine.

Precautions for Use by Those over 60 Years of Age
The natural changes in body composition and function that occur after 60 may increase your susceptibility to the more serious adverse effects of the sulfonamide drugs.

Small doses taken at longer intervals often achieve adequate blood and tissue drug levels.

Report promptly the development of reduced urine volume, fever, sore throat, unusual bleeding or bruising, or skin irritation with itching, particularly in the genital or anal regions.

Advisability of Use During Pregnancy
Pregnancy Category: C (tentative). See Pregnancy Code inside back cover.

Animal reproduction studies in mice and rats reveal significant birth defects due to drugs of this class.

Information from adequate studies in pregnant women is not available.
It is advisable to avoid use of this drug during first 3 months and just prior
  to termination of pregnancy.
Ask physician for guidance.

Advisability of Use While Nursing Infant

Drug known to be present in milk and known to have adverse effects on
infant. Avoid use. Ask physician for guidance.

Habit-Forming Potential

None.

Effects of Overdosage

With Moderate Overdose: Nausea, vomiting, abdominal pain, possibly diarrhea.

With Large Overdose: Blood in urine, reduced urine formation.

Possible Effects of Extended Use

Development of thyroid gland enlargement (goiter) with or without reduced
  thyroid function (hypothyroidism).
An orange-yellow discoloration of the skin has been reported. This is not
  jaundice.

Suggested Periodic Examinations While Taking This Drug (at physician's discretion)

Complete blood cell counts, weekly for the first 8 weeks.
Liver and kidney function tests.

While Taking This Drug, Observe the Following

Foods: Follow prescribed diet. Sulfasalazine does not require any specific
food restriction. Drug may be taken immediately after eating to minimize
irritation of stomach.

Beverages: Ask physician for guidance regarding the intake of milk. Sulfasalazine does not require any specific beverage restriction. Total liquid
intake should be no less than 3 pints every 24 hours.

Alcohol: Use with caution until combined effect is determined. Some sulfonamide drugs can *increase* the intoxicating effects of alcohol. Colitis may
react unfavorably to alcohol.

Tobacco Smoking: No interactions expected.

Marijuana Smoking: No interactions expected.

Other Drugs

Sulfasalazine may *increase* the effects of
  • methotrexate.
  • oral anticoagulants (see Drug Class, Section Three). Dosage adjustments
    may be necessary to prevent abnormal bleeding or hemorrhage.
  • oral anti-diabetic preparations (see Drug Class, Section Three). Dosage
    adjustments may be necessary to prevent hypoglycemia (see Glossary).
  • phenytoin (Dantoin, Dilantin, etc.). Dosage adjustments may be necessary to prevent toxic effects on the brain.

Sulfasalazine may *decrease* the effects of
- penicillin.

Sulfasalazine *taken concurrently* with
- methenamine, may cause crystal formation and kidney blockage.
- isoniazid, may cause hemolytic anemia (see Glossary).

The following drugs may *increase* the effects of sulfasalazine
- aspirin
- oxyphenbutazone (Oxalid, Tandearil)
- phenylbutazone (Azolid, Butazolidin, etc.)
- probenecid (Benemid)
- promethazine (Phenergan, etc.)
- sulfinpyrazone (Anturane)
- trimethoprim (Syraprim)

The following drugs may *decrease* the effects of sulfasalazine
- antibiotic drugs
- iron preparations
- paraldehyde (Paral)
- para-aminosalicylic acid (PAS)

Driving a Vehicle, Operating Machinery, Engaging in Hazardous Activities: No restrictions unless dizziness or disturbance of balance occurs.

Aviation Note: The use of this drug *may be a disqualification* for the piloting of aircraft. Consultation with a designated Aviation Medical Examiner is advised.

Exposure to Sun: Use caution until sensitivity is determined. Some sulfonamide drugs can cause photosensitivity (see Glossary).

Discontinuation: Dosage adjustment may be necessary for the following drugs if taken concurrently with sulfasalazine: oral anticoagulants, oral anti-diabetic preparations, phenytoin.

After (not during) treatment with a sulfonamide drug, ask physician for guidance regarding the need for supplemental Vitamin C to correct any deficiency due to therapy.

Special Storage Instructions
Keep in a tightly closed, light-resistant container.

SULFINPYRAZONE

Year Introduced: 1959

Brand Names

USA	Canada
Anturane (CIBA)	Antazone (ICN)
	Anturan (Geigy)
	Apo-Sulfinpyrazone
	(Apotex)
	Novopyrazone
	(Novopharm)
	Zynol (Horner)

Common Synonyms ("Street Names"):   Gout pills

Drug Class: Anti-gout, Blood platelet inhibitor

Prescription Required: USA: Yes   Canada: No

Available for Purchase by Generic Name: USA: No   Canada: Yes

Available Dosage Forms and Strengths
Tablets — 100 mg.
Capsules — 200 mg.

Tablet May Be Crushed or Capsule Opened for Administration: Yes

How This Drug Works
  Intended Therapeutic Effect(s)
    Reduction in the frequency and severity of acute attacks of gout; *not* intended for the relief of symptoms during the acute attack.
    Reduction in the severity of recurrent heart attack (repeated coronary thrombosis).
    Note: This use has not yet been sanctioned by the U. S. Food and Drug Administration.* Informed consent advised.
  Location of Drug Action(s)
    • the tubular systems of the kidney that regulate the uric acid content of the urine.
    • the blood platelets.
  Method of Drug Action(s)
    By acting on the tubular systems of the kidney to increase the amount of uric acid excreted in the urine, this drug reduces the level of uric acid in the blood and body tissues.
    By preventing blood platelet aggregation (see Glossary), this drug reduces the tendency to blood clot formation and thereby lessens the extent of heart muscle damage in recurrent coronary thrombosis (heart attack).

*This use is approved in Canada.

Principal Uses of This Drug

As a Single Drug Product: This drug is used in the management of two unrelated conditions. Its original use was to prevent the occurrence of acute episodes of joint pain and swelling in the treatment of chronic gout. A more recent use is the prevention of recurrence (or extension) of heart damage during the first six months of treatment following a heart attack (myocardial infarction).

THIS DRUG SHOULD NOT BE TAKEN IF

—you have had an allergic reaction to any dosage form of it previously.
—you are experiencing an attack of acute gout at the present time.
—you have an active stomach or duodenal ulcer, enteritis, or ulcerative colitis.
—you have a blood cell disorder.

INFORM YOUR PHYSICIAN BEFORE TAKING THIS DRUG IF

—you are allergic to oxyphenbutazone (Tandearil, etc.) or phenylbutazone (Butazolidin, etc.).
—you have a history of kidney disease or impaired kidney function.
—you have a history of stomach or duodenal ulcer, recurrent enteritis or colitis.
—you have a history of a blood cell disorder.
—you are taking any form of aspirin, oral anticoagulant drugs, oral antidiabetic drugs, insulin or "sulfa" drugs (see respective Drug Classes, Section Three).

Time Required for Apparent Benefit

Uric acid levels in the blood begin to decrease within the first week.
Continuous use on a regular schedule (and with proper dosage adjustments) for several months is needed to prevent acute attacks of gout and to remove deposits of uric acid (tophi) from body tissues.
Significant reduction in blood platelet aggregation is thought to occur within 1 week.

Possible Side-Effects *(natural, expected, and unavoidable drug actions)*

Development of kidney stones (composed of uric acid). This tendency can be reduced significantly by drinking 2 to 3 quarts of water daily and by making the urine alkaline (non-acid). Ask physician for guidance.

Possible Adverse Effects *(unusual, unexpected, and infrequent reactions)*

IF ANY OF THE FOLLOWING DEVELOP, DISCONTINUE DRUG AND NOTIFY YOUR PHYSICIAN AS SOON AS POSSIBLE

Mild Adverse Effects
Allergic Reactions: Skin rashes.
Other Reactions: Stomach irritation, nausea, vomiting, abdominal pain.
Serious Adverse Effects
Bone marrow depression (see Glossary)—fatigue, weakness, fever, sore throat, unusual bleeding or bruising.
Stomach and/or intestinal bleeding.

CAUTION

1. During the first few days of treatment this drug may *increase* the blood level of uric acid and cause an acute attack of gout or kidney stone. Careful

monitoring of blood levels of uric acid and appropriate adjustment of dosage are necessary to minimize this response.

2. Aspirin may cause unpredictable and serious prolongation of the bleeding time and if taken in combination with this drug may cause episodes of undue bleeding. Also, aspirin decreases the ability of this drug to promote the excretion of uric acid, reducing its effectiveness in the management of chronic gout.
3. A closely related drug, phenylbutazone (Butazolidin, etc.), has been reported to reduce the effectiveness of oral contraceptives and to increase the incidence of "breakthrough" bleeding.
4. The total intake of this drug should not exceed 1000 mg. per day.

Precautions for Use by Those over 60 Years of Age

The natural decline in kidney function that occurs after 60 makes it advisable to initiate treatment with one-half the standard dose used for younger adults.

Advisability of Use During Pregnancy

Pregnancy Category: C (tentative). See Pregnancy Code inside back cover. Animal reproduction studies are inconclusive.

Information from adequate studies in pregnant women is not available. Ask physician for guidance.

Advisability of Use While Nursing Infant

Presence of drug in milk is not known. Avoid use if possible.

Habit-Forming Potential

None.

Effects of Overdosage

With Moderate Overdose: Nausea, vomiting, stomach pain.

With Large Overdose: Loss of balance, staggering gait, labored breathing, convulsions, coma.

Possible Effects of Extended Use

Development of kidney damage in sensitive individuals.

Suggested Periodic Examinations While Taking This Drug (at physician's discretion)

Uric acid blood levels to evaluate the effectiveness of the drug and to regulate dosage.

Complete blood cell counts.

Kidney function studies, especially in the presence of known kidney disease or reduced kidney function.

While Taking This Drug, Observe the Following

Foods: Follow physician's advice regarding the need for a low purine diet. This drug should be taken with food or immediately after eating to reduce stomach irritation.

Beverages: This drug may be taken with milk. A large intake of coffee, tea, or cola beverages may reduce the effectiveness of treatment. It is advisable to drink no less than 2 to 3 quarts of liquids every 24 hours. Some "herbal teas" (promoted as being beneficial for arthritis) contain phenylbutazone and other potentially toxic ingredients. Avoid "herbal teas" if you are not certain of their source, content and medicinal effects.

Alcohol: No interactions expected with this drug. However, alcohol may raise the blood level of uric acid and impair management of chronic gout.

Tobacco Smoking: No interactions expected.

Marijuana Smoking

Occasional (once or twice weekly):   No significant interactions expected. Daily: Possible increase in blood uric acid level.

Other Drugs

Sulfinpyrazone may *increase* the effects of
- anticoagulants of the coumarin family (see Drug Class, Section Three), and increase the risk of bleeding. Careful dosage adjustment is necessary.
- anti-diabetic drugs of the sulfonylurea family (Diabinese, Dymelor, Orinase, Tolinase).
- cephalexin (Keflex) and cephradine (Anspor, Velosef).
- insulin.
- the penicillins.
- the "sulfa" drugs (Gantrisin, sulfadiazine, etc.).

Sulfinpyrazone may *decrease* the effects of
- oral contraceptives, increase the frequency of break-through bleeding.

Sulfinpyrazone *taken concurrently* with
- aspirin, may cause episodes of undue bleeding.

The following drug may *increase* the effects of sulfinpyrazone
- probenecid (Benemid) may increase its effectiveness in the management of chronic gout.

The following drug may *decrease* the effects of sulfinpyrazone
- aspirin may block its therapeutic effect and reduce its effectiveness in the management of chronic gout.

Driving a Vehicle, Operating Machinery, Engaging in Hazardous Activities: Usually no restrictions. Be alert to the possible occurrence of nausea; restrict activities accordingly.

Aviation Note: The use of this drug *may be a disqualification* for the piloting of aircraft. Consultation with a designated Aviation Medical Examiner is advised.

Exposure to Sun: No restrictions.

Heavy Exercise or Exertion: Ask physician for specific guidance.

Occurrence of Unrelated Illness: Consult your physician if you develop an illness that causes nausea and/or vomiting and makes it impossible to continue this drug on a regular schedule.

Discontinuation: Sudden discontinuation of this drug may cause a prompt rise in blood uric acid levels resulting in an acute attack of gout. Do not discontinue without consulting your physician. At the time of discontinuation, consult the Other Drugs section (above) to see if you are taking any drugs which may require dosage adjustments.

Special Storage Instructions

Keep in a dry, tightly closed container.

SULFISOXAZOLE

Year Introduced: 1949

Brand Names

USA		Canada
Barazole (Barry Martin)	Sosol (McKesson)	Apo-Sulfisoxazole (Apotex)
Chemovag (Fellows)	Soxa (Vita Elixir)	Gantrisin (Roche)
Gantrisin (Roche)	Sulfium (Alcon)	Novosoxazole
G-Sox (Scrip)	Sulfizin (Tutag)	(Novopharm)
Lipo Gantrisin (Roche)	Azo Gantrisin [CD] (Roche)	Azo Gantrisin [CD] (Roche)
SK-Soxazole (Smith Kline & French)		

Common Synonyms ("Street Names"):   Sulfa drug

Drug Class: Antimicrobial (Anti-infective), Sulfonamides

Prescription Required: Yes

Available for Purchase by Generic Name: Yes

Available Dosage Forms and Strengths

Tablets — 500 mg.
Syrup — 500 mg. per teaspoonful (5 ml.)
Pediatric suspension — 500 mg. per teaspoonful (5 ml.)
Emulsion — 1 gm. per teaspoonful (5 ml.)
Suppositories — 500 mg.

Tablet May Be Crushed or Capsule Opened for Administration: Yes

How This Drug Works

Intended Therapeutic Effect(s):   The elimination of infections responsive to the action of this drug.

Location of Drug Action(s):   Any body tissue or fluid in which sufficient concentration of the drug can be achieved.

Method of Drug Action(s):   This drug prevents the growth and multiplication of susceptible bacteria by interfering with their formation of folic acid, an essential nutrient.

Principal Uses of This Drug

As a Single Drug Product: This short-acting member of the sulfonamide class ("sulfa" drugs) is used to treat a variety of bacterial and protozoal infections. It is used most commonly to treat certain infections of the urinary tract.

As a Combination Drug Product [CD]:   This drug is available in combination with phenazopyridine, an analgesic drug that relieves the discomfort associated with acute infections of the urinary bladder and urethra. This combination provides early symptomatic relief while the underlying infection is being eradicated.

THIS DRUG SHOULD NOT BE TAKEN IF

—you are allergic to any sulfonamide ("sulfa") drug (see Drug Class, Section Three).

—you are in the ninth month of pregnancy.

—it is prescribed for an infant under 2 months of age.

INFORM YOUR PHYSICIAN BEFORE TAKING THIS DRUG IF

—you are allergic to any of the drugs chemically related to the sulfonamide ("sulfa") drugs: acetazolamide (Diamox), oral anti-diabetics, and thiazide diuretics (see Drug Classes, Section Three).

—you are allergic by nature and have a history of hayfever, asthma, hives or eczema.

—you have a history of serious liver or kidney disease.

—you have a history of acute intermittent porphyria.

—you have ever had anemia caused by a drug.

—you are now taking any of the following drugs:
methotrexate
oral anticoagulants
oral anti-diabetic preparations
oxyphenbutazone (Oxalid, Tandearil)
phenylbutazone (Azolid, Butazolidin, etc.)
phenytoin (Dantoin, Dilantin, etc.)
probenecid (Benemid)

—you plan to have surgery under pentothal anesthesia while taking this drug.

Time Required for Apparent Benefit

Varies with nature of infection under treatment; usually 2 to 5 days.

Possible Side-Effects *(natural, expected, and unavoidable drug actions)*

Brownish discoloration of urine, of no significance.

Superinfections (see Glossary).

Possible Adverse Effects *(unusual, unexpected, and infrequent reactions)*

IF ANY OF THE FOLLOWING DEVELOP, DISCONTINUE DRUG AND NOTIFY YOUR PHYSICIAN AS SOON AS POSSIBLE

Mild Adverse Effects

Allergic Reactions: Skin rashes (various kinds), hives, itching, swelling of face, redness of eyes.

Other Reactions

Reduced appetite, nausea, vomiting, abdominal pain, diarrhea, irritation of mouth.

Headache, impaired balance, dizziness, ringing in ears, numbness and tingling of extremities, acute mental or behavioral disturbance.

Serious Adverse Effects

Allergic Reactions: Anaphylactic reaction (see Glossary), fever, swollen glands, swollen painful joints.

Idiosyncratic Reactions: Hemolytic anemia (see Glossary).

Other Reactions

Bone marrow depression (see Glossary)—fatigue, weakness, fever, sore throat, unusual bleeding or bruising.

Hepatitis with or without jaundice (see Glossary).

Kidney damage with reduction of urine formation.

CAUTION

1. A large intake of water (up to 2 quarts daily) is mandatory to ensure an adequate volume of dilute urine.
2. Shake liquid dosage forms thoroughly before measuring each dose.

Precautions for Use by Those over 60 Years of Age

The natural changes in body composition and function that occur after 60 may increase your susceptibility to the more serious adverse effects of the sulfonamide drugs.

Small doses taken at longer intervals often achieve adequate blood and tissue drug levels.

Report promptly the development of reduced urine volume, fever, sore throat, unusual bleeding or bruising, or skin irritation with itching, particular in the genital or anal regions.

Advisability of Use During Pregnancy

Pregnancy Category: C (tentative). See Pregnancy Code inside back cover.

Animal reproduction studies in mice and rats reveal significant birth defects due to drugs of this class.

Information from studies in pregnant women indicates no increase in defects in 4287 exposures to this drug. It is advisable to avoid use of this drug during first 3 months and just prior to termination of pregnancy. Ask physician for guidance.

Advisability of Use While Nursing Infant

Drug known to be present in milk and known to have adverse effects on infant. Avoid use. Ask physician for guidance.

Habit-Forming Potential

None.

Effects of Overdosage

With Moderate Overdose: Nausea, vomiting, abdominal pain, possibly diarrhea.

With Large Overdose: Blood in urine, reduced urine formation.

Possible Effects of Extended Use

Development of thyroid gland enlargement (goiter) with or without reduced thyroid function (hypothyroidism).
Superinfections.

Suggested Periodic Examinations While Taking This Drug (at physician's discretion)

Complete blood cell counts, weekly for the first 8 weeks.
Liver and kidney function tests.

While Taking This Drug, Observe the Following

Foods: No restrictions of food selection. Drug may be taken immediately after eating to minimize irritation of stomach.

Beverages: No restriction of beverage selection. However, total liquid intake should be no less than 4 pints every 24 hours while taking a sulfonamide.

Alcohol: Use with caution until combined effect is determined. Sulfonamide drugs can *increase* the intoxicating effects of alcohol.

Tobacco Smoking: No interactions expected.

Marijuana Smoking: No interactions expected.

Other Drugs

Sulfisoxazole may *increase* the effects of

- methotrexate.
- oral anticoagulants (see Drug Class, Section Three). Dosage adjustments may be necessary to prevent abnormal bleeding or hemorrhage.
- oral anti-diabetic preparations (see Drug Class, Section Three). Dosage adjustment may be necessary to prevent hypoglycemia (see Glossary).
- phenytoin (Dantoin, Dilantin, etc.). Dosage adjustments may be necessary to prevent toxic effects on the brain.

Sulfisoxazole may *decrease* the effects of

- penicillin.

Sulfisoxazole *taken concurrently* with

- methenamine, may cause crystal formation and kidney blockage.
- isoniazid, may cause hemolytic anemia (see Glossary).

The following drugs may *increase* the effects of sulfisoxazole

- aspirin
- oxyphenbutazone (Oxalid, Tandearil)
- phenylbutazone (Azolid, Butazolidin, etc.)
- probenecid (Benemid)
- promethazine (Phenergan, etc.)
- sulfinpyrazone (Anturane)
- trimethoprim (Syraprim)

The following drugs may *decrease* the effects of sulfisoxazole

- paraldehyde (Paral)
- para-aminosalicylic acid (PAS)

Driving a Vehicle, Operating Machinery, Engaging in Hazardous Activities: No restrictions unless dizziness or disturbance of balance occurs.

Aviation Note: The use of this drug *may be a disqualification* for the piloting of aircraft. Consultation with a designated Aviation Medical Examiner is advised.

Exposure to Sun: Use caution until sensitivity is determined. Some sulfonamide drugs can cause photosensitivity (see Glossary).

Discontinuation: Dosage adjustment may be necessary for the following drugs if taken concurrently with sulfisoxazole: oral anticoagulants, oral anti-diabetic preparations, phenytoin.

After (not during) treatment with a sulfonamide drug, ask physician for guidance regarding the need for supplemental Vitamin C to correct any deficiency due to therapy.

Special Storage Instructions
Keep in a tightly closed, light-resistant container.

SULINDAC

Year Introduced: 1978

Brand Names

USA	Canada
Clinoril (Merck Sharp & Dohme)	Clinoril (Frosst)

Common Synonyms ("Street Names"):   Arthritis medicine, aspirin substitute

Drug Class: Analgesic, Mild, Anti-inflammatory, Fever Reducer (Antipyretic)

Prescription Required: Yes

Available for Purchase by Generic Name: No

Available Dosage Forms and Strengths
Tablets — 150 mg., 200 mg.

Tablet May Be Crushed or Capsule Opened for Administration: Yes

How This Drug Works
Intended Therapeutic Effect(s):   Relief of joint pain, stiffness, inflammation, and swelling associated with arthritis.

Location of Drug Action(s):   Not completely established. This drug may act in the brain (at the level of the hypothalamus) as well as in the inflamed tissues of arthritic joints.

Method of Drug Action(s):   Not completely known. It is thought that this drug reduces the tissue concentration of prostaglandins, chemicals involved in the production of inflammation and pain.

Principal Uses of This Drug

As a Single Drug Product: This "aspirin substitute" is used primarily to provide symptomatic relief in acute and chronic arthritis, including gout. It is also used to relieve the pain associated with acute bursitis and tendinitis of the shoulder.

THIS DRUG SHOULD NOT BE TAKEN IF

—you have had an allergic reaction to any dosage form of it previously.
—you are allergic to aspirin (hives, nasal polyps, and/or asthma caused by aspirin).
—you have a bleeding disorder.
—you have an active stomach ulcer or active ulcerative colitis.
—you have severe impairment of liver or kidney function.

INFORM YOUR PHYSICIAN BEFORE TAKING THIS DRUG IF

—you have a history of peptic ulcer disease, ulcerative colitis, or previous stomach or intestinal bleeding.
—you are taking any kind of anticoagulant drug (see Drug Class, Section Three).
—you are presently under treatment for an active infection of any kind.

Time Required for Apparent Benefit

Drug action begins within 1 to 2 hours and persists for 6 to 8 hours.
Significant improvement may require continuous use on a regular schedule for 1 to 2 weeks.

Possible Side-Effects *(natural, expected, and unavoidable drug actions)*

Drowsiness in sensitive individuals.

Possible Adverse Effects *(unusual, unexpected, and infrequent reactions)*

IF ANY OF THE FOLLOWING DEVELOP, DISCONTINUE DRUG AND NOTIFY YOUR PHYSICIAN AS SOON AS POSSIBLE

Mild Adverse Effects
  Allergic Reactions: Skin rash (various kinds), hives, itching.
  Other Reactions
    Headache, dizziness, confusion, mild numbness or tingling, ringing in the ears.
    Indigestion, nausea, vomiting, constipation.
Serious Adverse Effects
  Allergic Reactions: Anaphylactic reaction (see Glossary).
  Idiosyncratic Reactions: None reported.
  Other Reactions
    Stomach and/or intestinal bleeding.
    Impaired formation of white blood cells (granulocytes) with resulting reduction in resistance to infections. Blurred vision, impaired hearing.
    Acute pancreatitis—abdominal pain, nausea, vomiting.

Possible Delayed Adverse Effects

Mild anemia due to "silent" blood loss from the stomach (less than that caused by aspirin).

CAUTION

1. The optimal dosage schedule must be determined for each person individually. Dosage should always be limited to the smallest amount that produces reasonable improvement.
2. This drug's anti-inflammatory and antipyretic effects can make it more difficult to recognize the presence of infection. If you develop any symptoms that suggest an active infection, inform your physician promptly.

Precautions for Use by Those over 60 Years of Age

It is advisable to begin treatment with small doses until individual tolerance and response have been determined. Limit dosage to the smallest amount that produces reasonable improvement.

Sudden gain in weight or the development of swelling of the feet and ankles may indicate the excessive retention of water in body tissues. Inform your physician promptly of these developments.

You may be more susceptible to the development of headache, dizziness, confusion, impairment of memory, stomach bleeding, and constipation.

Advisability of Use During Pregnancy

Pregnancy Category: C (tentative). See Pregnancy Code inside back cover. Animal reproduction studies are inconclusive.

Information from adequate studies in pregnant women is not available. Ask physician for guidance.

Advisability of Use While Nursing Infant

The presence of this drug in milk is not known. Ask physician for guidance.

Habit-Forming Potential

None apparent to date.

Effects of Overdosage

With Moderate Overdose: Stomach irritation, nausea, vomiting, diarrhea.

With Large Overdose: No serious or threatening effects reported to date.

Possible Effects of Extended Use

Cataracts have been reported with the use of similar drugs, but a definite cause-and-effect relationship (see Glossary) has not been established.

Suggested Periodic Examinations While Taking This Drug (at physician's discretion)

Complete blood cell counts.

Kidney function tests.

Liver function tests.

Eye examinations for possible changes in the lens.

While Taking This Drug, Observe the Following

Foods: This drug should be taken with or immediately following food if stomach irritation occurs. However, it is more effective if it is taken 1 hour before or 2 hours after eating.

Beverages: This drug may be taken with milk. Some "herbal teas" (promoted as being beneficial for arthritis) contain phenylbutazone and other potentially toxic ingredients. Avoid "herbal teas" if you are not certain of their source, content and medicinal effects.

Alcohol: Use with caution. The irritant action of alcohol on the stomach lining, added to the irritant action of sulindac in sensitive individuals, can increase the risk of stomach bleeding and/or ulceration.

Tobacco Smoking: No interactions expected.

Marijuana Smoking

Occasional (once or twice weekly):   No effect to mild increase in pain relief from this drug.

Daily: Moderate increase in pain relief from this drug.

Other Drugs

Sulindac may *increase* the effects of

- oral anticoagulant drugs, and increase the risk of unwanted bleeding. Consult your physician regarding the frequency of prothrombin time testing.
- phenytoin (Dantoin, Dilantin, etc.), and cause symptoms of overdosage.
- "sulfa" drugs, and make it advisable to reduce their dosage.

The following drugs may *decrease* the effects of sulindac

- aspirin and aspirin-containing compounds.
- phenobarbital.

Driving a Vehicle, Operating Machinery, Engaging in Hazardous Activities: This drug can cause dizziness and confusion in sensitive individuals. Use caution until its full effects have been determined.

Aviation Note: The use of this drug *may be a disqualification* for the piloting of aircraft. Consultation with a designated Aviation Medical Examiner is advised.

Exposure to Sun: No restrictions.

Heavy Exercise or Exertion: Follow physician's instructions.

Occurrence of Unrelated Illness: This drug may mask the usual symptoms that indicate the presence of infection. Consult your physician promptly if you suspect that you may be developing an infection of any kind.

Discontinuation: This drug may be discontinued abruptly without danger. However, it may be necessary to adjust the doses of other drugs taken concurrently with it. Consult your physician.

Special Storage Instructions

Keep in a dry, tightly closed container.

TERBUTALINE

Year Introduced: 1974

Brand Names

USA	Canada
Brethine (Geigy)	Bricanyl (Astra)
Bricanyl (Merrell Dow)	

Common Synonyms ("Street Names"):   Asthma pills

Drug Class: Anti-asthmatic (Bronchodilator)

Prescription Required: Yes

Available for Purchase by Generic Name: No

Available Dosage Forms and Strengths
Tablets — 2.5 mg., 5 mg.
Injection — 1.0 mg. per ml.

Tablet May Be Crushed or Capsule Opened for Administration: Yes

How This Drug Works
Intended Therapeutic Effect(s):   Relief of difficult breathing associated with acute attacks of bronchial asthma and with other disorders characterized by spasm of the bronchial tubes, such as bronchitis and emphysema.
Location of Drug Action(s):   Those nerve terminals of the sympathetic nervous system that activate the muscles in the walls of bronchial tubes to produce dilation.
Method of Drug Action(s):   By stimulating certain sympathetic nerve terminals, this drug acts to dilate those bronchial tubes that are in sustained constriction, thereby increasing the size of the airways and improving the ability to breathe.

Principal Uses of This Drug
As a Single Drug Product: Used primarily to provide symptomatic relief in the treatment of bronchial asthma. It is also used to relieve asthmatic-like symptoms (bronchial spasm) associated with some types of bronchitis and emphysema.

THIS DRUG SHOULD NOT BE TAKEN IF
—you have had an allergic reaction to any dosage form of it previously.
—you have a serious heart rhythm disorder.
—you are taking, or have taken during the past 2 weeks, any monoamine oxidase (MAO) inhibitor drug (see Drug Class, Section Three).

INFORM YOUR PHYSICIAN BEFORE TAKING THIS DRUG IF
—you are overly sensitive to drugs that stimulate the sympathetic nervous system.
—you are currently using epinephrine (Adrenalin, etc.) to relieve asthmatic breathing.

—you have high blood pressure.
—you have diabetes.
—you have a history of heart disease, especially angina (coronary insufficiency).
—you have a history of overactivity of the thyroid gland (hyperthyroidism).
—you are taking any form of digitalis (digitoxin, digoxin).

Time Required for Apparent Benefit
By mouth (tablet)—drug action begins within 30 minutes and reaches a peak in 2 to 3 hours.
By injection—drug action begins within 5 minutes and reaches a peak in 30 to 60 minutes.

Duration of Drug Effects After Last Dose
By mouth (tablet) — 4 to 8 hours.
By injection — 1 and one-half to 4 hours.

Possible Side-Effects *(natural, expected, and unavoidable drug actions)*
In sensitive individuals—nervousness, anxiety, tremor, palpitation.

Possible Adverse Effects *(unusual, unexpected, and infrequent reactions)*

IF ANY OF THE FOLLOWING DEVELOP, DISCONTINUE DRUG AND NOTIFY YOUR PHYSICIAN AS SOON AS POSSIBLE

Mild Adverse Effects
Headache, dizziness, drowsiness. Nausea, vomiting, sweating.
Serious Adverse Effects
None reported.

CAUTION
1. Do not exceed a total dose of 15 mg. per 24 hours.
2. Discoloration or cloudiness of terbutaline solution indicates drug deterioration. Discard it promptly; do not use.
3. The frequently repeated use of this drug at short intervals can produce a condition of unresponsiveness and result in medication failure. If this develops, avoid use completely for 12 hours at which time normal response should return.

Precautions for Use by Those over 60 Years of Age
If you have hardening of the arteries (arteriosclerosis), heart disease, or high blood pressure, use this drug with caution. It can precipitate episodes of angina and disturbances of heart rhythm; it can cause sudden elevation of the blood pressure and induce stroke.
If you have difficulty with urination due to enlargement of the prostate gland (prostatism), this drug may increase the difficulty. Ask physician for guidance.
If you have Parkinson's disease, this drug may temporarily increase the rigidity and tremor in your extremities.

Advisability of Use During Pregnancy

Pregnancy Category: B (tentative). See Pregnancy Code inside back cover. Animal reproduction studies reveal no birth defects due to this drug. Information from adequate studies in pregnant women is not available. Ask physician for guidance.

Advisability of Use While Nursing Infant

Presence of drug in milk is not known. Ask physician for guidance.

Habit-Forming Potential

None.

Effects of Overdosage

With Moderate Overdose: Excessive nervousness, anxiety, headache, dizziness, palpitation, tremor.

With Large Overdose: Severe palpitation, chest pain in heart region, rapid heart rate, prolonged tremor.

Possible Effects of Extended Use

None reported.

Suggested Periodic Examinations While Taking This Drug (at physician's discretion)

None.

While Taking This Drug, Observe the Following

Foods: No restrictions.

Beverages: No restrictions.

Alcohol: No interactions expected.

Tobacco Smoking: No interactions expected. Follow physician's advice regarding smoking as it affects the condition under treatment.

Marijuana Smoking

Occasional (once or twice weekly):   Mild and transient improvement in anti-asthmatic effect of this drug.

Daily: More persistent improvement in anti-asthmatic effect of this drug.

Other Drugs

Terbutaline may *increase* the effects of

• ephedrine, and cause excessive stimulation of the heart.

Terbutaline *taken concurrently with*

• epinephrine (by injection), may cause excessive stimulation of the heart. Avoid concurrent use.

• mono-amine oxidase (MAO) inhibitor drugs, may be dangerous. Avoid concurrent use. (See Drug Class, Section Three).

The following drug may *decrease* the effects of terbutaline

• propranolol (Inderal) may impair its effectiveness in the treatment of asthma.

Driving a Vehicle, Operating Machinery, Engaging in Hazardous Activities: Usually no restrictions. Use caution if excessive nervousness or dizziness occurs.

Aviation Note: The use of this drug *may be a disqualification* for the piloting of aircraft. Consultation with a designated Aviation Medical Examiner is advised.

Exposure to Sun: No restrictions.

Exposure to Cold: No restrictions. Protect hands and feet from prolonged exposure to excessive cold.

Heavy Exercise or Exertion: No interactions with drug. However, excessive exertion can induce asthma in sensitive individuals.

Occurrence of Unrelated Illness: The development of acute respiratory infections—head and/or chest colds—can increase the frequency and severity of asthma, and reduce the effectiveness of this drug. Obtain evaluation and treatment of such illness promptly.

Discontinuation: If this drug fails to provide relief after adequate trial, discontinue it and consult your physician regarding alternate drug therapy. Do not increase the dosage or the frequency of use. To do so could be dangerous.

Special Storage Instructions

Tablets: Keep in a dry, tightly closed container at room temperature.

Solution: Keep vials in original carton at room temperature. Protect from light and excessive heat.

TETRACYCLINE

Year Introduced: 1953

Brand Names

USA

Achromycin (Lederle)
Achromycin V
   (Lederle)
Bicycline (Knight)
Centet (Central)
Cycline-250 (Scrip)
Cyclopar
   (Parke-Davis)
Desamycin
   (Pharmics)
G-Mycin (Coast)
Nor-Tet (Vortech)
Panmycin (Upjohn)
Piracaps (Tutag)
Retet
   (Reid-Provident)
Robitet (Robins)
Sarocycline (Saron)
Scotrex (Scott/Cord)
SK-Tetracycline
   (Smith Kline &
   French)

Sumycin (Squibb)
T-250 (Elder)
Tet-Cy (Metro)
Tetra-C (Century)
Tetrachel (Rachelle)
Tetraclor (Kenyon)
Tetra-Co (Coastal)
Tetracyn
   (Pfipharmecs)
Tetralan (Lannett)
Tetram (Dunhall)
Tetramax (Rand)
Tetrex (Bristol)
Trexin (A.V.P.
   Pharm.)
Mysteclin-F [CD]
   (Squibb)
Tetrastatin [CD]
   (Pfipharmecs)

Canada

Achromycin (Lederle)
Achromycin V
   (Lederle)
Cefracycline (Frosst)
Medicycline (Medic)
Neo-Tetrine (Neolab)
Novotetra
   (Novopharm)
Tetracyn (Pfizer)
Tetralean (Organon)

Common Synonyms ("Street Names"):   None

Drug Class: Antibiotic (Anti-infective), Tetracyclines

Prescription Required: Yes

Available for Purchase by Generic Name: Yes

Available Dosage Forms and Strengths
    Tablets — 250 mg., 500 mg.
    Capsules — 100 mg., 250 mg., 500 mg.
Oral suspension — 125 mg. per teaspoonful (5 ml.)
    Eye ointment — 1%, 3%
    Eye suspension — 1%
Topical Solution — 2.2 mg per ml.

Tablet May Be Crushed or Capsule Opened for Administration: Yes

How This Drug Works
    Intended Therapeutic Effect(s):   The elimination of infections responsive to
    the action of this drug.

Location of Drug Action(s):   Any body tissue or fluid in which sufficient concentration of the drug can be achieved.

Method of Drug Action(s):   This drug prevents the growth and multiplication of susceptible bacteria by interfering with their formation of essential proteins.

Principal Uses of This Drug

As a Single Drug Product: This broad spectrum antibiotic is used to treat a large variety of infections. In some instances it can be used as a substitute when the patient is allergic to penicillin. It is usually used on a short-term basis to control acute infections. However, it is commonly used for the long-term management of chronic acne.

As a Combination Drug Product [CD]:   This drug is available in combination with amphotericin B or with nystatin, antifungal antibiotics that are provided to reduce the risk of developing an overgrowth of yeast organisms (superinfection) of the gastrointestinal tract.

THIS DRUG SHOULD NOT BE TAKEN IF
—you are allergic to any tetracycline drug (see Drug Class, Section Three).
—you are pregnant or breast feeding.

INFORM YOUR PHYSICIAN BEFORE TAKING THIS DRUG IF
—you have a history of liver or kidney disease.
—you have systemic lupus erythematosus.
—you are taking any penicillin drug.
—you are taking any anticoagulant drug.
—you plan to have surgery under general anesthesia in the near future.
—it is prescribed for a child under 9 years of age.

Time Required for Apparent Benefit
Varies with nature of infection under treatment; usually 2 to 5 days.

Possible Side-Effects *(natural, expected, and unavoidable drug actions)*
Superinfections (see Glossary), often due to yeast organisms. These can occur in the mouth, intestinal tract, rectum, and/or vagina, resulting in rectal and vaginal itching.

Possible Adverse Effects *(unusual, unexpected, and infrequent reactions)*

IF ANY OF THE FOLLOWING DEVELOP, DISCONTINUE DRUG AND NOTIFY YOUR PHYSICIAN AS SOON AS POSSIBLE

Mild Adverse Effects
Allergic Reactions: Skin rash (various kinds), hives, itching of hands and feet, swelling of face or extremities.

Photosensitivity (see Glossary) Reactions: Exaggerated sunburn or skin irritation occurs commonly with some tetracyclines.

Other Reactions
   Loss of appetite, nausea, vomiting, diarrhea.
   Irritation of mouth or tongue, "black tongue," sore throat, abdominal pain or cramping.

Serious Adverse Effects

Allergic Reactions: Anaphylactic reaction (see Glossary), asthma, fever, painful swollen joints, unusual bleeding or bruising, jaundice (see Glossary).

Other Reactions: Permanent discoloration and/or malformation of teeth when taken under 9 years of age, including unborn child and infant.

CAUTION

1. Antacids, dairy products, and iron preparations will prevent adequate absorption of this drug and reduce its effectiveness significantly.
2. Troublesome and persistent diarrhea can develop in sensitive individuals. If diarrhea persists more than 24 hours, discontinue this drug and consult your physician for guidance.
3. If your kidney function is reduced significantly, dosage schedule must be adjusted accordingly.
4. If surgery under general anesthesia is planned while taking this drug, the choice of anesthetic agent must be considered carefully to prevent serious kidney damage.

Precautions for Use by Those over 60 Years of Age

The natural decline in kidney function that occurs after 60 may require significant reduction in dosage and lengthening of dosage intervals. Dosage must be carefully individualized and based upon measurements of kidney function.

Natural changes in the skin after 60 may predispose to severe and prolonged itching reactions in the genital and anal regions. This reaction should be reported promptly.

Advisability of Use During Pregnancy

Pregnancy Category: D (tentative). See Pregnancy Code inside back cover. Animal reproduction studies reveal significant birth defects due to this drug. Information from studies in pregnant women indicates that this drug can cause impaired development and discoloration of teeth and other developmental defects.

It is advisable to avoid this drug completely during entire pregnancy.

Ask physician for guidance.

Advisability of Use While Nursing Infant

Tetracyclines can be present in milk and can have adverse effects on infant. Avoid use.

Habit-Forming Potential

None.

Effects of Overdosage

Possible nausea, vomiting, diarrhea.

Acute liver damage (rare).

Possible Effects of Extended Use

Impairment of bone marrow, liver, or kidney function (all rare).

Superinfections.

Suggested Periodic Examinations While Taking This Drug (at physician's discretion)

Complete blood cell counts.

Liver and kidney function tests.

During extended use, sputum and stool examinations may detect early super-infections due to yeast organisms.

While Taking This Drug, Observe the Following

Foods: Dairy products can interfere with absorption. Tetracyclines should be taken 1 hour before or 2 hours after eating.

Beverages: Avoid milk for 1 hour before and after each dose of a tetracycline.

Alcohol: Avoid while taking a tetracycline if you have a history of liver disease.

Tobacco Smoking: No interactions expected.

Marijuana Smoking: No interactions expected.

Other Drugs

Tetracyclines may *increase* the effects of

• oral anticoagulants, and make it necessary to reduce their dosage.
• lithium (Lithane, Eskalith, Lithotabs, etc.), and increase the risk of lithium toxicity.

Tetracyclines may *decrease* the effects of

• the oral contraceptives, and impair their effectiveness in preventing pregnancy.
• the penicillins, and impair their effectiveness in treating infections.

The following drugs may *decrease* the effects of tetracyclines

• antacids may reduce drug absorption.
• iron and mineral preparations may reduce drug absorption.

Driving a Vehicle, Operating Machinery, Engaging in Hazardous Activities: Usually no restrictions. Be alert to the possible occurrence of nausea and/or diarrhea; restrict activities accordingly.

Aviation Note: The use of this drug *may be a disqualification* for the piloting of aircraft. Consultation with a designated Aviation Medical Examiner is advised.

Exposure to Sun: Avoid as much as possible. Photosensitivity (see Glossary) is common with some tetracyclines.

Special Storage Instructions

Keep in a tightly closed, light-resistant container.

THEOPHYLLINE
(Aminophylline, Oxtriphylline)

Year Introduced: 1930

Brand Names

USA

Accurbron (Merrell Dow)
Amesec [CD] (Glaxo)
Aminodur (Berlex)
Amodrine [CD] (Searle)
Brondecon [CD] (Parke-Davis)
Bronkaid [CD] (Winthrop)
Bronkodyl (Breon)
Bronkodyl S-R (Breon)
Bronkolixir [CD] (Breon)
Bronkotabs [CD] (Breon)
Choledyl (Parke-Davis)
Choledyl SA (Parke-Davis)
Elixicon (Berlex)
Elixophyllin (Berlex)
Elixophyllin SR (Berlex)
Isuprel Compound Elixir [CD] (Breon)
LaBID (Norwich Eaton)
Lodrane (Poythress)
Marax [CD] (Roerig)
Mudrane [CD] (Poythress)
Quadrinal [CD] (Knoll)
Quibron [CD] (Mead Johnson)
Quibron Plus [CD] (Mead Johnson)

Quibron-T Dividose (Mead Johnson)
Quibron-T/SR Dividose (Mead Johnson)
Respbid (Boehringer Ingleheim)
Slo-bid Gyrocaps (Rorer)
Slo-Phyllin Gyrocaps (Rorer)
Slo-Phyllin 80 (Rorer)
Somophyllin (Fisons)
Somophyllin-CRT (Fisons)
Somophyllin-DF (Fisons)
Somophyllin-T (Fisons)
Sustaire (Roerig)
Tedral [CD] (Parke-Davis)
Theobid Duracaps (Glaxo)
Theobid Jr. Duracaps (Glaxo)
Theo-Dur (Key)
Theo-Dur Sprinkles (Key)
Theolair (Riker)
Theolair-SR (Riker)
Theophyl (McNeil)
Theophyl-SR (McNeil)
Theophyl-225 (McNeil)
Theovent (Schering)
Verequad [CD] (Knoll)

Canada

Amesec [CD] (Lilly)
Elixophyllin (Pentagone)
Marax [CD] (Pfizer)
Pulmophylline (Riva)
Quibron [CD] (Bristol)
Quibron-T (Bristol)
Quibron-T/SR (Bristol)
Respbid (Boehringer)
Somophyllin-T (Fisons)
Somophyllin-12 (Fisons)
Tedral [CD] (P.D.)
Theo-Dur (Astra)
Theolair (Riker)
Theolixir (Pharmascience)

Common Synonyms ("Street Names"): Asthma medicine

Drug Class: Anti-asthmatic (Bronchodilator)

Prescription Required: USA: Yes   Canada: No

Available for Purchase by Generic Name: Yes

Available Dosage Forms and Strengths

Tablets —	100 mg., 125 mg., 200 mg., 225 mg., 250 mg., 300 mg.
Chewable tablets —	100 mg.
Prolonged-action tablets —	100 mg., 130 mg., 200 mg., 250 mg., 300 mg., 400 mg., 500 mg., 600 mg.
Capsules —	100 mg., 200 mg., 250 mg.
Prolonged-action capsules —	50 mg., 65 mg., 130 mg., 260 mg., 300 mg.
Elixir —	80 mg., 112.5 mg. per tablespoonful (15 ml.); 100 mg. per teaspoonful (5 ml.)
Suppositories —	120 mg., 250 mg., 500 mg.
Syrup —	80 mg. per tablespoonful (15 ml.).
Pediatric Syrup —	50 mg. per teaspoonful (5 ml.)
Suspension —	300 mg. per tablespoonful (15 ml.).

Also marketed in a variety of tablets, capsules, and liquids in combination with other drugs.

Tablet May Be Crushed or Capsule Opened for Administration

Regular tablets and capsules —	Yes
Prolonged-action tablets and capsules —	No
Aminodur-Duratab —	No
Elixophyllin-SR capsules, Slo-Phyllin Gyrocap, and Theophyl-SR capsules —	Yes, but do not crush or chew contents

How This Drug Works

Intended Therapeutic Effect(s):   Symptomatic relief in the management of bronchial asthma.

Location of Drug Action(s):   The muscles of the bronchial tubes.

Method of Drug Action(s):   This drug increases the activity of the chemical system within the muscle cell that causes relaxation and expansion of the bronchial tube, thus reversing the constriction responsible for asthma.

Principal Uses of This Drug

As a Single Drug Product: Used primarily to relieve the shortness of breath and wheezing characteristic of acute bronchial asthma, and to prevent the recurrence of asthmatic episodes. It is also useful in relieving the asthmatic-like symptoms associated with some types of chronic bronchitis and emphysema.

As a Combination Drug Product [CD]:   This drug is available in combination with several other drugs that are beneficial in the overall management of bronchial asthma and related conditions. Ephedrine is added to enhance the bronchodilator effects; guaifenesin is added to provide an expectorant effect that thins the mucus secretions in the bronchial tubes; mild sedatives such as barbiturates or hydroxyzine are added to allay the anxiety that often accompanies acute attacks of asthma.

THIS DRUG SHOULD NOT BE TAKEN IF
—you have had an allergic reaction to any dosage form of it previously.
—you have an active peptic ulcer.

INFORM YOUR PHYSICIAN BEFORE TAKING THIS DRUG IF
—you have a history of kidney disease or impaired kidney function.
—you have a history of gastritis or peptic ulcer.
—you have high blood pressure or heart disease.
—you are taking any medication for gout.

Time Required for Apparent Benefit
Drug action begins in 15 to 30 minutes, reaches a maximum in 1 to 2 hours, and subsides in 7 to 10 hours (depending upon dosage form and size of dose).

Possible Side-Effects *(natural, expected, and unavoidable drug actions)*
Nervousness, insomnia.

Possible Adverse Effects *(unusual, unexpected, and infrequent reactions)*

IF ANY OF THE FOLLOWING DEVELOP, DISCONTINUE DRUG AND NOTIFY YOUR PHYSICIAN AS SOON AS POSSIBLE

Mild Adverse Effects
Allergic Reactions: Skin rash.
Other Reactions
Stomach irritation, nausea, vomiting, diarrhea.
Headache, dizziness, rapid or irregular heart action.
Serious Adverse Effects
Idiosyncratic Reactions: Severe anxiety, confusion, behavioral disturbances.

CAUTION
This drug should not be taken concurrently with other anti-asthmatic drugs unless you are directed to do so by your physician. Serious overdosage could result.

Precautions for Use by Those over 60 Years of Age
The natural decline in liver function that occurs after 60 may require that you use smaller doses of this drug.
You may be more susceptible to the development of nausea, stomach irritation, vomiting, and diarrhea.

Advisability of Use During Pregnancy
Pregnancy Category: C (tentative). See Pregnancy Code inside back cover.
Animal reproduction studies in mice reveal significant birth defects due to this drug.
Information from adequate studies in pregnant women is not available.
It is advisable to avoid use of this drug during first 3 months if possible.
Ask physician for guidance.

Advisability of Use While Nursing Infant
Drug is present in milk in small amounts. Ask physician for guidance.

Habit-Forming Potential
None.

Effects of Overdosage
With Moderate Overdose: Nausea, vomiting, restlessness, irritability, confusion, thirst, increased urination.

With Large Overdose: Delirium, convulsions, high fever, weak and rapid pulse, collapse of circulation.

Possible Effects of Extended Use
Stomach irritation.

Suggested Periodic Examinations While Taking This Drug (at physician's discretion)
None required.

While Taking This Drug, Observe the Following
Foods: No restrictions. Drug is more effective if taken on empty stomach, but antacids may be necessary to reduce stomach irritation.

Beverages: Large intake of coffee or tea may increase the nervousness and insomnia caused by this drug in sensitive individuals.

Alcohol: No interactions expected.

Tobacco Smoking: No interactions expected with this drug. However, smoking may aggravate asthma, bronchitis, or emphysema. Follow physician's advice.

Marijuana Smoking

Occasional (once or twice weekly): Mild and transient improvement in anti-asthmatic effect of this drug.

Daily: More persistent improvement in anti-asthmatic effect of this drug.

Other Drugs

Theophylline may *increase* the effects of

- other drugs used to treat asthma, especially epinephrine (Adrenalin) and ephedrine. The combined effects are beneficial when dosages are adjusted properly.
- furosemide (Lasix) resulting in increased diuresis.

Theophylline may *decrease* the effects of

- drugs commonly used to treat gout; these include allopurinol (Zyloprim), probenecid (Benemid), sulfinpyrazone (Anturan). Consult physician regarding tests of uric acid blood levels and adjustment of dosage schedules for control of gout.
- lithium (Eskalith, Lithane, etc.), by hastening its elimination in the urine.

Theophylline *taken concurrently* with

- reserpine (Serpasil, Ser-Ap-Es, etc.) may cause rapid heart action.

The following drugs may *increase* the effects of theophylline:

- clindamycin (Cleocin)

- erythromycin (E.E.S., E-Mycin, Erythrocin, etc.)
- troleandomycin (Tao)

Driving a Vehicle, Operating Machinery, Engaging in Hazardous Activities:
No restrictions unless lightheadedness or dizziness occurs.

Aviation Note: The use of this drug *may be a disqualification* for the piloting of aircraft. Consultation with a designated Aviation Medical Examiner is advised.

Exposure to Sun: No restrictions.

Special Storage Instructions
Keep in a dry, tightly closed container.

THIORIDAZINE

Year Introduced: 1959

Brand Names

USA	Canada
Mellaril (Sandoz)	Apo-Thioridazine
Mellaril-S (Sandoz)	(Apotex)
	Mellaril (Sandoz)
	Novoridazine
	(Novopharm)
	Thioril (Pharmascience)

Common Synonyms ("Street Names"): None

Drug Class: Tranquilizer, Strong (Anti-psychotic), Phenothiazines

Prescription Required: Yes

Available for Purchase by Generic Name: Yes

Available Dosage Forms and Strengths
Tablets — 10 mg., 15 mg., 25 mg., 50 mg., 100 mg., 150 mg., 200 mg.
Concentrate — 30 mg. per ml., 100 mg. per ml.
Suspension — 25 mg., 100 mg. per teaspoonful (5 ml.)

Tablet May Be Crushed or Capsule Opened for Administration: Yes

How This Drug Works
Intended Therapeutic Effect(s): Restoration of emotional calm. Relief of severe anxiety, agitation, and psychotic behavior.
Location of Drug Action(s): Those nerve pathways in the brain that utilize the tissue chemical dopamine for the transmission of nerve impulses.

Method of Drug Action(s):   Not completely established. Present theory is that by inhibiting the action of dopamine, this drug acts to correct an imbalance of nerve impulse transmissions that is thought to be responsible for certain mental disorders.

Principal Uses of This Drug

As a Single Drug Product: This major tranquilizer is used in the management of the following psychotic conditions: moderate to marked depression with significant anxiety and nervous tension; agitation, anxiety, depression, and exaggerated fears in the elderly; severe behavioral problems in children characterized by hyperexcitability, combativeness, short attention span, rapid swings in mood.

THIS DRUG SHOULD NOT BE TAKEN IF
—you have had an allergic reaction to any dosage form of it previously.
—you have severe heart disease.
—it is prescribed for a child under 2 years of age.

INFORM YOUR PHYSICIAN BEFORE TAKING THIS DRUG IF
—you are allergic or sensitive to any phenothiazine drug (see Drug Class, Section Three).
—you are taking any sedatives, sleep-inducing drugs, other tranquilizers, antidepressants, antihistamines, or narcotic drugs of any kind.
—you have epilepsy.
—you plan to have surgery under general or spinal anesthesia in the near future.

Time Required for Apparent Benefit
Some benefit usually apparent in first week. Maximal benefit may require regular dosage for several weeks.

Possible Side-Effects *(natural, expected, and unavoidable drug actions)*
Drowsiness, lethargy, blurred vision, nasal congestion, dryness of the mouth, constipation, impaired urination.

Possible Adverse Effects *(unusual, unexpected, and infrequent reactions)*

IF ANY OF THE FOLLOWING DEVELOP, DISCONTINUE DRUG AND NOTIFY YOUR PHYSICIAN AS SOON AS POSSIBLE

Mild Adverse Effects
Allergic Reactions: Skin rash (various kinds), hives, swelling of the salivary glands, fever.
Other Reactions
   Headache, lightheadedness and faintness in upright position (see orthostatic hypotension in Glossary).
   Confusion, agitation, restlessness.
   Breast congestion, milk formation, menstrual irregularity.
   Nausea, vomiting, loss of appetite.
Serious Adverse Effects
Allergic Reactions: Hepatitis with jaundice (see Glossary), very rare with this drug.

Other Reactions
> Bone marrow depression (see Glossary), usually mild.
>
> Convulsions.
>
> Parkinson-like disorders (see Glossary), less frequent than with other phenothiazines.

CAUTION

1. Many over-the-counter (OTC) medications (see Glossary) for allergies, colds, and coughs contain drugs that can interact unfavorably with this drug. Ask your physician or pharmacist for guidance before using any such medications.
2. Antacids that contain aluminum and/or magnesium can prevent the absorption of this drug and reduce its effectiveness.
3. Obtain prompt evaluation of any disturbance or change in vision.

Precautions for Use by Those over 60 Years of Age

You may be more sensitive to all of the actions of this drug. Small doses are advisable until your individual response has been determined.

You may be more susceptible to the development of drowsiness, lethargy, constipation, lowering of body temperature (hypothermia), and excessive drop in blood pressure on arising from a lying or sitting position (see orthostatic hypotension in Glossary).

This drug can increase the degree of impaired urination associated with prostate gland enlargement (prostatism)

You may also be more susceptible to the development of Parkinson-like disorders and/or tardive dyskinesia (see discussion of these terms in Glossary). These conditions must be recognized early since they may become unresponsive to treatment and irreversible. Consult your physician promptly if suggestive symptoms develop.

Advisability of Use During Pregnancy

Pregnancy Category: C (tentative). See Pregnancy Code inside back cover.

Animal reproduction studies are conflicting.

Information from adequate studies in pregnant women is not available.

Ask physician for guidance.

Advisability of Use While Nursing Infant

Safety not established. Ask physician for guidance.

Habit-Forming Potential

None.

Effects of Overdosage

With Moderate Overdose: Marked drowsiness, confusion, disorientation, blurred vision, nasal congestion, marked dryness of mouth, weakness.

With Large Overdose: Deep sleep, coma, convulsions, drop in body temperature, shallow breathing.

Possible Effects of Extended Use

Pigmentation of the retina of the eye, causing impairment of vision, brownish coloration of vision, reduced night vision.

Tardive dyskinesia (see Glossary).

Suggested Periodic Examinations While Taking This Drug (at physician's discretion)

Complete eye examinations for changes in vision and pigment deposits in the retina.

Complete blood cell counts and liver function tests.

Periodic electrocardiograms.

Periodic examination of the tongue for the appearance of fine, involuntary, wave-like movements that could indicate the development of tardive dyskinesia.

While Taking This Drug, Observe the Following

Foods: No restrictions.

Beverages: No restrictions.

Alcohol: Use extreme caution until combined effects have been determined. Alcohol can increase the sedative action of thioridazine and accentuate its depressant effects on brain function. Thioridazine can increase the intoxicating effects of alcohol.

Tobacco Smoking: No interactions expected.

Marijuana Smoking

Occasional (once or twice weekly):   No effect to mild and transient increase in drowsiness and accentuation of orthostatic hypotension (see Glossary); some risk of precipitating latent psychoses (in predisposed individuals).

Daily: Moderate increase in drowsiness, significant accentuation of orthostatic hypotension; increased risk of precipitating latent psychoses, confusing interpretation of mental status and of drug responses.

Other Drugs

Thioridazine may *increase* the effects of

• all sedatives, sleep-inducing drugs, other tranquilizers, antidepressants, antihistamines, and narcotic drugs, and produce oversedation. Ask physician for guidance regarding dosage adjustments.

• all drugs containing atropine or having atropine-like actions (see Drug Class, Section Three).

Thioridazine may *decrease* the effects of

• levodopa (Dopar, Larodopa, etc.), and reduce its effectiveness in the treatment of Parkinson's disease (shaking palsy).

• appetite suppressant drugs (Pre-Sate, Preludin, Benzedrine, Dexedrine, etc.).

Thioridazine *taken concurrently* with

• quinidine, may impair heart function. Avoid the use of these two drugs at the same time.

The following drugs may *increase* the effects of thioridazine

• tricyclic antidepressants (see Drug Class, Section Three).

Driving a Vehicle, Operating Machinery, Engaging in Hazardous Activities: This drug can impair mental alertness, judgment, and physical coordination. Avoid hazardous activities.

Aviation Note: The use of this drug *is a disqualification* for the piloting of aircraft. Consultation with a designated Aviation Medical Examiner is advised.

Exposure to Sun: Use caution until sensitivity has been determined. This drug may produce photosensitivity (see Glossary).

Exposure to Heat: Use caution and avoid excessive heat. This drug may impair the regulation of body temperature and increase the risk of heat stroke.

Heavy Exercise or Exertion: Use caution and follow your physician's instructions if you have any form of heart disease.

Discontinuation: If it has been necessary to use this drug for an extended period of time, do not discontinue it suddenly. Ask physician for guidance regarding dosage reduction and withdrawal. Upon discontinuation of this drug, it may also be necessary to adjust the dosages of other drugs taken concurrently with it.

Special Storage Instructions
Store liquid concentrate in a tightly closed, amber glass container, at temperatures below 86°F. (30°C.).

THIOTHIXENE

Year Introduced: 1967

Brand Names

USA	Canada
Navane (Roerig)	Navane (Pfizer)

Common Synonyms ("Street Names"):   None

Drug Class: Tranquilizer, Strong (Anti-psychotic), Thioxanthines

Prescription Required: Yes

Available for Purchase by Generic Name: No

Available Dosage Forms and Strengths
Capsules — 1 mg., 2 mg., 5 mg., 10 mg., 20 mg.
Concentrate — 5 mg. per ml.
Injection — 2 mg. per ml., 5 mg. per ml.

Tablet May Be Crushed or Capsule Opened for Administration: Yes

How This Drug Works
Intended Therapeutic Effect(s):   Restoration of emotional calm. Relief of severe anxiety, agitation, and psychotic behavior.

Location of Drug Action(s):   Those nerve pathways in the mesolimbic area of the brain that utilize the tissue chemical dopamine for the transmission of nerve impulses.

Method of Drug Action(s):   Not completely established. Present theory is that by inhibiting the action of dopamine, this drug acts to correct an imbalance of nerve impulse transmissions that is thought to be responsible for certain mental disorders.

Principal Uses of This Drug

As a Single Drug Product: This major tranquilizer is used to ameliorate the psychotic thinking and behavior associated with acute psychoses of unknown nature, episodes of mania and paranoia, and acute schizophrenia.

THIS DRUG SHOULD NOT BE TAKEN IF
—you have had an allergic reaction to any dosage form of it previously.
—you have a serious blood disorder.
—you have any form of Parkinson's disease.
—it is prescribed for a child under 12 years of age.

INFORM YOUR PHYSICIAN BEFORE TAKING THIS DRUG IF
—you have had an allergic reaction to any phenothiazine drug in the past (see Drug Class, Section Three).
—you have a history of liver or kidney disease, or impaired liver or kidney function.
—you have epilepsy.
—you have glaucoma.
—you have any form of heart disease, especially angina (coronary insufficiency).
—you have high blood pressure.
—you drink alcoholic beverages daily.
—you are taking sedatives, sleep-inducing drugs, tranquilizers, antidepressants, antihistamines, or narcotic drugs of any kind.
—you plan to have surgery under general or spinal anesthesia in the near future.

Time Required for Apparent Benefit
Significant benefit may occur within 3 weeks. However, maximal benefit may require continuous use on a regular basis for several months.

Possible Side-Effects *(natural, expected, and unavoidable drug actions)*
Drowsiness, lethargy, blurred vision, dryness of the mouth, impaired urination, constipation, transient drop in blood pressure.

Possible Adverse Effects *(unusual, unexpected, and infrequent reactions)*

IF ANY OF THE FOLLOWING DEVELOP, DISCONTINUE DRUG AND NOTIFY YOUR PHYSICIAN AS SOON AS POSSIBLE

Mild Adverse Effects
Allergic Reactions: Itching, skin rash, hives, drug fever (see Glossary).
Other Reactions
Lightheadedness, fainting, rapid heart rate.
Insomnia, restlessness, agitation.

Nausea, vomiting, diarrhea.
Increased appetite, gain in weight.
Change in menstrual pattern.
Breast fullness, tenderness, and milk production.

Serious Adverse Effects
Allergic Reactions: Anaphylactic reaction (see Glossary).
Other Reactions
Parkinson-like disorders (see Glossary).
Muscle spasms affecting the jaw, neck, back, hands, or feet.
Eye-rolling, muscle twitching, convulsions.
Sexual impotence.
Fluctuations in number of white blood cells.

CAUTION

1. Many over-the-counter (OTC) medications (see Glossary) for allergies, colds, and coughs contain drugs that can interact unfavorably with this drug. Ask your physician or pharmacist for guidance before using any such medications
2. Antacids that contain aluminum and/or magnesium can prevent the absorption of this drug and reduce its effectiveness.
3. Obtain prompt evaluation of any disturbance or change in vision

Precautions for Use by Those over 60 Years of Age

You may be more sensitive to all of the actions of this drug. Small doses are advisable until your individual response has been determined.

You may be more susceptible to the development of drowsiness, lethargy, constipation, lowering of body temperature (hypothermia), and excessive drop in blood pressure on arising from a lying or sitting position (see orthostatic hypotension in Glossary).

This drug can increase the degree of impaired urination associated with prostate gland enlargement (prostatism).

You may also be more susceptible to the development of Parkinson-like disorders and/or tardive dyskinesia (see discussion of these terms in Glossary). These conditions must be recognized early since they may become unresponsive to treatment and irreversible. Consult your physician promptly if suggestive symptoms develop.

Advisability of Use During Pregnancy

Pregnancy Category: B (tentative). See Pregnancy Code inside back cover.
Animal reproduction studies reveal no birth defects due to this drug.
Information from adequate studies in pregnant women is not available.
Ask physician for guidance.

Advisability of Use While Nursing Infant

The presence of this drug in milk is not known. Ask your physician for guidance.

Habit-Forming Potential

None.

Effects of Overdosage
With Moderate Overdose: Marked drowsiness, dizziness, weakness, muscle rigidity and twitching, tremors, confusion, dryness of mouth, blurred or double vision.

With Large Overdose: Deep sleep progressing to coma, weak and rapid pulse, shallow and slow breathing, very low blood pressure, convulsions.

Possible Effects of Extended Use
Eye changes, such as pigment deposits in the lens and retina.
Tardive dyskinesia (see Glossary).

Suggested Periodic Examinations While Taking This Drug (at physician's discretion)
Complete blood cell counts.
Liver function tests.
Complete eye examinations, including eye structures and visual acuity.
Careful inspection of the tongue for early evidence of fine, involuntary, wave-like movements that could indicate the beginning of tardive dyskinesia.

While Taking This Drug, Observe the Following
Foods: No restrictions.

Beverages: No restrictions. The liquid concentrate form of this drug may be taken in water, in fruit or vegetable juices, or in milk.

Alcohol: Avoid completely. Alcohol can increase this drug's sedative action and accentuate its depressant effects on brain function. Thiothixene can increase the intoxicating effects of alcohol.

Tobacco Smoking: No interactions expected.

Marijuana Smoking
Occasional (once or twice weekly): No effect to mild and transient increase in drowsiness and accentuation of orthostatic hypotension (see Glossary); some risk of precipitating latent psychoses (in predisposed individuals).

Daily: Moderate increase in drowsiness, significant accentuation of orthostatic hypotension; increased risk of precipitating latent psychoses, confusing interpretation of mental status and of drug responses.

Other Drugs
Thiothixene may *increase* the effects of
- atropine-like drugs, and cause an increase in internal eye pressure in the presence of glaucoma (see Drug Class, Section Three).
- sedatives, sleep-inducing drugs, other tranquilizers, antihistamines, and narcotic drugs, and cause excessive sedation.

Thiothixene may *decrease* the effects of
- bethanidine.
- guanethidine.
- levodopa.

Thiothixene *taken concurrently* with
- anti-convulsant drugs, may cause a change in the pattern of seizures. Dosage adjustment of the anti-convulsant may be necessary.
- anti-hypertensive drugs (some), may cause excessive lowering of the blood pressure.

The following drugs may *increase* the effects of thiothixene
- barbiturates may cause excessive sedation.
- other tranquilizers may cause excessive sedation.
- tricyclic antidepressants may cause excessive sedation.

Driving a Vehicle, Operating Machinery, Engaging in Hazardous Activities: This drug can impair mental alertness, judgment, and physical coordination. Avoid all hazardous activities if you experience such drug effects.

Aviation Note: The use of this drug *is a disqualification* for the piloting of aircraft. Consultation with a designated Aviation Medical Examiner is advised.

Exposure to Sun: Use caution until full effect is known. This drug can cause photosensitivity.

Exposure to Heat: Use caution in hot environments. This drug may contribute to the development of heat stroke.

Heavy Exercise or Exertion: Use caution until tolerance for physical activity and exercise are determined. This drug may alter normal adaptive responses in perspiration and blood pressure adjustment.

Discontinuation: If this drug has been taken for an extended period of time, do not discontinue it abruptly. Ask your physician for guidance regarding gradual reduction of dosage over a period of several weeks to prevent possible withdrawal symptoms of tremors, dizziness, nausea, and vomiting.

Special Storage Instructions
Keep all forms of this drug in airtight containers. Protect from light.

THYROID

Year Introduced: 1896

Brand Names

USA		Canada
Armour Thyroid (Armour)	S-P-T (Fleming)	Proloid (P.D.)
Proloid (Parke-Davis)	Thyrar (Armour)	
	Thyrobrom (Mills)	

Common Synonyms ("Street Names"):   None

Drug Class: Thyroid Hormones

Prescription Required: Yes

Available for Purchase by Generic Name: Yes

Available Dosage Forms and Strengths:

Tablets — 15 mg. (0.25 gr.), 30 mg. (0.5 gr.), 65 mg. (1 gr.),
100 mg. (1.5 gr.), 130 mg. (2 gr.), 150 mg. (2.5 gr.)
200 mg. (3 gr.), 260 mg. (4 gr.), 325 mg. (5 gr.)

Enteric-coated tablets — 32 mg. (0.5 gr.), 65 mg. (1 gr.), 130 mg. (2 gr.), 195
mg. (3 gr.).

Capsules — 65 mg. (1 gr.), 130 mg. (2 gr.), 200 mg. (3 gr.), 325
mg. (5 gr.)

Sugar-coated tablets — 32 mg. (0.5 gr.), 65 mg. (1 gr.), 130 mg. (2 gr.), 195
mg. (3 gr.).

Tablet May Be Crushed or Capsule Opened for Administration
Regular tablets and capsules — Yes
Prolonged-Action capsules — No

How This Drug Works
Intended Therapeutic Effect(s):   Correction of thyroid hormone deficiency
(hypothyroidism) by replacement therapy.

Location of Drug Action(s):   Affects the biochemical activity of all tissues
throughout the body.

Method of Drug Action(s):   By altering the processes of cellular chemistry
that store energy in an inactive (reserve) form, this drug makes more
energy available for biochemical activity and increases the rate of cellular
metabolism.

Principal Uses of This Drug
As a Single Drug Product: Used solely to correct a deficiency of thyroid
hormone (hypothyroidism). In the absence of true thyroid deficiency, the
use of this drug to reduce weight is inappropriate and possibly harmful.

THIS DRUG SHOULD NOT BE TAKEN IF
—you have had an allergic reaction to any dosage form of it previously.
—you are recovering from a recent heart attack (ask physician for guidance).
—you are using it to lose weight and you do not have a thyroid deficiency (your
thyroid function is normal).

INFORM YOUR PHYSICIAN BEFORE TAKING THIS DRUG IF
—you have any form of heart disease.
—you have high blood pressure.
—you have diabetes.
—you have Addison's disease or a history of adrenal gland deficiency.
—you are using Adrenalin, ephedrine, or isoproterenol to treat asthma.
—you are taking any anticoagulant drugs.

Time Required for Apparent Benefit
Drug action begins within 48 hours and reaches a maximum in 8 to 10 days.
Full effectiveness requires continuous use on a regular schedule for several
weeks.

Possible Side-Effects *(natural, expected, and unavoidable drug actions)*
None if dosage is adjusted correctly.

Possible Adverse Effects *(unusual, unexpected, and infrequent reactions)*

IF ANY OF THE FOLLOWING DEVELOP, DISCONTINUE DRUG AND NOTIFY YOUR PHYSICIAN AS SOON AS POSSIBLE

Mild Adverse Effects
Allergic Reactions: Skin rash, hives.
Other Reactions
Headache in sensitive individuals, even with proper dosage adjustment.
Changes in menstrual pattern, during dosage adjustments.
Serious Adverse Effects
Increased frequency or intensity of angina in the presence of coronary artery disease.

CAUTION
1. Thyroid hormones are used to correct conditions due to thyroid deficiency and to treat thyroid gland enlargement (goiter) and thyroid cancer. They should not be used to treat obesity if diagnostic studies indicate that there is no thyroid deficiency contributing to the obesity.
2. The need for and response to thyroid hormone treatment varies greatly from person to person. Careful supervision of individual response is necessary to determine correct dosage. Do not change your dosage schedule without consulting your physician.

Precautions for Use by Those over 60 Years of Age
Natural changes in body composition and function after 60 usually increase sensitivity to thyroid hormone action. It is anticipated that you will respond well to small doses. Report promptly any indications that suggest overdosage.

Advisability of Use During Pregnancy
Pregnancy Category: C (tentative). See Pregnancy Code inside back cover.
Animal reproduction studies: No data available.
Information from limited studies in pregnant women is inconclusive.
Ask physician for guidance.
Thyroid hormones do not reach the fetus (cross the placenta) in significant amounts. This drug is safe to use in pregnancy but *only* if given to correct a true thyroid deficiency, and with properly adjusted dosage.

Advisability of Use While Nursing Infant
Thyroid hormones are present in milk. Nursing is safe when the mother's dose of thyroid hormones is correctly adjusted to maintain normal thyroid activity.

Habit-Forming Potential
None.

Effects of Overdosage
With Moderate Overdose: Sense of increased body heat, heart palpitation, nervousness, increased sweating, hand tremors, insomnia.

With Large Overdose: Rapid and irregular pulse, fever, headache, marked nervousness and irritability, diarrhea, weight loss, muscle spasm and cramping.

Possible Effects of Extended Use
None with correct dosage adjustment.

Suggested Periodic Examinations While Taking This Drug (at physician's discretion)
Physician's assessment of response to treatment, with evaluation of subjective and objective changes due to thyroid hormone activity.

Measurement of thyroid hormone levels in the blood.

While Taking This Drug, Observe the Following
Foods: To improve absorption this drug should be taken on arising and before eating. Avoid heavy use of soybean preparations because of their ability to interfere with thyroid function.

Beverages: No restrictions.

Alcohol: No interactions expected.

Tobacco Smoking: No interactions expected.

Marijuana Smoking: No interactions expected.

Other Drugs

Thyroid may *increase* the effects of
- stimulants such as Adrenalin, ephedrine, the amphetamines (Dexedrine), methylphenidate (Ritalin), etc., and cause excessive stimulation. Dosage adjustment may be necessary.
- oral anticoagulants of the coumarin family (see Drug Class, Section Three), and cause bleeding or hemorrhage. Reduction in dosage of the anticoagulant is usually necessary.
- tricyclic antidepressants (see Drug Class, Section Three).
- digitalis preparations (digitoxin, digoxin). Careful dosage adjustment is necessary to prevent digitalis toxicity.

Thyroid may *decrease* the effects of
- barbiturates, making larger doses necessary for effective sedation.

Thyroid *taken concurrently* with
- all anti-diabetic drugs (insulin and oral anti-diabetic medications), may require an increase in the dosage of the anti-diabetic agent to obtain proper control of blood sugar levels. After correct doses of both drugs have been determined, a reduction in the dose of thyroid will require a simultaneous reduction in the dose of the anti-diabetic drug to prevent hypoglycemia.
- cortisone-like drugs, requires careful dosage adjustment to prevent the development of cortisone deficiency.

The following drugs may *increase* the effects of thyroid
- aspirin (in large doses and with continuous use)
- phenytoin (Dantoin, Dilantin, etc.)

The following drugs may *decrease* the effects of thyroid
- cholestyramine (Cuemid, Questran) may reduce its absorption. Intake of the two drugs should be 5 hours apart.

Driving a Vehicle, Operating Machinery, Engaging in Hazardous Activities: No restrictions or precautions.

Aviation Note: The use of this drug *may be a disqualification* for the piloting of aircraft. Consultation with a designated Aviation Medical Examiner is advised.

Exposure to Sun: No restrictions.

Exposure to Heat: This drug may decrease individual tolerance to warm environments, increasing the discomfort due to heat. Avoid excessive sweating. Consult your physician if you develop symptoms of overdosage during the warm months of the year.

Exposure to Cold: This drug may increase individual tolerance to cold, decreasing the discomfort due to cold.

Heavy Exercise or Exertion: Use caution in the presence of angina and known coronary artery disease. This drug may increase the frequency of angina during physical activity.

Discontinuation: This drug must be taken continuously on a regular schedule to correct thyroid deficiency. Do not discontinue it without consulting your physician.

Special Storage Instructions

Keep in a dry, tightly closed container at room temperature. Protect from light.

THYROXINE
(Levothyroxine, T–4)

Year Introduced: 1953

Brand Names

USA		Canada
Levoid (Nutrition Control)	Euthroid [CD] (Parke-Davis)	Eltroxin (Glaxo)
Levothroid (Armour)	Thyrolar [CD] (Armour)	Synthroid (Flint)
Synthroid (Flint)		Thyrolar [CD] (USV)

Common Synonyms ("Street Names"):   Thyroid pills

Drug Class: Thyroid Hormones

Prescription Required: Yes

Available for Purchase by Generic Name: Yes

Available Dosage Forms and Strengths
Tablets — 0.025 mg., 0.05 mg., 0.1 mg., 0.125 mg., 0.15 mg., 0.175 mg., 0.2 mg., 0.3 mg., 0.5 mg.
Injection — 0.05 mg. per ml., 0.1 mg. per ml.

Tablet May Be Crushed or Capsule Opened for Administration: Yes

How This Drug Works
Intended Therapeutic Effect(s):   Correction of thyroid hormone deficiency (hypothyroidism) by replacement therapy.
Location of Drug Action(s):   Affects the biochemical activity of all tissues throughout the body.
Method of Drug Action(s):   By altering the processes of cellular chemistry that store energy in an inactive (reserve) form, this drug makes more energy available for biochemical activity and increases the rate of cellular metabolism.

Principal Uses of This Drug
As a Single Drug Product: Used solely to correct a deficiency of thyroid hormone (hypothyroidism). In the absence of true thyroid deficiency, the use of this drug to reduce weight is inappropriate and possibly harmful.
As a Combination Drug Product [CD]:   This thyroid hormone is available in combination with the other principal thyroid hormone, liothyronine, in a preparation that resembles as closely as possible the natural hormone material produced by the thyroid gland.

THIS DRUG SHOULD NOT BE TAKEN IF
—you have had an allergic reaction to any dosage form of it previously.
—you are recovering from a recent heart attack (ask physician for guidance).
—you are using it to lose weight and you do not have a thyroid deficiency (your thyroid function is normal).

INFORM YOUR PHYSICIAN BEFORE TAKING THIS DRUG IF
—you have any form of heart disease.
—you have high blood pressure.
—you have diabetes.
—you have Addison's disease or a history of adrenal gland deficiency.
—you are using Adrenalin, ephedrine, or isoproterenol to treat asthma.
—you are taking any anticoagulant drugs.

Time Required for Apparent Benefit
Drug action begins within 48 hours and reaches a maximum in 8 to 10 days. Full effectiveness requires continuous use on a regular schedule for several weeks.

Possible Side-Effects (*natural, expected, and unavoidable drug actions*)
None if dosage is adjusted correctly.

Possible Adverse Effects *(unusual, unexpected, and infrequent reactions)*

IF ANY OF THE FOLLOWING DEVELOP, DISCONTINUE DRUG AND NOTIFY
YOUR PHYSICIAN AS SOON AS POSSIBLE

Mild Adverse Effects
Allergic Reactions: Skin rash, hives.
Other Reactions
Headache in sensitive individuals, even with proper dosage adjustment.
Changes in menstrual pattern, during dosage adjustments.

Serious Adverse Effects
Increased frequency or intensity of angina in the presence of coronary
artery disease.

CAUTION
1. Thyroid hormones are used to correct conditions due to thyroid deficiency
   and to treat thyroid gland enlargement (goiter) and thyroid cancer. They
   should not be used to treat obesity if diagnostic studies indicate that there
   is no thyroid deficiency contributing to the obesity.
2. The need for and response to thyroid hormone treatment varies greatly
   from person to person. Careful supervision of individual response is necessary to determine correct dosage. Do not change your dosage schedule
   without consulting your physician.

Precautions for Use by Those over 60 Years of Age
Natural changes in body composition and function after 60 usually increase
sensitivity to thyroid hormone action. It is anticipated that you will respond
well to small doses. Report promptly any indications that suggest overdosage.

Advisability of Use During Pregnancy
Pregnancy Category: C (tentative). See Pregnancy Code inside back cover.
Animal reproduction studies in rats, rabbits, and guinea pigs reveal signif-
icant birth defects due to this drug.
Information from limited studies in pregnant women is inconclusive.
Ask physician for guidance.
Thyroid hormones do not reach the fetus (cross the placenta) in significant
amounts. This drug is safe to use in pregnancy but only if given to correct
a true thyroid deficiency and with properly adjusted dosage.

Advisability of Use While Nursing Infant
Thyroid hormones are present in milk. Nursing is safe when the mother's
dose of thyroid hormones is correctly adjusted to maintain normal thyroid
activity.

Habit-Forming Potential
None.

Effects of Overdosage
With Moderate Overdose: Sense of increased body heat, heart palpitation,
nervousness, increased sweating, hand tremors, insomnia.

With Large Overdose: Rapid and irregular pulse, fever, headache, marked nervousness and irritability, diarrhea, weight loss, muscle spasm and cramping.

Possible Effects of Extended Use
None with correct dosage adjustment.

Suggested Periodic Examinations While Taking This Drug (at physician's discretion)
Physician's assessment of response to treatment, with evaluation of subjective and objective changes due to thyroid hormone activity.

Measurement of thyroid hormone levels in the blood.

While Taking This Drug, Observe the Following
Foods: To improve absorption this drug should be taken on arising and before eating. Avoid heavy use of soybean preparations because of their ability to interfere with thyroid function.

Beverages: No restrictions.

Alcohol: No interactions expected.

Tobacco Smoking: No interactions expected.

Marijuana Smoking: No interactions expected.

Other Drugs

Thyroxine may *increase* the effects of

- stimulants such as Adrenalin, ephedrine, the amphetamines (Dexedrine), methylphenidate (Ritalin), etc., and cause excessive stimulation. Dosage adjustments may be necessary.
- oral anticoagulants of the coumarin family (see Drug Class, Section Three), and cause bleeding or hemorrhage. Reduction in dosage of the anticoagulant is usually necessary.
- tricyclic antidepressants (see Drug Class, Section Three).
- digitalis preparations (digitoxin, digoxin). Careful dosage adjustment is necessary to prevent digitalis toxicity.

Thyroxine may *decrease* the effects of
- barbiturates, making larger doses necessary for effective sedation.

Thyroxine *taken concurrently* with
- all anti-diabetic drugs (insulin and oral anti-diabetic medications), may require an increase in the dosage of the anti-diabetic agent to obtain proper control of blood sugar levels. After correct doses of both drugs have been determined, a reduction in the dose of thyroid will require a simultaneous reduction in the dose of the anti-diabetic drug to prevent hypoglycemia.
- cortisone-like drugs, requires careful dosage adjustment to prevent the development of cortisone deficiency.

The following drugs may *increase* the effects of thyroxine
- aspirin (in large doses and with continuous use)
- phenytoin (Dantoin, Dilantin, etc.)

The following drug may *decrease* the effects of thyroxine
- cholestyramine (Cuemid, Questran) may reduce its absorption. Intake of the two drugs should be 5 hours apart.

Driving a Vehicle, Operating Machinery, Engaging in Hazardous Activities: No restrictions or precautions.

Aviation Note: The use of this drug *may be a disqualification* for the piloting of aircraft. Consultation with a designated Aviation Medical Examiner is advised.

Exposure to Sun: No restrictions.

Exposure to Heat: This drug may decrease individual tolerance to warm environments, increasing discomfort due to heat. Avoid excessive sweating. Consult your physician if you develop symptoms of overdosage during the warm months of the year.

Exposure to Cold: This drug may increase individual tolerance to cold, decreasing the discomfort due to cold.

Heavy Exercise or Exertion: Use caution in the presence of angina and known coronary artery disease. This drug may increase the frequency of angina during physical activity.

Discontinuation: This drug must be taken continuously on a regular schedule to correct thyroid deficiency. Do not discontinue it without consulting your physician.

Special Storage Instructions

Keep in a dry, tightly closed container at room temperature. Protect from light.

TIMOLOL

Year Introduced: 1972

Brand Names

USA	Canada
Blocadren (Merck Sharp & Dohme)	Blocadren (Frosst)
Timoptic (Merck Sharp & Dohme)	Timoptic (MSD)
Timolide [CD] (Merck Sharp & Dohme)	Timolide [CD] (Frosst)

Common Synonyms ("Street Names"): Blood pressure pills, Glaucoma eye drops

Drug Class: Anti-glaucoma, Anti-hypertensive, Beta-Adrenergic Blocker

Prescription Required: USA: Yes   Canada: Yes

Available for Purchase by Generic Name: USA: No   Canada: No

Available Dosage Forms and Strengths
        Tablets — 5 mg., 10 mg., 20 mg.
  Ophthalmic solution — 0.25%, 0.5%

Tablet May Be Crushed or Capsule Opened for Administration: Yes

How This Drug Works
  Intended Therapeutic Effect(s):   Reduction of high blood pressure; reduction of high internal eye pressure.
  Location of Drug Action(s):   Not completely established.
  The principal sites are thought to include
  • the heart muscle.
  • the vasomotor center in the brain that influences the control of the sympathetic nervous system over blood vessels (principally arterioles) throughout the body.
  • sympathetic nerve terminals in blood vessel walls.
  • possibly the kidneys.
  • tissues in the front chamber of the eye that produce the internal fluid (aqueous humor).
  Method of Drug Action(s):   Not completely established. It is thought that by blocking certain actions of the sympathetic nervous system, this drug
  • reduces the degree of contraction of blood vessel walls, resulting in their relaxation and expansion and lowering of the blood pressure.
  • inhibits the release of renin by the kidneys, resulting in further lowering of the blood pressure.
  • reduces the rate of production of fluid in the front chamber of the eye, resulting in less volume and a lower pressure within the eye.

Principal Uses of This Drug
  As a Single Drug Product: This member of the "beta-blocker" class is used primarily to treat high blood pressure and glaucoma. It is used alone or as a "step 2" antihypertensive in the management of mild to moderate high blood pressure. In addition, it is used to prevent classical effort-induced angina pectoris, and to provide protection against certain complications during recovery from heart attack (myocardial infarction).
  As a Combination Drug Product [CD]:   This drug is available in combination with hydrochlorothiazide, a "step 1" antihypertensive that utilizes a different method of action. The combined actions of these two drugs are more effective in the long-term management of hypertension.

THIS DRUG SHOULD NOT BE TAKEN IF
—you have had an allergic reaction to any dosage form of it previously.
—you have Prinzmetal's variant type of angina (coronary artery spasm).
—you currently have congestive heart failure.
—you are subject to acute bronchial asthma.
—you are presently experiencing seasonal allergic rhinitis.
—your heart rate is below 50 beats per minute.

—you are currently taking, or have taken within the past 2 weeks, any monoamine oxidase (MAO) inhibitor drug (see Drug Class, Section Three).

INFORM YOUR PHYSICIAN BEFORE TAKING THIS DRUG IF
—you have a history of prior heart disease, with or without episodes of heart failure.
—you have a history of hay fever, bronchial asthma, chronic bronchitis, or emphysema.
—you have a history of over-active thyroid function (hyperthyroidism).
—you have diabetes or myasthenia gravis.
—you are subject to hypoglycemia.
—you have impaired liver or kidney function.
—you are currently taking any form of reserpine, digitalis or quinidine, or a "calcium blocker" drug (see Drug Class, Section Three).
—you plan to have surgery under general anesthesia in the near future.

Time Required for Apparent Benefit
Drug action usually begins in 30 minutes and reaches its peak in 1 to 3 hours. Continuous use on a regular schedule for 10 to 14 days is usually necessary to determine this drug's effectiveness in lowering the blood pressure or controlling glaucoma.

Possible Side-Effects (natural, expected, and unavoidable drug actions)
Lethargy, fatiguability, cold hands and feet, slow heart rate, low blood pressure.

Possible Adverse Effects (unusual, unexpected, and infrequent reactions)

IF ANY OF THE FOLLOWING DEVELOP, DISCONTINUE DRUG AND NOTIFY YOUR PHYSICIAN AS SOON AS POSSIBLE

Mild Adverse Effects
Allergic Reactions: Skin rash, itching.
Other Reactions: Headache, drowsiness, lightheadedness, dizziness, vertigo, orthostatic hypotension (see Glossary), fainting, ringing in the ears, visual disturbances.
Loss of appetite, nausea, vomiting, diarrhea, stomach pains.
Numbness, tingling, and/or pains in the extremities.

Serious Adverse Effects
Allergic Reactions: Severe dermatitis with peeling of skin, spasm of the vocal cords.
Idiosyncratic Reactions: Acute behavioral disturbances: confusion, disorientation, hallucinations, loss of memory—all reported for propranolol, but not for timolol to date.
Other Reactions: Reduced heart reserve, with precipitation of congestive heart failure (3%).
Mental depression, anxiety, vivid dreams, nightmares.
Induction of bronchial asthma, shortness of breath.
Reduced libido, impotence, impaired urination.
Masking of the warning signs of impending low blood sugar (hypoglycemia) in drug-treated diabetes.

Adverse Effects That May Mimic Natural Diseases or Disorders
Reduced blood flow into the extremities may resemble Raynaud's disease.

Natural Diseases or Disorders That May Be Activated By This Drug
Prinzmetal's variant form of angina, Raynaud's disease, circulatory deficiency in the legs (muscle cramping with exercise), myasthenia gravis (?).

CAUTION
1. If you are being treated for angina, *do not discontinue this drug suddenly.*
2. If you develop any of the following symptoms, inform your physician promptly: angina pain that occurs at rest (without exertion), shortness of breath with exertion, swelling of the feet and ankles, leg cramps while walking, disturbances of sleep, emotional depression.

Precautions for Use by Those over 60 Years of Age
The basic rule in treating high blood pressure after 60 is to proceed *cautiously.* The elevated systolic blood pressure often present after 60 is not necessarily a threat to health, and can serve as an adaptive and compensatory change with age that should not be altered drastically. The goals of treatment must be adjusted to the natural changes in body function that occur with aging. Unacceptably high blood pressure should be reduced without creating the risks associated with excessively low blood pressure.

It is advisable to start treatment with small doses and to monitor the blood pressure response frequently. Sudden, rapid, and excessive reduction of blood pressure can predispose to stroke or heart attack.

You may be more susceptible to the development of orthostatic hypotension with resultant lightheadedness, dizziness, unsteadiness, fainting, and falling. Report such symptoms to your physician promptly.

Advisability of Use During Pregnancy
Pregnancy Category: C (tentative). See Pregnancy Code inside back cover.

Animal reproduction studies reveal no birth defects.

Information from adequate studies in pregnant women is not available.

Use this drug only if clearly needed. Avoid it during labor and delivery because of its possible effects on the newborn infant.

Advisability of Use While Nursing Infant
This drug is probably present in human milk. If drug is necessary, monitor the nursing infant for slow heart rate and low blood sugar.

Habit-Forming Potential
None.

Effects of Overdosage
With Moderate Overdose: General weakness, slow pulse, orthostatic hypotension.

With Large Overdose: Marked drop in blood pressure, fainting, slow and weak pulse, cold and sweaty skin, convulsions.

Possible Effects of Extended Use

Reduced reserve of heart muscle strength, with predisposition to congestive heart failure in susceptible individuals.

Suggested Periodic Examinations While Taking This Drug (at physician's discretion)

Complete blood cell counts, including platelet counts. Evaluation of blood pressure status and heart function.

While Taking This Drug, Observe the Following

Foods: No restrictions. Avoid excessive salt intake.
Preferably taken 1 hour before eating to maximize absorption.

Beverages: No restrictions. May be taken with milk.

Alcohol: Use with caution until the combined effect has been determined. Alcohol may exaggerate this drug's ability to lower the blood pressure and may increase its mild sedative action.

Tobacco Smoking: Follow physician's advise regarding smoking. Nicotine may reduce this drug's effectiveness in treating angina and high blood pressure.

Marijuana Smoking

Occasional (once or twice weekly): No effect to mild and transient cooling of hands and/or feet.

Daily: More marked and persistent coldness of hands and/or feet.

Other Drugs

Timolol may *increase* the effects of

- other antihypertensive drugs and cause excessive lowering of the blood pressure. Careful dosage adjustments are necessary.
- sedatives, tranquilizers, sleep-inducing drugs, narcotics, and cause excessive sedation.
- digitalis preparations and cause excessive slowing of the heart rate.
- ergot preparations (Cafergot, etc.) and cause excessive constriction of blood vessels.
- phenothiazines and cause excessive lowering of the blood pressure (see Drug Class, Section Three).
- reserpine (Ser-Ap-Es, etc.) and cause excessive lowering of the blood pressure, sedation, and emotional depression.

Timolol may *decrease* the effects of

- aminophylline and theophylline and reduce their anti-asthmatic effects.
- isoproterenol and reduce its anti-asthmatic effect.

Timolol *taken concurrently* with

- anti-diabetic drugs requires close monitoring to avoid undetected drops in blood sugar levels (hypoglycemia).
- clonidine (Catapres) requires close monitoring for rebound hypertension if clonidine is withdrawn while timolol is still being taken.
- disopyramide (Norpace) can cause excessive depression of heart function.
- mono-amine oxidase (MAO) inhibitor drugs may cause uncertain consequences. This combination should be avoided on theoretical grounds.

• methyldopa (Aldomet) may result in hypertensive episodes during periods of severe physiological stress.

The following drugs may *decrease* the effects of timolol

• antacids containing aluminum hydroxide may impair its absorption.

• indomethacin (Indocin) and other "aspirin substitutes" may reduce timolol's antihypertensive effect.

Driving a Vehicle, Operating Machinery, Engaging in Hazardous Activities: Use caution until the full extent of drowsiness or lethargy has been determined.

Aviation Note: The use of this drug and the disorder for which this drug is prescribed *may be disqualifications* for the piloting of aircraft. Consultation with a designated Aviation Medical Examiner is advised.

Exposure to Sun: No restrictions.

Exposure to Heat: Use caution. Hot environments can induce low blood pressure.

Exposure to Cold: Use caution. Cold environments can enhance the circulatory deficiency in the extremities induced by this drug. The elderly should dress warmly and avoid situations conducive to hypothermia. Raynaud's disorder may be exaggerated.

Heavy Exercise or Exertion: It is advisable to avoid exertion that causes lightheadedness, excessive fatigue, muscle cramping, or angina. Isometric exercises—the "overload" technique for strengthening individual muscles —can raise the blood pressure significantly. The use of this drug may intensify the hypertensive response to isometric exercises. Ask your physician for guidance.

Occurrence of Unrelated Illness: The fever that may accompany systemic infections can lower the blood pressure. Dosage adjustments of this drug may be necessary. Illnesses that cause nausea or vomiting may prohibit regular or continuous use of this drug. Monitor closely for adverse effects if regular use is interrupted.

Discontinuation: It is advisable to avoid sudden discontinuation of this drug in all situations. Abrupt withdrawal in the presence of coronary artery disease can cause a marked increase in the frequency and severity of angina and can increase the risk of heart attack (myocardial infarction). If possible, dosage should be reduced gradually over a period of 2 or more weeks.

Special Storage Instructions

Keep tablets in a dry, tightly closed container at room temperature.
Keep eye solution at room temperature. Protect from light.

TOLAZAMIDE

Year Introduced: 1966

Brand Names

USA	Canada
Tolinase (Upjohn)	None

Common Synonyms ("Street Names"):   Diabetes pills

Drug Class: Anti-diabetic, Oral (Hypoglycemic), Sulfonylureas

Prescription Required: Yes

Available for Purchase by Generic Name: No

Available Dosage Forms and Strengths
  Tablets — 100 mg., 250 mg., 500 mg.

Tablet May Be Crushed or Capsule Opened for Administration: Yes

How This Drug Works
  Intended Therapeutic Effect(s):   The correction of insulin deficiency in adult (maturity-onset) diabetes of moderate severity.
  Location of Drug Action(s):   The insulin-producing tissues of the pancreas.
  Method of Drug Action(s):   It is well established that sulfonylurea drugs stimulate the secretion of insulin (by a pancreas capable of responding to stimulation). Therapeutic doses may increase the amount of available insulin.

Principal Uses of This Drug
  As a Single Drug Product: To assist in the control of mild to moderately severe diabetes mellitus of the adult (maturity-onset) type that does not require insulin by injection, but that cannot be adequately controlled by diet alone.

THIS DRUG SHOULD NOT BE TAKEN IF
—you have had an allergic reaction to any dosage form of it previously.
—you have a history of impaired liver function or kidney function.

INFORM YOUR PHYSICIAN BEFORE TAKING THIS DRUG IF
—your diabetes has been difficult to control in the past ("brittle type").
—you have a history of peptic ulcer of the stomach or duodenum.
—you have a history of porphyria.
—you do not know how to recognize or treat hypoglycemia (see Glossary).

Time Required for Apparent Benefit
  A single dose may lower the blood sugar within 4 to 6 hours. Regular use for 1 to 2 weeks may be needed to determine this drug's effectiveness in controlling your diabetes.

Possible Side-Effects *(natural, expected, and unavoidable drug actions)*
Usually none. If drug dosage is excessive or food intake is inadequate, abnormally low blood sugar (hypoglycemia) will occur as a predictable drug effect.

Possible Adverse Effects *(unusual, unexpected, and infrequent reactions)*
IF ANY OF THE FOLLOWING DEVELOP, DISCONTINUE DRUG AND NOTIFY YOUR PHYSICIAN AS SOON AS POSSIBLE
Mild Adverse Effects
Allergic Reactions: Skin rashes (various kinds), hives, itching, drug fever.
Other Reactions
Headache, ringing in ears.
Indigestion, heartburn, nausea, diarrhea.
Serious Adverse Effects
Allergic Reactions: Hepatitis with jaundice (see Glossary).
Idiosyncratic Reactions: Hemolytic anemia in susceptible individuals (see Glossary).
Other Reactions: Bone marrow depression (see Glossary)—fatigue, weakness, fever, sore throat, unusual bleeding or bruising.

CAUTION
1. This drug must be looked upon as only one part of the total program for the management of your diabetes. It is not a substitute for a properly prescribed diet.
2. Over a period of time (usually several months), this drug may lose its effectiveness in controlling blood sugar levels. Periodic follow-up examinations are necessary to monitor all aspects of response to drug treatment.
3. Individual response to this drug varies widely. The effects of overdosage—hypoglycemia—can occur in sensitive individuals taking doses well within the recommended range.
4. Do not begin treatment with a large or "loading" dose. This is unnecessary and can be dangerous.
5. The total daily dose should not exceed 1000 mg.

Precautions for Use by Those over 60 Years of Age
The natural decline in kidney function that occurs after 60, together with the duration of this drug's action, requires that both initial and maintenance dosage be less than that normally used in the younger adult. Do not exceed a total dosage of 1000 mg. in 24 hours.
The aging brain adapts well to the higher blood sugar levels associated with diabetes. Attempts to achieve "normal" blood sugar levels can result in unrecognized hypoglycemia that is manifested by confusion and abnormal behavior. Repeated episodes of hypoglycemia in the elderly can cause brain damage.

Advisability of Use During Pregnancy
Pregnancy Category: B (tentative). See Pregnancy Code inside back cover.
Animal reproduction studies reveal no birth defects due to this drug.
Information from adequate studies in pregnant women is not available.
Use during pregnancy is not recommended by manufacturer.

Advisability of Use While Nursing Infant
Drug is known to be present in milk. Ask physician for guidance.

Habit-Forming Potential
None.

Effects of Overdosage
With Moderate Overdose: Symptoms of mild to moderate hypoglycemia: headache, lightheadedness, faintness, nervousness, confusion, tremor, sweating, heart palpitation, weakness, and hunger.

With Large Overdose: Hypoglycemic coma (see hypoglycemia in Glossary).

Possible Effects of Extended Use
Reduced function of the thyroid gland (hypothyroidism), resulting in lowered metabolism.

Reports of increased frequency and severity of heart and blood vessel diseases associated with long-term use of the members of this drug family are highly controversial and inconclusive. A direct cause-and-effect relationship (see Glossary) has not been established to date. Ask your physician for guidance regarding extended use.

Suggested Periodic Examinations While Taking This Drug (at physician's discretion)
Complete blood cell counts.
Liver function tests.
Thyroid function tests.
Periodic evaluation of heart and circulatory system.

While Taking This Drug, Observe the Following
Foods: Follow the diabetic diet prescribed by your physician.

Beverages: As directed in the diabetic diet prescribed by your physician.

Alcohol: Use with extreme caution until the combined effect has been determined. This drug can cause a marked intolerance to alcohol resulting in a disulfiram-like reaction (see Glossary).

Tobacco Smoking: No interactions expected. No restrictions unless imposed as part of your overall treatment program. Ask physician for guidance.

Marijuana Smoking
Occasional (once or twice weekly): No significant interactions expected.
Daily: Possible increase in blood sugar.

Other Drugs
Tolazamide may *increase* the effects of

- sedatives and sleep-inducing drugs, by slowing their elimination from the body.
- "sulfa" drugs, by slowing their elimination from the body.

Tolazamide *taken concurrently* with

- oral anticoagulants, may cause unpredictable changes in anticoagulant drug actions. Ask physician for guidance regarding prothrombin blood tests and dosage adjustment.
- propranolol (Inderal), may allow hypoglycemia to develop without adequate warning. Follow diet and dosage schedules very carefully.

The following drugs may *increase* the effects of tolazamide
- bishydroxycoumarin (Dicumarol, Dufalone)
- chloramphenicol (Chloromycetin, etc.)
- clofibrate (Atromid-S)
- mono-amine oxidase (MAO) inhibitors (see Drug Class, Section Three)
- oxyphenbutazone (Tandearil)
- phenformin (DBI)
- phenylbutazone (Azolid, Butazolidin, etc.)
- phenyramidol (Analexin)
- probenecid (Bememid)
- propranolol (Inderal)
- salicylates (aspirin, sodium salicylate)
- sulfaphenazole (Orisul, Sulfabid)
- sulfisoxazole (Gantrisin, Novosoxazole, etc.)

The following drugs may *decrease* the effects of tolazamide
- chlorpromazine (Thorazine, Largactil, etc.)
- cortisone and related drugs (see Drug Class, Section Three)
- estrogens (Premarin, Menotrol, Ogen, etc.)
- isoniazid (INH, Isozide, etc.)
- nicotinic acid (Niacin, etc.)
- oral contraceptives
- pyrazinamide (Aldinamide)
- thiazide diuretics (see Drug Class, Section Three)
- thyroid preparations

Driving a Vehicle, Operating Machinery, Engaging in Hazardous Activities: Regulate your dosage schedule, eating schedule and physical activities very carefully to prevent hypoglycemia. Be able to recognize the early symptoms of hypoglycemia and avoid hazardous activities if you suspect that hypoglycemia is developing.

Aviation Note: Diabetes *is a disqualification* for the piloting of aircraft. Consultation with a designated Aviation Medical Examiner is advised.

Exposure to Sun: Use caution until sensitivity has been determined. This drug can cause photosensitivity (see Glossary).

Heavy Exercise or Exertion: Use caution. Excessive exercise may result in hypoglycemia.

Occurrence of Unrelated Illness: Acute infections, illnesses causing vomiting or diarrhea, serious injuries, and the need for surgery can interfere with diabetic control and may require a change in medication. If any of these conditions occur, ask your physician for guidance regarding the continued use of this drug.

Discontinuation: If you find it necessary to discontinue this drug for any reason, notify your physician and ask for guidance regarding necessary changes in your treatment program for diabetic control.

Special Storage Instructions
Keep in a dry, tightly closed container.

TOLBUTAMIDE

Year Introduced: 1956

Brand Names

USA	Canada
Orinase (Upjohn)	Apo-Tolbutamide
SK-Tolbutamide (Smith	(Apotex)
Kline & French)	Mobenol (Horner)
	Novobutamide
	(Novopharm)
	Orinase (Hoechst)

Common Synonyms ("Street Names"):   Diabetes pills

Drug Class: Anti-diabetic, Oral (Hypoglycemic), Sulfonylureas

Prescription Required: Yes

Available for Purchase by Generic Name: Yes

Available Dosage Forms and Strengths
Tablets — 250 mg., 500 mg.

Tablet May Be Crushed or Capsule Opened for Administration: Yes

How This Drug Works
Intended Therapeutic Effect(s):   The correction of insulin deficiency in adult (maturity-onset) diabetes of moderate severity.
Location of Drug Action(s):   The insulin-producing tissues of the pancreas.
Method of Drug Action(s):   It is well established that sulfonylurea drugs stimulate the secretion of insulin (by a pancreas capable of responding to stimulation). Therapeutic doses may increase the amount of available insulin.

Principal Uses of This Drug
As a Single Drug Product: To assist in the control of mild to moderately severe diabetes mellitus of the adult (maturity-onset) type that does not require insulin by injection, but that cannot be adequately controlled by diet alone.

THIS DRUG SHOULD NOT BE TAKEN IF
—you are allergic to any of the drugs bearing the brand names listed above.
—you have severe impairment of liver function or kidney function.

INFORM YOUR PHYSICIAN BEFORE TAKING THIS DRUG IF
—your diabetes has been difficult to control in the past ("brittle type").
—you have a history of peptic ulcer of the stomach or duodenum.
—you have a history of porphyria.
—you do not know how to recognize or treat hypoglycemia (see Glossary).

Time Required For Apparent Benefit

A single dose may lower the blood sugar within 3 to 6 hours. Regular use for 1 to 2 weeks may be needed to determine this drug's effectiveness in controlling your diabetes.

Possible Side-Effects *(natural, expected, and unavoidable drug actions)*

Usually none. If drug dosage is excessive or food intake is inadequate, abnormally low blood sugar (hypoglycemia; see Glossary) will occur as a predictable drug effect.

Possible Adverse Effects *(unusual, unexpected, and infrequent reactions)*

IF ANY OF THE FOLLOWING DEVELOP, DISCONTINUE DRUG AND NOTIFY YOUR PHYSICIAN AS SOON AS POSSIBLE

Mild Adverse Effects
Allergic Reactions: Skin rashes (various kinds), hives, itching, drug fever.
Other Reactions
Headache, ringing in ears.
Indigestion, heartburn, nausea, diarrhea.
Serious Adverse Effects
Allergic Reactions: Hepatitis with jaundice (see Glossary).
Idiosyncratic Reactions: Hemolytic anemia (see Glossary).
Other Reactions: Bone marrow depression (see Glossary)—fatigue, weakness, fever, sore throat, unusual bleeding or bruising.

CAUTION

1. This drug must be looked upon as only one part of the total program for the management of your diabetes. It is not a substitute for a properly prescribed diet.
2. Over a period of time (usually several months), this drug may lose its effectiveness in controlling blood sugar levels. Periodic follow-up examinations are necessary to monitor all aspects of response to drug treatment.
3. Individual response to this drug varies widely. The effects of overdosage—hypoglycemia—can occur in sensitive individuals taking doses well within the recommended range.
4. Do not begin treatment with a large or "loading" dose. This is unnecessary and can be dangerous.
5. The total daily dose should not exceed 2000 mg.

Precautions for Use by Those over 60 Years of Age

The natural decline in kidney function that occurs after 60, together with the duration of this drug's action, requires that both initial and maintenance dosage be less than that normally used in the younger adult. Do not exceed a total dosage of 2000 mg. in 24 hours.

The aging brain adapts well to the higher blood sugar levels associated with diabetes. Attempts to achieve "normal" blood sugar levels can result in unrecognized hypoglycemia that is manifested by confusion and abnormal behavior.

Repeated episodes of hypoglycemia in the elderly can cause brain damage.

Advisability of Use During Pregnancy

Pregnancy Category: C (tentative). See Pregnancy Code inside back cover. Animal reproduction studies reveal significant birth defects due to this drug.

Information from adequate studies in pregnant women is not available.

Use during pregnancy is not recommended by manufacturer.

Advisability of Use While Nursing Infant

Drug is known to be present in milk. Ask physician for guidance.

Habit-Forming Potential

None.

Effects of Overdosage

With Moderate Overdose: Symptoms of mild to moderate hypoglycemia: headache, lightheadedness, faintness, nervousness, confusion, tremor, sweating, heart palpitation, weakness and hunger.

With Large Overdose: Hypoglycemic coma (see hypoglycemia in Glossary).

Possible Effects of Extended Use

Reduced function of the thyroid gland (hypothyroidism), resulting in lowered metabolism.

Reports of increased frequency and severity of heart and blood vessel diseases associated with long-term use of the members of this drug family are highly controversial and inconclusive. A direct cause-and-effect relationship (see Glossary) has not been established to date. Ask your physician for guidance regarding extended use.

Suggested Periodic Examinations While Taking This Drug (at physician's discretion)

Complete blood cell counts.

Liver function tests.

Thyroid function tests.

Periodic evaluation of heart and circulatory system.

While Taking This Drug, Observe the Following

Foods: Follow the diabetic diet prescribed by your physician.

Beverages: As directed in the diabetic diet prescribed by your physician.

Alcohol: Use with extreme caution until the combined effect has been determined. This drug can cause a marked intolerance to alcohol, resulting in a disulfiram-like reaction (see Glossary).

Tobacco Smoking: No restrictions unless imposed as part of your overall treatment program. Ask physician for guidance.

Marijuana Smoking

Occasional (once or twice weekly): No significant interactions expected.

Daily: Possible increase in blood sugar.

Other Drugs

Tolbutamide may *increase* the effects of

• sedatives and sleep-inducing drugs, by slowing their elimination from the body.

• "sulfa" drugs, by slowing their elimination from the body.

Tolbutamide *taken concurrently* with
- oral anticoagulants, may cause unpredictable changes in anticoagulant drug actions. Ask physician for guidance regarding prothrombin blood tests and dosage adjustments.
- propranolol (Inderal), may allow hypoglycemia to develop without adequate warning. Follow diet and dosage schedules very carefully.

The following drugs may *increase* the effects of tolbutamide
- anabolic drugs (Adroyd, Anavar, Dianabol, etc.)
- oral anticoagulants of the coumarin type (see Drug Class, Section Three)
- chloramphenicol (Chloromycetin, etc.)
- clofibrate (Atromid-S)
- fenfluramine (Pondimin)
- guanethidine (Ismelin)
- mono-amine oxidase (MAO) inhibitors (see Drug Class, Section Three)
- oxyphenbutazone (Oxalid, Tandearil)
- phenformin (DBI)
- phenylbutazone (Azolid, Butazolidin, etc.)
- phenyramidol (Analexin)
- probenecid (Benemid)
- propranolol (Inderal)
- salicylates (aspirin, sodium salicylate)
- sulfaphenazole (Orisul, Sulfabid)
- sulfinpyrazone (Anturane)
- sulfisoxazole (Gantrisin, Novosoxazole, etc.)

The following drugs may *decrease* the effects of tolbutamide
- chlorpromazine (Thorazine, Largactil, etc.)
- cortisone and related drugs (see Drug Class, Section Three)
- ethacrynic acid (Edecrin)
- estrogens (Premarin, Menotrol, Ogen, etc.)
- furosemide (Lasix)
- isoniazid (INH, Isozide, etc.)
- nicotinic acid (Niacin, etc.)
- oral contraceptives
- pyrazinamide (Aldinamide)
- thiazide diuretics (see Drug Class, Section Three)
- thyroid preparations

Driving a Vehicle, Operating Machinery, Engaging in Hazardous Activities: Regulate your dosage schedule, eating schedule, and physical activities very carefully to prevent hypoglycemia. Be able to recognize the early symptoms of hypoglycemia and avoid hazardous activities if you suspect that hypoglycemia is developing.

Aviation Note: Diabetes *is a disqualification* for the piloting of aircraft. Consultation with a designated Aviation Medical Examiner is advised.

Exposure to Sun: Use caution until sensitivity has been determined. This drug can cause photosensitivity (see Glossary).

Heavy Exercise or Exertion: Use caution. Excessive exercise may result in hypoglycemia.

Occurrence of Unrelated Illness: Acute infections, illnesses causing vomiting or diarrhea, serious injuries, and the need for surgery can interfere with diabetic control and may require a change in medication. If any of these conditions occur, ask your physician for guidance regarding the continued use of this drug.

Discontinuation: If you find it necessary to discontinue this drug for any reason, notify your physician and ask for guidance regarding necessary changes in your treatment program for diabetic control.

Special Storage Instructions

Keep in a dry, tightly closed container.

TOLMETIN

Year Introduced: 1976

Brand Names

USA	Canada
Tolectin (McNeil)	Tolectin (McNeil)
Tolectin DS (McNeil)	

Common Synonyms ("Street Names"):   Arthritis medicine, aspirin substitute

Drug Class: Analgesic, Mild, Anti-inflammatory, Fever Reducer (Antipyretic)

Prescription Required: Yes

Available for Purchase by Generic Name: No

Available Dosage Forms and Strengths
Tablets — 200 mg.
Capsules — 400 mg.

Tablet May Be Crushed or Capsule Opened for Administration: Yes

How This Drug Works
Intended Therapeutic Effect(s):   Relief of joint pain, stiffness, inflammation, and swelling associated with arthritis.

Location of Drug Action(s):   Not completely established. This drug may act in the brain (at the level of the hypothalamus) as well as in the inflamed tissues of arthritic joints.

Method of Drug Action(s):   Not completely known. It is thought that this drug reduces the tissue concentration of prostaglandins, chemicals involved in the production of inflammation and pain.

Principal Uses of This Drug

As a Single Drug Product: This "aspirin substitute" is used primarily to provide symptomatic relief in acute and chronic arthritis, including juvenile arthritis. It is also used to relieve the pain associated with bursitis and tendinitis of the shoulder and similar inflammatory conditions.

THIS DRUG SHOULD NOT BE TAKEN IF

—you have had an allergic reaction to any dosage form of it previously.
—you are allergic to aspirin (hives, nasal polyps, and/or asthma caused by aspirin).
—you have a bleeding disorder.
—you have an active stomach ulcer or active ulcerative colitis.
—you have severe impairment of liver or kidney function.
—it has been prescribed for a child under 12 years of age.

INFORM YOUR PHYSICIAN BEFORE TAKING THIS DRUG IF

—you are allergic to fenoprofen (Nalfon), ibuprofen (Motrin), indomethacin (Indocin), or naproxen (Naprosyn).
—you have a history of peptic ulcer disease or ulcerative colitis.
—you have a history of heart disease.
—you have impaired kidney function.
—you are taking any kind of anticoagulant drug (see Drug Class, Section Three).
—you are presently under treatment for an active infection of any kind.

Time Required for Apparent Benefit

Drug action begins within 30 to 60 minutes and persists for 2 to 4 hours. Significant improvement may require continuous use on a regular schedule for 1 to 2 weeks.

Possible Side-Effects *(natural, expected, and unavoidable drug actions)*

Drowsiness in sensitive individuals.

Possible Adverse Effects *(unusual, unexpected, and infrequent reactions)*

IF ANY OF THE FOLLOWING DEVELOP, DISCONTINUE DRUG AND NOTIFY YOUR PHYSICIAN AS SOON AS POSSIBLE

Mild Adverse Effects
Allergic Reactions: Skin rashes (various kinds), hives, itching.
Other Reactions
Headache, lightheadedness, dizziness, ringing in the ears.
Indigestion, heartburn, nausea, vomiting, constipation.
Serious Adverse Effects
Stomach and/or intestinal bleeding.
Impaired formation of white blood cells (granulocytes) with resulting reduction in resistance to infections.
Possible Delayed Adverse Effects
Mild anemia due to "silent" blood loss from the stomach (less than that caused by aspirin).

CAUTION
1. Do not exceed a dose of 2.0 grams (2000 mg.) per 24 hours.
2. The optimal dosage schedule must be determined for each person individually. Dosage should always be limited to the smallest amount that produces reasonable improvement.
3. This drug's anti-inflammatory and antipyretic effects can make it more difficult to recognize the presence of infection. If you develop any symptoms that suggest an active infection, inform your physician promptly.

Precautions for Use by Those over 60 Years of Age
It is advisable to begin treatment with small doses until individual tolerance and response have been determined. Limit dosage to the smallest amount that produces reasonable improvement.

Sudden gain in weight or the development of swelling of the feet and ankles may indicate the excessive retention of water in body tissues (edema). Inform your physician promptly of these developments.

You may be more susceptible to the development of headache, dizziness, stomach ulcer, stomach bleeding, and constipation.

Advisability of Use During Pregnancy
Pregnancy Category: B (tentative). See Pregnancy Code inside back cover. Animal reproduction studies reveal no birth defects due to this drug. Information from adequate studies in pregnant women is not available. Ask physician for guidance.

Advisability of Use While Nursing Infant
The presence of this drug in milk is not known. Ask physician for guidance.

Habit-Forming Potential
None apparent to date.

Effects of Overdosage
With Moderate Overdose: Stomach irritation, nausea, vomiting, diarrhea.

With Large Overdose: No serious or threatening effects reported to date.

Possible Effects of Extended Use
None reported.

Suggested Periodic Examinations While Taking This Drug (at physician's discretion)
Complete blood cell counts.
Kidney function tests.
Liver function tests.
Eye examinations for possible changes in the lens.

While Taking This Drug, Observe the Following
Foods: This drug should be taken with or immediately following food if stomach irritation occurs. However, it is more effective if it is taken 1 hour before or 2 hours after eating.

Beverages: This drug may be taken with milk. Some "herbal teas" (promoted as being beneficial for arthritis) contain phenylbutazone and other potentially toxic ingredients. Avoid "herbal teas" if you are not certain of their source, content, and medicinal effects.

Alcohol: Use with caution. The irritant action of alcohol on the stomach lining, added to the irritant action of tolmetin in sensitive individuals, can increase the risk of stomach bleeding and/or ulceration.

Tobacco Smoking: No interactions expected.

Marijuana Smoking

Occasional (once or twice weekly):   No effect to mild increase in pain relief from this drug.

Daily: Moderate increase in pain relief from this drug.

Other Drugs

Tolmetin may *increase* the effects of

• anticoagulant drugs (see Drug Class, Section Three), because it prolongs the bleeding time. (Tolmetin does *not* increase the prothrombin time.)

The following drugs may *decrease* the effects of tolmetin

• aspirin and aspirin-containing compounds. (Tolmetin and aspirin should *not* be taken concurrently.)

Driving a Vehicle, Operating Machinery, Engaging in Hazardous Activities: This drug can cause lightheadedness and/or dizziness in sensitive individuals. Use caution until its full effects have been determined.

Aviation Note: The use of this drug *may be a disqualification* for the piloting of aircraft. Consultation with a designated Aviation Medical Examiner is advised.

Exposure to Sun: No restrictions.

Heavy Exercise or Exertion: Follow physician's instructions.

Occurrence of Unrelated Illness: This drug may mask the usual symptoms that indicate the presence of infections. Consult your physician promptly if you suspect that you may be developing an infection of any kind.

Discontinuation: This drug may be discontinued abruptly without danger. However, it may be necessary to adjust the doses of other drugs taken concurrently with it. Consult your physician.

Special Storage Instructions

Keep in a dry, tightly closed container. Protect from light.

TRANYLCYPROMINE

Year Introduced: 1961

Brand Names

USA	Canada
Parnate (Smith Kline & French)	Parnate (SK&F)

Common Synonyms ("Street Names"):   None

Drug Class: Antidepressant, Mono-amine Oxidase Inhibitors

Prescription Required: Yes

Available for Purchase by Generic Name: No

Available Dosage Forms and Strengths
Tablets — 10 mg.

Tablet May Be Crushed or Capsule Opened for Administration: Yes

How This Drug Works
   Intended Therapeutic Effect(s):   Gradual relief of emotional depression and improvement of mood.
   Location of Drug Action(s):   Those areas of the brain that determine mood and emotional stability.
   Method of Drug Action(s):   Not completely established. It is thought that by inhibiting the action of a certain enzyme (mono-amine oxidase) in brain tissue, this drug produces an increase of those nerve impulse transmitters that maintain normal mood and emotional stability.

Principal Uses of This Drug
   As a Single Drug Product: This potent MAO inhibitor drug is used exclusively to treat severe situational (reactive) depression and severe spontaneous (endogenous) depression. Because of the supervision required during its use and its potential for adverse effects, this drug is usually reserved to treat depressions that have not responded satisfactorily to other antidepressant therapy.

THIS DRUG SHOULD NOT BE TAKEN IF
—you have had an allergic reaction to it previously.
—you have advanced heart disease.
—you have liver disease or impaired liver function.
—you have an adrenalin-producing tumor (pheochromocytoma).
—you are now taking any of the following drugs:

amitriptyline (Elavil, etc.)
amitriptyline + perphenazine (Etrafon)
carbamazepine (Tegretol, etc.)
desipramine (Norpramin, Pertofrane)
doxepin (Adapin, Sinequan)
furazolidone (Furoxone)
imipramine (Imavate, Presamine, SK-Pramine, Tofranil, etc.)

isocarboxazid (Marplan)
nialamide (Niamid)
nortriptyline (Aventyl, Pamelor)
pargyline (Eutonyl)
pargyline + methyclothiazide (Eutron)
phenylzine (Nardil)
protriptyline (Vivactil)

INFORM YOUR PHYSICIAN BEFORE TAKING THIS DRUG IF
—you have high blood pressure.
—you have had a stroke, or have impaired circulation to the brain.
—you have coronary heart disease, with or without angina.

—you have frequent or severe headaches.
—you have diabetes.
—you have epilepsy.
—you have schizophrenia.
—you have overactive thyroid function (hyperthyroidism).
—you have impaired kidney function.
—you plan to have surgery under general or spinal anesthesia in the near future.

Time Required for Apparent Benefit

Improvement can occur within 2 days, or it may require continuous treatment on a regular schedule for up to 3 weeks.

Possible Side-Effects *(natural, expected, and unavoidable drug actions)*

Insomnia if taken in the evening.

Lightheadedness, dizziness, weakness, feeling of impending faint in upright position (see orthostatic hypotension in Glossary).

Possible Adverse Effects *(unusual, unexpected, and infrequent reactions)*

IF ANY OF THE FOLLOWING DEVELOP, DISCONTINUE DRUG AND NOTIFY YOUR PHYSICIAN AS SOON AS POSSIBLE

Mild Adverse Effects
Allergic Reactions: Skin rash.
Other Reactions
  Headache, vertigo, agitation, confusion, impaired memory, tremors, muscle twitching, blurred vision.
  Dryness of mouth, loss of appetite, indigestion, constipation.

Serious Adverse Effects
Allergic Reactions: Hepatitis with jaundice (see Glossary).
Other Reactions
  Rapid and extreme rise in blood pressure (hypertensive crisis)—severe throbbing headache, palpitation, nausea, vomiting, sweating, risk of brain hemorrhage.
  Disturbances of heart rate and rhythm.
  Impairment of red-green color vision.
  Impairment of sexual potency and performance.

Natural Diseases or Disorders That May Be Activated by This Drug
Latent schizophrenia.
This drug may convert a depression into the manic phase of a manic-depressive psychosis.

CAUTION

1. Careful dosage adjustment is mandatory. Determine the lowest effective dose and do not exceed it.
2. The development of headache or palpitation may indicate a dangerous elevation of blood pressure. Discontinue this drug immediately and consult your physician.
3. This drug may suppress angina pain that would normally serve as a warning of excessive demand on the heart.

4. This drug may increase the possibility of hypoglycemic reactions if used concurrently with insulin or oral anti-diabetic drugs (see Drug Class, Section Three). It can also delay recovery from hypoglycemia (see Glossary).
5. This drug can alter the threshold for convulsions in anyone with epilepsy or a seizure disorder. The dosage of any anticonvulsant drug taken concurrently may require adjustment.
6. This drug should be discontinued 1 to 2 weeks before elective surgery under general or spinal anesthesia.
7. Many over-the-counter (OTC) drugs (see Glossary) contain ingredients that can cause serious interactions if taken concurrently with this drug. Avoid the use of OTC cold remedies, hay fever remedies, and weight-reducing preparations until you have consulted your physician regarding their safe use with this drug.
8. It is advisable to carry a card of personal identification with a notation that you are taking this drug (see Table 19 and Section Six).

Precautions for Use by Those over 60 Years of Age
Not recommended for use by anyone over 60 years of age. However, if poor response to other treatment justifies consideration of a trial with this drug, it is inadvisable to use it in the presence of high blood pressure, hardening of the arteries, impaired circulation to the brain, or coronary heart disease.

If you have an enlarged prostate gland that is impairing your ability to urinate (prostatism), this drug may cause an inability to empty the bladder.

Sensitive individuals in this age group may develop marked swelling of the feet, ankles, and lower legs while taking this drug.

Advisability of Use During Pregnancy
Pregnancy Category: B (tentative). See Pregnancy Code inside back cover. Animal reproduction studies reveal no birth defects due to this drug. Information from adequate studies in pregnant women is not available. Ask physician for guidance.

Advisability of Use While Nursing Infant
This drug is known to be present in milk. Ask physician for guidance.

Habit-Forming Potential
This drug is related to amphetamine and can produce a mild euphoriant effect. A few instances of dependence have been reported.

Effects of Overdosage
With Moderate Overdose: Overstimulation, agitation, restlessness, anxiety, excessive activity and talking, insomnia, rapid heart rate.

With Large Overdose: Mental confusion, delirium, hallucinations, twitching, convulsions, high fever, labored breathing, circulatory collapse, coma.

Possible Effects of Extended Use
The conversion of mental depression into a state of hypomania—excessive mental and physical activity, excitement, agitation, loud and rapid talking, delusional thinking.

Suggested Periodic Examinations While Taking This Drug (at physician's discretion)

Frequent measurements of blood pressure in lying, sitting, and standing positions.

White blood cell counts.

Blood sodium levels.

Liver function tests.

While Taking This Drug, Observe the Following

Foods: The following tyramine-rich foods should be avoided completely (see tyramine in Glossary):

Aged cheeses of all kinds*

Avocado

Banana skins

Beef liver (unless fresh and used at once)

"Bovril" extract

Broad bean pods

Chicken liver (unless fresh and used at once)

Chocolate

Figs, canned

Fish, dried and salted

Herring, pickled

"Marmite" extract

Meat extracts

Meat tenderizers

Raisins

Raspberries

Soy sauce

Yeast extracts

Note: Any high-protein food that is aged or has undergone breakdown by putrefaction probably contains tyramine and could produce a hypertensive crisis in anyone taking this drug.

Beverages: The following tyramine-rich beverages should be avoided completely:

Beer (unpasteurized)

Chianti wine

Sherry wine

Sour cream

Vermouth

Note: Limit coffee, tea, and cola beverages to one serving daily.

Alcohol: Use extreme caution until combined effect has been determined. Alcohol can increase the depressant effect of this drug on brain function in sensitive individuals.

Tobacco Smoking: No interactions expected.

Marijuana Smoking

Occasional (once or twice weekly):   No interactions expected.

Daily: Increased tendency to orthostatic hypotension (see Glossary); possible reduced effectiveness of this drug.

Other Drugs

Tranylcypromine may *increase* the effects of

• acetazolamide (Diamox).

• amphetamine and amphetamine-like drugs.

• oral anticoagulants (see WARFARIN *Drug Profile*).

*Cottage cheese, cream cheese, and processed cheese are safe to eat.

- oral anti-diabetic drugs (Diabinese, Dymelor, Orinase, Tolinase).
- antihistamines.
- anti-hypertensives (some).
- barbiturates, and cause excessive sedation.
- carisoprodol (Rela, Soma), and cause excessive relaxation.
- chloral hydrate (Noctec, Somnos, etc), and cause excessive sedation.
- chlordiazepoxide (Librium), and cause excessive sedation.
- clorazepate (Tranxene), and cause excessive sedation.
- diazepam (Valium), and cause excessive sedation.
- ephedrine, and cause excessive stimulation.
- epinephrine (Adrenalin) by injection, and cause excessive rise in blood pressure.
- ethchlorvynol (Placidyl), and cause excessive sedation.
- flurazepam (Dalmane), and cause excessive sedation.
- narcotic analgesics: codeine, meperidine (Demerol), morphine, etc., and cause excessive depression of vital brain functions.
- oxazepam (Serax), and cause excessive sedation.
- phenothiazines, and increase their ability to lower the blood pressure.
- phenylephrine (Neo-Synephrine, etc.), and cause excessive rise in blood pressure.
- phenylpropanolamine (Propadrine, etc.), and cause excessive rise in blood pressure.
- primidone (Mysoline), and require adjustment of dosage to prevent toxicity.
- pseudoephedrine (Sudafed), and cause excessive stimulation.

Tranylcypromine *taken concurrently* with
- anti-parkinsonism drugs, may cause tremors and heavy sweating.
- atropine and atropine-like drugs, may increase their potential for toxicity.
- carbamazepine (Tegretol), may cause severe toxic reactions.
- chloroquine (Aralen), may enhance its toxic effects.
- chlorphentermine (Pre-Sate), may cause excessive stimulation.
- diethylpropion (Tenuate, Tepanil), may cause excessive stimulation.
- fenfluramine (Pondimin), may cause excessive stimulation.
- glutethimide (Doriden, etc.), may cause excessive sedation, coma, and respiratory arrest.
- guanethidine (Ismelin), may cause acute hypertensive crisis.
- haloperidol (Haldol), may cause excessive depression of vital brain functions.
- levodopa (Dopar, Larodopa, etc.), may cause a dangerous rise in blood pressure.
- methyldopa (Aldomet), may cause a dangerous rise in blood pressure.
- methylphenidate (Ritalin), may cause severe headache, weakness, and numbness in extremities.
- other mono-amine oxidase inhibitor (MAO) drugs (see Drug Class, Section Three) can cause acute hypertensive crisis, high fever, respiratory failure, and death.

Allow a drug-free interval of 2 weeks between discontinuing one MAOI and starting another.
- phenmetrazine (Preludin), may cause excessive stimulation.
- quinacrine (Atabrine), may enhance its toxic effects—skin eruptions, bone marrow depression, eye damage.
- reserpine (Ser-Ap-Es, Serpasil, etc.), may cause a dangerous rise in blood pressure.
- tricyclic antidepressants (see Drug Class, Section Three), may cause severe toxic reactions including high fever, delirium, tremor, convulsions, coma.

The following drugs may *increase* the effects of tranylcypromine:
- over-the-counter (OTC) cold and hayfever remedies that contain decongestants.
- over-the-counter (OTC) appetite-control (weight reduction) preparations containing phenylpropanolamine.
- propranolol (Inderal).

Driving a Vehicle, Operating Machinery, Engaging in Hazardous Activities: This drug can cause a drop in blood pressure, dizziness, and blurred vision. Avoid hazardous activities if these drug effects occur.

Aviation Note: The use of this drug and the disorder for which this drug is prescribed *are disqualifications* for the piloting of aircraft. Consultation with a designated Aviation Medical Examiner is advised.

Exposure to Sun: Use caution until sensitivity has been determined. Some drugs of this family have been reported to cause photosensitivity (see Glossary).

Heavy Exercise or Exertion: If you have angina or coronary heart disease, avoid excessive exertion. This drug can suppress the development of angina that would normally serve as a warning that you have exceeded your heart's tolerance for physical activity.

Occurrence of Unrelated Illness: Because of the very serious and life-threatening interactions that can occur between this drug and many others, it is mandatory that you inform each physician and dentist you consult that you are taking a mono-amine oxidase inhibiting drug.

Discontinuation: If this drug is not effective after 4 weeks of continuous use, it should be discontinued. If it is effective, continue to take it in proper dosage until advised to stop. It is inadvisable to discontinue it abruptly. If another mono-amine oxidase inhibitor or a tricyclic antidepressant is to be tried, a drug-free waiting period of 14 days must elapse between the discontinuation of this drug and initiation of the new one.

Special Storage Instructions
Keep in a dry, tightly closed container at room temperature.

TRAZODONE

Year Introduced: 1967

Brand Names

USA	Canada
Desyrel (Mead Johnson)	Desyrel (Bristol)

Common Synonyms ("Street Names"):   Depression pills

Drug Class: Antidepressants

Prescription Required: USA: Yes   Canada: Yes

Available for Purchase by Generic Name: USA: No   Canada: No

Available Dosage Forms and Strengths
Tablets — 50 mg., 100 mg.

Tablet May Be Crushed or Capsule Opened for Administration: Yes

How This Drug Works
Intended Therapeutic Effect(s):   Gradual improvement of mood and relief of emotional depression.
Location of Drug Action(s):   Those areas of the brain that determine mood and emotional stability.
Method of Drug Action(s):   Not fully established. It is thought that this drug increases the availability of the nerve impulse transmitter serotonin in the brain and thereby relieves the symptoms of depression.

Principal Uses of This Drug
As a Single Drug Product: To provide symptomatic relief in all types of depression, with or without anxiety; to initiate the restoration of normal mood.

THIS DRUG SHOULD NOT BE TAKEN IF
—you have had an allergic reaction to it previously.
—you are taking or have taken within the past 14 days any mono-amine oxidase (MAO) inhibitor drug (see Drug Class, Section Three).
—you are recovering from a recent heart attack.
—it is prescribed for a child under 18 years of age.

INFORM YOUR PHYSICIAN BEFORE TAKING THIS DRUG IF
—you have a history of any of the following: alcoholism, epilepsy, heart disease (especially heart rhythm disturbances), impaired liver or kidney function.
—you plan to have surgery under general anesthesia in the near future.
—you are taking any anti-hypertensive drug for high blood pressure.

Time Required for Apparent Benefit
Drug action usually begins in 30 minutes and reaches its peak in 1 hour if fasting, and 2 hours if taken with food. Continuous use on a regular schedule for 14 to 21 days is usually necessary to determine this drug's effectiveness

in relieving depression. However, benefit may be apparent within 1 week in some individuals.

Possible Side-Effects *(natural, expected, and unavoidable drug actions)*
Drowsiness, lightheadedness, blurring of vision, dryness of mouth, constipation.

Possible Adverse Effects *(unusual, unexpected, and infrequent reactions)*

IF ANY OF THE FOLLOWING DEVELOP, DISCONTINUE DRUG AND NOTIFY YOUR PHYSICIAN AS SOON AS POSSIBLE

Mild Adverse Effects
  Allergic Reactions: Skin rash.
  Other Reactions: Headache, dizziness, fatigue, decreased concentration, nervousness, tremors.
    Rapid heart beat, palpitations.
    Peculiar taste, stomach discomfort, nausea, vomiting, diarrhea.
    Altered libido, muscular aches and pains.
Serious Adverse Effects
  Behavioral effects: Confusion, anger, hostility, disorientation, impaired memory, delusions, nightmares.
  Irregular heart rhythms, fainting.
  Altered menstrual pattern; prolonged, painful erection of penis (priapism).

CAUTION
1. The dosage of this drug should be adjusted carefully for each person individually.
2. It is advisable to withhold this drug if electroconvulsive therapy (ECT) is to be used.

Precautions for Use by Infants and Children
Safety and effectiveness in children below 18 years of age have not been established.

Precautions for Use by Those over 60 Years of Age
During the first 2 weeks of treatment observe for the development of confusional reactions—restlessness, agitation, excitement, forgetfulness, confusion, disorientation. Reduction of dosage or discontinuation may be necessary.
Observe for unsteadiness and incoordination which may predispose to falling and injury.
This drug may increase the degree of impaired urination associated with prostate gland enlargement (prostatism).

Advisability of Use During Pregnancy
Pregnancy Category: C (tentative). See Pregnancy Code inside back cover.
  Animal reproduction studies reveal fetal death and birth defects in the newborn.
  Information from adequate studies in pregnant women is not available.
  Avoid completely during the first 3 months.
  Ask physician for guidance.

Advisability of Use While Nursing Infant
This drug is probably present in human milk. Nursing may be permitted with careful observation of the infant for drowsiness or failure to feed. Ask physician for guidance.

Habit-Forming Potential
None.

Effects of Overdosage
With Moderate Overdose: Marked drowsiness, confusion, weakness, low blood pressure, tremors.

With Large Overdose: Stupor, coma, possible convulsions, rapid heart rate, possible heart rhythm irregularity, low blood pressure.

Possible Effects of Extended Use
None reported.

Suggested Periodic Examinations While Taking This Drug (at physician's discretion)
Complete blood cell counts. (This drug may cause slight reductions in white blood cell counts. This should be monitored closely if infection, sore throat or fever develops.)

Serial blood pressure readings and electrocardiograms.

While Taking This Drug, Observe the Following
Foods: No restrictions. Best taken with food to improve absorption.

Beverages: No restrictions. May be taken with milk.

Alcohol: Avoid completely. This drug can increase markedly the intoxicating effects of alcohol and accentuate its depressant action on brain function.

Tobacco Smoking: No interactions expected.

Marijuana Smoking

Occasional (once or twice weekly): Transient increase in drowsiness and dryness of the mouth.

Daily: Persistent drowsiness, increased dryness of the mouth, possible reduced effectiveness of this drug.

Other Drugs

Trazodone may *increase* the effects of

- anti-hypertensive drugs and cause excessive lowering of the blood pressure. Dosage adjustments may be necessary.
- atropine-like drugs (see Drug Class, Section Three).
- digoxin (Lanoxin) by raising its blood level. Observe closely for digitalis toxicity.
- phenytoin (Dilantin) by raising its blood level. Observe closely for phenytoin toxicity.
- sedatives, sleep-inducing drugs, tranquilizers, antihistamines, and narcotic drugs, and cause oversedation. Dosage adjustments may be necessary.

Driving a Vehicle, Operating Machinery, Engaging in Hazardous Activities:
This drug may impair mental alertness, judgment, physical coordination and reaction time. Avoid hazardous activities.

Aviation Note: The use of this drug *is a disqualification* for the piloting of aircraft. Consultation with a designated Aviation Medical Examiner is advised.

Exposure to Sun: No restrictions.

Exposure to Heat: Caution advised until the combined effect has been determined. This drug may inhibit sweating in some individuals and impair the body's adaptation to hot environments, increasing the risk of heat stroke. Use saunas cautiously.

Exposure to Cold: The elderly should use caution to avoid conditions that could cause hypothermia.

Occurrence of Unrelated Illness: In any condition that tends to lower the blood pressure, this drug may exaggerate the response and cause additional reduction of pressure beyond the expected.

Discontinuation: It is advisable to discontinue this drug gradually. Ask physician for guidance in dosage reduction over an appropriate period of time. When this drug is discontinued, it may be necessary to adjust the doses of other drugs taken concurrently.

Special Storage Instructions

Keep tablets in a dry, tightly closed container at room temperature. Protect from light.

TRIAMCINOLONE

Year Introduced: 1958

Brand Names

USA	Canada
Aristocort (Lederle)	Aristocort (Lederle)
Kenacort (Squibb)	Aristospan (Lederle)
	Kenacort (Squibb)
	Trialean (Organon)
	Triamacort (ICN)

Common Synonyms ("Street Names"):   Cortisone medicine

Drug Class: Cortisone-like Drug, Adrenocortical Steroids

Prescription Required: Yes

Available for Purchase by Generic Name: USA: Yes   Canada: No

Available Dosage Forms and Strengths

Tablets — 1 mg., 2 mg., 4 mg., 8 mg., 16 mg.
Syrup — 2 mg. and 4 mg. per teaspoonful (5 ml.)
Cream — 0.025%, 0.1%, 0.5%
Ointment — 0.1%, 0.5%

Tablet May Be Crushed or Capsule Opened for Administration: Yes

How This Drug Works

Intended Therapeutic Effect(s):   The symptomatic relief of inflammation (swelling, redness, heat and pain) in any tissue, and from many causes. (Cortisone-like drugs do not correct the underlying disease process).

Location of Drug Action(s):   Significant biological effects occur in most tissues throughout the body. The principal actions of therapeutic doses occur at sites of inflammation and/or allergic reaction, regardless of the nature of the causative injury or illness.

Method of Drug Action(s):   Not completely established. Present thinking is that cortisone-like drugs probably inhibit several mechanisms within the tissues that induce inflammation. Well-regulated dosage aids the body in restoring normal stability. However, prolonged use or excessive dosage can impair the body's defense mechanisms against infectious disease.

Principal Uses of This Drug

As a Single Drug Product: This member of the cortisone class of drugs is used to treat a wide variety of allergic and inflammatory conditions. It is used primarily in the management of serious skin disorders, bronchial asthma, regional enteritis, ulcerative colitis, and all types of major rheumatic disorders including most forms of arthritis, bursitis, tendinitis, and related conditions.

THIS DRUG SHOULD NOT BE TAKEN IF

—you have had an allergic reaction to any dosage form of it previously.
—you have an active peptic ulcer (stomach or duodenum).
—you have an active infection of the eye caused by the herpes simplex virus (ask your eye doctor for guidance).
—you have active tuberculosis.

INFORM YOUR PHYSICIAN BEFORE TAKING THIS DRUG IF

—you have had an unfavorable reaction to any cortisone-like drug in the past.
—you have a history of tuberculosis.
—you have diabetes or a tendency to diabetes.
—you have a history of peptic ulcer disease.
—you have glaucoma or a tendency to glaucoma.
—you have a deficiency of thyroid function (hypothyroidism).
—you have high blood pressure.
—you have myasthenia gravis.
—you have a history of thrombophlebitis.
—you plan to have surgery of any kind in the near future, especially if under general anesthesia.

Time Required for Apparent Benefit

Evidence of beneficial drug action is usually apparent in 24 to 48 hours. Dosage must be individualized to give reasonable improvement. This is usually accomplished in 4 to 10 days. It is unwise to demand complete relief of all symptoms. The effective dose varies with the nature of the disease and with the patient. During long-term use it is essential that the smallest effective dose be determined and maintained.

Possible Side-Effects *(natural, expected, and unavoidable drug actions)*
Flushing of the face, increased sweating, increased susceptibility to infection.

Possible Adverse Effects *(unusual, unexpected, and infrequent reactions)*

IF ANY OF THE FOLLOWING DEVELOP, DISCONTINUE DRUG AND NOTIFY YOUR PHYSICIAN AS SOON AS POSSIBLE

Mild Adverse Effects
Allergic Reactions: Skin rash.
Other Reactions
Headache, dizziness, insomnia.
Acid indigestion, abdominal distention.
Muscle cramping and weakness.
Irregular menstrual periods.
Acne, excessive growth of facial hair.

Serious Adverse Effects
Mental and emotional disturbances of serious magnitude.
Reactivation of latent tuberculosis.
Development of peptic ulcer.
Increased blood pressure.
Development of inflammation of the pancreas.
Thrombophlebitis (inflammation of a vein with the formation of blood clot)
—pain or tenderness in thigh or leg, with or without swelling of the foot, ankle, or leg.
Pulmonary embolism (movement of blood clot to the lung)—sudden shortness of breath, pain in the chest, coughing, bloody sputum.

CAUTION

1. It is advisable to carry a card of personal identification with a notation that you are taking this drug if your course of treatment is to exceed 1 week (see Table 19 and Section Six).
2. Do not discontinue this drug abruptly.
3. While taking this drug, immunization procedures should be given with caution. If vaccination against measles, smallpox, rabies, or yellow fever is required, discontinue this drug 72 hours before vaccination and do not resume for at least 14 days after vaccination.

Precautions for Use by Those over 60 Years of Age
The "cortisone-related" drugs should be used very sparingly after 60, and only when the disorder under treatment is unresponsive to adequate trials of non-cortisone drugs. Prolonged use should be avoided.
The continuous use of this drug (even in small doses) can increase the severity of diabetes, enhance fluid retention (edema), raise the blood pressure, weaken resistance to infection, induce stomach ulcer, and accelerate the development of cataract and softening of the bones (osteoporosis).
In sensitive individuals, cortisone-related drugs can cause serious emotional disturbance and disruptive behavior.

Advisability of Use During Pregnancy

Pregnancy Category: C (tentative). See Pregnancy Code inside back cover.

Animal reproduction studies in mice, rats, rabbits, and monkeys reveal significant birth defects due to this drug.

Information from adequate studies in pregnant women is not available. Ask physician for guidance.

If use of this drug is considered necessary, limit dosage and duration of use as much as possible. Following birth, the infant should be examined for possible defective function of the adrenal glands (deficiency of adrenal cortical hormones).

Advisability of Use While Nursing Infant

Drug is known to be present in milk. Ask physician for guidance.

Habit-Forming Potential

Use of this drug to suppress symptoms over an extended period of time may produce a state of functional dependence (see Glossary). In the treatment of conditions like rheumatoid arthritis and asthma, it is advisable to try alternate-day drug administration to keep the daily dose as small as possible, and to attempt drug withdrawal after periods of reasonable improvement. Such procedures may reduce the degree of "steroid rebound"—the return of symptoms as the drug is withdrawn.

Effects of Overdosage

With Moderate Overdose: Fatigue, muscle weakness, stomach irritation, acid indigestion, excessive sweating.

With Large Overdose: Marked flushing of the face, muscle cramping, emotional depression, erratic behavior.

Possible Effects of Extended Use

Development of increased blood sugar, possibly diabetes.

Increased fat deposits on the trunk of the body ("buffalo hump"), rounding of the face ("moon face"), and thinning of the arms and legs.

Thinning and fragility of the skin, easy bruising.

Loss of texture and strength of the bones, resulting in spontaneous fractures.

Development of increased internal eye pressure, possibly glaucoma.

Development of cataracts.

Retarded growth and development in children.

Suggested Periodic Examinations While Taking This Drug (at physician's discretion)

Measurement of blood potassium levels.

Measurement of blood sugar levels 2 hours after eating.

Measurement of blood pressure at regular intervals.

Complete eye examination at regular intervals.

Chest X-ray if history of previous tuberculosis.

Determination of the rate of development of the growing child to detect retardation of normal growth.

While Taking This Drug, Observe the Following

Foods: No interactions. Consult physician regarding need to restrict salt intake or to eat potassium-rich foods. During long-term use of this drug it is advisable to have a high protein diet.

Beverages: No restrictions.

Alcohol: No interactions expected.

Tobacco Smoking: Nicotine increases the blood levels of naturally-produced cortisone and related hormones. Heavy smoking may add to the expected actions of this drug and requires close observation for excessive effects.

Marijuana Smoking

Occasional (once or twice weekly):   No interactions expected.

Daily: Additional impairment of immunity due to this drug.

Other Drugs

Triamcinolone may *increase* the effects of

- barbiturates and other sedatives and sleep-inducing drugs, causing over-sedation.

Triamcinolone may *decrease* the effects of

- insulin and oral anti-diabetic drugs, by raising the level of blood sugar. Doses of anti-diabetic drugs may have to be raised.
- anticoagulants of the coumarin family. Monitor prothrombin times closely and adjust dosage accordingly.
- choline-like drugs (Mestinon, pilocarpine, Prostigmin), and reduce their effectiveness in treating glaucoma and myasthenia gravis.

Triamcinolone *taken concurrently* with

- thiazide diuretics, may cause excessive loss of potassium. Monitor blood levels of potassium on physician's advice.
- atropine-like drugs (see Drug Class, Section Three), may cause increased internal eye pressure and initiate or aggravate glaucoma.
- digitalis preparations, requires close monitoring of body potassium stores to prevent digitalis toxicity.
- stimulant drugs (Adrenalin, amphetamines, ephedrine, etc.), may increase internal eye pressure and initiate or aggravate glaucoma.

The following drugs may *increase* the effects of triamcinolone:

- indomethacin (Indocin, Indocid)
- aspirin

The following drugs may *decrease* the effects of triamcinolone:

- barbiturates
- phenytoin (Dantoin, Dilantin, etc.)
- antihistamines
- chloral hydrate (Noctec, Somnos)
- glutethimide (Doriden)
- phenylbutazone (Azolid, Butazolidin, etc.) may reduce its effectiveness following a brief, initial increase in effectiveness.
- propranolol (Inderal)

Driving a Vehicle, Operating Machinery, Engaging in Hazardous Activities:
Usually no restrictions. Be alert to the rare occurrence of dizziness; restrict
activities accordingly.

Aviation Note: The use of this drug *is a disqualification* for the piloting of
aircraft. Consultation with a designated Aviation Medical Examiner is advised.

Exposure to Sun: No restrictions.

Occurrence of Unrelated Illness

This drug may decrease natural resistance to infection. Notify your physician if you develop an infection of any kind.

This drug may reduce your body's ability to respond appropriately to the
stress of acute illness, injury, or surgery. Keep your physician fully informed of any significant changes in your state of health.

Discontinuation

If you have been taking this drug for an extended period of time, do not
discontinue it abruptly. Ask physician for guidance regarding gradual
withdrawal.

For a period of 2 years after discontinuing this drug, it is essential in the
event of illness, injury, or surgery that you inform attending medical
personnel that you used this drug in the past. The period of inadequate
response to stress following the use of cortisone-like drugs may last for
1 to 2 years.

Special Storage Instructions
Keep in a tightly closed container. Protect from light.

TRIAMTERENE

Year Introduced: 1964

Brand Names

USA	Canada
Dyrenium (Smith Kline & French)	Dyrenium (SK&F)
Dyazide [CD] (Smith Kline & French)	Dyazide [CD] (SK&F)

Common Synonyms ("Street Names"):   Water pills

Drug Class: Anti-hypertensive (Hypotensive); Diuretic

Prescription Required: Yes

Available for Purchase by Generic Name: No

Available Dosage Forms and Strengths
Capsules — 50 mg., 100 mg.

Tablet May Be Crushed or Capsule Opened for Administration: Yes

How This Drug Works
Intended Therapeutic Effect(s):   Elimination of excessive fluid retention
(edema) without loss of potassium from the body.
Location of Drug Action(s):   The tubular systems of the kidney that determine the final composition of the urine.
Method of Drug Action(s):   By increasing the elimination of salt and water
but not potassium from the body (through increased urine production), this
drug reduces the volume of fluid in the blood and body tissues and lowers
the sodium content throughout the body.

Principal Uses of This Drug
As a Single Drug Product: This relatively mild diuretic is used primarily to
relieve water retention (edema) associated with congestive heart failure,
certain types of liver and kidney disease, cortisone-induced edema, and
other less common conditions. It is used in conjunction with other forms
of appropriate therapy.
As a Combination Drug Product [CD]:   This drug is avaialble in combination with hydrochlorothiazide, another diuretic. Both of these drugs have
a mild antihypertensive effect, and the combination is used as a "step 1"
medication in the treatment of mild to moderate high blood pressure.
Triamterene, which retains potassium in the body, is combined with hydrochlorothiazide to counteract the latter's tendency to cause potassium loss
from the body.

THIS DRUG SHOULD NOT BE TAKEN IF
—you have had an allergic reaction to any dosage form of it previously.
—you have a history of severe liver or kidney disease with impaired function
of either.

INFORM YOUR PHYSICIAN BEFORE TAKING THIS DRUG IF
—you have a history of gout.
—you have diabetes.
—you are taking any form of digitalis.

Time Required for Apparent Benefit
Increased volume of urine begins in 2 hours and persists for 8 to 12 hours.
Maximal effectiveness in removing fluid from the body may require 2 to 3
days. Usefulness in treatment of high blood pressure may require regular use
for 2 to 3 weeks.

Possible Side-Effects (natural, expected, and unavoidable drug actions)
Blue coloration of the urine, of no significance. Usually no other side-effects,
unless there is *excessive* loss of salt and water from the body or *excessive*
retention of potassium (see Effects of Overdosage, below).

Possible Adverse Effects *(unusual, unexpected, and infrequent reactions)*

IF ANY OF THE FOLLOWING DEVELOP, DISCONTINUE DRUG AND NOTIFY
YOUR PHYSICIAN AS SOON AS POSSIBLE

Mild Adverse Effects
   Allergic Reactions: Skin rash.
   Other Reactions
      Nausea, vomiting, diarrhea, dryness of mouth.
      Headache, weakness, dizziness.
Serious Adverse Effects
   Allergic Reactions: Anaphylactic reaction (see Glossary).
   Other Reactions: Bone marrow depression (see Glossary), resulting in
   anemia.

CAUTION
It is not advisable to use potassium supplements or to deliberately increase
your intake of potassium-rich foods while using this diuretic drug.

Precautions for Use by Those over 60 Years of Age
The natural decline in kidney function that occurs after 60 may predispose
to excessive retention of potassium in the body. It is advisable to limit the
use of this drug to periods of 2 to 3 weeks.
You may be more sensitive to the actions of this drug. Small doses are advisable until your individual response has been determined.
If you are taking this drug to treat high blood pressure, remember that warm
weather and fever can reduce your blood pressure and make it necessary
to adjust your dosage.
Overdosage and extended use of this drug can cause excessive loss of body
water, thickening (increased viscosity) of the blood, and an increased tendency of the blood to clot, predisposing to stroke, heart attack, or thrombophlebitis.

Advisability of Use During Pregnancy
Pregnancy Category: B (tentative). See Pregnancy Code inside back cover.
Animal reproduction studies reveal no birth defects due to this drug.
Information from adequate studies in pregnant women is not available.
Ask physician for guidance.

Advisability of Use While Nursing Infant
Drug is known to be present in milk. Ask physician for guidance.

Habit-Forming Potential
None.

Effects of Overdosage
With Moderate Overdose: Imbalance of body water, salt, and potassium,
causing drowsiness, fatigue, weakness, nausea, vomiting, thirst.
With Large Overdose: Marked lethargy, irregular heart action.

Possible Effects of Extended Use

Retention of potassium in the body, resulting in blood potassium levels above the normal range. This can have an adverse effect on the regulation of heart rhythm and performance.

Suggested Periodic Examinations While Taking This Drug (at physician's discretion)

Complete blood cell counts.
Liver function tests.
Kidney function tests.
Measurement of blood sodium, chloride, and potassium levels.

While Taking This Drug, Observe the Following

Foods: Do not restrict the intake of salt (or salted foods) unless directed to do so by your physician.

Beverages: No restrictions.

Alcohol: No interactions expected.

Tobacco Smoking: No interactions expected.

Marijuana Smoking

Occasional (once or twice weekly):   No effect to mild increase in thirst and/or urinary frequency.

Daily: Moderate increase in thirst and/or urinary frequency; possible accentuation of orthostatic hypotension (see Glossary).

Other Drugs

Triamterene may *increase* the effects of

• other anti-hypertensive drugs. Dosage adjustments are necessary to avoid excessive lowering of blood pressure.

Triamterene may *decrease* the effects of

• oral anti-diabetic drugs. Ask for guidance regarding dosage adjustments to insure proper diabetic control.

• digitalis preparations, if excessive potassium is retained in the body.

Triamterene *taken concurrently* with

• spironolactone, may cause excessive (dangerous) retention of potassium in the body. Concurrent use of these two drugs should be avoided.

Driving a Vehicle, Operating Machinery, Engaging in Hazardous Activities: No restrictions unless drowsiness or dizziness occurs.

Aviation Note: Serious cardiovascular disorders *are a disqualification* for the piloting of aircraft. Consultation with a designated Aviation Medical Examiner is advised.

Exposure to Sun: Use caution until sensitivity has been determined. This drug may cause photosensitivity (see Glossary).

Heavy Exercise or Exertion: Isometric exercises—the "overload" technique for strengthening individual muscles—can raise the blood pressure significantly. Ask your physician for guidance regarding participation in this form of exercise.

Discontinuation: This drug should be discontinued gradually to prevent a rapid loss of potassium from the body that could occur with sudden discontinuation. Consult physician for guidance regarding the need to adjust the dosage schedule of the following drugs taken concurrently with triamterene: anti-diabetic drugs, anti-hypertensives, digitalis preparations.

Special Storage Instructions
Keep in a dry, tightly closed, light-resistant container.

TRIFLUOPERAZINE

Year Introduced: 1958

Brand Names

USA		Canada
Stelazine (Smith Kline & French)	Apo-Trifluoparazine (Apotex)	Stelazine (SK&F)
Suprazine (Major)	Novoflurazine (Novopharm)	Terfluzine (ICN)
	Solazine (Horner)	Triflurin (Technilab)

Common Synonyms ("Street Names"):   None

Drug Class: Tranquilizer, Strong (Anti-psychotic), Phenothiazines

Prescription Required: Yes

Available for Purchase by Generic Name: Yes

Available Dosage Forms and Strengths
Tablets — 1 mg., 2 mg., 5 mg., 10 mg.
Concentrate — 10 mg. per ml.
Injection — 2 mg. per ml.

Tablet May Be Crushed or Capsule Opened for Administration: Yes

How This Drug Works
Intended Therapeutic Effect(s):   Restoration of emotional calm. Relief of severe anxiety, agitation, and psychotic behavior.

Location of Drug Action(s):   Those nerve pathways in the brain that utilize the tissue chemical dopamine for the transmission of nerve impulses.

Method of Drug Action(s):   Not completely established. Present theory is that by inhibiting the action of dopamine, this drug acts to correct an imbalance of nerve impulse transmissions that is thought to be responsible for certain mental disorders.

Principal Uses of This Drug
As a Single Drug Product: This phenothiazine drug is used primarily in the management of patients with schizophrenic or manic psychoses. It is most effective in those who are withdrawn and apathetic and in those with delusions, hallucinations, and agitation.

THIS DRUG SHOULD NOT BE TAKEN IF
—you have had an allergic reaction to any dosage form of it previously.
—you have a blood or bone marrow disorder.
—you have impaired liver function.

INFORM YOUR PHYSICIAN BEFORE TAKING THIS DRUG IF
—you are allergic or sensitive to any phenothiazine drug (see Drug Class, Section Three).
—you are taking any sedatives, sleep-inducing drugs, other tranquilizers, antidepressants, antihistamines, or narcotic drugs of any kind.
—you have angina (coronary heart disease).
—you have epilepsy.
—you have glaucoma.
—you have a lung disorder, especially asthma or emphysema.
—you plan to have surgery under general or spinal anesthesia in the near future.

Time Required for Apparent Benefit
Approximately 1 to 2 hours. In treating nervous and mental disorders, maximal benefit may require regular use for several weeks.

Possible Side-Effects *(natural, expected, and unavoidable drug actions)*
Drowsiness, blurring of vision, nasal congestion, dryness of mouth, constipation, impaired urination.

Possible Adverse Effects *(unusual, unexpected, and infrequent reactions)*
IF ANY OF THE FOLLOWING DEVELOP, DISCONTINUE DRUG AND NOTIFY YOUR PHYSICIAN AS SOON AS POSSIBLE

Mild Adverse Effects
  Allergic Reactions: Skin rashes (various kinds), hives, low-grade fever.
  Other Reactions
    Dizziness, fatigue, weakness.
    Agitation, restlessness, insomnia.
    Menstrual irregularity, breast congestion, milk formation.
Serious Adverse Effects
  Parkinson-like disorders (see Glossary).
  Spasms of the muscles of the face, neck, back, and extremities, causing rolling of the eyes, grimacing, clamping of the jaw, protrusion of the tongue, difficulty in swallowing, arching of the back, cramping of the hands and feet.

CAUTION
1. Many over-the-counter (OTC) medications (see Glossary) for allergies, colds, and coughs contain drugs that can interact unfavorably with this drug. Ask your physician or pharmacist for guidance before using any such medications.
2. Antacids that contain aluminum and/or magnesium can prevent the absorption of this drug and reduce its effectiveness.
3. Obtain prompt evaluation of any disturbance or change in vision.

Precautions for Use by Those over 60 Years of Age

You may be more sensitive to all of the actions of this drug. Small doses are advisable until your individual response has been determined.

You may be more susceptible to the development of drowsiness, lethargy, constipation, lowering of body temperature (hypothermia), and excessive drop in blood pressure on arising from lying or sitting position (see orthostatic hypotension in Glossary).

This drug can increase the degree of impaired urination associated with prostate gland enlargement (prostatism).

You may also be more susceptible to the development of Parkinson-like disorders and/or tardive dyskinesia (see discussion of these terms in Glossary). These conditions must be recognized early since they may become unresponsive to treatment and irreversible. Consult your physician promptly if suggestive symptoms develop.

Advisability of Use During Pregnancy

Pregnancy Category: C (tentative). See Pregnancy Code inside back cover.

Animal reproduction studies in mice and rats reveal significant birth defects due to this drug.

Information from studies in pregnant women indicates no increase in defects in 700 exposures to this drug.

It is advisable to avoid use of this drug during first 3 months.

Ask physician for guidance.

Advisability of Use While Nursing Infant

Drug is known to be present in milk. Ask physician for guidance.

Habit-Forming Potential

None.

Effects of Overdosage

With Moderate Overdose: Marked drowsiness, weakness, tremor, restlessness, agitation.

With Large Overdose: Stupor, deep sleep, coma, convulsions.

Possible Effects of Extended Use

Tardive dyskinesia (see Glossary).

Suggested Periodic Examinations While Taking This Drug (at physician's discretion)

Complete blood cell counts, especially during first 3 months of treatment.

Careful inspection of the tongue for early evidence of fine, involuntary, wave-like movements that could indicate the beginning of tardive dyskinesia.

While Taking This Drug, Observe the Following

Foods: No restrictions.

Beverages: No restrictions.

Alcohol: Use with extreme caution until combined effect has been determined. Alcohol can increase the sedative action of trifluoperazine and accentuate its depressant effects on brain function. Trifluoperazine may increase the intoxicating effects of alcohol.

Tobacco Smoking: No interactions expected.

Marijuana Smoking

Occasional (once or twice weekly):   No effect to mild and transient increase in drowsiness and accentuation of orthostatic hypotension (see Glossary); some risk of precipitating latent psychoses (in predisposed individuals).

Daily: Moderate increase in drowsiness, significant accentuation of orthostatic hypotension; increased risk of precipitating latent psychoses, confusing interpretation of mental status and of drug responses.

Other Drugs

Trifluoperazine may *increase* the effects of

• all sedatives, sleep-inducing drugs, other tranquilizers, antihistamines, and narcotic drugs, and produce oversedation. Ask physician for guidance regarding dosage adjustment.

• all drugs containing atropine or having an atropine-like action (see Drug Class, Section Three).

• phenytoin (Dantoin, Dilantin, etc.).

Trifluoperazine may *decrease* the effects of

• levodopa (Dopar, Larodopa, etc.), and reduce its effectiveness in the treatment of Parkinson's disease (shaking palsy).

• appetite suppressant drugs (Pre-Sate, Preludin, Benzedrine, Dexedrine, etc.).

Trifluoperazine *taken concurrently* with

• quinidine, may impair heart function. Avoid the combined use of these two drugs.

The following drugs may *increase* the effects of trifluoperazine

• tricyclic antidepressants (see Drug Class, Section Three)

Driving a Vehicle, Operating Machinery, Engaging in Hazardous Activities: This drug can impair mental alertness, judgment, and physical coordination. Avoid hazardous activities.

Aviation Note: The use of this drug *is a disqualification* for the piloting of aircraft. Consultation with a designated Aviation Medical Examiner is advised.

Exposure to Sun: Use caution. Drugs closely related to trifluoperazine are known to produce photosensitivity (see Glossary).

Exposure to Heat: Use caution and avoid excessive heat. This drug may impair the regulation of body temperature and increase the risk of heat stroke.

Heavy Exercise or Exertion: Use caution and follow your physician's instructions if you have angina.

Discontinuation: If it has been necessary to use this drug for an extended period of time, do not discontinue it suddenly. Ask physician for guidance regarding dosage reduction and withdrawal. Upon discontinuation of this drug, it may also be necessary to adjust the dosages of other drugs taken concurrently with it.

Special Storage Instructions
Keep in a tightly closed, light-resistant container.

TRIMEPRAZINE

Year Introduced: 1958

Brand Names

USA	Canada
Temaril (Smith Kline & French)	Panectyl (Rhône-Poulenc)

Common Synonyms ("Street Names"):   None

Drug Class: Anti-itching (Antipruritic), Phenothiazines

Prescription Required: Yes

Available for Purchase by Generic Name: USA: Yes   Canada: No

Available Dosage Forms and Strengths
Tablets — 2.5 mg.
Prolonged-action capsules — 5 mg.
Syrup — 2.5 mg. per teaspoonful (5 ml.)

Tablet May Be Crushed or Capsule Opened for Administration
Tablets — Yes
Prolonged-action capsules (Temaril spansule) — Yes, but do not crush or chew contents

How This Drug Works
Intended Therapeutic Effect(s):   Relief of itching associated with hives, allergic dermatitis, chicken pox, and other skin disorders.
Location of Drug Action(s):   Those hypersensitive areas of the skin that release excessive histamine as part of an allergic reaction.
Method of Drug Action(s):   This drug reduces the intensity of the allergic response by blocking the action of histamine after it has been released from sensitized tissue cells. In addition, it produces a mild sedative effect.

Principal Uses of This Drug
As a Single Drug Product: This member of the phenothiazine class has predominantly antihistaminic effects. It is used primarily to relieve itching in a large variety of conditions. It provides symptomatic relief in most allergic skin rashes, hives, neurodermatitis, pityriasis rosea, eczema, and poison ivy dermatitis.

THIS DRUG SHOULD NOT BE TAKEN IF
—you have had an allergic reaction to any dosage form of it previously.
—you have a blood or bone marrow disorder.
—it is prescribed for an infant under 6 months of age.
—the prolonged action capsule is prescribed for a child under 6 years of age.

INFORM YOUR PHYSICIAN BEFORE TAKING THIS DRUG IF
—you are allergic or sensitive to any phenothiazine drug (see Drug Class, Section Three).
—you are taking any sedatives, sleep-inducing drugs, tranquilizers, other antihistamines, antidepressants, or narcotic drugs of any kind.
—you have a history of recurring peptic ulcer.
—you have a history of prostate gland enlargement.
—you plan to have surgery under general anesthesia in the near future.

Time Required for Apparent Benefit
Usually 1 to 2 hours.

Possible Side-Effects *(natural, expected, and unavoidable drug actions)*
Drowsiness, blurred vision, dryness of the mouth, inability to concentrate.

Possible Adverse Effects *(unusual, unexpected, and infrequent reactions)*

IF ANY OF THE FOLLOWING DEVELOP, DISCONTINUE DRUG AND NOTIFY YOUR PHYSICIAN AS SOON AS POSSIBLE
Mild Adverse Effects
  Allergic Reactions: Skin rash (very rare).
  Other Reactions: Dizziness, weakness.
Serious Adverse Effects
  Paradoxical Reactions: hyperexcitability, abnormal movements of arms and legs, nightmares.
  Other Reactions
  Parkinson-like disorders (see Glossary).
  Muscle spasms of the face, neck, back, and extremities, causing rolling of the eyes, twisting of the neck, arching of the back, spasms of the hands and feet.
  Bone marrow depression (see Glossary), mild and very rare.
  Hepatitis with jaundice (see Glossary), very rare.

CAUTION
1. Many over-the-counter (OTC) medications (see Glossary) for allergies, colds, and coughs contain drugs that can interact unfavorably with this drug. Ask your physician or pharmacist for guidance before using any such medications.
2. Antacids that contain aluminum and/or magnesium can prevent the absorption of this drug and reduce its effectiveness.
3. Obtain prompt evaluation of any disturbance or change in vision.
4. Children with acute illness ("flu"-like infections, measles, chickenpox, etc.) are very susceptible to adverse effects involving muscular spasms of the

face, neck, back, or extremities when this drug is used to control nausea and vomiting. Observe closely and notify physician if such reactions occur.

Precautions for Use by Those over 60 Years of Age

You may be more sensitive to all of the actions of this drug. Small doses are advisable until your individual response has been determined.

You may be more susceptible to the development of drowsiness, lethargy, constipation, lowering of body temperature (hypothermia), and excessive drop in blood pressure on arising from a lying or sitting position (see orthostatic hypotension in Glossary).

This drug can increase the degree of impaired urination associated with prostate gland enlargement (prostatism).

You may also be more susceptible to the development of Parkinson-like disorders and/or tardive dyskinesia (see discussion of these terms in Glossary). These conditions must be recognized early since they may become unresponsive to treatment and irreversible. Consult your physician promptly if suggestive symptoms develop.

Advisability of Use During Pregnancy

Pregnancy Category: C (tentative). See Pregnancy Code inside back cover.
Animal reproduction studies: No data available.
Information from adequate studies in pregnant women is not available.
Ask physician for guidance.

Advisability of Use While Nursing Infant

Apparently safe; ask physician for guidance regarding dosage schedule. Observe infant for evidence of sedation.

Habit-Forming Potential

None.

Effects of Overdosage

With Moderate Overdose: Marked drowsiness, weakness, unsteady stance and gait, agitation, delirium.

With Large Overdose: Deep sleep, coma, convulsions.

Possible Effects of Extended Use

Bone marrow depression (see Glossary).

Suggested Periodic Examinations While Taking This Drug (at physician's discretion)

Complete blood cell counts.

While Taking This Drug, Observe the Following

Foods: Drug may be taken with or following food if it causes stomach irritation.

Beverages: No restrictions.

Alcohol: Use with caution until combined effect has been determined. Alcohol can increase the sedative action of trimeprazine. Trimeprazine can increase the intoxicating action of alcohol.

Tobacco Smoking: No interactions expected.

Marijuana Smoking

Occasional (once or twice weekly):   Mild increase in drowsiness and dryness of mouth.

Daily: Moderate to marked increase in drowsiness and dryness of mouth; possible accentuation of impaired thinking.

Other Drugs

Trimeprazine may *increase* the effects of

- all sedatives, sleep-inducing drugs, pain-relieving drugs, other antihistamines, tranquilizers, and narcotic drugs, and cause oversedation. Ask physician for guidance regarding dosage adjustment.
- atropine and drugs with an atropine-like action (see Drug Class, Section Three).

Driving a Vehicle, Operating Machinery, Engaging in Hazardous Activities: This drug can cause drowsiness and dizziness. Avoid hazardous activities until its full effect has been determined.

Aviation Note: The use of this drug *may be a disqualification* for the piloting of aircraft. Consultation with a designated Aviation Medical Examiner is advised.

Exposure to Sun: Use caution until sensitivity has been determined. This drug can cause photosensitivity (see Glossary).

Special Storage Instructions

Keep in a tightly closed container. Protect from light.

TRIMETHOBENZAMIDE

Year Introduced: 1959

Brand Names

USA	**Canada**
Tigan (Beecham)	Tigan (Roche)

Common Synonyms ("Street Names"):   Nausea medicine

Drug Class: Antinausea (Anti-emetic)

Prescription Required: USA: Yes   Canada: No

Available for Purchase by Generic Name: USA: Yes   Canada: No

Available Dosage Forms and Strengths

Capsules — 100 mg., 250 mg.
Suppositories — 100 mg., 200 mg.
Injection — 100 mg. per ml.

Tablet May Be Crushed or Capsule Opened for Administration: Yes

How This Drug Works

Intended Therapeutic Effect(s):   Relief of nausea and vomiting.

Location of Drug Action(s):   Those nerve pathways within the brain that activate the vomiting centers.

Method of Drug Action(s):   Not completely established. It is thought that this drug relieves nausea and prevents vomiting by blocking the action of the tissue chemicals that transmit nerve impulses to the vomiting centers.

Principal Uses of This Drug

As a Single Drug Product: Used exclusively for the control of nausea and vomiting. It is not as effective as the phenothiazines in relieving nausea and preventing vomiting, but it is significantly safer to use for long-term therapy.

THIS DRUG SHOULD NOT BE TAKEN IF

—you have had an allergic reaction to any dosage form of it previously.

Note: The suppositories contain benzocaine.

INFORM YOUR PHYSICIAN BEFORE TAKING THIS DRUG IF

—you have had any unfavorable reaction to antihistamine drugs in the past. (This drug resembles antihistamines in its pharmacological actions.)

Time Required for Apparent Benefit

Drug action begins in 20 to 40 minutes and persists for approximately 3 to 4 hours.

Possible Side-Effects *(natural, expected, and unavoidable drug actions)*

Drowsiness.

Temporary drop in blood pressure, when given by injection.

Possible Adverse Effects *(unusual, unexpected, and infrequent reactions)*

IF ANY OF THE FOLLOWING DEVELOP, DISCONTINUE DRUG AND NOTIFY YOUR PHYSICIAN AS SOON AS POSSIBLE

Mild Adverse Effects

Allergic Reactions: Skin rash.

Other Reactions: Headache, dizziness, blurring of vision, muscle spasm, and cramping.

Serious Adverse Effects

Parkinson-like disorders (see Glossary).

Liver damage with jaundice (see Glossary).

CAUTION

Use with extreme caution in children with acute infections characterized by fever, vomiting, and dehydration. Such children may be very susceptible to the adverse effects of this drug.

Precautions for Use by Those over 60 Years of Age

You may be more susceptible to the sedative and blood pressure-lowering effects of this drug. Report the development of drowsiness, lightheadedness, dizziness, weakness, or sense of impending faint. Use caution to prevent falls.

Advisability of Use During Pregnancy
Pregnancy Category: B (tentative). See Pregnancy Code inside back cover.

Animal reproduction studies reveal no birth defects due to this drug.

Information from studies in pregnant women indicates no increase in defects in 700 exposures to this drug.

Ask physician for guidance.

Advisability of Use While Nursing Infant
Presence of drug in milk is not known. Safety for infant not established. Ask physician for guidance.

Habit-Forming Potential
None.

Effects of Overdosage
With Moderate Overdose: Drowsiness, weakness, incoordination, muscle spasms in neck and extremities.

With Large Overdose: Confusion, disorientation, convulsions, coma.

Possible Effects of Extended Use
None reported.

Suggested Periodic Examinations While Taking This Drug (at physician's discretion)
Liver function tests.

While Taking This Drug, Observe the Following
Foods: No restrictions. Follow prescribed diet.

Beverages: No restrictions. As allowed by prescribed diet.

Alcohol: Best avoided. Alcohol may increase the sedative response which some individuals experience with this drug.

Tobacco Smoking: No interactions expected.

Marijuana Smoking

Occasional (once or twice weekly): No effect to mild increase in anti-nausea effect of this drug.

Daily: Moderate increase in anti-nausea effect of this drug.

Other Drugs

Trimethobenzamide may *increase* the effects of

• all other drugs with sedative effects, and cause oversedation. Dosage adjustments may be necessary.

Driving a Vehicle, Operating Machinery, Engaging in Hazardous Activities: This drug may cause drowsiness. Avoid hazardous activities until full effect has been determined.

Aviation Note: The use of this drug *is a disqualification* for the piloting of aircraft. Consultation with a designated Aviation Medical Examiner is advised.

Exposure to Sun: No restrictions.

Special Storage Instructions
Keep in a dry, tightly closed container. Keep suppositories refrigerated.

TRIMETHOPRIM

Year Introduced: 1967

Brand Names

USA	Canada
Proloprim (Burroughs Wellcome)	Proloprim (Calmic)
Trimpex (Roche)	Bactrim [CD] (Roche)
Bactrim [CD] (Roche)	Bactrim DS [CD] (Roche)
Bactrim DS [CD] (Roche)	Septra [CD] (B.W. Ltd.)
Septra [CD] (Burroughs Wellcome)	Septra DS [CD] (B.W. Ltd.)
Septra DS [CD] (Burroughs Wellcome)	

Common Synonyms ("Street Names"):   None

Drug Class: Antimicrobial (Anti-infective)

Prescription Required: Yes

Available for Purchase by Generic Name: USA: Yes   Canada: No

Available Dosage Forms and Strengths
            Tablets — 100 mg.
            Tablets — 80 mg. (+ 400 mg. sulfamethoxazole)*
                   — 160 mg. (+ 800 mg. sulfamethoxazole)
      Oral suspension — 40 mg. (+ 200 mg. sulfamethoxazole) per teaspoonful (5 ml.)

Tablet May Be Crushed or Capsule Opened for Administration: Yes

How This Drug Works
   Intended Therapeutic Effect(s):   The elimination of infections responsive to the action of this drug.
   Location of Drug Action(s):   Those body tissues and fluids in which adequate concentration of the drug can be achieved.
   Method of Drug Action(s):   This drug prevents the growth and multiplication of susceptible infecting organisms by interfering with the enzyme systems essential to the formation of proteins.

*In some countries the generic name co-trimoxazole is used to designate the combination of trimethoprim and sulfamethoxazole in a single drug product.

Principal Uses of This Drug

As a Single Drug Product: Used primarily to treat the initial episode of certain infections of the urinary tract that are not complicated by the presence of kidney stones or obstructions to the normal flow of urine. It is sometimes used to prevent the recurrence of such infections.

As a Combination Drug Product [CD]:   This drug is available in combination with sulfamethoxazole for the treatment of certain urinary tract infections. Each drug has a slightly different mechanism of action against the infecting organism; the combined actions are more effective in treating infections that are resistant to therapy.

THIS DRUG SHOULD NOT BE TAKEN IF

—you have had an allergic reaction to any dosage form of it previously (see also the SULFAMETHOXAZOLE Drug Profile).

INFORM YOUR PHYSICIAN BEFORE TAKING THIS DRUG IF

—you are pregnant or nursing an infant.
—you have a history of liver or kidney disease.

Time Required for Apparent Benefit

Varies with nature of infection under treatment; usually 2 to 5 days.

Possible Side-Effects *(natural, expected, and unavoidable drug actions)*
None.

Possible Adverse Effects *(unusual, unexpected, and infrequent reactions)*

IF ANY OF THE FOLLOWING DEVELOP, DISCONTINUE DRUG AND NOTIFY YOUR PHYSICIAN AS SOON AS POSSIBLE

Mild Adverse Effects
Allergic Reactions: Skin rashes (various kinds), nausea, vomiting.
Serious Adverse Effects
Idiosyncratic Reactions: Interference with red blood cell production.

Precautions for Use by Those over 60 Years of Age

The natural decline in liver and kidney function that occurs after 60 may require reduction in dosage and lengthening of dosage intervals. Dosage must be carefully individualized and based upon measurements of kidney funtion.

Natural changes in the skin after 60 may predispose to severe and prolonged itching reactions in the genital and anal regions. This reaction should be reported promptly.

You may be more susceptible to the development of bone marrow depression (see Glossary). Comply with your physician's requests for periodic blood cell counts.

Advisability of Use During Pregnancy

Pregnancy Category: "C" (Tentative). See Pregnancy Code inside back cover.

Animal reproduction studies in rats reveal significant birth defects due to this drug.

Information from adequate studies in pregnant women is not available. It is advisable to avoid this drug completely during first 3 months. Ask physician for guidance.

Advisability of Use While Nursing Infant
Safety for infant not established. Avoid use if possible. Ask physician for guidance. (See also the SULFAMETHOXAZOLE Drug Profile.)

Habit-Forming Potential
None.

Effects of Overdosage
With Moderate Overdose: Nausea, vomiting, diarrhea.

Possible Effects of Extended Use
Bone marrow depression (see Glossary), with impaired red blood cell production resulting in anemia.

Suggested Periodic Examinations While Taking This Drug (at physician's discretion)
Complete blood cell counts.

While Taking This Drug, Observe the Following
Foods: No restrictions of food selection. May be taken with food to minimize stomach irritation.

Beverages: No restrictions.

Alcohol: No interactions expected with trimethoprim. However, see SULFAMETHOXAZOLE Drug Profile if you are taking a combination of these two drugs.

Tobacco Smoking: No interactions expected.

Marijuana Smoking: No interactions expected.

Other Drugs

Trimethoprim may *increase* the effects of
- sulfamethoxazole, making it more effective in the treatment of certain infections.

Trimethoprim *taken concurrently* with
- thiazide diuretics, may cause unusual bleeding or bruising (see Drug Class, Section Three). This is more likely to occur in the elderly.

Driving a Vehicle, Operating Machinery, Engaging in Hazardous Activities: No restrictions regarding trimethoprim. However, see SULFAMETHOXAZOLE Drug Profile if you are taking a combination of these two drugs.

Aviation Note: The use of this drug *may be a disqualification* for the piloting of aircraft. Consultation with a designated Aviation Medical Examiner is advised.

Exposure to Sun: No restrictions regarding trimethoprim (see SULFAMETHOXAZOLE Drug Profile).

Special Storage Instructions
Keep in a dry, tightly closed, light-resistant container.

TRIPELENNAMINE

Year Introduced: 1945

Brand Names

USA	Canada
PBZ (Geigy)	Pyribenzamine (CIBA)
PBZ-SR (Geigy)	
Ro-Hist (Robinson)	

Common Synonyms ("Street Names"):   Allergy pills

Drug Class: Antihistamines

Prescription Required: USA: Yes   Canada: No

Available for Purchase by Generic Name: Yes

Available Dosage Forms and Strengths
Tablets — 25 mg., 50 mg.
Prolonged-action tablets — 50 mg., 100 mg.
Elixir — 37.5 mg. per teaspoonful (5 ml.)

Tablet May Be Crushed or Capsule Opened for Administration
Tablets — Yes
Prolonged-action tablets — No

How This Drug Works
Intended Therapeutic Effect(s):   Relief of symptoms associated with hayfever (allergic rhinitis) and with allergic reactions in the skin, such as itching, swelling, hives, and rash.
Location of Drug Action(s):   Those hypersensitive tissues that release excessive histamine as part of an allergic reaction. The principal tissue sites are
the eyes, the nose, and the skin.
Method of Drug Action(s):   This drug reduces the intensity of the allergic
response by blocking the action of histamine after it has been released from
sensitized tissue cells.

Principal Uses of This Drug
As a Single Drug Product: Used primarily to provide symptomatic relief in
allergic and related disorders: seasonal and perennial allergic rhinitis (hay
fever), allergic conjunctivitis, and vasomotor rhinitis; also used in hives and
localized swellings (angioedema) of allergic origin. This drug is not effective
in the treatment of allergically-induced bronchial asthma.

THIS DRUG SHOULD NOT BE TAKEN IF
—you have had an allergic reaction to any dosage form of it previously.
—you are subject to acute attacks of asthma.
—you have glaucoma (narrow-angle type).
—you have difficulty emptying the urinary bladder.
—you are taking, or have taken during the past 2 weeks, any mono-amine
oxidase (MAO) inhibitor drug (see Drug Class, Section Three).
—it has been prescribed for a newborn infant.

INFORM YOUR PHYSICIAN BEFORE TAKING THIS DRUG IF
—you have had an unfavorable reaction to any antihistamine drug in the past.
—you have a history of peptic ulcer disease.
—you plan to have surgery under general anesthesia in the near future.

Time Required for Apparent Benefit
Drug action begins in approximately 30 minutes, reaches a maximum in 1 hour, and subsides in 4 to 6 hours.

Possible Side-Effects *(natural, expected, and unavoidable drug actions)*
Drowsiness, sense of weakness, dryness of nose, mouth, and throat, constipation.

Possible Adverse Effects *(unusual, unexpected, and infrequent reactions)*

IF ANY OF THE FOLLOWING DEVELOP, DISCONTINUE DRUG AND NOTIFY YOUR PHYSICIAN AS SOON AS POSSIBLE

Mild Adverse Effects
Allergic Reactions: Skin rash, hives.
Other Reactions
   Headache, dizziness, inability to concentrate, nervousness, blurring of vision, double vision, difficulty in urination.
   Nausea, vomiting, diarrhea.
   Reduced tolerance for contact lenses.

Serious Adverse Effects
Allergic Reactions: Anaphylactic reaction (see Glossary).
Idiosyncratic Reactions: Acute behavioral disturbances—excitement, confusion, hallucinations, insomnia (more common in children).
Other Reactions
   Hemolytic anemia (see Glossary).
   Bone marrow depression (see Glossary)—fatigue, weakness, fever, sore throat, unusual bleeding or bruising.

Precautions for Use by Those over 60 Years of Age
You may be more susceptible to the development of drowsiness, dizziness, and lethargy and to impairment of thinking, judgment, and memory.
This drug can increase the degree of impaired urination associated with prostate gland enlargement (prostatism).

Advisability of Use During Pregnancy
Pregnancy Category: B (tentative). See Pregnancy Code inside back cover.
   Animal reproduction studies reveal no birth defects due to this drug.
   Information from studies in pregnant women indicates no increase in defects in 490 exposures to this drug.
   Ask physician for guidance.

Advisability of Use While Nursing Infant
This drug may impair milk formation and make nursing difficult. The drug is thought to be present in milk. Ask physician for guidance.

Habit-Forming Potential
None.

Effects of Overdosage
With Moderate Overdose: Marked drowsiness, confusion, incoordination, unsteady gait, muscle tremors. In children: excitement, hallucinations, overactivity, convulsions.

With Large Overdose: Stupor progressing to coma, fever, flushed face, dilated pupils, weak pulse, shallow breathing.

Possible Effects of Extended Use
Bone marrow depression.
Emotional and behavioral abnormalities.

Suggested Periodic Examinations While Taking This Drug (at physician's discretion)
Complete blood cell counts.

While Taking This Drug, Observe the Following
Foods: No restrictions. Stomach irritation can be reduced if drug is taken after eating.

Beverages: Coffee and tea may help to reduce the drowsiness caused by most antihistamines.

Alcohol: Use with extreme caution until combined effect has been determined. The combination of alcohol and antihistamines can cause rapid and marked sedation.

Tobacco Smoking: No interactions expected.

Marijuana Smoking

Occasional (once or twice weekly):   Mild increase in drowsiness and dryness of mouth.

Daily: Moderate to marked increase in drowsiness and dryness of mouth; possible accentuation of impaired thinking.

Other Drugs

Tripelennamine may *increase* the effects of

• sedatives, sleep-inducing drugs, tranquilizers, antidepressants, pain relievers, and narcotic drugs, and result in oversedation. Careful dosage adjustments are necessary.

• atropine and drugs with atropine-like action (see Drug Class, Section Three).

The following drugs may *increase* the effects of tripelennamine

• all sedatives, sleep-inducing drugs, tranquilizers, pain relievers, and narcotic drugs may exaggerate its sedative action and cause oversedation.

• mono-amine oxidase (MAO) inhibitor drugs (see Drug Class, Section Three) may delay its elimination from the body, thus exaggerating and prolonging its action.

The following drugs may *decrease* the effects of tripelennamine

• amphetamines (Benzedrine, Dexedrine, Desoxyn, etc.) may reduce the drowsiness caused by most antihistamines.

Driving a Vehicle, Operating Machinery, Engaging in Hazardous Activities:
This drug may impair mental alertness, judgment, physical coordination, and reaction time. Avoid hazardous activities until full sedative effect has been determined.

Aviation Note: The use of this drug *is a disqualification* for the piloting of aircraft. Consultation with a designated Aviation Medical Examiner is advised.

Exposure to Sun: No restrictions.

Special Storage Instructions
Keep in a dry, tightly closed, light-resistant container.

TRIPROLIDINE

Year Introduced: 1958

Brand Names

USA	Canada
Actidil (Burroughs Wellcome)	Actidil (B.W.)
Actifed [CD] (Burroughs Wellcome)	Actifed [CD] (B.W.)
Actifed-C Expectorant [CD] (Burroughs Wellcome)	Actifed-A [CD] (B.W.)
	Actifed-Plus [CD] (B.W.)
	Actifed DM [CD] (B.W.)

Common Synonyms ("Street Names"):   Allergy pills

Drug Class: Antihistamines

Prescription Required: USA: Yes (Actifed-C is a Controlled Drug, U.S. Schedule V)*
Canada: No

Available for Purchase by Generic Name: USA: Yes   Canada: No

Available Dosage Forms and Strengths
Tablets — 2.5 mg.
Syrup — 1.25 mg. per teaspoonful (5 ml.)

Tablet May Be Crushed or Capsule Opened for Administration: Yes

How This Drug Works
Intended Therapeutic Effect(s):   Relief of symptoms associated with hayfever (allergic rhinitis) and with allergic reactions in the skin, such as itching, swelling, hives, and rash.

*See Schedules of Controlled Drugs inside back cover.

Location of Drug Action(s):   Those hypersensitive tissues that release excessive histamine as part of an allergic reaction. The principal tissue sites are the eyes, the nose, and the skin.

Method of Drug Action(s):   This drug reduces the intensity of the allergic response by blocking the action of histamine after it has been released from sensitized tissue cells.

Principal Uses of This Drug

As a Single Drug Product: Used primarily to provide symptomatic relief in allergic and related disorders: seasonal and perennial allergic rhinitis (hay fever), allergic conjunctivitis, and vasomotor rhinitis; also in hives and localized swellings (angioedema) of allergic origin. This drug is not effective in the treatment of allergically-induced bronchial asthma.

As a Combination Drug Product [CD]:   This drug is available in combination with pseudoephedrine, a decongestant that enhances the drying effect of the antihistamine. The combination is used to reduce tissue swelling and secretions in allergic and infectious disorders of the nose and sinuses. It is also combined with decongestants, expectorants, and codeine to increase their effectiveness in providing symptomatic relief of allergic and infectious disorders of the lower respiratory tract, often with associated coughing.

THIS DRUG SHOULD NOT BE TAKEN IF

—you have had an allergic reaction to any dosage form of it previously.

—you are taking, or have taken within the past 2 weeks, any mono-amine oxidase (MAO) inhibitor drug (see Drug Class, Section Three).

—it has been prescribed for a newborn infant.

INFORM YOUR PHYSICIAN BEFORE TAKING THIS DRUG IF

—you have had an unfavorable reaction to any antihistamine in the past.

—you have glaucoma (narrow-angle type).

—you have difficulty emptying the urinary bladder.

—you plan to have surgery under general anesthesia in the near future.

Time Required for Apparent Benefit

Drug action begins in approximately 30 minutes, reaches a maximum in 3 and one-half hours, and subsides in 12 hours.

Possible Side-Effects *(natural, expected, and unavoidable drug actions)*

Drowsiness, lassitude, dryness of nose, mouth and throat.

Possible Adverse Effects *(unusual, unexpected, and infrequent reactions)*

IF ANY OF THE FOLLOWING DEVELOP, DISCONTINUE DRUG AND NOTIFY YOUR PHYSICIAN AS SOON AS POSSIBLE

Mild Adverse Effects

Allergic Reactions: Skin rash (rare).

Other Reactions

Dizziness, incoordination, unsteadiness, inability to concentrate.

Indigestion, nausea.

Serious Adverse Effects

Idiosyncratic Reactions: Acute behavioral disturbances—excitement, irritability, insomnia.

Precautions for Use by Those over 60 Years of Age

You may be more susceptible to the development of drowsiness, dizziness, and lethargy and to impairment of thinking, judgment, and memory.

This drug can increase the degree of impaired urination associated with prostate gland enlargement (prostatism).

Advisability of Use During Pregnancy

Pregnancy Category: C (tentative). See Pregnancy Code inside back cover.

Animal reproduction studies: No data available.

Information from adequate studies in pregnant women is not available. Ask physician for guidance.

Advisability of Use While Nursing Infant

Presence of drug in milk is not known. Other antihistamine drugs are known to be present in milk. Ask physician for guidance.

Habit-Forming Potential

None.

Effects of Overdosage

With Moderate Overdose: Marked drowsiness, confusion, delirium, excitement and agitation; in the young, hallucinations, muscle tremors.

With Large Overdose: Stupor progressing to coma, convulsions.

Possible Effects of Extended Use

None reported.

Suggested Periodic Examinations While Taking This Drug (at physician's discretion)

Complete blood cell counts. Some antihistamines have caused bone marrow depression and hemolytic anemia (see Glossary) with extended use.

While Taking This Drug, Observe the Following

Foods: No restrictions.

Beverages: Coffee and tea may offset the drowsiness caused by some antihistamines.

Alcohol: Use with extreme caution until combined effect has been determined. The combination of alcohol and antihistamines can produce rapid and marked sedation.

Tobacco Smoking: No interactions expected.

Marijuana Smoking

Occasional (once or twice weekly): Mild increase in drowsiness and dryness of mouth.

Daily: Moderate to marked increase in drowsiness and dryness of mouth; possible accentuation of impaired thinking.

Other Drugs

Triprolidine may *increase* the effects of

- all sedatives, sleep-inducing drugs, tranquilizers, antidepressants, pain relievers, and narcotic drugs, and cause oversedation. Dosage adjustments may be necessary.

The following drugs may *increase* the effects of triprolidine

- all sedatives, sleep-inducing drugs, tranquilizers, antidepressants, pain relievers, and narcotic drugs. Dosage adjustments may be necessary to prevent oversedation.

Driving a Vehicle, Operating Machinery, Engaging in Hazardous Activities: This drug may impair mental alertness, judgment, physical coordination, and reaction time. Avoid hazardous activities until its full sedative effect has been determined.

Aviation Note: The use of this drug *may be a disqualification* for the piloting of aircraft. Consultation with a designated Aviation Medical Examiner is advised.

Exposure to Sun: Use caution until sensitivity has been determined. This drug has caused photosensitivity (see Glossary).

Special Storage Instructions

Keep in a dry, tightly closed, light-resistant container.

VALPROIC ACID

Year Introduced: 1967

Brand Names

USA	Canada
Depakene (Abbott)	Depakene (Abbott)
Depakote (Abbott)	

Common Synonyms ("Street Names"):   Epilepsy medicine

Drug Class: Anti-epileptic, Anticonvulsant

Prescription Required: USA: Yes   Canada: Yes

Available for Purchase by Generic Name: USA: No   Canada: No

Available Dosage Forms and Strengths
Tablets (enteric-coated) — 250 mg., 500 mg.
Capsules — 250 mg., 500 mg.
Syrup — 250 mg. per teaspoonful (5 ml.)

Tablet May Be Crushed or Capsule Opened for Administration: No

How This Drug Works

Intended Therapeutic Effect(s):   Reduction in the frequency and severity of seizures associated with all major types of epilepsy.

Location of Drug Action(s):   Thought to be those specific sites in the outer layer of the brain that initiate abnormal electrical impulses which spread through brain tissue to produce seizures.

Method of Drug Action(s):   Not fully established. It is thought that by increasing the availability of the nerve impulse transmitter gamma-aminobutyric acid (GABA), this drug suppresses the spread of abnormal electrical impulses responsible for epileptic seizures.

Principal Uses of This Drug

As a Single Drug Product: Used effectively in the management of the following types of epilepsy: simple and complex absence seizures (petit mal), tonic-clonic seizures (grand mal), myoclonic seizures, complex partial seizures (psychomotor, temporal lobe epilepsy). It is sometimes used adjunctively with other anticonvulsants as needed.

THIS DRUG SHOULD NOT BE TAKEN IF
—you have had an allergic reaction to any dosage form of it previously.
—you have active liver disease.
—you have an active bleeding disorder.

INFORM YOUR PHYSICIAN BEFORE TAKING THIS DRUG IF
—you have a history of liver disease or impaired liver function.
—you have a history of any type of bleeding disorder.
—you are currently taking any type of anticoagulant drug ("blood thinner").
—you are currently taking any other anticonvulsant drugs.
—you are currently taking any antidepressant drugs, either tricyclic type drugs or mono-amine oxidase (MAO) inhibitors (see Drug Classes, Section Three).
—you have myasthenia gravis.
—you plan to have surgery or dental extraction in the near future.

Time Required for Apparent Benefit

Drug action usually begins in 30 to 60 minutes and reaches its peak in 1 to 4 hours. Continuous use on a regular schedule for 2 weeks is usually necessary to determine this drug's effectiveness in reducing the frequency and severity of seizures.

Possible Side-Effects *(natural, expected, and unavoidable drug actions)*
Drowsiness and lethargy (5%).

Possible Adverse Effects *(unusual, unexpected, and infrequent reactions)*

IF ANY OF THE FOLLOWING DEVELOP, DISCONTINUE DRUG AND NOTIFY YOUR PHYSICIAN AS SOON AS POSSIBLE

Mild Adverse Effects
Allergic Reactions: Skin rash (rare).
Other Reactions: Headache, dizziness, confusion, unsteadiness, slurred speech.

Nausea, indigestion, stomach cramps, diarrhea.

Temporary loss of scalp hair.

Serious Adverse Effects

Idiosyncratic Reactions: Bizarre behavior, hallucinations.

Other Reactions: Possible drug-induced hepatitis or pancreatitis.

Possible Reye's syndrome.

Reduced formation of blood platelets and impaired platelet function, with increased risk of abnormal bleeding.

Adverse Effects That May Mimic Natural Diseases or Disorders

Liver toxicity may suggest viral hepatitis.

CAUTION

1. The capsules and tablets should be swallowed without chewing to avoid irritation of the mouth and throat.
2. This drug can impair normal blood clotting mechanisms. In the event of injury, dental extraction, or need for surgery, inform your physician or dentist that you are taking this drug.
3. Because this drug can impair the normal function of blood platelets, it is advisable to avoid aspirin (which has the same effect).
4. Over-the-counter drug products that contain antihistamines (allergy and cold remedies, sleep aids) can enhance the sedative effects of this drug.

Precautions for Use by Infants and Children

The concurrent use of aspirin with this drug may cause abnormal bruising or bleeding.

Children with mental retardation, organic brain disease, or severe seizure disorders may be at increased risk for severe liver toxicity while taking this drug.

Monitor closely for the development of fever that could indicate the onset of a drug-induced Reye's syndrome.

Concurrent use of clonazepam (Clonopin) may result in continuous petit mal episodes.

Precautions for Use by Those over 60 Years of Age

Impaired liver and/or kidney function may delay the elimination of this drug and require adjustment of dosage and administration schedule. Start with small doses and increase cautiously as needed and tolerated.

Monitor closely for excessive sedation, confusion, and/or unsteadiness in stance and gait.

Advisability of Use During Pregnancy

Pregnancy Category: C (tentative). See Pregnancy Code inside back cover.

Animal reproduction studies in mice, rats, and rabbits reveal birth defects in the palate and skeleton.

Information from adequate studies in pregnant women is not available.

Avoid use of this drug during the first 3 months if possible. Use this drug during the last 6 months only if clearly needed.

Advisability of Use While Nursing Infant
This drug is present in human milk. Observe nursing infant for drowsiness and ability to obtain adequate nourishment.

Habit-Forming Potential
None.

Effects of Overdosage
With Moderate Overdose: Increased drowsiness, weakness, unsteadiness, and confusion.

With Large Overdose: Stupor progressing to coma, shallow breathing.

Possible Effects of Extended Use
None identified.

Suggested Periodic Examinations While Taking This Drug (at physician's discretion)
Complete blood cell counts and liver function studies to be done before and during treatment.

While Taking This Drug, Observe the Following
Foods: No restrictions. Preferably taken 1 hour before meals. However, it may be taken with or following food to reduce stomach irritation.

Beverages: *Do not* administer the syrup in carbonated beverages. This can liberate valproic acid and irritate the mouth and throat. The capsules and tablets may be taken with milk.

Alcohol: Use caution until the combined effect has been determined. Alcohol can enhance the sedative effect of this drug. Also, this drug can increase the depressant effect of alcohol on brain function.

Tobacco Smoking: No interactions expected.

Marijuana Smoking

Occasional (once or twice weekly): Possible mild and transient increase in drowsiness.

Daily: Moderate increase in drowsiness and unsteadiness. Possible decrease in therapeutic effects of valproic acid.

Other Drugs

Valproic acid may *increase* the effects of

- anticoagulants ("blood thinners") and increase the risk of abnormal bleeding.
- other drugs that depress brain function and cause excessive sedation.
- mono-amine oxidase (MAO) inhibitor drugs (see Drug Class, Section Three).
- primidone (Mysoline) and cause excessive sedation.
- tricyclic antidepressants (see Drug Class, Section Three).

Valproic acid *taken concurrently* with

- antiplatelet drugs—aspirin, dipyridamole (Persantine), sulfinpyrazone (Anturane)—may enhance the inhibition of platelet function and increase the risk of abnormal bleeding.

- clonazepam (Clonopin) may increase the occurrence of absence seizures (petit mal).
- phenytoin (Dilantin) can cause unpredictable fluctuations of blood levels; therapeutic monitoring of the blood levels of both drugs is advised.

The following drugs may *increase* the effects of valproic acid
- antihistamines, both prescription and over-the-counter preparations, may increase its sedative effects.

The following drugs may *decrease* the effects of valproic acid
- phenobarbital may hasten its elimination from the body.

Driving a Vehicle, Operating Machinery, Engaging in Hazardous Activities: This drug may cause drowsiness, dizziness, confusion, and impaired vision. If these drug effects occur, avoid all hazardous activities.

Aviation Note: The use of this drug and the disorder for which this drug is prescribed *are disqualifications* for the piloting of aircraft. Consultation with a designated Aviation Medical Examiner is advised.

Exposure to Sun: No restrictions.

Heavy Exercise or Exertion: Use caution. Hyperventilation can precipitate seizures in sensitive individuals.

Occurrence of Unrelated Illness: Intercurrent infections with fever can alter the body's disposition of this drug and reduce its anticonvulsant effect with some loss of seizure control.

Discontinuation: This drug should not be discontinued abruptly. Sudden withdrawal may cause repetitive seizures that are difficult to control.

Special Storage Instructions
Keep in a dry, tightly closed container at room temperature. Protect from moisture and direct light.

VERAPAMIL
(Iproveratril)

Year Introduced: 1967

Brand Names

USA	Canada
Calan (Searle)	Isoptin (Searle)
Isoptin (Knoll)	

Common Synonyms ("Street Names"):   Angina pills, heart pills

Drug Class: Anti-anginal, Calcium channel blocker

Prescription Required: USA: Yes   Canada: Yes

Available for Purchase by Generic Name: USA: No   Canada: No

Avaialble Dosage Forms and Strengths
Tablets — 80 mg., 120 mg.
Injection — 2.5 mg. per ml.

Tablet May Be Crushed or Capsule Opened for Administration: Yes

How This Drug Works
Intended Therapeutic Effect(s):   Reduction in the frequency and severity of pain associated with angina pectoris.

Location of Drug Action(s):   Specific sites (the calcium channels) in the walls of cells that comprise the heart muscle and the muscular layers of small arteries.

Method of Drug Action(s):   By blocking the flow of calcium through certain cell walls, this drug impairs the ability of the heart muscle to contract and the ability of the muscular walls of small arteries to constrict. The consequences are (1) the relaxation and prevention of coronary artery constriction, and (2) the reduction of the work load on the heart muscle. The net effects of improved coronary artery blood flow and reduced oxygen demand by the heart muscle are responsible for the reduction in the frequency and severity of angina pain.

Principal Uses of This Drug
As a Single Drug Product: Used primarily to treat both types of angina, the classical effort-induced angina associated with coronary artery disease (atherosclerosis), and the variant type of angina due to spasm of the coronary artery (Prinzmetal's angina). It is also used by injection to correct certain rhythm disturbances of the heart. In addition to these "approved" uses, this drug is also used experimentally to treat high blood pressure and migraine headache.

THIS DRUG SHOULD NOT BE TAKEN IF
—you have had an allergic reaction to it previously.
—you have active liver disease.
—you have severe congestive heart failure.
—you have severe low blood pressure (systolic blood pressure below 90).
—you have 2nd or 3rd degree heart block.
—you have a "sick sinus" syndrome (ask your physician).

INFORM YOUR PHYSICIAN BEFORE TAKING THIS DRUG IF
—you are taking *any* other drugs at this time.
—you have had a recent stroke or heart attack.
—you have a history of heart disease, especially heart rhythm disturbances.
—you have impaired liver or kidney function.
—you have constitutionally low blood pressure.

Time Required for Apparent Benefit
Drug action usually begins in 1 to 2 hours and reaches its peak in about 5 hours. Continuous use on a regular schedule for 1 to 2 weeks is usually necessary to determine this drug's effectiveness in preventing angina.

Possible Side-Effects *(natural, expected, and unavoidable drug actions)*
Low blood pressure (2.9%), fluid retention (1.7%).

Possible Adverse Effects *(unusual, unexpected, and infrequent reactions)*

IF ANY OF THE FOLLOWING DEVELOP, DISCONTINUE DRUG AND NOTIFY YOUR PHYSICIAN AS SOON AS POSSIBLE

Mild Adverse Effects

Allergic Reactions: Skin rash, itching, hives, aching joints.

Other Reactions: Headache (1.8%), dizziness (3.6%), fatigue (1.1%). Nausea (1.6%), constipation (6.3%).

Serious Adverse Effects

Allergic Reactions: Possible drug-induced hepatitis without jaundice (very rare).

Other Reactions: Excessively slow heart rate—less than 50 beats per minute (1.1%).

Third-degree heart block (0.8%).

Congestive heart failure (0.9%).

CAUTION

1. If this drug is used concurrently with a "beta-blocker" drug, you may develop excessively low blood pressure.
2. This drug may cause swelling of the feet and ankles. This is not indicative of heart or kidney trouble.
3. If you notice any increase in the frequency, duration, or severity of angina pain, inform your physician promptly.

Precautions for Use by Those over 60 Years of Age

It is advisable to begin treatment with small doses and to increase the dosage gradually if needed.

Observe carefully for any tendency to lightheadedness or dizziness that could cause falling and injury.

Advisability of Use During Pregnancy

Pregnancy Category: C (tentative). See Pregnancy Code inside back cover.

Animal reproduction studies in rats reveal toxic effects on the embryo and retarded growth of the fetus, but no birth defects.

Information from adequate studies in pregnant women is not available.

Avoid this drug during the first 3 months if possible.

Use it during the last 6 months only if clearly needed.

Advisability of Use While Nursing Infant

The presence of this drug in human milk is not known. If this drug is used, monitor the nursing infant for poor feeding and possible low blood pressure. Ask physician for guidance.

Habit-Forming Potential

None.

Effects of Overdosage

With Moderate Overdose: Flushed and warm skin, sweating, lightheadedness, irritability, rapid heart rate, low blood pressure.

With Large Overdose: Marked low blood pressure, loss of consciousness.

Possible Effects of Extended Use
None identified.

Suggested Periodic Examinations While Taking This Drug (at physician's discretion)
Measurements of blood pressure in lying, sitting, and standing positions. Liver function tests.

While Taking This Drug, Observe the Following
Foods: No specific restrictions. Avoid excessive salt.
May be taken with or following food to reduce stomach irritation.

Beverages: No restrictions. May be taken with milk.

Alcohol: Use caution until the combined effect has been determined. Alcohol can enhance the blood pressure-lowering effects of this drug.

Tobacco Smoking: To be avoided. Nicotine can inhibit the potential benefits of this drug significantly.

Marijuana Smoking
Occasional (once or twice weekly): No effect to mild and transient additional lowering of the blood pressure.
Daily: Possible increase in heart rate and further lowering of the blood pressure.

Other Drugs
Verapamil may *increase* the effects of
- anti-hypertensive drugs and cause excessive lowering of the blood pressure.
- digitalis preparations (digoxin, Lanoxin) by raising their blood level. Monitor carefully to prevent digitalis toxicity.
- nitroglycerin and the long-acting nitrates in the treatment of angina (improved anti-anginal effects).

Verapamil *taken concurrently* with
- beta-blocking drugs (see Drug Class, Section Three) may increase the risk of worsening angina, inducing low blood pressure, or initiating congestive heart failure.

Driving a Vehicle, Operating Machinery, Engaging in Hazardous Activities: Usually no restrictions. However, it is advisable to observe for the possible occurrence of excessively low blood pressure with dizziness and weakness; restrict activities accordingly.

Aviation Note: Angina pectoris *is a disqualification* for the piloting of aircraft. Consultation with a designated Aviation Medical Examiner is advised.

Exposure to Sun: No restrictions unless a skin rash develops.

Exposure to Heat: Use caution. Hot environments can enhance the blood pressure-lowering effects of this drug.

Exposure to Cold: Use caution. Cold environments can induce angina and reduce the effectiveness of this drug.

Heavy Exercise or Exertion: Use caution. This drug can increase your tolerance for exercise. Avoid exertion that causes angina or shortness of breath.

Occurrence of Unrelated Illness: The fever associated with serious infections can lower the blood pressure. Observe carefully for the combined effects while taking this drug.

Discontinuation: It is advisable to reduce the dose gradually over a period of 7 to 10 days, and to observe for the possible development of rebound angina.

Special Storage Instructions

Keep tablets in a dry, tightly closed container at room temperature. Protect from light, moisture, and excessive heat.

VITAMIN C
(Ascorbic Acid)

Year Introduced: 1933 (Chemical identity established)

Brand Names

USA	Canada
Ascorbajen (Jenkins)	Apo-C (Apotex)
Ascorbicap (ICN)	Ce-Vi-Sol (Mead Johnson)
Cecon (Abbott)	Redoxon (Roche)
Cetane (O'Neal)	
Cevalin (Lilly)	
Cevi-Bid (Geriatric)	
Ce-Vi-Sol (Mead Johnson)	
(Numerous others)	

Common Synonyms ("Street Names"):   None

Drug Class: Vitamins

Prescription Required: No

Available for Purchase by Generic Name: Yes

Available Dosage Forms and Strengths

Tablets — 25 mg., 50 mg., 100 mg., 250 mg., 500 mg., 1000 mg.

Chewable Tablets — 100 mg., 250 mg., 500 mg., 1000 mg.

Prolonged-action tablets — 250 mg., 500 mg., 750 mg.

Capsules — 25 mg., 100 mg., 250 mg., 500 mg.

Prolonged-action capsules — 500 mg.

Oral drops — 35 mg. per 0.6 ml., 100 mg. per ml.

Syrup — 100 mg. per teaspoonful (5 ml.)

Injection — 50 mg. per ml., 100 mg. per ml., 200 mg. per ml., 250 mg. per ml., 500 mg. per ml.

Tablet May Be Crushed or Capsule Opened for Administration

Regular tablets and capsules — Yes

Prolonged-action tablets and capsules — No

How This Drug Works

Intended Therapeutic Effect(s)

Prevention and treatment of scurvy, a disease resulting from deficiency of Vitamin C.

Treatment of some types of anemia.

Maintenance of an acid urine (using a dose of 1 gram [1000 mg.] every 6 hours).

Location of Drug Action(s)

Tissues throughout the body that require Vitamin C for the formation of collagen, a principal structural protein of skin, tendon, bone, teeth, cartilage, and connective tissue.

The intestinal tract and bone marrow.

The kidneys, ureters, and bladder.

Method of Drug Action(s)

Not established. It is thought that Vitamin C plays an essential role in the enzyme activity involved in the formation of collagen.

Vitamin C increases the absorption of iron from the intestine and contributes to the formation of hemoglobin and red blood cells in the bone marrow.

By acidifying the urine, Vitamin C (ascorbic acid) creates an environment which is unfavorable to the growth of certain bacteria that commonly infect the urinary tract. This action also enhances the therapeutic effects of some widely used anti-infective drugs.

Note: There is insufficient scientific evidence to establish that Vitamin C is significantly beneficial in the prevention or treatment of the common cold. Individual experience varies greatly. For those who find that the benefits of using Vitamin C in large doses clearly outweigh the small risks involved, no significant toxicity is anticipated.

Principal Uses of This Drug

As a Single Drug Product: Used most commonly at this time in large doses to reduce the frequency, severity, and duration of head colds. It is used less frequently to acidify the urine in those individuals who are susceptible to recurrent infections of the urinary tract.

As a Combination Drug Product [CD]: This drug is available in a large variety of combinations that include multiple vitamins and minerals. These preparations are used as nutritional supplements.

THIS DRUG SHOULD NOT BE TAKEN IF

—you have had an allergic reaction to a Vitamin C drug product previously (ask physician for guidance).

INFORM YOUR PHYSICIAN BEFORE TAKING THIS DRUG IF

—you have sickle cell anemia.

—you have a history of kidney stones.

—you are taking an oral anticoagulant drug.

Time Required for Apparent Benefit
In the treatment of Vitamin C deficiency, significant improvement is apparent within 1 week.

Possible Side-Effects *(natural, expected, and unavoidable drug actions)*
None.

Possible Adverse Effects *(unusual, unexpected, and infrequent reactions)*

IF ANY OF THE FOLLOWING DEVELOP, DISCONTINUE DRUG AND NOTIFY YOUR PHYSICIAN AS SOON AS POSSIBLE

Mild Adverse Effects
Diarrhea, with large doses.
Serious Adverse Effects
Idiosyncratic Reactions: Hemolytic anemia (see Glossary).
Other Reactions
Formation of kidney stones, with large doses.
Precipitation of crisis in individuals with sickle cell anemia.

CAUTION
1. Some Vitamin C preparations for oral use contain sodium ascorbate as the principal component. For individuals on a low-sodium diet, the intake of sodium could be significant, depending upon daily dosage. Consult your physician.
2. It is advisable to avoid large doses of Vitamin C while taking any sulfonamide ("sulfa") drug.
3. Large doses of Vitamin C may cause a *false positive* test result for urine sugar when testing with Benedict's solution, and a *false negative* test result when testing with Clinistix or Tes-Tape.
4. Large doses of Vitamin C may cause a *false negative* test result for blood in the stool (fecal blood) when testing with the Hemoccult slide method.

Precautions for Use by Those over 60 Years of Age
If you use large doses of Vitamin C (1000 mg. or more) daily, it is advisable to drink 2 quarts of water daily to ensure a dilute urine and thus reduce the risk of kidney stone formation. Consult your physician regarding the advisability and safety of a large fluid intake.

Advisability of Use During Pregnancy
Pregnancy Category: B (tentative). See Pregnancy Code inside back cover.
Animal reproduction studies reveal no birth defects due to this drug.
Information from adequate studies in pregnant women is not available.
Ask physician for guidance.
Adhere to recommended dose of 100 mg. daily. Avoid large doses.

Advisability of Use While Nursing Infant
Adhere to recommended dose of 150 mg. daily. Avoid large doses.

Habit-Forming Potential
None.

Effects of Overdosage
With Moderate Overdose: Diarrhea.
With Large Overdose: No toxic effects reported.

Possible Effects of Extended Use
Formation of kidney stones, when taken in large doses.

Suggested Periodic Examinations While Taking This Drug (at physician's discretion)
Urine analyses.

While Taking This Drug, Observe the Following
Foods: No restrictions.
Beverages: No restrictions.
Alcohol: No interactions expected.
Tobacco Smoking: Smoking appears to increase the requirement for Vitamin C. The reasons for this are not known.
Marijuana Smoking: No interactions expected.
Other Drugs

Vitamin C (in large doses) may *increase* the effects of
- aspirin. (Vitamin C, taken as ascorbic acid and in large doses, may acidify the urine in some individuals and cause aspirin accumulation and toxicity.)
- barbiturates (see Drug Class, Section Three).
- iron preparations.
- sulfonamide ("sulfa") drugs (see Drug Class, Section Three).

Vitamin C (in large doses) may *decrease* the effects of
- oral anticoagulants (see Drug Class, Section Three).
- atropine and atropine-like drugs (see Drug Class, Section Three).
- quinidine.

Vitamin C (in large doses) *taken concurrently* with
- sulfonamide drugs, may cause crystal formation in the kidneys, resulting in kidney damage and impaired kidney function.

The following drugs may *decrease* the effects of Vitamin C
- barbiturates
- mineral oil
- salicylates (principally aspirin)
- sulfonamide drugs

Aviation Note: Usually no restrictions.
Exposure to Sun: No restrictions.
Occurrence of Unrelated Illness: Vitamin C requirements are increased during pregnancy, nursing, peptic ulcer, infections, and overactive thyroid states; also following surgery, injuries, and burns. Consult your physician about the advisability of supplementary Vitamin C prior to surgery.

Special Storage Instructions

Keep all forms of Vitamin C in tightly closed, nonmetallic containers. Protect from light.

WARFARIN
(and other Coumarin Anticoagulants*)

Year Introduced: 1954

Brand Names

USA	Canada
Athrombin-K (Purdue-Frederick)	Athrombin-K (Purdue-Frederick)
Coumadin (Endo)	Coumadin (Endo)
Panwarfin (Abbott)	Warfilone (Frosst)
	Warnerin (P.D.)

Common Synonyms ("Street Names"):   Blood thinner

Drug Class: Anticoagulant, Coumarins

Prescription Required: Yes

Available for Purchase by Generic Name: No

Available Dosage Forms and Strengths

Tablets — 2 mg., 2.5 mg., 5 mg., 7.5 mg., 10 mg.
Injection — 50 mg. per vial

Tablet May Be Crushed or Capsule Opened for Administration: Yes

How This Drug Works

Intended Therapeutic Effect(s):   A deliberate reduction in the ability of the blood to clot. This effect is often beneficial in the management of stroke, heart attack, abnormal clotting in arteries and veins (thrombosis), and the movement of a blood clot from vein to lung (pulmonary embolism).

Location of Drug Action(s):   Those tissues in the liver that use Vitamin K to produce prothrombin (and other factors) essential to the clotting of blood.

Method of Drug Action(s):   The coumarin anticoagulants interfere with the production of four essential blood-clotting factors by blocking the action of Vitamin K. This leads to a deficiency of these clotting factors in circulating blood and inhibits blood-clotting mechanisms.

---

*Other members of the coumarin anticoagulant drug family available in the United States are Dicumarol, Liquamar, Sintrom, and Tromexan. Dicumarol and Sintrom are also available in Canada. The major characteristics of warfarin are shared by all coumarin anticoagulants (see Drug Class, Section Three).

Principal Uses of This Drug

As a Single Drug Product: Used exclusively for its anticoagulant effect in treating the following conditions: (1) acute thrombosis (clot) or thrombophlebitis of the deep veins; (2) acute pulmonary embolism, resulting from blood clots that originate anywhere in the body; (3) atrial fibrillation, to prevent clotting of blood inside the heart that could result in embolization of small clots to any part of the body; (4) acute myocardial infarction (heart attack), to prevent clotting and embolization; (5) transient ischemic attack (TIA)—temporary reduction of blood flow to part of the brain; used here to reduce the risk of repeated attacks or possible stroke. Other possible uses include the long-term prevention of recurrent heart attack, and prevention of embolization from the heart in those individuals with artificial heart valves.

THIS DRUG SHOULD NOT BE TAKEN IF

—you are allergic to any of the drugs bearing the brand names listed above.
—you have a history of a bleeding disorder.
—you have an active peptic ulcer.
—you have ulcerative colitis.

INFORM YOUR PHYSICIAN BEFORE TAKING THIS DRUG IF

—you are now taking *any other drugs*—either drugs prescribed by another physician or non-prescription drugs you purchased over-the-counter (see OTC drugs in Glossary).
—you have high blood pressure.
—you have abnormally heavy or prolonged menstrual bleeding.
—you have diabetes.
—you are using an indwelling catheter.
—you have a history of serious liver or kidney disease, or impaired liver or kidney function.
—you plan to have a surgical or dental procedure in the near future.

Time Required for Apparent Benefit

Drug action begins in 24 to 36 hours, produces desired effects within 36 to 72 hours, and persists for 4 to 5 days. Continuous use on a regular schedule for up to 2 weeks (with daily prothrombin testing and dosage adjustment) is needed to determine the correct maintenance dose for each individual.

Possible Side-Effects *(natural, expected, and unavoidable drug actions)*

Minor episodes of bleeding may occur even when dosage is well within the recommended range. If in doubt regarding its significance, consult your physician regarding the need for prothrombin testing.

Possible Adverse Effects *(unusual, unexpected, and infrequent reactions)*

IF ANY OF THE FOLLOWING DEVELOP, DISCONTINUE DRUG AND NOTIFY YOUR PHYSICIAN AS SOON AS POSSIBLE

Mild Adverse Effects
   Allergic Reactions: Skin rash, hives, loss of scalp hair, drug fever.
   Other Reactions: Nausea, vomiting, diarrhea.

Serious Adverse Effects

Abnormal bruising, major bleeding, or hemorrhage. Notify physician of nosebleeds, bleeding gums, bloody sputum, blood-tinged urine, bloody or tarry stools. (The incidence of significant bleeding is 2% to 4%.)

CAUTION

1. Always carry with you a card of personal identification that includes a statement indicating that *you are using an anticoagulant* (see Table 19 and Section Six).
2. While you are taking an anticoagulant drug, always consult your physician *before* starting any new drug, changing the dosage schedule of any drug, or discontinuing any drug.

Precautions for Use by Those over 60 Years of Age

You may be more sensitive to the action of this drug. Small doses are mandatory until your individual response has been determined.

Observe regularly for indications of excessive drug effects such as prolonged bleeding from shaving cuts, bleeding gums, bloody urine, rectal bleeding, or excessive bruising.

Advisability of Use During Pregnancy

Pregnancy Category: X (tentative). See Pregnancy Code inside back cover.
Animal reproduction studies in mice reveal fetal hemorrhage and death due to this drug.

Information from studies in pregnant women indicates fetal defects and fetal hemorrhage due to this drug. The manufacturers state that this drug is contraindicated during entire pregnancy.

Ask physician for guidance.

Advisability of Use While Nursing Infant

This drug is present in milk and may cause bleeding or hemorrhage in the nursing infant. Ask physician for guidance.

Habit-Forming Potential

None.

Effects of Overdosage

With Moderate Overdose: Episodes of minor bleeding: blood spots in white portion of eye, nosebleeds, gum bleeding, small bruises, prolonged bleeding from minor cuts received while shaving or from other small lacerations.

With Large Overdose: Episodes of major internal bleeding: vomiting of blood, grossly bloody urine or stools.

Possible Effects of Extended Use

None reported.

Suggested Periodic Examinations While Taking This Drug (at physician's discretion)

Regular determination of prothrombin time is essential to safe dosage and proper control.

Occasional urine analysis for red blood cells.

While Taking This Drug, Observe the Following

Foods: A larger intake than usual of foods high in Vitamin K may reduce the effectiveness of this drug and make larger doses necessary. Foods rich in Vitamin K include: cabbage, cauliflower, fish, kale, liver, spinach.

Beverages: No restrictions.

Alcohol: Use with caution until combined effect has been determined. Alcohol can either increase or decrease the effect of this drug. It is advisable to use alcohol sparingly while taking anticoagulants.

Note: Heavy users of alcohol with liver damage may be very sensitive to anticoagulants and require smaller than usual doses.

Tobacco Smoking: No interactions expected. Follow physician's advice regarding smoking (based upon condition under treatment).

Marijuana Smoking: No interactions expected.

Other Drugs: Refer to individual Drug Profiles and to Drug Classes (Section Three) for brand names of the drugs listed below.

Warfarin may *increase* the effects of

- insulin.
- phenytoin (Dantoin, Dilantin, etc.).
- oral anti-diabetics of the sulfonylurea Drug Class (Dymelor, Orinase, Tolinase).

The following drugs *taken concurrently* with warfarin may cause *either an increase or a decrease* in anticoagulant effect

- antihistamines.
- benzodiazepines (Dalmane, Librium, Serax, Valium).
- chloral hydrate (Noctec, Somnos, Chloralixir, etc.).
- cholestyramine (Cuemid, Questran).
- clofibrate (Atromid-S).
- cortisone and related drugs.
- oral contraceptives.
- reserpine (Ser-Ap-Es, Serpasil, Neo-Serp, etc.).

The following drugs may *increase* the effects of warfarin

- acetaminophen (Tempra, Tylenol, etc.), in doses of 2 to 6 grams daily (slight increase only).
- allopurinol (Zyloprim).
- anabolic drugs (Adroyd, Anavar, Dianabol, etc.).
- androgens (Android, Metandren, Oreton, etc.).
- antibiotics (Kantrex, the penicillins, tetracyclines, etc.).
- chloramphenicol (Chloromycetin, etc.).
- cimetidine (Tagamet).
- disulfiram (Antabuse).
- ethacrynic acid (Edecrin).
- glucagon.
- guanethidine (Ismelin).
- hydroxyzine (Atarax, Vistaril).
- indomethacin (Indocin, Indocid).

- isocarboxazid (Marplan).
- isoniazid (INH, Isozide, Niconyl, etc.).
- mefenamic acid (Ponstel, Ponstan).
- mercaptopurine (Purinethol).
- methyldopa (Aldomet, Dopamet).
- methylphenidate (Ritalin, Methidate).
- metronidazole.
- nalidixic acid (NegGram).
- nortriptyline (Aventyl).
- oxyphenbutazone (Oxalid, Tandearil).
- para-aminosalycylic acid (P.A.S., Pamisyl, etc.).
- phenelzine (Nardil).
- phenylbutazone (Butazolidin, Phenbutazone, etc.)—increase with initial use only.
- phenyramidol (Analexin).
- probenecid (Benemid).
- propoxyphene (Darvon).
- propylthiouracil (Propacil, Propyl-Thyracil).
- quinidine (Quinidex, Cardioquin).
- salicylates (aspirin, aspirin combinations).
- sulfinpyrazone (Anturane).
- sulfonamides (certain short- and long-acting "sulfa" drugs).
- sulfonylureas (Diabinese, Dymelor, Orinase, Tolinase).
- tetracycline (Achromycin, Panmycin, Sumycin, etc.).
- thyroid preparations (Cytomel, Proloid, Synthroid, Thyroxine, etc.).
- tricyclic antidepressants (Elavil, Sinequan, Tofranil).
- trimethoprim (Bactrim, Septra, etc.).
- vitamin E (in large doses).

The following drugs may *decrease* the effects of warfarin
- antacids (when used in large doses).
- barbiturates (Amytal, Butisol, Seconal, etc.).
- carbamazepine (Tegretol).
- chlorpromazine (Thorazine, Largactil, etc.).
- digitalis preparations.
- estrogens (Premarin, Milprem, Formatrix, etc.).
- ethchlorvynol (Placidyl).
- furosemide (Lasix).
- glutethimide (Doriden, Somide).
- griseofulvin (Fulvicin, Grisactin, Grifulvin).
- haloperidol (Haldol).
- meprobamate (Equanil, Miltown, etc.).
- oral contraceptives.
- phenylbutazone (Butazolidin, Phenbutazone, etc.)—subsequent decrease following initial increase.
- phenylpropanolamine (Propadrine, Allerest, Naldecon, Triaminic, etc.).
- phenytoin (Dantoin, Dilantin, etc.).
- Vitamin C (when used in large doses).

Driving a Vehicle, Operating Machinery, Engaging in Hazardous Activities: Usually no restrictions. Avoid unnecessary hazardous activities that could cause injury and result in excessive bleeding. Consult your physician for assessment of individual risk and for guidance regarding specific restrictions.

Aviation Note: Thrombo-embolic disorders *are a disqualification* for the piloting of aircraft. Consultation with a designated Aviation Medical Examiner is advised.

Exposure to Sun: No restrictions.

Exposure to Heat: Prolonged hot weather may increase the prothrombin time and make it advisable to reduce anticoagulant dosage. Ask physician for guidance.

Occurrence of Unrelated Illness: Any acute illness that causes fever, vomiting, or diarrhea can alter your response to this drug. Notify your physician so corrective action can be taken.

Discontinuation: Do not discontinue this drug abruptly unless abnormal bleeding occurs. Ask physician for guidance regarding gradual reduction of dosage over a period of 3 to 4 weeks.

Special Storage Instructions
Keep in a dry, tightly closed container. Protect from light.

SECTION THREE

DRUG CLASSES

Drug Classes

Throughout the Drug Profiles in Section Two reference is made to various drug classes. The reader may be advised to consult Section Three to become familiar with the drugs which belong to a particular class of drugs that share important characteristics in their chemical composition or in their actions within the body. Often it is important to know that *any* drug (or *all* drugs) within a given class can be expected to behave in a particular way. Such information may be useful in preventing interactions that could reduce the effectiveness of the drugs in use or result in unanticipated and sometimes hazardous adverse effects.

The presentation of each Drug Class is divided into two listings. The upper list contains the more widely recognized brand names of the drugs within the class, the lower list contains the generic names of the class members. In some instances the number of brand names in use is so large that a complete listing is not possible. In such cases, to be certain that you are consulting the correct drug class, determine the generic name of the drug that concerns you and consult the lower list to see if it is included there. The generic name listing is sufficiently complete to serve the scope of this book.

The following page lists the names of all the Drug Classes included in this section.

LIST OF DRUG CLASSES

Amphetamine-like Drugs
Analgesics, Mild
Analgesics, Strong (Narcotic Drugs)
Anti-acne Drugs
Anti-allergic Drugs
Anti-anginal Drugs
Anti-arthritic/Anti-inflammatory Drugs (Aspirin Substitutes)
Anti-asthmatic Drugs
Antibiotics
Anticoagulants
Antidepressants
Anti-diabetics, Oral
Anti-diarrheal Drugs
Anti-epileptic Drugs (Anticonvulsants)
Anti-Glaucoma Drugs
Anti-Gout Drugs
Antihistamines
Anti-hypertensives
Anti-itching Drugs (Antipruritics)
Antimicrobial Drugs (Non-antibiotic)
Anti-Motion Sickness/Anti-Nausea Drugs (Anti-emetics)
Anti-parkinsonism Drugs
Antispasmodics, Synthetic
Appetite Suppressants (Anorexiants)
Atropine-like Drugs
Barbiturates
Benzodiazepines
Beta-Adrenergic Blocking Drugs ("Beta-Blockers")
Calcium Channel Blocking Drugs ("Calcium Blockers")

Cephalosporins
Cholesterol Reducing Drugs
Cortisone-like Drugs (Adrenocortical Steroids)
Cough Suppressants (Antitussives)
Decongestants
Digitalis Preparations
Diuretics
Female Sex Hormones
Fever-reducing Drugs (Antipyretics)
Heart Rhythm Regulators (Anti-arrhythmic Drugs)
Histamine (H-2) Blocking Drugs ("H-2 Blockers")
Male Sex Hormones (Androgens)
Mono-amine Oxidase (MAO) Inhibitor Drugs
Muscle Relaxants
Nitrates
Penicillins
Phenothiazines
Salicylates
Sedatives/Sleep Inducers (Hypnotics), Non-barbiturate
Sulfonamides ("Sulfa" Drugs)
Sulfonylureas
Tetracyclines
Thiazide Diuretics
Tranquilizers, Mild (Anti-anxiety Drugs)
Tranquilizers, Strong (Antipsychotic Drugs)
Vasodilators
Xanthines

AMPHETAMINE-LIKE DRUGS

BRAND NAMES

Amodex	Fastin	Ritalin
Benzedrine	Ionamin	Tenuate
Biphetamine	Obalan	Tepanil
Desoxyn	Plegine	Tora
Dexedrine	Preludin	Wilpowr
Didrex		

GENERIC NAMES

amphetamine	methamphetamine
benzphetamine	methylphenidate
dextroamphetamine	phendimetrazine
diethylpropion	phenmetrazine
levamphetamine	phentermine

ANALGESICS, MILD

BRAND NAMES

Anaprox	Indocin	Talwin
A.S.A. Preparations	Motrin	Taper
Darvocet	Nebs	Tempra
Darvon	Percodan	Tylenol
Datril	Ponstel	Valadol

GENERIC NAMES

acetaminophen	naproxen
aspirin	oxycodone
codeine	paregoric
ibuprofen	pentazocine
indomethacin	propoxyphene
mefenamic acid	

ANALGESICS, STRONG (NARCOTIC DRUGS)

BRAND NAMES

GENERIC NAMES

Demerol	anileridine
Dilaudid	hydromorphone
Dolophine	meperidine
Leritine	methadone
	morphine

ANTI-ACNE DRUGS

BRAND NAMES	GENERIC NAMES
Accutane	benzoyl peroxide
Achromycin V	erythromycin
Eryderm	isotretinoin
Lucidol	tetracycline
Retin-A	tretinoin

ANTI-ALLERGIC DRUGS

See: Antihistamines
Cortisone-like Drugs

ANTI-ANGINAL DRUGS

BRAND NAMES

Calan	Isordil
Cardizem	Nitrostat
Corgard	Peritrate
Inderal	Persantine
Isoptin	Procardia

GENERIC NAMES

diltiazem	nitrates (see Class)
dipyridamole	propranolol
nadolol	verapamil
nifedipine	

ANTI-ARTHRITIC/ANTI-INFLAMMATORY DRUGS
(Aspirin Substitutes)

BRAND NAMES

Clinoral	Nalfon
Indocin	Naprosyn
Motrin	Tolectin

GENERIC NAMES

fenoprofen	naproxen
ibuprofen	sulindac
indomethacin	tolmetin

ANTI-ASTHMATIC DRUGS

Aarane	Bronkotabs	Neothylline
Adrenalin	Choledyl	Norisodrine
Aminodur	Elixophyllin	Proternol
Brethine	Intal	Slo-Phyllin
Bricanyl	Isuprel	Somophylline
Bronkodyl	Lufyllin	Sus-Phrine
Bronkometer	Medihaler-Epi	Theolair
Bronkosol	Medihaler-Iso	Vaponefrin

aminophylline	isoetharine
cromolyn	isoproterenol
dyphylline	oxtriphylline
ephedrine	terbutaline
epinephrine	theophylline

ANTIBIOTICS

See respective Classes listed under Generic Names

cephalosporins	lincomycin
chloramphenicol	penicillins
clindamycin	rifampin
erythromycins	tetracyclines

ANTICOAGULANTS

Coumarin Family

BRAND NAMES	GENERIC NAMES
Coumadin	acenocoumarol
Dicumarol	dicumarol
Liquamar	phenprocoumon
Panwarfin	warfarin
Sintrom	
Tromexan	

Indandione Family

BRAND NAMES	GENERIC NAMES
Danilone	anisindione
Dipaxin	diphenadione
Eridione	phenindione
Hedulin	
Miradon	

ANTIDEPRESSANTS

BRAND NAMES

Anafranil	Pertofrane
Asendin	Presamine
Aventyl	Sinequan
Elavil	Surmontil
Ensidon	Tofranil
Ludiomil	Vivactil
Norpramin	

GENERIC NAMES

amitriptyline	maprotiline
amoxapine	nortriptyline
clomipramine	opipramol
desipramine	protriptyline
doxepin	trimipramine
imipramine	

ANTI-DIABETICS, ORAL

Sulfonylurea Family

BRAND NAMES

Chloronase	Euglucon
Diabeta	Mobenol
Diabinese	Orinase
Dimelor	Stabinol
Dymelor	Tolinase

GENERIC NAMES

acetohexamide
chlorpropamide
glyburide
tolazamide
tolbutamide

Biguanide Family

BRAND NAMES	GENERIC NAMES
DBI	metformin
Glucophage	phenformin
	(limited availability)

ANTI-DIARRHEAL DRUGS

BRAND NAMES	GENERIC NAMES
Donnagel	atropine
Imodium	diphenoxylate
Kaopectate	kaolin
Lomotil	loperimide
Parepectolin	paregoric
	pectin

ANTI-EPILEPTIC DRUGS
(Anticonvulsants)

BRAND NAMES

Clonopin	Mysoline
Depakene	Tegretol
Diamox	Valium
Dilantin	Zarontin
Luminal	

GENERIC NAMES

acetazolamide	phenobarbital
carbamazepine	phenytoin
clonazepam	primidone
diazepam	valproic acid
ethosuximide	

ANTI-GLAUCOMA DRUGS

BRAND NAMES	GENERIC NAMES
Diamox	acetazolamide
Glaucon	epinephrine
Isopto-carpine	pilocarpine
Timoptic	timolol

ANTI-GOUT DRUGS

BRAND NAMES	GENERIC NAMES
Anturane	allopurinol
Benemid	colchicine
Zyloprim	probenecid
	sulfinpyrazone

ANTIHISTAMINES

BRAND NAMES

Actidil	Dimetane	Neo-Antergan
Atarax	Dramamine	Norflex
Benadryl	Hispril	Periactin
Bonine	Histadyl	Phenergan
Chlor-Trimeton	Histalon	Pyribenzamine
Clistin	Inhiston	Trimeton
Decapryn	Marezine	Vistaril

GENERIC NAMES

brompheniramine	diphenhydramine	orphenadrine
carbinoxamine	diphenylpyraline	pheniramine
chlorpheniramine	doxylamine	promethazine
cyclizine	hydroxyzine	pyrilamine
cyproheptadine	meclizine	tripelennamine
dimenhydrinate	methapyrilene	triprolidine

ANTI-HYPERTENSIVES

BRAND NAMES

Aldomet	Esidrix	Loniten
Anhydron	Eutonyl	Lopressor
Apresoline	Exna	Minipress
Capoten	HydroDiuril	Naqua
Catapres	Hygroton	Naturetin
Corgard	Inderal	Renese
Diuril	Inversine	Saluron
Enduron	Ismelin	Serpasil
Esbaloid	Lasix	

GENERIC NAMES

bendroflumethiazide	guanethidine	minoxidil
benzthiazide	hydralazine	nadolol
bethanidine	hydrochlorothiazide	pargyline
captopril	hydroflumethiazide	polythiazide
chlorothiazide	mecamylamine	prazosin
chlorthalidone	methyclothiazide	propranolol
clonidine	methyldopa	reserpine
cyclothiazide	metoprolol	trichlormethiazide
furosemide		

ANTI-ITCHING DRUGS
(Antipruritics)

BRAND NAMES	GENERIC NAMES
Atarax	cortisone-like drugs (see Class)
Cortaid	cyproheptadine
Dermolate	hydroxyzine
Periactin	trimeprazine
Temaril	
Vistaril	

ANTIMICROBIAL DRUGS
(Non-antibiotic)

BRAND NAMES

Bactrim	Macrodantin
Flagyl	NegGram
Furadantin	Septra
Gantrisin	

GENERIC NAMES

metronidazole
nalidixic acid
nitrofurantoin
sulfonamides (see Class)
trimethoprim

ANTI-MOTION SICKNESS/ANTI-NAUSEA DRUGS
(Anti-emetics)

BRAND NAMES

Antivert   Dramamine
Atarax   Marezine
Benadryl   Phenergan
Bonine   Thorazine
Compazine   Tigan
Dexedrine   Vistaril

GENERIC NAMES

chlorpromazine   meclizine
cyclizine   prochlorperazine
dextroamphetamine   promethazine
dimenhydrinate   scopolamine
diphenhydramine   trimethobenzamide
hydroxyzine

ANTI-PARKINSONISM DRUGS

BRAND NAMES

Akineton   Kemadrin   Parlodel
Artane   Larodopa   Parsidol
Bendopa   Levodopa   Phenoxene
Biodopa   Norflex   Pipanol
Cogentin   Pagitane   Symmetrel
Disipal   Parda   Tremin
Dopar

GENERIC NAMES

amantadine   ethopropazine
benztropine   levodopa
biperiden   orphenadrine
bromocriptine   procyclidine
chlorphenoxamine   trihexyphenidyl
cycrimine

ANTISPASMODICS, SYNTHETIC

BRAND NAMES

Antrenyl	Nacton	Quarzan
Banthine	Pamine	Robinul
Bentyl	Pathilon	Tral
Cantil	Prantal	Trocinate
Darbid	Pro-Banthine	

GENERIC NAMES

clidinium	isopropamide	poldine
dicyclomine	mepenzolate	propantheline
diphemanil	methantheline	thiphenamil
glycopyrrolate	methscopolamine	tridihexethyl
hexocyclium	oxyphenonium	

APPETITE SUPPRESSANTS
(Anorexiants)

BRAND NAMES

Dexedrine	Preludin
Dietac	Pre-Sate
Fastin	Sanorex
Ionamin	Tenuate
Plegine	Tepanil
Pondimin	

GENERIC NAMES

chlorphentermine	phendimetrazine
dextroamphetamine	phenmetrazine
diethylpropion	phentermine
fenfluramine	phenylpropanolamine
mazindol	

ATROPINE-LIKE DRUGS

The drugs included in the following groups may exhibit atropine-like (anticholinergic) action. This can be important in the management of certain diseases and in potential interactions with other drugs used concurrently.

All drugs containing:

atropine	Antidepressants
belladonna	Antihistamines (some)
hyoscyamine	Anti-parkinsonism Drugs
scopolamine	Antispasmodics, Synthetic
	Muscle Relaxants (some)

BARBITURATES

BRAND NAMES

Alurate	Mebaral
Amytal	Nembutal
Butisol	Sandoptal
Lotusate	Seconal
Luminal	Sombulex

GENERIC NAMES

amobarbital	mephobarbital
aprobarbital	pentobarbital
butabarbital	phenobarbital
butalbital	secobarbital
hexobarbital	talbutal

BENZODIAZEPINES

BRAND NAMES

Ativan	Restoril
Clonopin	Serax
Dalmane	Tranxene
Libritabs	Valium
Librium	Verstran
Paxipam	Xanax

GENERIC NAMES

alprazolam	halazepam
chlorazepate	lorazepam
chlordiazepoxide	oxazepam
clonazepam	prazepam
diazepam	temazepam
flurazepam	

BETA-ADRENERGIC BLOCKING DRUGS
("Beta-Blockers")

BRAND NAMES

Blocadren	Lopressor
Corgard	Tenormin
Inderal	Visken

GENERIC NAMES

atenolol	pindolol
metoprolol	propranolol
nadolol	timolol

CALCIUM CHANNEL BLOCKING DRUGS
("Calcium Blockers")

BRAND NAMES	GENERIC NAMES
Calan	diltiazem
Cardizem	nifedipine
Isoptin	verapamil
Procardia	

CEPHALOSPORINS

BRAND NAMES

Anspor   Keflex
Ceclor   Novolexin
Ceporex   Ultracef
Duricef   Velosef

GENERIC NAMES

cefaclor
cefadroxil
cephalexin
cephradine

CHOLESTEROL REDUCING DRUGS

BRAND NAMES

Atromid S   Lorelco
Choloxin   Nicobid
Colestid   Questran
Cytellin

GENERIC NAMES

cholestyramine   nicotinic acid (niacin)
clofibrate   probucol
colestipol   sitosterols
dextrothyroxine

CORTISONE-LIKE DRUGS
(Adrenocortical Steroids)

BRAND NAMES

Aristocort
Colisone
Cortef
Cortril
Decadron
Delta-Cortef
Deltasone
Deltra
Deronil
Dexameth

Dexamethadrone
Dexasone
Gammacorten
Hexadrol
Hydeltra
Hydrocortone
Inflamase
Kenacort
Maxidex
Medrol

Meticorten
Novadex
Novapred
Paracort
Prednis
Servisone
Sterane
Valisone
Vanceril
Wescopred

GENERIC NAMES

beclomethasone
betamethasone
cortisone
dexamethasone
hydrocortisone

methylprednisolone
prednisolone
prednisone
triamcinolone

COUGH SUPPRESSANTS
(Antitussives)

BRAND NAMES

Benylin
Benylin DM
Dilaudid
Hycodan

Phenergan
Tessalon
Tussionex

GENERIC NAMES

benzonatate
codeine
dextromethorphan
diphenhydramine

hydrocodone
hydromorphone
promethazine

DECONGESTANTS

<u>BRAND NAMES</u>

Afrin

Gluco-Fedrin

Neo-Synephrine

Novafed

Otrivin

Privine

Propadrine

Sudafed

Tyzine

<u>GENERIC NAMES</u>

ephedrine

naphazoline

oxymetazoline

phenylephrine

phenylpropanolamine

pseudoephedrine

tetrahydrozoline

xylometazoline

DIGITALIS PREPARATIONS

<u>BRAND NAMES</u>

Crystodigin

Digifortis

Digiglusin

Gitaligin

Lanoxicaps

Lanoxin

Purodigin

<u>GENERIC NAMES</u>

digitalis

digitoxin

digoxin

gitalin

DIURETICS

BRAND NAMES

Aldactone
Bumex
Diamox
Diuril
Dyrenium
Edecrin
Hygroton
Lasix
(See Thiazide Brand Names)
Zaroxolyn

GENERIC NAMES

acetazolamide
bumetanide
chlorthalidone
ethacrynic acid
furosemide
metolazone
spironolactone
thiazides (see Class)
triamterene

FEMALE SEX HORMONES

BRAND NAMES

Estrogens
DES
Delestrogen
Estinyl
Estrace
Estrovis
Evex
Feminone
Ogen
Premarin
TACE

Progestogens
Amen
Curretab
Megace
Micronor
Norlutin
Ovrette
Provera

GENERIC NAMES

Estrogens
chlorotrianisene
diethylstilbestrol
estradiol
estrogens, conjugated
estrogens, esterified
estropipate
ethinyl estradiol
quinestrol

Progestogens
medroxyprogesterone
megestrol
norethindrone
norgestrel

FEVER-REDUCING DRUGS
(Antipyetics)

BRAND NAMES

Anaprox	Naprosyn
Clinoril	Ponstel
Indocin	Rufen
Motrin	Tolectin
Nalfon	Tylenol

GENERIC NAMES

acetaminophen	mefenamic acid
aspirin	naproxen
fenoprofen	sulindac
ibuprofen	tolmetin
indomethacin	

HEART RHYTHM REGULATORS
(Anti-arrhythmic Drugs)

BRAND NAMES

Calan	Procan SR
Crystodigin	Pronestyl
Inderal	Purodigin
Isoptin	Quinaglute
Lanoxin	Quinidex
Norpace	Quinora

GENERAL NAMES

digitoxin	propranolol
digoxin	quinidine
disopyramide	verapamil
procainamide	

HISTAMINE (H-2) BLOCKING DRUGS
("H-2 Blockers")

BRAND NAMES	GENERIC NAMES
Tagamet	cimetidine
Zantac	ranitidine

MALE SEX HORMONES
(Androgens)

BRAND NAMES

Android   Oratestin
Android F   Ora-Testryl
Depo-Testosterone   Oreton
Halotestin   Oreton Methyl
Metandren   Testred

GENERIC NAMES

fluoxymesterone
methyltestosterone
testosterone

MONO-AMINE OXIDASE (MAO) INHIBITOR DRUGS

BRAND NAMES

Actomol   Marsilid
Catron   Nardil
Drazine   Niamid
Eutonyl   Parnate
Furoxone   Tersavid
Marplan

GENERIC NAMES

furazolidone   phenelzine
iproniazid   pheniprazine
isocarboxazid   phenoxypropazine
mebanazine   piohydrazine
nialamide   tranylcypromine
pargyline

MUSCLE RELAXANTS

BRAND NAMES

Equanil
Flexeril
Lioresal
Norflex
Paraflex
Parafon Forte
Rela
Robaxin
Skelaxin
Soma
Valium

GENERIC NAMES

baclofen
carisoprodol
chlorzoxazone
cyclobenzaprine
diazepam
meprobamate
metaxalone
methocarbamol
orphenadrine

NITRATES

BRAND NAMES

Cardilate
Isordil
Laserdil
Neo-Corovas
Nitro-Bid
Nitroglyn
Nitrospan
Nitrostat
Peritrate
SK-Petn
Sorbide
Sorbitrate

GENERIC NAMES

erythrityl tetranitrate
isosorbide dinitrate
nitroglycerin
pentaerythritol tetranitrate

PENICILLINS

BRAND NAMES

Alpen	Omnipen	Principen
Amcill	Orbenin	Prostaphlin
Amoxil	Pathocil	Spectrobid
Bactocil	Penbritin	Tegopen
Dynapen	Pentids	Unipen
Geocillin	Pen-Vee K	V-Cillin K
Geopen	Polycillin	Veracillin
Larotid	Polymox	

GENERIC NAMES

amoxicillin	nafcillin
ampicillin	oxacillin
bacampicillin	penicillin G
carbenicillin	penicillin V
cloxacillin	
dicloxacillin	

PHENOTHIAZINES

BRAND NAMES

Chlor-PZ	Proketazine	Tacaryl
Compazine	Prolixin	Temaril
Largon	Promatar	Thorazine
Levoprome	Quide	Tindal
Mellaril	Repoise	Torecan
Parsidol	Sparine	Trilafon
Permitil	Serentil	Vesprin
Phenergan	Stelazine	

GENERIC NAMES

acetophenazine	methdilazine	propiomazine
butaperazine	methotrimeprazine	thiethylperazine
carphenazine	perphenazine	thioridazine
chlorpromazine	piperacetazine	trifluoperazine
ethopropazine	prochlorperazine	triflupromazine
fluphenazine	promazine	trimeprazine
mesoridazine	promethazine	

SALICYLATES

BRAND NAMES

Arthropan   Empirin
Bufferin   Magan
Causalin   Neocylate
Ecotrin   Uracel

GENERIC NAMES

aspirin
choline salicylate
magnesium salicylate
potassium salicylate
sodium salicylate

SEDATIVES/SLEEP INDUCERS (HYPNOTICS), NON-BARBITURATE

BRAND NAMES

Carbrital   Noctec   Restoril
Dalmane   Noludar   Somnafac
Doriden   Parest   Sopor
Dorimide   Placidyl   Valmid
Felsules

GENERIC NAMES

carbromal   flurazepam
chloral hydrate   glutethimide
ethchlorvynol   methyprylon
ethinamate   temazepam

SULFONAMIDES ("SULFA" DRUGS)

BRAND NAMES

Azulfidine	Gantanol	Sonilyn
Coco-Diazine	Gantrisin	Suladyne
Cosulfa	Kynex	Thiosulfil
Dagenan	Madribon	Triple Sulfas
Diamox	Midicel	Urobiotic
Elkosin	Neotrizine	

GENERIC NAMES

acetazolamide	sulfamethazine	sulfasalazine
sulfachlorpyridazine	sulfamethizole	sulfisomidine
sulfadiazine	sulfamethoxazole	sulfisoxazole
sulfadimethoxine	sulfamethoxypyridazine	trisulfapyrimidines
sulfamerazine	sulfapyridine	

SULFONYLUREAS

BRAND NAMES

Chloronase	Novobutamide
Diabinese	Orinase
Dimelor	Tolbutone
Dymelor	Tolinase
Mobenol	

GENERIC NAMES

acetohexamide
chlorpropamide
tolazamide
tolbutamide

TETRACYCLINES

BRAND NAMES

Achromycin	Rondomycin	Tetracyn
Aureomycin	Steclin	Vectrin
Declomycin	Sumycin	Velacycline
Minocin	Terramycin	Vibramycin
Panmycin	Tetrachel	

GENERIC NAMES

chlortetracycline	minocycline
demeclocycline	oxytetracycline
doxycycline	rolitetracycline
methacycline	tetracycline

THIAZIDE DIURETICS

BRAND NAMES

Anhydron	Hydrazide	Naqua
Chemhydrazide	Hydrid	Naturetin
Diucardin	Hydrite	Neocodema
Diuchlor	Hydro-Aquil	Novohydrazide
Diuril	Hydrodiuretex	Oretic
Duretic	HydroDiuril	Renese
Edemol	Hydrosaluret	Saluron
Enduron	Hydrozide	Thiuretic
Esidrix	Metahydrin	Urozide
Exna		

GENERIC NAMES

bendroflumethiazide	hydroflumethiazide
benzthiazide	methyclothiazide
chlorothiazide	polythiazide
cyclothiazide	trichlormethiazide
hydrochlorothiazide	

TRANQUILIZERS, MILD

BRAND NAMES

Atarax	Miltown	Tybatran
Deprol	Paxipam	Ultran
Equanil	Serax	Valium
Fenarol	Trancopal	Vistaril
Librium	Tranxene	Xanax

GENERIC NAMES

alprazolam	halazepam
benactyzine	hydroxyzine
chlordiazepoxide	meprobamate
chlormezanone	oxazepam
clorazepate	phenaglycodol
diazepam	tybamate

TRANQUILIZERS, STRONG

BRAND NAMES

Carbolith	Lithonate	Serpasil
Eskalith	Lithotabs	Taractan
Haldol	Navane	(See Phenothiazines,
Lithane	Sandril	Brand Names)

GENERIC NAMES

chlorprothixene	phenothiazines (see Class)
haloperidol	reserpine
lithium	thiothixene

VASODILATORS

<u>BRAND NAMES</u>

Arlidin   Pavabid
Cerespan   Vasodilan
Cyclospasmol   Vasospan
Ethatab

<u>GENERIC NAMES</u>

cyclandelate
ethaverine
isoxsuprine
nylidrin
papaverine

XANTHINES

<u>BRAND NAMES</u>

Aminodur   Quibron-T
Bronkodyl   Slo-Phyllin
Choledyl   Theo-Dur
Droxine   Theolixir
Elixophylline   Theovent

<u>GENERIC NAMES</u>

aminophylline
dyphylline
oxtriphylline
theophylline

SECTION FOUR

A GLOSSARY
OF
DRUG-RELATED TERMS

Glossary

Addiction The traditional term used to identify the irresistible craving for and compulsive use of habit-forming drugs. The more recent preference for the term *dependence* has served to clarify the distinction between habituation and addiction. Drugs capable of producing addiction do so by interacting with the biochemistry of the brain in such a way that they assume a working role. This physical incorporation of the drug into the fundamental processes of brain tissue function is responsible for the agony of the "withdrawal syndrome"—the intense mental and physical pain experienced by the addict when intake of the drug is stopped abruptly. Thus addiction is a *physical dependence*. (See DEPENDENCE for a further account of physical and psychological dependence.)

   Example: The sedative and pain-relieving derivatives of opium—heroin, morphine, codeine—and their synthetic substitutes are all capable of producing addiction through physical dependence.

Adverse Effect or Reaction An abnormal, unexpected, infrequent and usually unpredictable injurious response to a drug. Used in this restrictive sense, the term adverse reaction does *not* include effects of a drug which are normally a part of its pharmacological action, even though such effects may be undesirable and unintended. (See SIDE-EFFECT.) Adverse reactions are of three basic types: those due to drug *allergy*, those caused by individual *idiosyncrasy*, and those representing *toxic* effects of drugs on tissue structure and function (see ALLERGY, IDIOSYNCRASY, and TOXICITY).

   Example: The possible interference with normal bone marrow function by phenylbutazone (Butazolidin), resulting in a serious reduction in formation of blood cells, is an adverse effect of a toxic nature. (See BONE MARROW DEPRESSION.)

Allergy (Drug) An abnormal mechanism of drug response that occurs in individuals who produce injurious antibodies* that react with foreign substances—in this instance, a drug. The person who is allergic by nature and has a history of hayfever, asthma, hives, or eczema is more likely to develop drug allergies. Allergic reactions to drugs take many forms: skin eruptions of various kinds, fever, swollen glands, painful joints, jaundice, interference with breathing, acute collapse of circulation, etc. Drug allergies can develop gradually over a long period of time, or they can appear with dramatic suddenness and require life-saving intervention.

---

*Antibodies are special tissue proteins that combine with substances foreign to the body. Protective antibodies destroy bacteria and neutralize toxins. Injurious antibodies, reacting with foreign substances, cause the release of histamine, the principal chemical responsible for allergic reactions.

Example: A 70-year-old woman developed a measles-like rash over her entire body. All diagnostic studies were normal. She left the city to attend a wedding and forgot her phenobarbital, which she had taken for epilepsy since she was in her late teens. The rash disappeared. Upon returning home she resumed the phenobarbital and the rash promptly reappeared. Her allergy to phenobarbital had developed after 50 years of continuous use.

Example: An 18-year-old girl developed a severe sore throat the day before her senior prom. She had taken penicillin once previously with no unfavorable effects. She was given an injection of penicillin to treat her infected throat. Within five minutes she complained of shortness of breath and shortly thereafter collapsed to the floor unconscious. Emergency resuscitation saved her life. She had experienced an acute reaction to penicillin, to which she had become allergic after a single exposure several years before (see ANAPHYLACTIC REACTION).

Anaphylactic (Anaphylactoid) Reaction A group of symptoms which represent (or resemble) a sometimes overwhelming and dangerous allergic reaction due to extreme hypersensitivity to a drug. Anaphylactic reactions, whether mild, moderate, or severe, often involve several body systems. Mild symptoms consist of itching, hives, nasal congestion, nausea, abdominal cramping, and/or diarrhea. Sometimes these precede more severe symptoms such as choking, shortness of breath, and sudden loss of consciousness (usually referred to as anaphylactic shock).

Characteristic features of anaphylactic reaction must be kept in mind. It can result from a very small dose of drug; it develops suddenly, usually within a few minutes after taking the drug; it can be rapidly progressive and can lead to fatal collapse in a short time if not reversed by appropriate treatment. A developing anaphylactic reaction is a true medical emergency. Any adverse effect that appears within 20 minutes after taking a drug should be considered the early manifestations of a possible anaphylactic reaction. Obtain medical attention immediately! (See ALLERGY, DRUG and HYPERSENSITIVITY.)

Example: A 40-year-old lawyer consulted his dentist (whose office was in the same building) for treatment of a gum abscess. Following surgical drainage of the abscess, the lawyer was given a prescription for penicillin tablets and instructed to begin medication immediately. The lawyer obtained the penicillin, returned to his office, and took the first tablet. Within 10 minutes his hands and feet began to itch, his face became swollen, and a choking sensation made it difficult to breathe. He rushed to his dentist's office, where he was given emergency treatment (Adrenalin and oxygen) to reverse the anaphylactic reaction to penicillin.

Anti-hypertensive A drug used to lower the blood pressure. The term "hypertension" denotes blood pressure above the normal range. It does not refer to excessive nervous or emotional tension. The term "anti-hypertensive" is sometimes used erroneously as if it had the same meaning as anti-anxiety (or tranquilizing) drug action.

Today there are more than 100 drug products in use for treating hypertension. Those most frequently prescribed for long-term use fall into three major groups:

drugs that increase urine production (the diuretics)
drugs that relax blood vessel walls
drugs that reduce the activity of the sympathetic nervous system.

Regardless of their mode of action, all these drugs share an ability to lower the blood pressure. It is important to remember that many other drugs can interact with anti-hypertensive drugs: some add to their effect and cause excessive reduction in blood pressure; others interfere with their action and reduce their effectiveness. Anyone who is taking medications for hypertension should consult with his or her physician whenever drugs are prescribed for the treatment of other conditions as well.

Example: A 45-year-old personnel officer was found to have a blood pressure of 185/115 during a routine examination by his company physician. Repeated examinations over the following week confirmed that his blood pressure was remaining unacceptably high. Although he felt well and had no symptoms indicative of hypertension, he followed his physician's urging and began a trial of chlorothiazide. Over the following 4 weeks his blood pressure gradually decreased to an average of 160/100, but it remained in this range in spite of maximal doses of chlorothiazide. By increasing the elimination of salt and water from the body through increased urine production, this thiazide diuretic had achieved a beneficial response but was unable to lower the pressure to the desired level. The physician then added methyldopa to the treatment program. Appropriate dosage adjustments of both drugs were made over the following 6 weeks. By reducing the activity of the sympathetic nervous system, the methyldopa provided additional anti-hypertensive effect. Through the combined actions of both drugs, the patient's blood pressure was maintained consistently below 145/95. Combining drugs with different actions made it possible to achieve satisfactory blood pressure control with reduced dosage of each drug and with fewer undesirable side effects.

Example: Some of the phenothiazine drugs (such as Compazine, Phenergan, and Thorazine) are used widely to treat nausea and vomiting. In some individuals these drugs are capable of causing a significant drop in blood pressure. In treating nausea and vomiting in a person on medication for high blood pressure, the selection of an antinausea (anti-emetic) drug should exclude those that could produce sudden and excessive reductions in blood pressure.

Example: The action of guanethidine (Ismelin) is significantly impaired by the oral contraceptives. In approximately 80% of hypertensive women taking guanethidine while they are using oral contraceptives concurrently, the dose of guanethidine has to be raised substantially to control their blood pressure.

Aplastic Anemia A form of bone marrow failure in which the production of all 3 types of blood cells is seriously impaired (also known as pancytopenia). Aplastic anemia can occur spontaneously from unknown causes, but about one-half of reported cases are induced by certain drugs or chemicals. The symptoms reflect the consequences of inadequate supplies of all 3 blood cell types: deficiency of red blood cells (anemia) results in fatigue, weakness, and pallor; deficiency of white blood cells (leukopenia) predisposes to infections; deficiency of blood platelets (thrombocytopenia) leads to spontaneous bruising and hemorrhage. Treatment is difficult and the outcome unpredictable. Even with the best of care, approximately 50% of cases end fatally.

These drugs and chemicals are known to be capable of inducing aplastic anemia:

acetazolamide	meprobamate
anti-cancer drugs	methimazole
aspirin	oxyphenbutazone
benzene (solvent)	penicillin
carbamazepine	phenacetin
carbon tetrachloride (solvent)	phenylbutazone
chlordane (insecticide)	phenytoin
chlordiazepoxide	primidone
chloromycetin	promazine
chlorothiazide	quinacrine
chlorpheniramine	sulfonamides
chlorpromazine	tetracyclines
chlorpropamide	thiouracil
colchicine	tolbutamide
DDT (insecticide)	triflupromazine
indomethacin	trimethadione
lithium	tripelennamine
mephenytoin	

Although aplastic anemia is a rare consequence of drug treatment (3 in 100,000 users of quinacrine, for example), anyone taking a drug capable of inducing it should have complete blood cell counts periodically if the drug is to be used over an extended period of time.

Bioavailability The measurable characteristics of a drug product (usually a tablet or a capsule) that represent how rapidly the active drug ingredient is absorbed into the bloodstream and to what extent it is absorbed. Two types of measurements—(1) blood levels of the drug at certain time intervals after administration, and (2) the duration of the drug's presence in the blood—indicate how much of the drug is available for biological activity and for how long.

Another method of determining a drug product's bioavailability is to measure (1) the cumulative amount of the drug (or any breakdown product after transformation) that is excreted in the urine, and (2) the rate of drug accumulation in the urine.

The two major factors that govern a drug product's bioavailability are the chemical and physical characteristics (the formulation) of the dosage form given, and the functional state of the digestive system of the individual who takes it. A drug product that disintegrates rapidly in a normally functioning stomach and small intestine produces blood levels of the absorbed drug quite promptly. Such a drug product can be demonstrated to possess good bioavailability.

Specially designed laboratory tests are now available to evaluate a drug product's potential bioavailability when taken by the "average" individual.

Bioequivalence It is generally accepted that the ability of a drug product to produce its intended therapeutic effect is directly related to its bioavailability. When a particular drug is marketed by several manufacturers, often in a variety of dosage forms, it is critically important that the drug product selected for use is one that possesses the bioavailability necessary to be effective therapeutically. Substantial variations occur among manufacturers in the formulation of their drug products. Although the principal drug ingredient of products from different firms may be identical chemically, it cannot be assumed that these products possess equal bioavailability and are therefore equal therapeutically.

The bioavailability of any drug product is governed to a large extent by the physical characteristics of its formulation; these in turn determine how rapidly and how completely the drug product disintegrates and releases its active drug component(s) for absorption into the bloodstream. Drug products that contain the same principal drug ingredient but are combined with different inert additives, are coated with different substances, or are enclosed in capsules of different composition, may or may not possess the same bioavailability. Those that do are said to be bioequivalent, and can be relied upon to be equally effective in achieving therapeutic results.

If you consider having your prescription filled with the generic equivalent of a brand name drug product, ask your physician *and* pharmacist for guidance. This decision requires professional judgment in each case. In many treatment situations, reasonable differences in the bioavailability patterns among drug products are acceptable. In some situations however, because of the serious nature of the illness, or because it is mandatory that blood levels of the drug be maintained within a narrowly defined range, it is essential to use a drug product that has been demonstrated to possess reliable bioavailability.

Blood Platelets The smallest of the three types of blood cells produced by the bone marrow. Platelets are normally present in very large numbers. Their primary function is to assist the process of normal blood clotting so as to prevent excessive bruising and bleeding in the event of injury. When present in proper numbers and functioning normally, platelets preserve the retaining power of the walls of the smaller blood vessels. By initiating appropriate clotting processes in the blood, platelets seal small points of leakage in the vessel walls, thereby preventing spontaneous bruising or bleeding (that which is unprovoked by trauma).

Certain drugs and chemicals may reduce the number of available blood platelets to abnormally low levels. Some of these drugs act by suppressing platelet formation; other drugs hasten their destruction. When the number of functioning platelets falls below a critical level, blood begins to leak through the thin walls of smaller vessels. The outward evidence of this leakage is the spontaneous appearance of scattered bruises in the skin of the thighs and legs. This is referred to as purpura. Bleeding may occur anywhere in the body, internally as well as superficially into the tissues immediately beneath the skin.

Example: A woman in her early forties developed a persistent bursitis in her shoulder. A popular form of buffered aspirin provided reasonable relief of pain. Certain that the bursitis would eventually disappear, she continued to use the aspirin in doses of 4 to 6 tablets daily over a period of 9 months. While bathing she noticed the appearance of a few small painless bruises scattered over her thighs. She could recall no injury to account for the bruising, so she dismissed the discovery as unimportant. As her recurrent bursitis required, she continued the intermittent use of aspirin. The areas of bruising became more numerous and extensive. On examination by her physician, blood studies revealed "a very low blood platelet count." She was advised to discontinue all drugs and was scheduled for bone marrow examination. Within a few days after discontinuing the use of aspirin, the bruises began to fade and no new bruising occurred. Bone marrow studies were normal and repeated examinations of the blood revealed that the blood platelets had returned to a normal level. She had experienced an allergic destruction of her blood platelets, a well-known adverse reaction to aspirin in sensitive individuals.

Bone Marrow Depression A serious reduction in the ability of the bone marrow to carry on its normal production of blood cells. This can occur as an adverse reaction to the toxic effect of certain drugs and chemicals on bone marrow components. When functioning normally, the bone marrow produces the majority of the body's blood cells. These consist of three types: the red blood cells (erythrocytes), the white blood cells (leukocytes), and the blood platelets (thrombocytes). Each type of cell performs one or more specific functions, all of which are indispensable to the maintenance of life and health.

Drugs that are capable of depressing bone marrow activity can impair the production of all types of blood cells simultaneously or of only one type selectively. Periodic examinations of the blood can reveal significant changes in the structure and number of the blood cells that indicate a possible drug effect on bone marrow activity.

Impairment of the production of red blood cells leads to anemia, a condition of abnormally low red cells and hemoglobin. This causes weakness, loss of energy and stamina, intolerance to cold environments, and shortness of breath on physical exertion. A reduction in the formation of white blood cells can impair the body's immunity and lower its resistance to infection. These changes may result in the development of fever, sore throat, or pneumonia. When the formation of blood platelets is suppressed to abnormally low levels, the blood loses its ability to quickly seal small points of leakage in blood vessel walls. This may lead to episodes of unusual and abnormal spontaneous bruising or to prolonged bleeding in the event of injury.

Any of these symptoms can occur in the presence of bone marrow depression. They should alert both patient and physician to the need for prompt studies of blood and bone marrow.

Example: A 10-year-old boy developed pneumonia while on a winter camping trip. He responded promptly to a course of chloramphenicol (Chloromycetin) and recovered without complication. Within a few weeks he began to experience a series of head and chest colds. Anxious to keep his absence from school to a minimum, and remembering how promptly he responded to earlier treatment for pneumonia, the boy's mother began to administer chloramphenicol whenever a head cold or chest cold began to develop. After several short courses of the drug over a period of 3 months, the boy's health began to fail noticeably. Concerned by his loss of weight, persistent fever, paleness, and fatigue, the mother arranged for medical evaluation. Routine blood studies disclosed a significant reduction of all three series of blood cells. A bone marrow examination confirmed the diagnosis of aplastic anemia due to the repeated use of chloramphenicol (see APLASTIC ANEMIA).

Brand Name The registered trade name given to a drug product by its manufacturer. Many drugs are marketed by more than one manufacturer or distributor. Each company adopts a distinctive trade name to identify its brand of the generic drug from that of its competitors. Thus a brand name designates a proprietary drug—one that is protected by patent or copyright. Generally brand names are shorter, easier to pronounce, and more readily remembered than their generic counterparts.

Example: The generic drug hydrochlorothiazide is marketed in the U.S. and Canada by sixteen manufacturers under the following *brand names:*

Chemhydrazide	Hydrodiuretex
Diuchlor H	HydroDiuril
Edemol	Hydrosaluret
Esidrix	Hydrozide
Hydrazide	Neo-Codema
Hydrid	Novohydrazide
Hydrite	Oretic
Hydro-Aquil	Urozide

Cause-and-Effect Relationship A possible causative association between a drug and an observed biologic event—most commonly a side-effect or an adverse effect. Knowledge of a drug's full spectrum of effects (wanted and unwanted) is highly desirable when weighing its benefits and risks in any treatment situation. However, it is often impossible to establish with certainty that a particular drug is the primary agent responsible for a suspected adverse effect. In the evaluation of every cause-and-effect relationship, therefore, meticulous consideration must be given to such factors as the time sequence of drug administration and possible reaction, the use of multiple drugs, possible interactions among these drugs, the effects of the disease under treatment, the physiological and psychological characteristics of the patient, and the possible influence of unrecognized disorders and malfunctions.

The majority of adverse drug reactions occur sporadically, unpredictably, and infrequently in the general population. A *definite* cause-and-effect relationship between drug and reaction is established when (1) the adverse effect immediately follows administration of the drug; or (2) the adverse effect disappears after the drug is discontinued (dechallenge) and promptly reappears when the drug is used again (rechallenge); or (3) the adverse effects are clearly the expected and predictable toxic consequences of drug overdosage.

In contrast to the obvious "causative" (definite) relationship, there exists a large gray area of "probable," "possible," and "coincidental" associations that are clouded by varying degrees of uncertainty. These classifications usually apply to alleged drug reactions that require a relatively long time to develop, are of low incidence, and for which there are no clear-cut objective means of demonstrating a causal mechanism that links drug and reaction. Clarification of cause-and-effect relationships in these uncertain groups requires carefully designed observation over a long period of time, followed by sophisticated statistical analysis. Occasionally the public is alerted to a newly found "relationship" based upon suggestive but incomplete data. Though early warning is clearly in the public interest, such announcements should make clear whether the presumed relationship is based upon definitive criteria or is simply inferred because the use of a drug and an observed event were found to occur together within an appropriate time frame.

The most competent techniques for evaluating cause-and-effect relationships of adverse drug reactions have been devised by the Division of Tissue Reactions to Drugs, a research unit of the Armed Forces Institute of Pathology. Based upon a highly critical examination of all available evidence, the Division's study of 2800 drug-related deaths yielded the following levels of certainty regarding cause-and-effect relationship:

No association	5.0%
Coincidental	14.5%
Possible	33.0%
Probable	30.0%
Causative	17.5%

It is significant that expert evaluation of 2800 drug-related cases concluded that only 47.5% could be substantiated as definitely or probably causative.

Example: A 48-year-old man went into anaphylactic shock within a few minutes after the administration of penicillin given to treat a large abscess on his neck. The almost immediate development of this overwhelming allergic reaction established a "causative" association between drug and adverse effect.

Example: A 50-year-old woman developed jaundice during the fourth week of chlorpromazine (Thorazine) treatment for chronic anxiety, raising the question of a possible drug reaction. A liver biopsy (tissue examination) and appropriate laboratory tests of liver function revealed a familiar pattern of results consistent with the type of liver disorder and jaundice generally associated with use of phenothiazine tranquilizers in sensitive individuals. The cause-and-effect relationship in this case was judged to be "probable."

Example: A 53-year-old man with a history of peptic ulcer (a stomach ulcer which bled 10 years earlier) was given phenylbutazone (Butazolidin) to treat acute bursitis of the shoulder. He took the drug after meals to reduce the possibility of indigestion. On the fifth day of treatment he awoke in the middle of the night acutely nauseated and vomiting blood. He required emergency hospitalization and blood transfusion. Subsequent X-ray studies revealed a prominent ulcer of the stomach. Although the mechanism of drug-induced peptic ulcer (in the stomach or duodenum) is not well understood, the association of ulcer reactivation with the use of certain drugs is well recognized. In the absence of definitive tests that could link his drug to stomach ulceration, the cause-and-effect relationship in this case was judged to be "possible."

Example: A husband and wife attended a community church supper and ate liberally of most foods served. Earlier the same day the husband had begun taking chlorthalidone (Hygroton), which had just been prescribed for his high blood pressure. Shortly after retiring, the husband developed abdominal cramping and diarrhea. He immediately concluded that he was probably experiencing a "reaction to the new medicine." An hour later his wife developed cramping and diarrhea. They learned the next day that most of their neighbors who ate chicken salad at the church supper also experienced cramping and diarrhea. The cause-and-effect relationship between drug and "reaction" in this case was judged to be "coincidental." Continued use of chlorthalidone was not accompanied by cramps or diarrhea.

Contraindication A condition or disease that precludes the use of a particular drug. Some contraindications are *absolute,* meaning that the use of the drug would expose the patient to extreme hazard and therefore cannot be justified. Other contraindications are *relative,* meaning that the condition or disease does not entirely bar the use of the drug but requires that, before the decision to use the drug is made, special consideration be given to factors which could aggravate existing disease, interfere with current treatment, or produce new injury.

Example: Severe allergy to penicillin is an *absolute contraindication* to its use for any reason.

Example: Reduced kidney function (such as that which results from chronic kidney disease) is a *relative contraindication* to the use of kanamycin (Kantrex) because the potential toxicity of kanamycin can be enhanced if kidney function is impaired.

Dependence The preferred term used to identify the drug-dependent states of *psychological dependence* (or *habituation*), and *physical dependence* (or *addiction*). In addition, a third kind of drug-dependence can be included under this term. This might be called *functional dependence*—the need to use a drug continuously in order to sustain a particular body function, the impairment of which causes annoying symptoms of varying degree and significance.

Psychological dependence is a form of neurotic behavior. Its principal characteristic is an obsession to satisfy a particular desire, be it one of self-gratification or one of escape from some real or imagined distress. Psychological dependence is a very human trait that is seen often in many socially acceptable patterns and practices such as entertainment, gambling, sports, and collecting. A common form of this dependence in today's culture is the increasing reliance upon drugs to help in coping with the every-day problems of living: pills for frustration, disappointment, nervous stom-ach, tension headache, and insomnia. The 20 million smokers of marijuana have found it to be a drug that eases their stress, one whose effectiveness fosters habit (psychological dependence) but not addiction.

Physical dependence, which is true addiction, includes two elements: habituation and tolerance. Addicting drugs provide relief from anguish and pain swiftly and effectively; they also induce a physiological tolerance that requires increasing dosage or repeated use if they are to remain effective. These two features foster the continued need for the drug and lead to its becoming a functioning component in the biochemistry of the brain. As this occurs, the drug assumes an "essential" role in ongoing chemical pro-cesses. (Thus some authorities prefer the term *chemical dependence.*) Sud-den removal of the drug from the system causes a major upheaval in body chemistry and provokes a withdrawal syndrome—the intense mental and physical pain experienced by the addict when intake of the drug is stopped abruptly—that is the hallmark of addiction.

Functional dependence differs significantly from both psychological and physical dependence. It occurs when a drug effectively relieves an annoying or distressing condition and the particular body function in-volved becomes increasingly dependent upon the action of the drug to provide a sense of well-being. Drugs which are capable of inducing func-tional dependence are used primarily for the relief of symptoms. They do not act on the brain to produce alteration of mood or consciousness as do those drugs with potential for either psychological or physical dependence. The most familiar example of functional dependence is the "laxative habit." Some types of constipation are made worse by the wrong choice of laxative, and natural function gradually fades as the colon becomes more and more dependent upon the action of certain laxative drugs.

Disulfiram-like (Antabuse-like) Reaction The symptoms that result from the interaction of alcohol and any drug that is capable of provoking the pattern of response typical of the "Antabuse effect." The interacting drug inter-rupts the normal decomposition of alcohol by the liver and thereby permits the accumulation of a toxic by-product that enters the bloodstream. When sufficient levels of both alcohol and drug are present in the blood the reaction occurs. It consists of intense flushing and warming of the face, a severe throbbing headache, shortness of breath, chest pains, nausea, re-peated vomiting, sweating, and weakness. If the amount of alcohol ingested has been large enough, the reaction may progress to blurred vision, vertigo, confusion, marked drop in blood pressure, and loss of consciousness. Severe reactions may lead to convulsions and death. The reaction can last from 30 minutes to several hours, depending upon the amount of alcohol in the body. As the symptoms subside, the individual is exhausted and usually sleeps for several hours.

Example: A 52-year-old business executive was found to have diabetes during his annual physical examination. His blood sugar levels remained above the normal range in spite of his careful adherence to a prescribed diet. To obtain better control of the blood sugar, his physician started him on a trial of chlorpropamide (Diabinese) but failed to mention that some individuals taking anti-diabetic drugs of the sulfonylurea family experience a disulfiram-like reaction following the use of alcohol. On the third day after starting his medication, the executive invited an associate to join him for a business lunch. As was his custom on such occasions, he drank two cocktails before starting to eat. Ten minutes later he began to experience a sense of warmth and fullness in his head. This was soon followed by pounding of his heart, shortness of breath, and profuse sweating. Alarmed and puzzled by this sudden development, he asked his associate to take him to the nearest hospital emergency room. When the attending physician obtained a history of current chlorpropamide therapy and luncheon cocktails, he readily identified the resulting disulfiram-like reaction.

Dosage Forms and Strengths This information category in the individual Drug Profiles (Section Two) uses several abbreviations to designate measurements of weight and volume. These are:

mcg. = microgram = 1,000,000th of a gram (weight)
mg. = milligram = 1000th of a gram (weight)
ml. = milliliter = 1000th of a liter (volume)
gm. = gram = 1000 milligrams (weight)

There are approximately 65 mg. in 1 grain.
There are approximately 5 ml. in 1 teaspoonful.
There are approximately 15 ml. in 1 tablespoonful.
There are approximately 30 ml. in 1 ounce.
1 milliliter of water weighs 1 gram.
There are approximately 454 grams in 1 pound.

Drug, Drug Product Terms often used interchangeably to designate a medicine (in any of its dosage forms) used in medical practice. Strictly speaking, the term *drug* refers to the single chemical entity that provokes a specific response when placed within a biological system—the "active" ingredient. A *drug product* is the manufactured dosage form—tablet, capsule, elixir, etc.—that contains the active drug intermixed with inactive ingredients to provide for convenient administration.

Drug products which contain only one active ingredient are referred to as single entity drugs. Drug products with two or more active ingredients are called combination drugs (designated [CD] in the lists of brand names in the Drug Profiles, Section Two).

Examples: Tylenol Elixir is a single entity *drug product;* acetaminophen is its only active *drug* ingredient.

Ser-Ap-Es is a combination *drug product;* it contains three active *drug* ingredients:

Serpasil (a brand name for reserpine)
Apresoline (a brand name for hydralazine)
Esidrix (a brand name for hydrochlorothiazide)

Drug Class A group of drugs that are similar in chemistry, method of action, and use in treatment. Because of their common characteristics, many drugs within a class will produce the same side-effects and have similar potential for provoking related adverse reactions and interactions. However, significant variations among members within a drug class can occur. This sometimes allows the physician an important degree of selectivity in choosing a drug if certain beneficial actions are desired or particular side-effects are to be minimized.

  Examples: Antihistamines, phenothiazines, tetracyclines (see Section Three).

Drug Fever The elevation of body temperature that occurs as an unwanted manifestation of drug action. Drugs can induce fever by several mechanisms; these include allergic reactions, drug-induced tissue damage, acceleration of tissue metabolism, constriction of blood vessels in the skin with resulting decrease in loss of body heat, and direct action on the temperature-regulating center in the brain.

  The most common form of drug fever is that associated with allergic reactions. It may be the only allergic manifestation apparent, or it may be part of a complex of allergic symptoms that can include skin rash, hives, joint swelling and pain, enlarged lymph glands, hemolytic anemia, or hepatitis. The fever usually appears about 7 to 10 days after starting the drug and may vary from low-grade to alarmingly high levels. It may be sustained or intermittent, but it usually persists for as long as the drug is taken. In previously sensitized individuals drug fever may occur within one or two hours after taking the first dose of medication.

  While many drugs are capable of producing fever, the following are more commonly responsible:

allopurinol	novobiocin
antihistamines	para-aminosalicylic acid
atropine-like drugs	penicillin
barbiturates	pentazocine
coumarin anticoagulants	phenytoin
hydralazine	procainamide
iodides	propylthiouracil
isoniazid	quinidine
methyldopa	rifampin
nadalol	sulfonamides

  Example: A 56-year-old man under treatment for high blood pressure was found to have an inadequate response to a trial of thiazide drugs used alone. His physician added methyldopa to his treatment routine and asked him to return for evaluation in 2 weeks. After 1 week of taking methyldopa daily, the patient experienced an abrupt onset of fever, chills, and fatigue. Believing he had the "flu," he stayed in bed, took aspirin and increased his intake of fluids. After 3 days of persistent fever (to levels of 103°), he discontinued all medication. Within 48 hours all symptoms disappeared. He called his physician, reported what had happened, and requested instructions regarding the resumption of medications for his high blood pressure. He was advised to resume the same medications he was taking before the episode of "flu." Within a few hours after restarting methyldopa, the patient experienced a sudden rise in temperature to 104°. By discontinuing the drug initially (dechallenge) and later resuming it (rechallenge), he inadvertently established the cause-and-effect relationship between methyldopa and his drug fever.

Extension Effect An unwanted but predictable drug response that is a logical consequence of mild to moderate overdosage. An extension effect is an exaggeration of the drug's normal pharmacological action; it can be thought of as a mild form of dose-related toxicity (see OVERDOSAGE and TOXICITY).

Example: The continued "hangover" of drowsiness and mental sluggishness that persists after arising in the morning is a common extension effect of a long-acting sleep-inducing drug (hypnotic) taken the night before.

Example: The persistent intestinal cramping and diarrhea that result from too generous a dose of laxative are extension effects of the drug's anticipated action.

Generic Name The official, common, or public name used to designate an active drug entity, whether in pure form or in dosage form. Generic names are coined by committees of officially appointed drug experts and are approved by governmental agencies for national and international use. Thus they are non-proprietary. Many drug products are marketed under the generic name of the principal active ingredient and bear no brand name of the manufacturer.

Though the total number of prescriptions written in the United States in 1975 declined by 1%, prescriptions specifying the *generic name* of the drug increased by 3.2%. Generically written prescriptions now account for 11.1% of all new prescriptions written in the United States. The drugs most commonly prescribed by generic name are listed below, ranked in descending order of the number of new prescriptions issued.

ampicillin	phenobarbital
tetracycline	penicillin G
erythromycin	meprobamate
penicillin V	digoxin
prednisone	thyroid

Example: Meprobamate is the generic name designating the active drug ingredient of two trademarked brands, Equanil and Miltown. *Diazepam* is the generic name that identifies the active drug entity of the widely used mild tranquilizer marketed as Valium.

Habituation A form of drug dependence based upon strong psychological gratification rather than the physical (chemical) dependence of addiction. The habitual use of drugs that alter mood or relieve minor discomforts results from a compulsive need to feel pleasure and satisfaction or to escape the manifestations of emotional distress. The abrupt cessation of habituating drugs does not produce the withdrawal syndrome seen in addiction. Thus habituation is a *psychological dependence.* (See DEPENDENCE for a further account of psychological and physical dependence.)

Example: Amphetamines (Benezedrine, Dexedrine) are capable of producing extreme psychological dependence but are not addicting. Many over-the-counter drugs used to relieve headaches, minor pains, nervous tension and insomnia can lead to psychological dependence if taken excessively. Regardless of the drug taken, its abusive use is a form of neurotic behavior.

Hemolytic Anemia A form of anemia (deficient red blood cells and hemoglobin) resulting from the premature destruction (hemolysis) of circulating
red blood cells. Several mechanisms can be responsible for the development of hemolytic anemia; among these is the action of certain drugs and
chemicals. Some individuals are susceptible to hemolytic anemia because
of a genetic deficiency in the makeup of their red blood cells. If such people
are given certain antimalarial drugs, sulfa drugs, or numerous other drugs,
some of their red cells will disintegrate on contact with the drug. (About
10% of American blacks have this genetic trait.)

Another type of drug-induced hemolytic anemia is a form of drug allergy. Many drugs in wide use (including quinidine, methyldopa, levodopa,
and chlorpromazine) are known to cause hemolytic destruction of red cells
as a hypersensitivity (allergic) reaction.

Hemolytic anemia can occur abruptly (with evident symptoms) or si-
lently. The acute form lasts about 7 days and is characterized by fever,
pallor, weakness, dark-colored urine, and varying degrees of jaundice (yellow coloration of eyes and skin). When drug-induced hemolytic anemia is
mild, involving the destruction of only a small number of red blood cells,
there may be no symptoms to indicate its presence. Such episodes are
detected only by means of laboratory studies (see IDIOSYNCRASY and AL-
LERGY, DRUG).

Hepatitis-like Reaction Changes in the liver, induced by certain drugs, which
closely resemble those produced by viral hepatitis. The symptoms of drug-
induced hepatitis and virus-induced hepatitis are often so similar that the
correct cause cannot be established without precise laboratory studies.

Hepatitis due to drugs may be a form of drug allergy (as in reaction to
many of the phenothiazines), or it may represent a toxic adverse effect (as
in reaction to some of the mono-amine oxidase inhibitor drugs). Liver
reactions of significance usually result in jaundice and represent serious
adverse effects (see JAUNDICE; see also Table 4 in Section Five).

Hypersensitivity A term subject to varying usages for many years. One common use has been to identify the trait of overresponsiveness to drug action,
that is, an intolerance to even small doses. Used in this sense, the term
indicates that the nature of the response is appropriate but the degree of
response is exaggerated.

The term is more widely used today to identify a state of allergy. To
have a *hypersensitivity* to a drug is to be *allergic* to it (see ALLERGY, DRUG).

Some individuals develop cross-hypersensitivity. This means that once
a person has developed an allergy to a certain drug, that person will experience an allergic reaction to other drugs which are closely related in chemical composition.

Example: The patient was known to be *hypersensitive* by nature, having a history of seasonal hay fever and asthma since childhood. His *allergy*
to tetracycline developed after his third course of treatment. This drug
hypersensitivity manifested itself as a diffuse, measles-like rash.

Hypoglycemia A condition in which the amount of glucose (a sugar) in the
blood is below the normal range. Since normal brain function is dependent
upon an adequate supply of glucose, reducing the level of glucose in the

blood below a critical point will cause serious impairment of brain activity. The resulting symptoms are characteristic of the hypoglycemic state. Early indications are headache, a sensation resembling mild drunkenness, and an inability to think clearly. These may be accompanied by hunger. As the level of blood glucose continues to fall, nervousness and confusion develop. Varying degrees of weakness, numbness, trembling, sweating, and rapid heart action follow. If sugar is not provided at this point and the blood glucose level drops further, impaired speech, incoordination, and unconsciousness, with or without convulsions, will follow.

Hypoglycemia in any stage requires prompt recognition and treatment. Because of the potential for injury to the brain, the mechanisms and management of hypoglycemia should be understood by all who use drugs capable of producing it.

Example: A 24-year-old traveling salesman required a morning dose of 65 units of an intermediate-acting insulin to control his diabetes. Late one afternoon, while driving between cities, he had a flat tire. During the process of changing wheels, he began to experience lightheadedness, weakness, trembling, and excessive perspiring. He felt flushed and noted rapid pounding of his heart. Recognizing these symptoms to be the early manifestations of an "insulin reaction," he immediately swallowed the cubes of table sugar he always carried with him for such an emergency. The concurrent effects of emotional stress, unusual physical exertion, a delayed evening meal, and unopposed insulin action had combined to induce a state of hypoglycemia; his prompt recognition of glucose deficiency and his timely corrective action prevented progression of his situation to a state of helplessness and coma.

Example: Upon returning home late one evening, a woman found her 61-year-old diabetic mother unconscious on the living room sofa. The family physician was summoned, and he promptly restored her to consciousness with an intravenous injection of glucose solution. She related that during her daughter's absence she had developed a headache, had taken two aspirin tablets along with her evening dose of tolbutamide (Orinase), and had lain down to rest before dinner. Apparently she fell asleep and slipped into hypoglycemic coma. The headache was probably an early manifestation of impending hypoglycemia. The interaction of aspirin with tolbutamide increased its ability to lower the blood glucose still further. Sleep prevented the intake of food that could have relieved the hypoglycemia.

(NOTE: The elderly are more susceptible to hypoglycemia from the use of oral antidiabetic drugs.)

Idiosyncrasy An abnormal mechanism of drug response that occurs in individuals who have a peculiar defect in their body chemistry (often hereditary) which produces an effect totally unrelated to the drug's normal pharmacological action. Idiosyncrasy is not a form of allergy. The actual chemical defects responsible for certain idiosyncratic drug reactions are well understood; others are not.

Example: Approximately 100 million people in the world (including 10% of American blacks) have a specific enzyme deficiency in their red blood cells that causes these cells to disintegrate when exposed to drugs such as sulfonamides (Gantrisin, Kynex), nitrofurantoin (Furadantin, Macrodantin), probenecid (Benemid), quinine, and quinidine. As a result of this reaction, these drugs (and others) can cause a significant anemia in susceptible individuals.

Example: Approximately 5% of the population of the United States is susceptible to the development of glaucoma on prolonged use of cortisone-related drugs (see Cortisone Drug Class in Section Three).

Interaction An unwanted change in the body's response to a drug that results when a second drug that is capable of altering the action of the first is administered at the same time. Some drug interactions can enhance the effect of either drug, producing an overresponse similar to overdosage. Other interactions may reduce drug effectiveness and cause inadequate response. A third type of interaction can produce a seemingly unrelated toxic response with no associated increase or decrease in the pharmacological actions of the interacting drugs.

Theoretically, many drugs can interact with one another, but in reality drug interactions are comparatively infrequent. Many interactions can be anticipated, and the physician can make appropriate adjustments in dosage to prevent or minimize unintended fluctuations in drug response.

Examples: Aspirin can *interact* with anticoagulant drugs (such as warfarin and dicumarol) to increase the anticoagulant effect. This may lead to abnormal bleeding, ranging from mild nose or gum bleeding to severe hemorrhage.

Barbiturates (such as phenobarbital) can *interact* with anticoagulants to decrease the anticoagulant effect. Larger than usual doses of the anticoagulant are then required to produce the desired response. Withdrawal of the barbiturate, without an appropriate reduction in the anticoagulant dose, may result in abnormal bleeding due to excessive (unopposed) anticoagulant effect.

A tricyclic antidepressant (amitriptyline, imipramine, etc.) given inadvertently to someone taking a mono-amine oxidase (MAO) inhibitor drug (furazolidone, pargyline, phenelzine, etc.) can produce a severe toxic reaction consisting of agitation, tremor, high fever, and coma.

Jaundice A yellow coloration of the skin (and the white portion of the eyes) that occurs when excessive bile pigments accumulate in the blood as a result of impaired liver function. Jaundice can be produced by several mechanisms. It may occur as a manifestation of a wide variety of diseases, or it may represent an adverse reaction to a particular drug. At times it is difficult to distinguish between disease-induced jaundice and drug-induced jaundice.

Jaundice due to a drug is always a serious adverse effect. Anyone taking a drug that is capable of causing jaundice should watch closely for any significant change in the color of urine or feces. Dark discoloration of the urine and paleness (lack of color) of the stool may be early indications of a developing jaundice. Should either of these symptoms occur, it is advisable to discontinue the drug and notify the prescribing physician promptly. Diagnostic tests are available to clarify the nature of the jaundice.

Example: A 30-year-old man was found to have converted from a negative to a positive tuberculin skin test after a fellow worker was hospitalized for active tuberculosis. As a preventive measure he was started on a one-year course of isoniazid (INH, Nydrazid). During the third week of treatment he began to feel ill. He lost his appetite and became aware of vague nausea. Within a few days he began to itch. His wife detected a yellowish tint in his eyes. The following day the skin of his chest and abdomen was found to be turning yellow when examined in daylight. Blood tests for viral hepatitis were negative. His physician discontinued the isoniazid and the jaundice cleared within 3 weeks. This type of drug-induced jaundice closely resembles viral hepatitis (an infection of the liver). It is thought to be allergic in nature and to represent a hypersensitivity reaction to the drug.

Lupus Erythematosus A serious disease of unknown cause that occurs in two forms, one limited to the skin (discoid LE) and the other involving several body systems (systemic LE). Both forms occur predominantly in young women. About 5% of cases of the discoid form convert to the systemic form. Basically, systemic LE is a disorder of the body's immune system which may result in chronic, progressive inflammation and destruction of the connective tissue framework of the skin, blood vessels, joints, brain, heart muscle, lungs, and kidneys. Altered proteins in the blood lead to the formation of antibodies which react with certain organ tissues to produce the inflammation and destruction characteristic of the disease. A reduction in the number of white blood cells and blood platelets often occurs. The course of systemic LE is usually quite protracted and unpredictable. While no cure is known, satisfactory management may be achieved in some cases by the judicious use of cortisone-like drugs.

Several drugs in wide use are capable of initiating a form of systemic LE quite similar to that which occurs spontaneously. (More than 100 cases due to the use of procainamide have been reported.) Suggestive symptoms may appear as early as 2 weeks or as late as 8 years after starting the responsible drug. The initial symptoms usually consist of low-grade fever, skin rashes of various kinds, aching muscles, and multiple joint pains. Chest pains (pleurisy) are fairly common. Enlargement of the lymph glands occurs less frequently. Symptoms usually subside following discontinuation of the responsible drug, but laboratory evidence of the reaction may persist for many months.

Drugs known to induce systemic LE include:

chlorpromazine	phenothiazines (some)
clofibrate	phenylbutazone
hydralazine	phenytoin
isoniazid	practolol
oral contraceptives	procainamide
penicillamine	thiouracil
phenolphthalein	

Example: A 48-year-old registered nurse with a history of premature heart beats since 18 years of age consulted her physician because of heart palpitation of increasing severity. As a result of multiple stresses, she had increased her cigarette consumption to 50 a day. She was found to have high blood pressure and a serious disorder of heart rhythm. She responded well to chlorothiazide and procainamide, and she resumed her professional activities. After 23 months of continuous use of procainamide she began to notice stiffness of her fingers on arising. This was soon followed by joint pain and tenderness in both hands and both elbows. A temperature of 99° to 99.4° was noted on several occasions. She interpreted her symptoms to be due to early rheumatoid arthritis (which her mother had quite severely) and treated herself for the next 3 months. When her hands became so painful she was unable to sleep, she was referred to a rheumatologist. Laboratory studies confirmed his suspicion of drug-induced systemic LE. The procainamide was discontinued and prednisone was started to treat the LE manifestations. Significant improvement occurred within 2 weeks, but complete clearance of all symptoms required 6 months of continuous treatment.

Orthostatic Hypotension A type of low blood pressure that is related to body position or posture (also called postural hypotension). The individual who is subject to orthostatic hypotension may have a normal blood pressure while lying down, but on sitting upright or standing he will experience sudden sensations of lightheadedness, dizziness, and a feeling of impending faint that compel him to return quickly to a lying position. These symptoms are manifestations of inadequate blood flow (oxygen supply) to the brain due to an abnormal delay in the rise in blood pressure that always occurs as the body adjusts the circulation to the erect position.

Many drugs (especially the stronger anti-hypertensives) may cause orthostatic hypotension. Individuals who experience this drug effect should report it to their physician so that appropriate dosage adjustment can be made to minimize it. Failure to correct or to compensate for these sudden drops in blood pressure can lead to severe falls and injury.

The tendency to orthostatic hypotension can be reduced by avoiding sudden standing, prolonged standing, vigorous exercise, and exposure to hot environments. Alcoholic beverages should be used cautiously until their combined effect with the drug in use has been determined.

Overdosage The meaning of this term should not be limited to the concept of doses that clearly exceed the normal dosage range recommended by the manufacturer. The optimal dose of many drugs (that amount which gives the greatest benefit with least distress) varies greatly from person to person. What may be an average dose for the majority of individuals will be an overdose for some and an underdose for others. Numerous factors, such as age, body size, nutritional status, and liver and kidney function, have significant influence on dosage requirements. Drugs with narrow safety margins often produce indications of overdosage if something delays the regular elimination of the customary daily dose. In this instance, overdosage results from accumulation of prescribed daily doses. Massive overdosage— as occurs with accidental ingestion of drugs by children or with suicidal intention by adults—is referred to as poisoning.

Example: The proper use of digitalis is based upon achieving a correct maintenance dose, one that provides a relatively stable level of the drug in blood and body tissues. The maintenance of this "steady state" requires a daily dose that very closely replaces the amount of the drug eliminated from the body each day in the urine and stool. The patient who is properly digitalized with digoxin (that is, on the correct maintenance dose) may develop manifestations of overdosage if his regular intake of liquids drops to a level that does not provide for adequate urine production.

Over-the-Counter (OTC) Drugs Drug products that can be purchased without prescription. Many are available in food stores, variety stores, and newsstands as well as in conventional drug stores. Because of the unrestricted availability of these drugs, many people do not look upon OTC medicines as drugs. But drugs they are! And like the more potent drug products that are sold only on prescription, they are chemicals that are capable of a wide variety of actions on biological systems. Within the last 30 years, many OTC drugs have assumed greater importance because of their ability to interact unfavorably with some widely used prescription drugs. Serious problems in drug management can arise when (1) the patient fails to inform the physician of the OTC drug(s) he is taking ("because they really aren't drugs") and (2) the physician fails to specify that his question about what medicines are being taken currently *includes all OTC drugs.* During any course of treatment, whether medical or surgical, the patient should consult with the physician regarding any OTC drug that he wishes to take.

The major classes of OTC drugs for internal use include:

allergy medicines (antihistamines)	laxatives
antacids	menstrual aids
anti-worm medicines	motion sickness remedies
aspirin and aspirin combinations	pain relievers
aspirin substitutes	reducing aids
asthma aids	salt substitutes
cold medicines (decongestants)	sedatives and tranquilizers
cough medicines	sleeping pills
diarrhea remedies	stimulants (caffeine)
digestion aids	sugar substitutes (saccharin)
diuretics	tonics
iron preparations	vitamins

Example: An insurance adjuster with a history of stress-induced indigestion used antacids occasionally during the day and always at bedtime in liberal amounts. During a period of chronic insomnia, his physician prescribed pentobarbital to be taken at bedtime. The habitual use of antacids at bedtime was never discussed by patient or physician. After a trial of pentobarbital for several nights, the patient reported no significant sedative effect. He was unaware that antacids can retard the absorption of pentobarbital and prevent the attainment of an effective blood level.

Example: A 42-year-old housewife was advised that she needed a hysterectomy (surgical removal of the womb). For the previous year she had been consuming large quantities of a popular aspirin-containing OTC preparation promoted to relieve headaches and nervous tension. When asked by her surgeon to name "the drugs" she was taking, she said she was not using any drugs. Since she did not consider an OTC preparation to be a "drug," her regular use of aspirin went undetected. During the course of her operation, the surgical team had considerable difficulty controlling her bleeding. She required a blood transfusion and intravenous Vitamin K to correct her impairment of normal blood clotting. The patient was unaware that large doses of aspirin can affect some of the clotting factors in the blood and predispose to abnormal bleeding.

Paradoxical Reaction   An unexpected drug response that is not consistent with the known pharmacology of the drug and may in fact be the opposite of the intended and anticipated response. Such reactions are due to individual sensitivity or variability and can occur in any age group. They are seen more commonly, however, in children and the elderly.

Example: An 80-year-old man was admitted to a nursing home following the death of his wife. He had difficulty adjusting to his new environment and was restless, agitated, and irritable. He was given a trial of the tranquilizer diazepam (Valium) to relax him, starting with small doses. On the second day of medication he became confused and erratic in behavior. The dose of diazepam was increased. On the third day he began to wander aimlessly, talked incessantly in a loud voice, and displayed anger and hostility when attempts were made to help him. Suspecting the possibility of a paradoxical reaction, the diazepam was discontinued. All behavioral disturbances gradually subsided within 3 days.

Parkinson-like Disorders (Parkinsonism)   A group of symptoms that resembles those caused by Parkinson's disease, a chronic disorder of the nervous system also known as shaking palsy. The characteristic features of Parkinsonism include a fixed, emotionless facial expression (mask-like in appearance), a prominent trembling of the hands, arms, or legs, and stiffness of the extremities that limits movement and produces a rigid posture and gait.

Parkinsonism is a fairly common adverse effect that occurs in about 15% of all patients who take large doses of strong tranquilizers (notably the phenothiazines) or use them over an extended period of time. If recognized early, the Parkinson-like features will lessen or disappear with reduced dosage or change in medication. In some instances, however, Parkinson-like changes may become permanent, requiring appropriate medication for their control.

Example: A 58-year-old woman was hospitalized for extreme agitation and depression following attempted suicide. She experienced remarkable improvement in the third week of treatment with high doses of chlorpromazine (Thorazine). To stabilize her condition, medication was continued at the same dosage. After 6 weeks of treatment she developed a constant shaking of her head and hands, a rigid, forward-bending posture, and a blank, apathetic expression. The dose of chlorpromazine was reduced by one-half, and an appropriate anti-Parkinsonism drug was started. All Parkinson-like features gradually disappeared and the anti-Parkinsonism drug was withdrawn. Parkinsonism did not reappear with a smaller maintenance dose of chlorpromazine.

Peripheral Neuritis (Peripheral Neuropathy) A group of symptoms that results from injury to nerve tissue in the extremities. A variety of drugs and chemicals are capable of inducing changes in nerve structure or function. The characteristic pattern consists of a sensation of numbness and tingling that usually begins in the fingers and toes and is accompanied by an altered sensation to touch and vague discomfort ranging from aching sensations to burning pain. Severe forms of peripheral neuritis may include loss of muscular strength and coordination.

A relatively common form of peripheral neuritis is that seen with the long-term use of isoniazid in the treatment of tuberculosis. If Vitamin B–6 (pyridoxine) is not given concurrently with isoniazid, peripheral neuritis may occur in sensitive individuals. Vitamin B–6 can be both preventive and curative in this form of drug-induced peripheral neuritis.

Since peripheral neuritis can also occur as a late complication following many viral infections, care must be taken to avoid assigning a cause-and-effect relationship to a drug which is not responsible for the nerve injury (see CAUSE-AND-EFFECT RELATIONSHIP).

Pharmacology The medical science that relates to the development and use of medicinal drugs, their composition and action in animals and man. Used in its broadest sense, pharmacology embraces the related sciences of medicinal chemistry, experimental therapeutics, and toxicology.

Example: The widely used sulfonylurea drugs (Diabinese, Dymelor, Orinase, Tolinase) are effective in the treatment of some forms of diabetes because of the accidental discovery that some of their parent "sulfa" drugs produced hypoglycemia (low blood sugar) during their early therapeutic trials as anti-infectives. Subsequent investigation of the mechanisms of action *(pharmacology)* of these drugs revealed that they are capable of stimulating the pancreas to produce more insulin.

Pharmacological studies on another group of "sulfa" related drugs—the thiazide diuretics—revealed that they could induce the kidney to excrete more water and salt in the urine. This drug action is of great value in treating high blood pressure and heart failure.

Photosensitivity A drug-induced change in the skin that results in the development of a rash or exaggerated sunburn on exposure to the sun or ultraviolet lamps. The reaction is confined to uncovered areas of skin, providing a clue to the nature of its cause. (See Table 6 in Section Five.)

Example: A patient receiving demeclocycline (Declomycin) for viral pneumonia decided to hasten his convalescence by sunbathing. Within 24 hours after his first sunbath, all exposed skin areas developed a severe sunburn far out of proportion to the intensity of the sun or the duration of the exposure.

Porphyria The name used to designate a group of hereditary disorders resulting from the excessive formation and excretion of certain tissue pigments known as porphyrins. The various porphyrias are characterized by unusual sensitivity of the skin to the sun (see PHOTOSENSITIVITY), by recurring episodes of severe abdominal pain, and by varying degrees of damage to the liver and the nervous system.

The following drugs have been reported to cause acute attacks of porphyria in predisposed individuals.

androgens	ethyl alcohol
anti-diabetic drugs*	griseofulvin
barbiturates*	meprobamate
chlordiazepoxide	oral contraceptives
chloroquine	phenytoin
estrogens	sulfonamides*

Secondary Effect A by-product or complication of drug use which does not occur as part of the drug's primary pharmacological activity. Secondary effects are unwanted consequences and may therefore be classified as adverse effects.

Example: The reactivation of dormant tuberculosis can be a *secondary effect* of long-term cortisone administration for arthritis. Cortisone and related drugs (see Drug Class, Section Three) suppress natural immunity and lower resistance to infection.

Example: The cramping of leg muscles can be a *secondary effect* of diuretic (urine-producing) drug treatment for high blood pressure. Excessive loss of potassium through increased urination renders the muscle vulnerable to painful spasm during exercise.

Side-Effect A normal, expected, and predictable response to a drug that accompanies the principal (intended) response sought in treatment. Side-effects are part of a drug's pharmacological activity and thus are unavoidable. Most side-effects are undesirable. The majority cause minor annoyance and inconvenience; some may cause serious problems in managing certain diseases; a few can be hazardous.

Example: The drug propantheline (Pro-Banthine) is used to treat peptic ulcer because one of the consequences of its pharmacological action is the reduction of acid formation in the stomach (an intended effect). Other consequences can include blurring of near vision, dryness of the mouth, and constipation. These are *side-effects*.

Superinfection (Suprainfection) The development of a second infection that is superimposed upon an initial infection currently under treatment. The superinfection is caused by organisms that are not susceptible to the killing action of the drug(s) used to treat the original (primary) infection. Superinfections usually occur during or immediately following treatment with a broad spectrum antibiotic—one that is capable of altering the customary balance of bacterial populations in various parts of the body. The disturbance of this balance permits the overgrowth of organisms that normally exist in numbers too small to cause disease. The superinfection may also require treatment, using those drugs that are effective against the offending organism.

*See Drug Class, Section Three.

Example: Recurrent infections of the kidney and bladder often require repeated courses of treatment with a variety of anti-infective drugs. When these are taken by mouth they can suppress the normally dominant types of bacteria present in the colon and rectum, encouraging the overgrowth of yeast organisms which are capable of causing *colitis.* When this occurs, colitis is a *superinfection.*

Tardive Dyskinesia A late-developing, drug-induced disorder of the nervous system characterized by involuntary bizarre movements of the jaws, lips, and tongue. It occurs after long-term treatment with the more potent drugs used in the management of serious mental illness. While it may occur in any age group, it is more common in the middle-aged and the elderly. Older, chronically ill women are particularly susceptible to this adverse drug effect. Once developed, the pattern of uncontrollable chewing, lip puckering, and repetitive tongue protruding (fly-catching movement) appears to be irreversible. No consistently satisfactory treatment or cure is available. To date, there is no way of identifying beforehand the individual who may develop this distressing reaction to drug treatment, and there is no known prevention. Fortunately, the persistent dyskinesia (abnormal movement) is not accompanied by further impairment of mental function or deterioration of intelligence. It is ironic, however, that the patient who shows significant improvement in his mental illness but is unfortunate enough to develop tardive dyskinesia may have to remain hospitalized because of a reaction to a drug that was given to make it possible for him to leave the hospital.

Example: A 39-year-old man with a diagnosis of schizophrenia developed a typical pattern of tardive dyskinesia in his third year of continuous treatment with a series of potent tranquilizing drugs. By actual count, he averaged 31 tongue protrusions, 32 chewing motions, and 24 lip-puckering movements per minute. Separate trials of treatment using four different drugs produced only a temporary reduction in the frequency of abnormal mouth and jaw movements. The patient is now in his fourth year of tardive dyskinesia and shows no indication of spontaneous recovery.

Tolerance An adaptation by the body that lessens responsiveness to a drug on continuous administration. Body tissues become accustomed to the drug's presence and react to it less vigorously. Tolerance can be beneficial or harmful in treatment.

Examples: Beneficial tolerance occurs when the hay fever sufferer finds that the side effect of drowsiness gradually disappears after four or five days of continuous use of antihistamines.

Harmful tolerance occurs when the patient with "shingles" (herpes zoster) finds that the usual dose of codeine is no longer sufficient to relieve pain and that the need for increasing dosage creates a risk of physical dependence or addiction.

Toxicity The capacity of a drug to dangerously impair body functions or to damage body tissues. Most drug toxicity is related to total dosage: the larger the overdose, the greater the toxic effects. Some drugs, however, can produce toxic reactions when used in normal doses. Such adverse effects are not due to allergy or idiosyncrasy; in many instances their mechanisms are not fully understood. Toxic effects due to overdosage are generally a harmful extension of the drug's normal pharmacological actions and—to some extent—are predictable and preventable. Toxic reactions which occur with normal dosage are unrelated to the drug's known pharmacology and for the most part are unpredictable and unexplainable.

Examples: Dose-related toxicity is seen quite commonly in the coma and death resulting from an overdose of "sleeping pills."

Toxicity unrelated to dosage is seen with some frequency in the occurrence of peptic ulcers (stomach and duodenum) shortly after starting treatment with indomethacin (Indocid, Indocin) or phenylbutazone (Butazolidin).

Tyramine A chemical present in many common foods and beverages that causes no difficulties to body functioning under normal circumstances. The main pharmacological action of tyramine is to raise the blood pressure. Normally, enzymes present in many body tissues neutralize this action of tyramine in the quantities in which it is consumed in the average diet. The principal enzyme responsible for neutralizing the blood-pressure-elevating action of tyramine (and chemicals related to it) is mono-amine oxidase (MAO). Mono-amine oxidase provides an important regulatory function that helps to balance several of the chemical processes in the body that control certain activities of the nervous system. Stabilization of the blood pressure is one of these activities. If the action of mono-amine oxidase is blocked, chemical substances like tyramine function unopposed, and relatively small amounts can cause alarming and dangerous elevations of blood pressure.

Several drugs in use today are capable of blocking the action of mono-amine oxidase. These drugs are commonly referred to as mono-amine oxidase inhibitors (see Drug Class, Section Three). If an individual is taking one of these drugs and his diet includes foods or beverages that contain a significant amount of tyramine, he may experience a sudden increase in blood pressure. Before this interaction of food and drug was understood, several deaths due to brain hemorrhage occurred in persons taking MAO inhibitor drugs as a result of an extreme elevation of blood pressure following a meal of tyramine-rich foods.

It should be noted also that MAO inhibitor drugs can interact with many other drugs and cause serious adverse effects. Consult your physician before taking *any* drug concurrently with one that can inhibit the action of mono-amine oxidase.

Any protein-containing food that has undergone partial decomposition may present a hazard because of its increased tyramine content. The following foods and beverages have been reported to contain varying amounts of tyramine. Unless their tyramine content is known to be insignificant, they should be avoided altogether while taking a MAO inhibitor drug (see Drug Class, Section Three). Consult your physician about the advisability of using any of the foods or beverages on these lists if you are taking such drugs.

FOODS	BEVERAGES
Aged cheeses of all kinds*	Beer (unpasteurized)
Avocado	Chianti wine
Banana skins	Sherry wine
Beef liver (unless fresh and used at once)	Sour cream
"Bovril" extract	Vermouth
Broad bean pods	
Chicken liver (unless fresh and used at once)	
Chocolate	
Figs, canned	
Fish, canned	
Fish, dried and salted	
Herring, pickled	
"Marmite" extract	
Meat extracts	
Meat tenderizers	
Raisins	
Raspberries	
Soy sauce	
Yeast extracts	

NOTE: *Any* high-protein food that is aged or has undergone breakdown by putrefaction probably contains tyramine and could produce a hypertensive crisis in anyone taking MAO inhibiting drugs.

*Cottage cheese, cream cheese, and processed cheese are safe to eat.

SECTION FIVE

TABLES OF DRUG INFORMATION

TABLE 1

A Checklist of Health Conditions That Can Influence the Choice of Drugs

Inform your physician if you have or have had any of the following health conditions. They could influence his or her choice of drugs, or the dosages of drugs, in planning any treatment you may require. In some instances these conditions may be *contraindications* to the use of certain drugs.

Addison's disease
Alcoholism
Allergies (hay fever, asthma, hives, eczema)
Allergies to specific drugs
Anemia (any type), especially
  Hemolytic anemia
  Sickle cell anemia
Angina
Arthritis (any type)
Asthma
Bleeding disorder
Bone marrow disorder
Bronchiectasis
Bronchitis, chronic
Cancer (any type)
Cataracts
Cirrhosis
Colitis
Constipation, chronic
Cystic breast disease
Diabetes
Drug dependence
Emotional depression
Endometriosis
Epilepsy
Fibroid tumors of the uterus
Gall bladder disease, gall stones
Gastritis
Glaucoma
Gout
Hay fever (allergic rhinitis)
Headaches (any type), especially
  Histamine headache

Migraine headache
Vascular headache
Hearing loss
Heart disease (any type)
Heart rhythm disorder
Hepatitis
Hiatal hernia
High blood calcium
High blood pressure
Hypoglycemia
Infection (any type)
Jaundice
Kidney disease, kidney stone
Liver disease
Low blood pressure
Low sperm count
Lung disease (any type)
Lung embolism
Lupus erythematosus
Malabsorption disorder
Manic type of mental disorder
Meniere's disease
Menstrual disorder
Multiple Sclerosis
Myasthenia gravis
Nervous tension (anxiety)
Neuritis (any type)
Pancreatitis
Parkinson's disease
Peptic ulcer disease
Pheochromocytoma
Phlebitis
Porphyria
Pregnancy

Prostate gland enlargement
Raynaud's phenomenon
Red blood cell disorder:
  Glucose-6-phosphate
  dehydrogenase deficiency
Schizophrenia
Sprue
Stroke

Sun sensitivity
Thyroid disorder
  Hyperthyroidism
  Hypothyroidism
Tuberculosis (any type)
Urinary tract infection (chronic or
  recurrent)
Vaginal bleeding (abnormal)

TABLE 2

Your Drugs, Your Anesthetic, and Your Surgery

Many drugs can affect the body's response to anesthetics and surgical procedures. If you are taking, or have taken recently, any of the drugs listed below,
and you plan to have an operation in the near future, consult your physician
regarding the need to modify your drug treatment *before* surgery.* It is essential that your anesthesiologist and surgeon be made aware of any of the listed
drugs you are taking. For some drugs, it may be advisable to adjust the dosage;
for others, it may be necessary to discontinue them altogether. The timing and
nature of such changes must be determined on an individual basis. Ask for
guidance at least one month before planned surgery. If it is necessary to have
emergency surgery, it is most important that your anesthesiologist and surgeon
be informed of any medications you are taking.

anti-arthritics (aspirin substitutes)**
anticoagulants**
antidepressants
antihistamines**
antihypertensives**
aspirin
atropine-like drugs**
barbiturates**
beta-blockers**
bethanidine
calcium blockers**
clindamycin
clonidine
codeine
colchicine
colistin
cortisone-like drugs**
cyclophosphamide
decongestants**
diethylstilbestrol
digitalis preparations
disulfiram
diuretics**
ecothiopate
emetine
ergotamine
estrogens
guanethidine
haloperidol
heart rhythm regulators
hydralazine

hypnotics (see Sedatives/Sleep
    Inducers)**
isoniazid
kanamycin
levodopa
lincomycin
meperidine
methadone
methyldopa
mono-amine oxidase inhibitor
    drugs**
neomycin
neostigmine
nitrates**
oral contraceptives
pentazocine
phenothiazines**
phenytoin
prazosin
primidone
procainamide
quinidine
reserpine
sodium salicylate
streptomycin
tetracyclines**
thiazides**
tranquilizers, mild**
tranquilizers, strong**
tranylcypromin
viomycin

*Consult the appropriate Drug Profile in Section Two to learn the class
designation of the drug you are taking.
**See Drug Class, Section Three.

TABLE 3

Specific Diseases and the Drugs That Can Interfere with Their Management

The management of most chronic diseases includes the use of drugs for an extended period of time. During such long-term treatment, a patient may develop other illnesses that require the use of additional drugs. The introduction of new medicines into a well-established treatment program may (1) adversely affect the course of the chronic disease, and/or (2) create a potential for interaction with the drugs already in use. The success of drug therapy is significantly greater when the patient realizes such treatment situations can be complex and shares with his or her physician the responsibility for monitoring the course of illnesses and evaluating responses to the drugs he or she is using.

If you are on drug therapy for a chronic disease, always consult your physician for specific guidance when a new drug is prescribed or if you intend to use a non-prescription drug. The Drug Profiles in Section Two will help you identify the effects drugs may have on certain diseases, as well as their possible interactions with foods, alcohol, and other drugs you may be taking.

If you have **DIABETES** and you intend to use any of the drugs listed below, it may be necessary to modify your treatment program in one or more of the following ways:

- increase the frequency of urine sugar testing to detect any change in the pattern of your diabetes.
- adjust the dosage of anti-diabetic drugs (insulin and/or oral medications) as directed to maintain proper control of blood sugar levels.
- adjust your diet and eating schedule as necessary to maintain proper control of blood sugar levels.
- adjust periodically the dosage schedule of the newly added drug, as your physician directs, to assure effectiveness, to prevent overdosage, and to avoid toxicity.

acenocoumarol	estrogen
amitriptyline	furosemide
amphetamines	haloperidol
anisindione	hydrocortisone
aspirin	imipramine
chlordiazepoxide	isoetharine
chlorthalidone	isoniazid
clofibrate	isoproterenol
desipramine	levodopa
dexamethasone	liothyronine
diazepam	lithium
dicumarol	medroxyprogesterone
disulfiram	methylprednisolone
doxepin	metoprolol
epinephrine	nicotinic acid

nortriptyline
oral contraceptives
oxymetazoline
phenindione
phenoxybenzamine
phenylephrine
phenylpropanolamine
potassium
prednisolone
prednisone
propranolol

protriptyline
pseudoephedrine
terbutaline
thiazides
thyroid
thyroxine
tranylcypromine
triamcinolone
triamterene
trimipramine

If you have **EPILEPSY** and you intend to use any of the drugs listed below, it may be necessary to modify your treatment program in one or more of the following ways:

- be alert for any increase in the frequency of seizures (reduced anti-convulsant effect) and for any toxic symptoms (excessive anti-convulsant effect).
- adjust the dosage schedule of anti-convulsant(s) as directed to increase protection or to decrease possible toxicity from overdosage.
- adjust periodically the dosage schedule of the newly added drug, as your physician directs, to assure effectiveness, to prevent overdosage, and to avoid toxicity.

amantadine
amitriptyline
amobarbital
amoxapine
bromocriptine
butabarbital
butalbital
caffeine
chlordiazepoxide
chlorpromazine
clorazepate
desipramine
diazepam
diethylpropion
disulfiram
doxepin
estrogen
fluphenazine
flurazepam
haloperidol
hydroxyzine
imipramine
indomethacin
isoniazid

levodopa
lithium
maprotiline
medroxyprogesterone
meperidine
meprobamate
mesoridazine
methocarbamol
methylphenidate
nalidixic acid
nortriptyline
oral contraceptives
oxazepam
para-aminosalicylic acid
pentazocine
pentobarbital
perphenazine
pethidine
phenobarbital/phenobarbitone
prochlorperazine
promazine
protriptyline
reserpine
secobarbital

thioridazine
thiothixene
tranylcypromine
trazodone

trifluoperazine
trimipramine
tybamate

If you have **GLAUCOMA** and you intend to use any of the drugs listed below, it may be necessary to modify your treatment program in one or more of the following ways:

- obtain measurement of internal eye pressures regularly to detect any significant increase.
- adjust the dosage schedule of anti-glaucoma medications as directed to maintain normal internal eye pressures.
- adjust periodically the dosage schedule of the newly added drug, as your physician directs, to assure effectiveness, to prevent overdosage, and to avoid toxicity.

amitriptyline
amphetamines
amoxapine
anisotropine
atropine
benztropine
biperiden
brompheniramine
carbamazepine
chlorpheniramine
chlorpromazine
clidinium
clorazepate
cyclandelate
cyproheptadine
desipramine
dexamethasone
diazepam
dicyclomine
diethylpropion
diphenhydramine
doxepin
doxylamine
epinephrine
erythrityl tetranitrate
haloperidol
hydrocortisone
imipramine
isopropamide
isosorbide dinitrate
levodopa

maprotiline
meperidine
methscopolamine
methylphenidate
methylprednisolone
mepyramine
nitroglycerin
nortriptyline
nylidrin
orphenadrine
papaverine
pentaerythritol tetranitrate
pheniramine
phentermine
prazepam
prednisolone
prednisone
prochlorperazine
procyclidine
promethazine
propantheline
protriptyline
pyrilamine
thiothixene
triamcinolone
tridihexethyl
trifluoperazine
trihexiphenidyl
trimipramine
tripelennamine
triprolidine

If you have **GOUT** and you intend to use any of the drugs listed below, it may be necessary to modify your treatment program in one or more of the following ways:

- obtain measurement of blood uric acid levels periodically to detect any significant change that could require adjustment of anti-gout medications.
- report attacks of acute gout so that all drug therapy can be reviewed and corrective adjustments can be made.

acetazolamide
aspirin
chlorthalidone
furosemide
ibuprofen

nicotinic acid
theophylline
thiazides
triamterene

If you have **HEART DISEASE** and you intend to use any of the drugs listed below, it may be necessary to modify your treatment program in one or more of the following ways:

- obtain periodic evaluation of heart performance to detect significant changes in rate, rhythm, and functional capacity that may be attributable to a newly added drug.
- adjust your intake of sodium and/or potassium, as your physician directs, to correct abnormalities produced by newly added drugs.
- report promptly the development of new and unexpected symptoms that could indicate derangement of heart function, such as chest pain, rapid or forceful heart action, irregular heart rhythm, shortness of breath (especially on exertion), and episodes of lightheadedness, weakness, or sense of impending faint.
- adjust periodically the dosage of newly added drugs, as your physician directs, to assure effectiveness, to prevent overdosage, and to avoid toxicity.

amantadine
amitriptyline
amphetamines
androgens
anisotropine
antacids (high sodium)
atropine
benztropine
biperiden
bromocriptine
caffeine
carbamazepine
chlorpromazine
clidinium
clonidine
colchicine
cyclandelate

desipramine
diethylpropion
disulfiram
doxepin
ephedrine
epinephrine
ergotamine
estrogen
guanethidine
haloperidol
hydralazine
imipramine
isoetharine
isopropamide
isoproterenol
levodopa
liothyronine

lithium
maprotiline
mesoridazine
metaproterenol
methscopolamine
methysergide
metoprolol
nortriptyline
oral contraceptives
orphenadrine
oxymetazoline
papaverine
phenoxybenzamine
phentermine
phenylbutazone
phenylephrine
phenylpropanolamine
potassium
prazosin

prochlorperazine
procyclidine
promazine
propantheline
propanolol
pseudoephedrine
terbutaline
theophylline
thioridazine
thiothixene
thyroid
thyroxine
tolmetin
tranylcypromine
trazodone
tridihexethyl
trifluoperazine
trihexiphenidyl
trimipramine

If you have **HIGH BLOOD PRESSURE** and you intend to use any of the drugs listed below, it may be necessary to modify your treatment program in one or more of the following ways:

• obtain measurement of blood pressure regularly to detect significant increases or decreases (without symptoms) that may be attributable to a newly added drug.
• adjust your intake of sodium and/or potassium, as your physician directs, to correct abnormalities produced by newly added drugs.
• report promptly the development of new and unexpected symptoms that could indicate excessive drop in blood pressure, such as lightheadedness, weakness, and faintness (see orthostatic hypotension in Glossary), or excessive rise in blood pressure, indicated by such symptoms as recurring headaches, forceful heart action, restlessness, and agitation.
• adjust periodically the dosage of newly added drugs, as your physician directs, to assure effectiveness, to prevent overdosage, and to avoid toxicity.

acenocoumarol
amphetamines
androgens
anisindione
antacids (high sodium)
benztropine
biperiden
bromocriptine
carbamazepine
dexamethasone
dicumarol

diethylpropion
diethylstilbestrol
ephedrine
epinephrine
ergotamine
estrogen
haloperidol
hydrocortisone
isoetharine
isoproterenol
isoxsuprine

levodopa
liothyronine
methylphenidate
methylprednisolone
methysergide
oral contraceptives
oxymetazoline
oxyphenbutazone
phenindione
phentermine
phenylbutazone
phenylephrine
phenypropanolamine

prednisolone
prednisone
procyclidine
protriptyline
pseudoephedrine
terbutaline
theophylline
thiothixene
thyroid
thyroxine
tranylcypromine
triamcinolone
trihexyphenidyl

If you have **PEPTIC ULCER DISEASE** and you intend to use any of the drugs listed below, it may be necessary to modify your treatment program in one or more of the following ways:

- consult your physician regarding the ulcer-producing potential of any new drug you intend to use.
- report, during the course of treatment for active peptic ulcer, any indications of continued or increased ulcer activity (possible delayed healing) that may be attributable to a newly added drug.
- be alert, during the quiescent phase of peptic ulcer disease (history of a "previous ulcer" or a "healed ulcer"), for symptoms that could indicate the development ("reactivation") of a new ulcer that may be attributable to a drug started recently for another condition.
- observe your stools regularly, if you have a history of peptic ulcer disease (currently active or inactive), for evidence of gastro-intestinal bleeding while taking any drug. Bleeding is indicated by dark coloration (gray to black) of the stool.
- consult your physician regarding the ability of any drug to cause obstruction if this condition is present:
  When repeated ulceration and healing of the stomach outlet result in scar tissue and narrowing (pyloric obstruction), the ability of the stomach to empty may be seriously impaired. Some of the drugs listed below can intensify this impairment.
- adjust periodically the dosage of newly added drugs, as your physician directs, to assure effectiveness, to prevent overdosage, and to avoid toxicity.

acenocoumarol
acetohexamide
amantadine
anisindione
anisotropine
aspirin
atropine
benztropine

caffeine
chlorpromazine
chlorpropamide
clidinium
clofibrate
colchicine
cyproheptadine
dexamethasone

dicumarol
dicyclomine
diphenhydramine
doxylamine
fluphenazine
glyburide
guanethidine
hydrocortisone
ibuprofen
indomethacin
isopropamide
levodopa
mepyramine
methotrexate
methscopolamine
methylprednisolone
methysergide
naproxen
nicotinic acid
nylidrin
orphenadrine
oxyphenbutazone
para-aminosalicylic acid
phenindione

pheniramine
phenylbutazone
piroxicam
potassium (wax matrix)
prednisolone
prednisone
probenecid
prochlorperazine
promethazine
propantheline
pyrilamine
reserpine
sulfinpyrazone
sulindac
theophylline
tolazamide
tolbutamide
tolmetin
triamcinolone
tridihexethyl
trihexyphenidyl
trimeprazine
tripelennamine
warfarin

TABLE 4

Symptoms That May Warn of Serious Adverse Effects

Symptoms that occur during a course of drug treatment may or may not be related to the drug(s) being taken. Occasionally, symptoms may appear that suggest the development of a serious adverse effect. On those occasions when a drug *is* responsible for the symptoms observed, early recognition of this association is essential. Often the drug can be discontinued before the harmful effect becomes irreversible. Therefore, whenever the symptoms listed below appear, it is advisable for you to discontinue the drug(s) in question and inform your physician promptly. He or she will be able to make a careful evaluation of the situation.

If you experience any of these symptoms:	And you are taking (generic names*):	It may indicate the development of:
Increased frequency or severity of headaches Throbbing or pulsating headaches Headaches more intense when lying down Awareness of forceful heart action	amphetamine-like drugs androgens cortisone-like drugs diethylstilbestrol levodopa medroxyprogesterone mono-amine oxidase inhibitor drugs oral contraceptives tranylcypromine	A significant increase in blood pressure
Pattern of sudden headaches Increased frequency or severity of migraine headaches Sudden dizziness Sudden changes in vision or hearing Difficulty in speaking Sudden weakness of any part of the body Sudden numbness, tingling, or loss of feeling of any part of the body	diethylstilbestrol estrogens oral contraceptives progestins	A stroke—a blood clot in the brain (cerebral thrombosis)

*Some drugs are represented by their Drug Class designation.

If you experience any of these symptoms:	And you are taking (generic names*):	It may indicate the development of:
Abrupt changes in vision in one or both eyes, without pain. "Spots" in front of the eyes Blank areas in the field of vision Flashes of light Reduced clarity of vision Poor vision in dim light	carisoprodol ibuprofen indomethacin isoniazid naproxen nicotinic acid (large doses) oral contraceptives oxyphenbutazone phenylbutazone thiothixene	Eye damage—retinal impairment, optic nerve impairment
Pain, discomfort, sense of pressure in the eyes Headache adjacent to the eyes Reduced clarity of vision Difficulty in focusing Loss of side vision "Halo" effect on looking at lights	antidepressants, tricyclic anti-Parkinsonism drugs chlordiazepoxide clorazepate cortisone-like drugs cyproheptadine dextroamphetamine diazepam haloperidol oral contraceptives orphenadrine thiothixene	Glaucoma—increasing internal eye pressure
Sudden pain or pressure in heart region, neck, jaws, shoulders, arms Shortness of breath, weakness, nausea, sweating, or sense of impending faint	diethylstilbestrol estrogens oral contraceptives	A heart attack (coronary thrombosis)
Soreness and tenderness of leg veins Swelling of foot, ankle or leg Sudden pain in the chest, worse with breathing Shortness of breath, with or without pain Cough, with or without bloody sputum	carbamazepine cortisone-like drugs diethylstilbestrol estrogens medroxyprogesterone oral contraceptives	Phlebitis—vein inflammation, vein thrombosis, lung embolism

*Some drugs are represented by their Drug Class designation.

If you experience any of these symptoms:	And you are taking (generic names*):	It may indicate the development of:
Acid indigestion Upper abdominal pain or distress Vomiting of blood ("coffee grounds" vomitus) Blood in stools (dark-colored or "tarry" stools) Progressive weakness due to "silent" blood loss from the stomach	aspirin caffeine cortisone-like drugs ethacrynic acid fenoprofen guanethidine ibuprofen indomethacin levodopa naproxen nicotinic acid oxyphenbutazone para-aminosalicylic acid phenylbutazone potassium (wax matrix) reserpine sulindac tolmetin	Peptic ulcer—stomach ulcer, duodenal ulcer, and/or Stomach/intestinal bleeding
Loss of appetite Nausea, with or without vomiting Fever, weakness, exhaustion Yellow coloration of eyes and skin Dark-colored urine Light-colored stools Itching	acetazolamide acetohexamide allopurinol anisindione antidepressants, tricyclic aspirin barbiturates carbamazepine chloramphenicol chlordiazepoxide chlorpromazine chlorpropamide chlorthalidone chlorzoxazone clindamycin clorazepate cyclophosphamide diazepam diethylstilbestrol erythromycin (estolate) ethchlorvynol fluoxymesterone flurazepam griseofulvin	Drug-induced hepatitis with jaundice

*Some drugs are represented by their Drug Class designation.

If you experience any of these symptoms:	And you are taking (generic names*):	It may indicate the development of:
Loss of appetite Nausea, with or without vomiting Fever, weakness, exhaustion Yellow coloration of eyes and skin Dark-colored urine Light-colored stools Itching	haloperidol hydralazine indomethacin isoniazid medroxyprogesterone methyldopa methyltestosterone nalidixic acid naproxen nicotinic acid nitrofurantoin oral contraceptives oxazepam oxyphenbutazone papaverine para-aminosalicylic acid phenazopyridine phenindione phenobarbital phenothiazines phenylbutazone phenytoin promethazine propoxyphene sulfonamides tetracyclines thiazides tolazamide tolbutamide tranylcypromine trimethobenzamide	Drug-induced hepatitis with jaundice
Pain or discomfort in upper right side of abdomen Swelling or enlargement in upper right side of abdomen (liver) Sudden abdominal pain, intense and persistent (internal bleeding)	oral contraceptives	Liver tumor, with threat of internal bleeding

*Some drugs are represented by their Drug Class designation.

If you experience any of these symptoms:	And you are taking (generic names*):	It may indicate the development of:
Progressive fatigue and weakness Paleness Susceptibility to infection Fever Sore throat Unusual, abnormal bleeding or bruising, nosebleeds, gum bleeding, bloody urine, extensive bruising unprovoked by trauma	acetaminophen acetazolamide acetohexamide allopurinol amitriptyline amoxicillin ampicillin anisindione aspirin brompheniramine carbamazepine carbenicillin cephalexin cephaloglycin cephradine chloramphenicol chlordiazepoxide chlorpheniramine chlorpromazine chlorpropamide chlorthalidone clofibrate clorazepate cloxacillin colchicine cyclophosphamide desipramine diazepam dicloxacillin diethylpropion doxepin fluphenazine furosemide glutethimide glyburide guanethidine haloperidol hydralazine ibuprofen imipramine indomethacin isoniazid levodopa lincomycin meprobamate	Bone marrow depression—low red blood cells (anemia), low white blood cells, low blood platelets (these can occur singly or in any combination)

*Some drugs are represented by their Drug Class designation.

If you experience any of these symptoms:	And you are taking (generic names*):	It may indicate the development of:
Progressive fatigue and weakness Paleness Susceptibility to infection Fever Sore throat Unusual, abnormal bleeding or bruising, nosebleeds, gum bleeding, bloody urine, extensive bruising unprovoked by trauma	mesoridazine methaqualone methyldopa methylphenidate methyprylon methysergide metronidazole nafcillin nalidixic acid naproxen nortriptyline oxacillin oxazepam oxyphenbutazone para-aminosalicylic acid penicillin G penicillin V pentazocine perphenazine phenacetin phenindione phenylbutazone phenytoin primidone probenecid procainamide prochlorperazine promazine promethazine propranolol protriptyline quinidine sulfinpyrazone sulfonamides thiazides thioridazine tolazamide tolbutamide triamterene trimeprazine trimethoprim trimipramine tripelennamine tybamate	Bone marrow depression—low red blood cells (anemia), low white blood cells, low blood platelets (these can occur singly or in any combination)

*Some drugs are represented by their Drug Class designation.

If you experience any of these symptoms:	And you are taking (generic names*):	It may indicate the development of:
Unusual and abnormal bleeding or bruising, without other symptoms Evidence of bleeding from any part of the body without apparent cause	acenocoumarol acetaminophen acetohexamide acetazolamide amitriptyline amoxicillin ampicillin anisindione aspirin barbiturates bethanidine carbenicillin chloramphenicol chlordiazepoxide chlorpromazine chlorpropamide chlortetracycline chlorthalidone chlorzoxazone cloxacillin demeclocycline desipramine dicloxacillin dicumarol digitoxin diphenhydramine doxepin doxycycline ethchlorvynol ethinamate fluphenazine furosemide glutethimide glyburide guanethidine hydralazine imipramine indomethacin	Impairment of normal blood coagulation, low prothrombin, low blood platelets

*Some drugs are represented by their Drug Class designation.

If you experience any of these symptoms:	And you are taking (generic names*):	It may indicate the development of:
Unusual and abnormal bleeding or bruising, without other symptoms Evidence of bleeding from any part of the body without apparent cause	isoniazid lincomycin meprobamate methacycline methaqualone methyldopa methylphenidate methyprylon minocycline nafcillin nortriptyline oxacillin oxyphenbutazone oxytetracycline para-aminosalicylic acid penicillin G penicillin V phenacetin phenindione phenylbutazone phenytoin procainamide probenecid promazine propranolol protriptyline quinidine rifampin sulfonamides tetracycline thiazides tolazamide tolbutamide trimipramine tripelennamine tybamate warfarin	Impairment of normal blood coagulation, low prothrombin, low blood platelets

*Some drugs are represented by their Drug Class designation.

If you experience any of these symptoms:	And you are taking (generic names*):	It may indicate the development of:
Fever, chills, fatigue, weakness, dark-colored urine, mild jaundice	acetazolamide acetohexamide aspirin chlorpropamide cyclophosphamide diphenhydramine furazolidone levodopa methyldopa methysergide nalidixic acid nitrofurantoin phenacetin phenazopyridine phenytoin procainamide probenecid quinidine sulfonamides tolazamide tolbutamide tripelennamine	Hemolytic anemia—destruction of red blood cells

*Some drugs are represented by their Drug Class designation.

TABLE 5

Your Drugs and Alcohol

Beverages containing alcohol may interact unfavorably with a wide variety of drugs. The most important (and most familiar) interaction occurs when the depressant action on the brain of sedatives, sleep-inducing drugs, tranquilizers, and narcotic drugs is intensified by alcohol. Alcohol may also reduce the effectiveness of some drugs, and it can interact with certain other drugs to produce toxic effects. Some drugs may increase the intoxicating effects of alcohol, producing further impairment of mental alertness, judgment, physical coordination, and reaction time.

While drug interactions with alcohol are generally predictable, the intensity and significance of these interactions can vary greatly from one individual to another and from one occasion to another. This is because many factors influence what happens when drugs and alcohol interact. These factors include individual variations in sensitivity to drugs (including alcohol), the chemistry and quantity of the drug, the type and amount of alcohol consumed, and the sequence in which drug and alcohol are taken. If you need to use any of the drugs listed in the following tables, you should ask your physician for guidance concerning the use of alcohol.

Drugs with which it is advisable to avoid alcohol completely

Drug name or class	Possible interaction with alcohol
amphetamines	excessive rise in blood pressure with alcoholic beverages containing tyramine**
barbiturates*	excessive sedation
bromides	confusion, delirium, increased intoxication
calcium carbamide	disulfiram-like reaction**
carbamazepine	excessive sedation
chlorprothixene	excessive sedation
chlorzoxazone	excessive sedation
disulfiram	disulfiram reaction**
ergotamine	reduced effectiveness of ergotamine
fenfluramine	excessive stimulation of nervous system with some beers and wines
furazolidone	disulfiram-like reaction**
haloperidol	excessive sedation
MAO inhibitor drugs*	excessive rise in blood pressure with alcoholic beverages containing tyramine**
meperidine	excessive sedation

*See Drug Class, Section Three.
**See Glossary.

Drug name or class	Possible interaction with alcohol
meprobamate	excessive sedation
metformin	increased lactic acidosis
methotrexate	increased liver toxicity and excessive sedation
metronidazole	disulfiram-like reaction**
narcotic drugs	excessive sedation
oxyphenbutazone	increased stomach irritation and/or bleeding
pentazocine	excessive sedation
pethidine	excessive sedation
phenformin	increased lactic acidosis
phenothiazines*	excessive sedation
phenylbutazone	increased stomach irritation and/or bleeding
procarbazine	disulfiram-like reaction**
propoxyphene	excessive sedation
reserpine	excessive sedation, orthostatic hypotension**

sleep-inducing drugs (hypnotics)
  carbromal
  chloral hydrate
  ethchlorvynol
  ethinamate
  glutethimide
  flurazepam
  methaqualone
  methyprylon
	excessive sedation

thiothixene	excessive sedation
tricyclic antidepressants*	excessive sedation, increased intoxication
trimethobenzamide	excessive sedation

Drugs with which alcohol should be used only in small amounts (use cautiously until combined effects have been determined)

Drug name or class	Possible interaction with alcohol
acetaminophen (Tylenol, etc.)	increased liver toxicity
amantadine	excessive lowering of blood pressure
anticoagulants (coumarins)*	increased anticoagulant effect
anti-diabetic drugs (sulfonylureas)*	increased anti-diabetic effect, excessive hypoglycemia**
antihistamines*	excessive sedation
anti-hypertensives*	excessive orthostatic hypotension**

*See Drug Class, Section Three.
**See Glossary.

Drug name or class	Possible interaction with alcohol
aspirin (large doses or continuous use)	increased stomach irritation and/or bleeding
carbamazepine	excessive sedation
carisoprodol	increased alcoholic intoxication
diethylpropion	excessive nervous system stimulation with alcoholic beverages containing tyramine**
dihydroergotoxine	excessive lowering of blood pressure
diphenoxylate	excessive sedation
dipyridamole	excessive lowering of blood pressure
diuretics*	excessive orthostatic hypotension**
ethionamide	confusion, delirium, psychotic behavior
fenoprofen	increased stomach irritation and/or bleeding
griseofulvin	flushing and rapid heart action
ibuprofen	increased stomach irritation and/or bleeding
indomethacin	increased stomach irritation and/or bleeding
insulin	excessive hypoglycemia**
iron	excessive absorption of iron
isoniazid	decreased effectiveness of isoniazid, increased incidence of hepatitis
lithium	increased confusion and delirium (avoid all alcohol if any indication of lithium overdosage)
methocarbamol	excessive sedation
methotrimeprazine	excessive sedation
methylphenidate	excessive nervous system stimulation with alcoholic beverages containing tyramine**
metoprolol	excessive orthostatic hypotension**
nalidixic acid	increased alcoholic intoxication
naproxen	increased stomach irritation and/or bleeding
nicotinic acid	possible orthostatic hypotension**
nitrates* (vasodilators)	possible orthostatic hypotension**
nylidrin	increased stomach irritation
orphenadrine	excessive sedation
phenoxybenzamine	possible orthostatic hypotension**
phentermine	excessive nervous system stimulation with alcoholic beverages containing tyramine**

*See Drug Class, Section Three.
**See Glossary.

Drug name or class	Possible interaction with alcohol
phenytoin	decreased effect of phenytoin
pilocarpine	prolongation of alcohol effect
prazosin	excessive lowering of blood pressure
primidone	excessive sedation
propranolol	excessive orthostatic hypotension**
sulfonamides*	increased alcoholic intoxication
sulindac	increased stomach irritation and/or bleeding
tolmetin	increased stomach irritation and/or bleeding
tranquilizers (mild) chlordiazepoxide clorazepate diazepam hydroxyzine meprobamate oxazepam phenaglycodol tybamate	excessive sedation
tranylcypromine	increased alcoholic intoxication

Drugs capable of producing a disulfiram-like reaction** when used concurrently with alcohol

anti-diabetic drugs (sulfonylureas)*
calcium carbamide
chloral hydrate
chloramphenicol
disulfiram
furazolidone
metronidazole

nifuroxine
nitrofurantoin
procarbazine
quinacrine
sulfonamides*
tinidazole
tolazoline

  *See Drug Class, Section Three.
**See Glossary.

TABLE 6

Photosensitivity: Your Drugs and the Sun

Some drugs are capable of sensitizing the skin of some individuals to the action of ultraviolet light. This can cause uncovered areas of the skin to react with a rash or exaggerated burn on exposure to sun or ultraviolet lamps. If you are taking any of the following drugs, ask your physician for guidance and use caution with regard to sun exposure.

acetohexamide
amitriptyline
amoxapine
barbiturates
bendroflumethiazide
carbamazepine
chlordiazepoxide
chloroquine
chlorothiazide
chlorpromazine
chlorpropamide
chlortetracycline
chlorthalidone
clindamycin
cyproheptadine
demeclocycline
desipramine
diethylstilbestrol
diltiazem
diphenhydramine
doxepin
doxycycline
estrogen
fluphenazine
gold preparations
glyburide
griseofulvin
hydrochlorothiazide
hydroflumethiazide
imipramine
isotretinoin

lincomycin
maprotiline
mesoridazine
methacycline
methotrexate
nalidixic acid
nortriptyline
oral contraceptives
oxyphenbutazone
oxytetracycline
perphenazine
phenobarbital
phenylbutazone
phenytoin
prochlorperazine
promazine
promethazine
protriptyline
pyrazinamide
sulfonamides
tetracycline
thioridazine
tolazamide
tolbutamide
tranylcypromine
triamterene
trifluoperazine
trimeprazine
trimipramine
triprolidine

TABLES 7–11

Drugs and the Fetus, Infant, and Child*

Our present knowledge of drug effects during the earliest periods of life is very limited. Recent research has established that the actions of drugs in the developing child (both before and after birth) differ significantly from the usual patterns seen in the older child and the adult. In these early periods of life, the growing tissues are extremely sensitive to the presence of such foreign chemicals as drugs, and interactions are more rapid and more unpredictable. The unborn child's mechanisms for neutralizing drugs and eliminating them from its body are immature and deficient, and they remain so for at least four weeks following full-term birth.

These factors make it essential that any drugs taken by the mother during pregnancy be selected with great care and given only when the benefit to the mother outweighs the possible harm to the fetus. It is now known that most drugs cross the placenta and enter the bloodstream of the developing fetus. While the risk of injury to the unborn child from most prescription and non-prescription drugs appears to be small, it is advisable to avoid **all** drugs during pregnancy unless there is unquestionable need and the effectiveness of the drug to be used is well established. When drug treatment during pregnancy is considered necessary, every attempt should be made to limit its use to the smallest effective dose and to the briefest possible period of time.

The successive periods of child development are defined as follows:

Embryo	from the second through the eighth weeks after conception
Fetus	from the ninth week after conception until birth
Premature Infant	one born from the 27th to the 38th weeks (full term) after conception
Newborn Infant	from the first through the fourth weeks following full-term birth
Infant	from birth to two years of age
Child	from two through eleven years of age

*See also Section Six.

TABLE 7

Drug Use During the First Trimester (First Three Months) of Pregnancy

The greatest risk of injury to the unborn child from exposure to drugs occurs during the first three months of pregnancy. The critical period of major organ development in the embryo occurs from the fourth through the eighth weeks. Drugs acting adversely upon the embryo during this period may cause permanent birth defects. For this reason, the use of any drug during early pregnancy must be considered hazardous. Based upon our present knowledge, it is advisable to observe the following guidelines.

Drugs to avoid completely (definitely harmful)	Drugs to use only if essential to mother's health (potentially harmful)	Drugs to avoid if possible or to use sparingly (may be harmful)
sex hormones	amphetamines	antacids
androgens	anti-cancer drugs	aspirin
estrogens	anticoagulants (oral)*	fenoprofen
diethylstilbestrol	barbiturates*	furosemide
oral contraceptives	carbamazepine	gentamicin
progesterone	chloramphenicol	indomethacin
anabolic drugs (male	chloroquine	iron
sex hormone-like	colistin	lithium
drugs used to	cortisone-like drugs*	nicotinamide
stimulate appetite	haloperidol	oral anti-diabetics
and weight gain)	kanamycin	(sulfonylureas)*
colchicine	metronidazole	sulfamethoxazole**
cyclophosphamide	nalidixic acid	tranquilizers (mild)*
tetracyclines*	nortriptyline	trimethoprim**
nicotine (tobacco)	phenytoin	Vitamin C (large doses)
	primidone	Vitamin D (large doses)
	propylthiouracil	
	quinidine	
	quinine	
	reserpine	
	streptomycin	
	thiazide diuretics*	
	thiothixene	
	vancomycin	
	viomycin	

*See Drug Class, Section Three.
**In some countries these two drugs in combination are designated generically as co-trimoxazole.

TABLE 8

Drug Use During the Second and Third Trimesters (Fourth Through Ninth Months) of Pregnancy

The developing fetus continues to be vulnerable to the adverse effects of drugs in various ways. Drugs may impair the normal development of the brain, the nervous system, and the external genital organs. The mother's use of drugs during the final weeks of pregnancy is of major concern because certain drugs within the fetus at the time of birth may have serious adverse effects. When the fetus becomes the newborn infant it must assume the full burden of drug metabolism and elimination. At that time, however, its incompletely developed metabolism is unable to process and eliminate drugs rapidly and effectively, and thus drugs may accumulate within the infant and produce manifestations of overdosage. For the premature infant, whose metabolism is even more immature, the hazards are proportionately greater.

Drugs to avoid completely	Drugs to use only on physician's orders
anabolic drugs (male sex hormone-like drugs used to stimulate appetite and weight gain)	amphetamines
	analgesics (strong)
	anesthetics
	antacids (containing sodium)
anticoagulants (oral)*	anti-thyroid drugs
aspirin (in large doses or for an extended period of time)	barbiturates*
	bromides
chloramphenicol	carbamazepine
diethylstilbestrol	chloroquine
iodides	colistin
nicotine (tobacco)	cortisone-like drugs*
nitrofurantoin	cyclophosphamide
oral anti-diabetics (sulfonylureas)* after 33 weeks	ergotamine
	kanamycin
sex hormones of any kind	laxatives
sulfonamides* (sulfa drugs)	lithium
tetracyclines*	nalidixic acid
	narcotic drugs
	nortriptyline
	phenothiazines*
	phenytoin
	primidone
	propranolol
	propylthiouracil
	quinidine
	quinine
	reserpine

*See Drug Class, Section Three.

Drugs to avoid completely	Drugs to use only on physician's orders
	streptomycin
	thiazide diuretics*
	tranquilizers (mild)*
	vancomycin
	viomycin
	Vitamin C (large doses)
	Vitamin K (synthetic form)

*See Drug Class, Section Three.

TABLE 9

Drug Use While Nursing an Infant

Most drugs taken by the nursing mother will be present to some degree in her milk. The amount of the drug in the milk and its effect on the nursing infant will vary greatly, depending on the chemical characteristics of the drug, the dosage, and the duration of use. The value of breast feeding is well established and it should not be compromised by the unwise or unnecessary use of drugs. Many drugs can be taken by the nursing mother without adverse effects on the infant, but it is advisable to consult your physician about the use of any drug while nursing an infant. It is important that the nursing infant be observed carefully and continuously for possible unwanted effects due to the presence of drugs in the milk.

Drugs to avoid completely	Drugs to use only on physician's orders (observing infant closely)
androgens	amphetamines
anti-cancer drugs	antacids (containing sodium)
anticoagulants (oral)*	aspirin (in large doses)
carbamazepine	atropine
carisoprodol	barbiturates*
chloramphenicol	bromides
cyclophosphamide	caffeine
ergotamine	chloral hydrate
erythromycin estolate	chlorpromazine
heroin	cortisone-like drugs*
iodine (radioactive)	diazepam
isoniazid	diethylstilbestrol
meprobamate	diphenhydramine
metronidazole	imipramine
nicotine (tobacco)	iodides
oral contraceptives	laxatives
penicillins*	lithium
propranolol	nalidixic acid
sulfonamides*	naproxen
tetracyclines*	oxyphenbutazone
thiouracil	phenytoin
	primidone
	pyrimethamine
	reserpine
	thiazide diuretics*

*See Drug Class, Section Three.

TABLE 10

Drug Use During Infancy (Birth to Two Years of Age)

This period includes the premature and newborn infant, to whom the special considerations on page 955 apply. Among the characteristics of infancy are the relative ease with which drugs enter the tissues of the brain and the fact that drugs applied to the skin (in the form of lotions and ointments) are absorbed more rapidly and to a greater degree than in older children, sometimes causing generalized (systemic) effects though they are intended only for local use. During infancy and childhood all drug use requires careful observation for possible impairment of normal growth and development.

Drugs to avoid completely if possible	Drugs to use with caution and under physician's close supervision
chloramphenicol	androgens
diphenoxylate	anti-worm drugs containing
erythromycin estolate	piperazine
isoniazid	aspirin
nalidixic acid, under 3 months of	colistin
age	cortisone-like drugs*
nitrofurantoin	nalidixic acid, over 3 months of age
sulfonamides* (sulfa drugs), under 2	phenacetin
months of age	phenothiazines*
tetracyclines*	sulfonamides* (sulfa drugs), over 2
	months of age
	Vitamin A (in large doses)

*See Drug Class, Section Three.

TABLE 11

Drug Use During Childhood (Two to Twelve Years of Age)

The child's ability to neutralize and eliminate drugs is significantly greater than the infant's, but it does not yet equal that of the adult. It is important that the selection and dosage of each drug be matched carefully to the individual child's age, weight, and sensitivity to medications. Accurate measurement of liquid doses can be greatly improved by shaking the bottle to ensure uniform mixing of drug components and by using a standard measuring device. (The common household "teaspoon" can vary in size from 2.5 to 9 milliliters.) It is important to follow exactly the physician's instructions concerning the duration of drug therapy and not to discontinue the drug as soon as symptoms subside. Children are susceptible to certain infections which can produce serious complications if drug therapy is stopped too soon.

Drugs to avoid completely if possible	Drugs to use with caution and under physician's close supervision
dextroamphetamine, under 3 years of age	androgens and androgen-like drugs
methylphenidate, under 6 years of age	anti-worm drugs containing piperazine
oxyphenbutazone	aspirin
phenylbutazone	cortisone-like drugs* (long-term use)
tetracyclines,* under 8 years of age	imipramine
	methylphenidate, over 6 years of age
	nalidixic acid
	para-aminosalicylic acid
	phenacetin
	phenothiazines*
	phenytoin
	reserpine
	sulfonamides* (sulfa drugs)

*See Drug Class, Section Three.

TABLE 12

Drugs and the Elderly (over 60 Years of Age)*

Advancing age brings changes in body structure and function that may alter significantly the action of drugs. An impaired digestive system may interfere with drug absorption. Reduced capacity of the liver and kidneys to metabolize and eliminate drugs may result in the accumulation of drugs in the body to toxic levels. By impairing the body's ability to maintain a "steady state" (homeostasis), the aging process may increase the sensitivity of many tissues to the actions of drugs, thereby altering greatly the responsiveness of the nervous and circulatory systems to standard drug doses. If aging should cause deterioration of understanding, memory, vision, or physical coordination, people with such impairments may not always use drugs safely and effectively.

Adverse reactions to drugs occur three times more frequently in the older population. An unwanted drug response can render a functioning and independent older person, whose health and reserves are at marginal levels, confused, incompetent, or helpless. For these reasons, drug treatment in the elderly must always be accompanied by the most careful consideration of the individual's health and tolerances, the selection of drugs and dosage schedules, and the possible need for assistance in treatment routines.

Guidelines for the use of drugs by the elderly

- Be certain that drug treatment is necessary. Many health problems of the elderly can be managed without the use of drugs.
- Avoid if possible the use of many drugs at one time. It is advisable to use not more than three drugs concurrently.
- Dosage schedules should be as uncomplicated as possible. When feasible, a single daily dose of each drug is preferable.
- In order to establish individual tolerance, treatment with most drugs is usually best begun by using smaller than standard doses. Maintenance doses should also be determined carefully. A maintenance dose is often smaller for persons over 60 years of age than for younger persons.
- Avoid large tablets and capsules if other dosage forms are available. Liquid preparations are easier for the elderly or debilitated to swallow.
- Have all drug containers labeled with the drug name and directions for use in large, easy-to-read letters.
- Ask the pharmacist to package drugs in easy-to-open containers. Avoid "childproof" caps and stoppers.
- Do not take any drug in the dark. Identify each dose of medicine carefully in adequate light to be certain you are taking the drug intended.
- To avoid taking the wrong drug or an extra dose, do not keep drugs on a bedside table. Drugs for emergency use, such as nitroglycerin, are an exception. It is advisable to have only one such drug at the bedside for use during the night.
- Drug use by older persons may require supervision. Observe drug effects continuously to ensure safe and effective use.

*See also Table 13, Your Drugs and Sexual Activity.

Drugs best avoided by the elderly because of increased possibility of adverse reactions

antacids (high sodium)*
barbiturates*
cyclophosphamide
diethylstilbestrol
estrogens
indomethacin

oxyphenbutazone
phenacetin
phenylbutazone
tetracyclines*
tranylcypromine

Drugs that should be used by the elderly in reduced dosages until full effect has been determined

anticoagulants (oral)*
antidepressants*
anti-diabetic drugs*
antihistamines*
anti-hypertensives*
barbiturates*
beta-blockers*
colchicine
cortisone-like drugs*
digitalis preparations*
diuretics* (all types)
ephedrine
epinephrine
fenoprofen
haloperidol

ibuprofen
isoetharine
metoprolol
nalidixic acid
naproxen
narcotic drugs
prazosin
propranolol
pseudoephedrine
quinidine
sleep inducers (hypnotics)*
sulindac
terbutaline
thyroid preparations
tolmetin

Drugs that may cause confusion and behavioral disturbances in the elderly

amantadine
antidepressants*
anti-diabetic drugs*
antihistamines*
atropine* (and drugs containing
  belladonna)
barbiturates*
benzodiazepines*
carbamazepine
cimetidine
digitalis preparations*
dihyroergotoxine
diuretics*
fenoprofen
ibuprofen

levodopa
meprobamate
methocarbamol
methyldopa
narcotic drugs
pentazocine
phenytoin
primidone
reserpine
sedatives
sleep inducers (hypnotics)*
sulindac
thiothixene
tranquilizers (mild)*
trihexyphenidyl

*See Drug Class, Section Three.

Drugs that may cause orthostatic hypotension in the elderly

antidepressants*
anti-hypertensives*
diuretics* (all types)
phenothiazines*

sedatives
tranquilizers (mild)*
vasodilators*

Drugs that may cause constipation and/or retention of urine in the elderly

amantadine
androgens
antidepressants*
anti-parkinsonism drugs*
atropine-like drugs*
dihydroergotoxine

epinephrine
isoetharine
narcotic drugs
phenothiazines*
terbutaline

Drugs that may cause loss of bladder control (urinary incontinence) in the elderly

diuretics* (all types)
sedatives

sleep inducers (hypnotics)*
tranquilizers (mild)*

*See Drug Class, Section Three.

TABLE 13

Your Drugs and Sexual Activity

The drugs listed below are capable of affecting some aspects of sexuality. As would be expected, the principal therapeutic effect of all of them is on the nervous or circulatory systems. As with any drug effect, the nature and degree of altered sexual function will vary greatly from one individual to another. While such effects may occur at any age, they are usually more frequent and more troublesome after the age of 50. If you suspect the possibility of such a drug response, consult your physician regarding the advisability of modifying your treatment program.

Drug name or class	Possible effects
acetazolamide	reduced libido and potency
alcohol	reduced potency in men, delayed orgasm in women
amphetamine	reduced libido and potency
antidepressants*	reduced libido and potency, impaired ejaculation
antihistamines	reduced libido and potency
atropine-like drugs (anticholinergics)	reduced potency, impaired ejaculation
beta-blockers*	reduced libido and potency
bethanidine	impaired ejaculation
cimetidine	reduced libido and potency
clofibrate	reduced libido and potency
clonidine	reduced libido and potency, impaired ejaculation
debrisoquine	reduced potency, impaired ejaculation
dextroamphetamine	reduced libido and potency
diazepam	reduced libido, impaired ejaculation
diethylstilbestrol	reduced libido and potency
digitalis preparations	reduced potency
disopyramide	reduced potency
disulfiram	reduced potency
estrogens	reduced libido in men
ethacrynic acid	reduced potency
fenfluramine	reduced libido and potency
furosemide	reduced potency
guanethidine	reduced potency; impaired ejaculation; prolonged, painful erections
haloperidol	reduced potency, painful ejaculation

*See Drug Class, Section Three.

Drug name or class	Possible effects
hydralazine	reduced potency; prolonged, painful erections
levodopa	increased libido (in some men and women)
lithium	reduced potency
methyldopa	reduced libido and potency, impaired ejaculation
metronidazole	reduced libido
oral contraceptives	reduced libido (in some women)
pargyline	impaired ejaculation
phenothiazines*	reduced libido and potency, impaired ejaculation (occasionally); prolonged, painful erections
phenoxybenzamine	impaired ejaculation
prazosin	reduced potency; prolonged, painful erections
primidone	reduced libido and potency
propantheline	reduced potency
propranolol	reduced libido and potency (infrequently)
reserpine	reduced libido and potency, impaired ejaculation
sedative and sleep-inducing drugs (hypnotics)* when used on a regular basis	reduced libido and potency
spironolactone	reduced libido and potency
thiazide diuretics*	reduced libido (occasionally, in some men), reduced potency
thiothixene	spontaneous ejaculations
tolbutamide	prolonged, painful erections
tranquilizers (mild)*	reduced libido and potency
tranylcypromine	reduced potency, spontaneous erections
trazodone	prolonged, painful erections

*See Drug Class, Section Three.

TABLE 14

Your Drugs and Vision

Approximately 3.5% of all adverse drug effects involve impairment of vision or damage to structures of the eye. Some effects, such as blurring of vision or double vision, may occur shortly after starting a drug. These quickly disappear with adjustment of dosage. More subtle and serious effects, such as the development of cataracts or damage to the retina or optic nerve, may not occur until a drug has been in continuous use for an extended period of time. Some of these changes are irreversible. If you are taking a drug that can affect the eye in any way, you are urged to report promptly any eye discomfort or change in vision so that appropriate evaluation can be made and corrective action taken as soon as possible.

Drugs reported to cause *blurring of vision*

acetazolamide
antidepressants*
antihistamines*
atropine-like drugs*
chlorthalidone
cortisone-like drugs*
diethylstilbestrol

fenfluramine
oral contraceptives
phenytoin
sulfonamides*
tetracyclines*
thiazide diuretics*

Drugs reported to cause *double vision*

antidepressants*
anti-diabetic drugs*
antihistamines*
aspirin
barbiturates*
benzodiazepines*
bromides
carbamazepine
carisoprodol
chloroquine
chlorprothixene
clomiphene
colchicine
colistin
cortisone-like drugs*
digitalis
digitoxin
digoxin
ethionamide
ethosuximide
guanethidine

hydroxychloroquine
indomethacin
isoniazid
levodopa
mephenesin
methocarbamol
methsuximide
morphine
nalidixic acid
nitrofurantoin
oral contraceptives
orphenadrine
oxyphenbutazone
pentazocine
phenothiazines*
phensuximide
phenylbutazone
phenytoin
primidone
propranolol

*See Drug Class, Section Three.

quinidine
sedative/sleep inducers*

thiothixene
tranquilizers*

Drugs reported to cause *farsightedness*

ergot
penicillamine

sulfonamides* (possibly)
tolbutamide (possibly)

Drugs reported to cause *nearsightedness*

acetazolamide
aspirin
carbachol
chlorthalidone
codeine
cortisone-like drugs*
ethosuximide
methsuximide
morphine

oral contraceptives
penicillamine
phenothiazines*
phensuximide
spironolactone
sulfonamides*
tetracyclines*
thiazide diuretics*

Drugs reported to *alter color vision*

acetaminophen
amodiaquine
amyl nitrite
aspirin
atropine
barbiturates*
belladonna
chloramphenicol
chloroquine
chlorpromazine
chlortetracycline
cortisone-like drugs*
digitalis
digitoxin
digoxin
disulfiram
epinephrine
ergotamine
erythromycin
ethchlorvynol
ethionamide
fluphenazine
furosemide

hydroxychloroquine
indomethacin
isocarboxazid
isoniazid
mephenamic acid
mesoridazine
methysergide
nalidixic acid
oral contraceptives
oxyphenbutazone
paramethadione
pargyline
penicillamine
pentylenetetrazol
perphenazine
phenacetin
phenylbutazone
primidone
prochlorperazine
promazine
promethazine
quinacrine
quinidine

*See Drug Class, Section Three.

quinine
reserpine
sodium salicylate
streptomycin
sulfonamides*
thioridazine

tranylcypromine
trifluoperazine
triflupromazine
trimeprazine
trimethadione

Drugs reported to cause *sensitivity to light* (photophobia)

anti-diabetic drugs*
atropine-like drugs*
bromides
chloraquine
clomiphene
digitoxin
doxepin
ethambutol
ethionamide
ethosuximide
hydroxychloroquine

mephenytoin
methsuximide
mono-amine oxidase inhibitor drugs*
nalidixic acid
oral contraceptives
paramethadione
phenothiazines*
quinidine
quinine
tetracyclines*
trimethadione

Drugs reported to cause *halos around lights*

amyl nitrite
chloroquine
cortisone-like drugs*
digitalis
digitoxin
digoxin
hydrochloroquine

nitroglycerin
oral contraceptives
paramethadione
phenothiazines*
quinacrine
trimethadione

Drugs reported to cause *visual hallucinations*

amantadine
amphetamine-like drugs*
amyl nitrite
antihistamines*
aspirin
atropine-like drugs*
barbiturates*
benzodiazepines*
bromides
carbamazepine
cephalexin
cephaloglycin
chloroquine
cycloserine

digitalis
digoxin
disulfiram
ephedrine
furosemide
griseofulvin
haloperidol
hydroxychloroquine
indomethacin
isosorbide
levodopa
nialamide
oxyphenbutazone
pargyline

*See Drug Class, Section Three.

pentazocine
phenothiazines*
phenylbutazone
phenytoin
primidone
propranolol

quinine
sedatives/sleep inducers*
sulfonamides*
tetracyclines*
tricyclic antidepressants*
tripelennamine

Drugs reported to impair the use of *contact lenses*

brompheniramine
carbinoxamine
chlorpheniramine
cyclizine
cyproheptadine
dexbrompheniramine
dexchlorpheniramine

dimethindene
diphenhydramine
diphenpyraline
furosemide
oral contraceptives
tripelennamine

Drugs reported to cause *cataracts* or *lens deposits*

allopurinol
busulfan
chlorpromazine
chlorprothixene
cortisone-like drugs*
fluphenazine
mesoridazine
methotrimeprazine
perphenazine
phenmetrazine

pilocarpine
prochlorperazine
promazine
promethazine
thioridazine
thiothixene
trifluoperazine
triflupromazine
trimeprazine

*See Drug Class, Section Three.

TABLE 15

Your Drugs and Hearing

Statistics indicate that approximately 3 per 1000 of hospitalized patients on drug therapy may develop some degree of hearing loss attributable to one or more drugs. In most instances the extent of ear damage and the associated hearing loss are related to drug dosage—the greatest loss occurring with higher drug doses.

It is now well recognized that certain conditions can significantly increase the risk of drug-induced hearing loss. These include reduced kidney function, severe thermal burns, and advanced age.

It is important to remember that drugs known to be toxic to the ear can also induce ear damage and impaired hearing in the fetus when taken during pregnancy.

Drugs reported to cause a *loss of hearing*

ampicillin (rare)
aspirin (11/1000)*
chloramphenicol
chloroquine
colistin (polymixin E)
erythromycin (intravenous)
ethacrynic acid (12/1000, intravenous)
fenoprofen
furosemide
gentamicin (12/1000)

indomethacin
kanamycin (16/1000)
neomycin (12/1000)
nortriptyline
propylthiouracil
quinidine (3/1000)
quinine
streptomycin (6/1000)
vancomycin
viomycin

Drugs reported to cause *exaggerated hearing*

carbamazepine

Drugs reported to cause *ringing in the ears* (tinnitus)

aspirin
carbamazepine
ethacrynic acid
furosemide
indomethacin
kanamycin
quinidine

quinine
streptomycin
thiabendazole
tobramycin
tolbutamide
vitamin A (in chronic overdosage)

Drugs reported to cause *auditory hallucinations*

amphetamines**
aspirin
digitalis preparations
diphenhydramine

indomethacin
morphine
pentazocine

*Figures in parentheses represent frequency of occurrence.
**See Drug Class, Section Three.

TABLE 16

Your Drugs and Sleep

In spite of years of research, the true nature and function of sleep are still poorly understood. Studies to date have provided the following observations about sleep and its most common disorder—insomnia. In turn, these observations underlie the principles that govern the prudent use of sleep-inducing drugs.

- The natural pattern of sleep changes with age, the longest periods of sleep occurring in infancy and childhood and the shortest in the elderly.
- There is marked variation in individual sleep patterns, with no clearly definable standard or norm. No two people sleep alike.
- With increasing age, sleep is characterized by frequent interruptions and shorter periods of continuous sleep. This has no apparent ill effect on general health or well-being.
- 15% of the general population and more than 20% of those over sixty experience insomnia.
- Insomnia is a purely subjective observation, not related to an established "sleep norm." It implies the existence of "poor" sleep combined with daytime fatigue.
- Occasional insomnia should be considered a normal experience. It does not justify use of hypnotic drugs under most circumstances.
- The average "chronic insomniac" characteristically misjudges how long it takes to fall asleep and the length of sleepless periods. Studies confirm that many self-diagnosed insomniacs often sleep 6 to 7 hours a night. The *real* problem is their faulty perception of their sleep experience—usually a result of chronic anxiety.
- A continuous pattern of unexplained insomnia requires careful medical and psychological evaluation to determine its cause. True insomnia is always a symptom of an underlying disorder.
- Insomnia characterized by early morning awakening is often a feature of emotional depression, a disorder which can be made worse by the use of hypnotic drugs.
- Sleep-inducing drugs—other than the benzodiazepines (flurazepam, Dalmane, etc.)—lose their effectiveness after 2 weeks of continuous use.
- Sleep-inducing drugs are, at best, only a temporary solution of limited usefulness. They should be used only occasionally and for short periods of time. Their continuous use can lead rapidly to the development of tolerance and psychological dependence—an inability to sleep without a medication (even a placebo).*
- Hypnotic drugs produce an "unnatural" sleep that does not provide the physiological and psychological restoration that accompanies natural sleep.
- The use of hypnotic drugs by the elderly often results in confusion, disorientation, agitation, delirium and combativeness.

*A placebo is a "dummy" dosage form made to appear identical to a specific drug but possessing no pharmacologic activity. Its ability to produce a desired effect is due to the power of suggestion.

- A barbiturate is not the drug of choice as a sedative or sleep-inducer for persons over 60.
- The benzodiazepine drugs (flurazepam, Dalmane, etc.) are the most satisfactory drugs currently available, producing a sleep that most closely approximates the natural state. However, these drugs can cause a "rebound insomnia" if they are discontinued abruptly.
- The occurrence of "hangover" is as much a function of individual response as of drug effect. The nature and degree of "hangover" is unpredictable in any individual and can only be determined by experience.

Drugs designed to induce *sleep* (sedatives/hypnotics)

*Barbiturates**
amobarbital
aprobarbital
butabarbital
butalbital
hexobarbital
mephobarbital
pentobarbital
phenobarbital
secobarbital
talbutal

Non-Barbiturates
carbromal
chloral hydrate
ethchlorvynol
ethinamate
flurazepam
glutethimide
methaqualone
methyprylon

Drugs not designed to induce sleep that may cause drowsiness and lethargy

acetazolamide
allopurinol
analgesics,* (mild and strong)
antidepressants*
antihistamines*
antispasmodics*
atropine-like drugs*
bromides
carbamazepine
carisoprodol
chlordiazepoxide
chlormezanone
chlorphenesin
chlorprothixene
chlorzoxazone
clofibrate
clonazepam
clonidine
clorazepate
diazepam

diphenoxylate
ethosuximide
griseofulvin
indomethacin
levodopa
lithium
lorazepam
mephenesin
meprobamate
metaxalone
methocarbamol
methsuximide
methyldopa
methysergide
nalidixic acid
orphenadrine
oxazepam
phenothiazines
phensuximide

*See Drug Class, Section Three.

phenytoin
prazepam
primidone
propoxyphene
pyrantel
reserpine

scopolamine
thiazide diuretics*
thiothixene
trimethadione
trimethobenzamide
tybamate

Drugs that may cause *insomnia*

amantadine
amphetamine-like drugs*
caffeine
cortisone-like drugs*
ephedrine
epinephrine
griseofulvin
isoproterenol
levodopa

methyldopa
methylphenidate
methysergide
oral contraceptives
oxymetazoline
propranolol
theophylline
xylometazoline

Drugs that may cause *nightmares* or *exaggerated dreaming*

antidepressants* (given as a single
    bedtime dose)
clonidine
folic acid (large doses)

methyldopa
pilocarpine (eye drops)
propranolol
reserpine

*See Drug Class, Section Three.

TABLE 17

Your Drugs and Your Mood (Emotions)

Drugs specifically designed to alter one's mood or emotional state in a particular way are among the most widely used medicinal agents in the developed world. Collectively, sedatives and tranquilizers have been the most frequently prescribed class of drugs for many years.*

Less apparent—but no less important—are the mood-altering *side-effects* of some drugs which are prescribed primarily for altogether unrelated conditions, with no intention of modifying emotional status. In keeping with the wide variation of individual response to the primary and intended effects of drugs, it is to be expected that the emotional and behavioral secondary effects will also be quite unpredictable and will vary enormously from person to person. However, the following experiences have been observed with sufficient frequency to establish recognizable patterns.

Drugs reported to cause *nervousness* (anxiety and irritability)

amantadine
amphetamine-like drugs* (appetite
  suppressants)
antihistamines*
caffeine
chlorphenesin
cortisone-like drugs*
ephedrine
epinephrine
isoproterenol

levodopa
liothyronine (in excessive dosage)
methylphenidate
methysergide
mono-amine oxidase inhibitor drugs*
nylidrin
oral contraceptives
theophylline
thyroid (in excessive dosage)
thyroxine (in excessive dosage)

Drugs reported to cause *emotional depression*

amantadine
amphetamine* (on withdrawal)
benzodiazepines*
carbamazepine
chloramphenicol
cortisone-like drugs*
cycloserine
digitalis
digitoxin
digoxin
diphenoxylate
estrogens
ethionamide
fenfluramine (on withdrawal)
fluphenazine
guanethidine

haloperidol
indomethacin
isoniazid
levodopa
methsuximide
methyldopa
methysergide
oral contraceptives
phenylbutazone
procainamide
progesterones
propranolol
reserpine
sulfonamides*
vitamin D (in excessive dosage)

*See Drug Class, Section Three.

Drugs reported to cause *euphoria*

amantadine
aminophylline
amphetamines
antihistamines* (some)
antispasmodics, synthetic*
aspirin
barbiturates*
benzphetamine
chloral hydrate
clorazepate
codeine
cortisone-like drugs*
diethylpropion
diphenoxylate

ethosuximide
flurazepam
haloperidol
levodopa
meprobamate
methysergide
mono-amine oxidase inhibitor drugs*
morphine
pargyline
pentazocine
phenmetrazine
propoxyphene
scopolamine
tybamate

Drugs reported to cause *excitement*

acetazolamide
amantadine
amphetamine-like drugs*
antidepressants*
antihistamines*
atropine-like drugs*
barbiturates* (paradoxical response)
benzodiazepines* (paradoxical response)
cortisone-like drugs
cycloserine
diethylpropion
digitalis
ephedrine
epinephrine

ethinamate (paradoxical response)
ethionamide
glutethimide (paradoxical response)
isoniazid
isoproterenol
levodopa
meperidine and MAO inhibitor drugs*
methyldopa and MAO inhibitor drugs*
methyprylon (paradoxical response)
nalidixic acid
orphenadrine
quinine
scopolamine

*See Drug Class, Section Three.

TABLE 18

Your Drugs and Mental Function

In addition to producing side-effects that can alter mood and disturb emotional stability, some drugs are capable of inducing unexpected and unpredictable patterns of abnormal thinking and behavior. Such responses are relatively infrequent, but the nature and degree of mental disturbance can, at times, be quite alarming and potentially dangerous for both patient and family. It is now well recognized that such paradoxical responses are often of an idiosyncratic nature, and that the individual with a history of a serious mental or emotional disorder is more likely to experience bizarre reactions involving disturbed behavior.

It is often difficult to judge whether a particular aberration of thought or behavior is primarily a feature of the disorder under treatment or an effect of one (or more) drugs the patient may be taking at the time. If in doubt, it is advisable to discontinue any drug with potential for such side-effects and observe for changes during a drug-free period.

Drugs reported to impair *concentration* and/or *memory*

antihistamines*
anti-Parkinsonism drugs*
barbiturates*
benzodiazepines*
isoniazid

mono-amine oxidase inhibitor drugs*
phenytoin
primidone
scopolamine

Drugs reported to cause *confusion, delirium,* or *disorientation*

acetazolamide
aminophylline
antidepressants*
antihistamines*
atropine-like drugs*
barbiturates*
benzodiazepines*
bromides
carbamazepine
chloroquine
cimetidine
cortisone-like drugs*
cycloserine
digitalis
digitoxin
digoxin
disulfiram

ethchlorvynol
ethinamate
fenfluramine
glutethimide
isoniazid
levodopa
meprobamate
para-amino salicylic acid
phenelzine
phenothiazines*
phenytoin
piperazine
primidone
propranolol
reserpine
scopolamine

*See Drug Class, Section Three.

Drugs reported to cause *paranoid thinking*

bromides
cortisone-like drugs*
diphenhydramine

disulfiram
isoniazid
levodopa

Drugs reported to cause *schizophrenic-like behavior*

amphetamines*
ephedrine

fenfluramine
phenmetrazine

Drugs reported to cause *manic-like behavior*

antidepressants*
cortisone-like drugs*

levodopa
mono-amine oxidase inhibitor drugs*

Drugs reported to cause *hallucinations*

See Table 14 for visual hallucinations.
See Table 15 for auditory hallucinations.

*See Drug Class, Section Three.

TABLE 19

Your Drugs and Personal Identification

Should you require emergency medical care, it is essential that those attending you be aware of certain health conditions that may warrant special attention. You are urged to carry with you (in wallet or purse) a card of personal identification that includes a statement of significant conditions and the names and dosages of the drugs you are taking. A model form for such a card will be found in Section Six. Listed below are those health conditions and drugs which should be noted on your identification card.

Significant Health Conditions

Addison's disease
Alcoholism
Allergic disorders
Allergies to drugs
Bleeding disorders
Cancer (any type)
Coronary heart disease
Depression
Diabetes
Epilepsy
Hemolytic anemia
Hemophilia
Hypertension (high blood pressure)

Kidney disease (chronic)
Lupus erythematosus
Manic disorder
Myasthenia gravis
Parkinson's disease
Peptic ulcer disease
Pernicious anemia
Phlebitis
Porphyria
Pregnancy
Rheumatic heart disease
Schizophrenia

Significant Medications

ambenonium
anti-cancer drugs
anticoagulant drugs*
antidepressants*
anti-diabetic drugs (oral)*
anti-hypertensive drugs*
anti-Parkinsonism drugs*
beta-blockers*
calcium blockers*
carbamazepine
clonidine
cortisone-like drugs*
digitalis
digitoxin
digoxin
disulfiram
haloperidol

insulin
lithium
mono-amine oxidase inhibitor drugs*
mephenytoin
neostigmine
penicillin (any type)*
phenacemide
phenobarbital (as an anti-convulsant)
phenothiazines*
phenytoin
primidone
procainamide
pyridostigmine
quinidine
reserpine
thiothixene
Vitamin B-12

*See Drug Class, Section Three.

SECTION SIX

PERSONAL DRUG HISTORIES

A written account of significant drug experiences is an important part of your family's medical record. This section provides the following forms to assist you in maintaining a file of appropriate drug information:

- Drugs Taken During Pregnancy
- Drugs Taken During Infancy and Childhood
- Drugs Taken by Adults
- Medical Alert

Drugs Taken During Pregnancy
(Record all prescription and non-prescription drugs)

Mother: _____
Residence: _____

Attending Physician: _____
Physician's Address: _____

Hospital: _____

Pregnancy Number: _____   Mother's Age: _____   Father's Age: _____
Estimated Date of Conception: _____   Drugs used by father at time of conception: _____
Estimated Date of Delivery: _____
Actual Date of Delivery: _____
Condition of Infant: _____

Complications During Pregnancy: _____

Drug Name Dosage Form & Strength	Prescribing Physician	Indication for Drug	Date Started	Date Stopped	Daily Dose	Drug Experience

Additional Notes: _____

Drugs Taken During Infancy and Childhood
(That Require Documentation)

Child's Name: _____   Date of Birth: _____

Residence: _____

Attending Physician: _____

Physician's Address: _____

Pharmacies Used: _____

Prescription #: _____

Drug Name Dosage Form & Strength	Prescribing Physician	Indication for Drug	Date Started	Date Stopped	Daily Dose	Drug Experience

Additional Notes:

Drugs Taken by Adults
(That Require Documentation)

Name: _____   Date of Birth: _____

Residence: _____

Attending Physician: _____

Physician's Address: _____

Pharmacies Used: _____

Prescription #: _____

Drug Name Dosage Form & Strength	Prescribing Physician	Indication for Drug	Date Started	Date Stopped	Daily Dose	Drug Experience

Additional Notes:

Card for Wallet or Purse

MEDICAL ALERT

Patient's Name: _____   Date of Birth: _____

Address: _____

Telephone: (Home) _____ (Business) _____

In Emergency Please Notify: (Name) _____

(Telephone) _____

Physician: _____ Employer: _____

(Telephone) _____ (Telephone) _____

Medical Conditions	Present Medications	Known Drug Allergies

(A copy of this form should be carried in wallet or purse at all times.)

SOURCES

Sources

The following sources were consulted in the compilation and revision of this book:

Adverse Drug Reaction Bulletin. Edited by D. M. Davies. Newcastle upon Tyne, England: Regional Postgraduate Institute for Medicine and Dentistry.

AMA Department of Drugs, *AMA Drug Evaluations,* 5th ed. Chicago: American Medical Association, 1983.

American Pharmaceutical Association. *Evaluations of Drug Interactions.* 2nd ed. Washington, D.C.: American Pharmaceutical Association, 1976.

Avery, Graeme S., ed., *Drug Treatment,* 2nd ed. Sydney, Australia: ADIS Press, 1980.

Azarnoff, Daniel L., *Steroid Therapy.* Philadelphia: W. B. Saunders Company, 1975.

Bassuk, E. L., Schoonover S. C., *The Practitioner's Guide to Psychoactive Drugs.* New York: Plenum, 1977.

Bevan, J. A., ed., *Essentials of Pharmacology.* Hagerstown, Maryland: Harper & Row, 1976.

Billups, N. F., ed., *American Drug Index 1984.* Philadelphia: J. B. Lippincott Co., 1978.

Bochner, F.; Carruthers, G.; and Kampmann, J., *Handbook of Clinical Pharmacology.* Boston: Little, Brown and Company, 1978.

Braude, M. C., Szara, S., eds., *Pharmacology of Marihuana,* Volumes 1 and 2. New York: Raven Press, 1976.

Canadian Pharmaceutical Association, *Compendium of Pharmaceuticals and Specialties,* 18th ed. Ottawa: Canadian Pharmaceutical Association, 1983.

Cape, Ronald, *Aging: Its Complex Management.* Hagerstown, Maryland: Harper & Row, 1978.

Clin-Alert. Louisville, Kentucky: Science Editors, Inc.

Clinical Pharmacology and Therapeutics. Edited by Walter Modell. St. Louis: The C. V. Mosby Co.

Cluff, Leighton E.; Caranasos, George J.; and Stewart, Ronald B., *Clinical Problems With Drugs.* Philadelphia: W. B. Saunders Company, 1975.

Cluff, L. E., and Petrie, J. C., eds., *Clinical Effects of Interaction Between Drugs.* New York: American Elsevier Publishing Co., Inc., 1974.

Davies, D. M., ed., *Textbook of Adverse Drug Reactions,* 2nd ed. New York: Oxford University Press, 1981.

Deichmann, William B., and Gerarde, Horace W., *Toxicology of Drugs and Chemicals.* New York: Academic Press, 1969.

Drug and Therapeutics Bulletin. Edited by Andrew Herxheimer. London: Consumers' Association.

Drug Intelligence and Clinical Pharmacy. Edited by Harvey A. K. Whitney, Jr. Hamilton, Illinois: Hamilton Press.

Dukes, M. N. G., ed., *Meyler's Side Effects of Drugs*, 9th ed. Amsterdam: Excerpta Medica, 1980.

Facts and Comparisons. Edited by James R. Boyd. St. Louis: Facts and Comparisons Division, J.B. Lippincott Co.

F.D.A. Drug Bulletin. Rockville, Maryland: Department of Health and Human Services, Food and Drug Administration.

Ferriss, G. S., ed., *Treatment of Epilepsy Today*. Oradell, N.J.: Medical Economics Co., 1978.

Fraunfelder, F. T., *Drug-Induced Ocular Side-Effects and Drug Interactions*. Philadelphia: Lea & Febiger, 1976.

Gershon, S., ed., *Lithium; Its Role in Psychiatric Research and Treatment*. New York: Plenum Press, 1973.

Gleason, Marion N.; Gosselin, Robert E.; Hodge, Howard C.; and Smith, Roger P., *Clinical Toxicology of Commercial Products*. 3rd ed. Baltimore: The Williams & Wilkins Co., 1969.

Goodman, Louis S., and Gilman, Alfred, *The Pharmacological Basis of Therapeutics*. 6th ed. New York: Macmillan, 1980.

Greenblatt, D. J., and Shader, R. I., *Benzodiazepines in Clinical Practice*. New York: Raven Press, 1974.

Hansten, Philip D., *Drug Interactions*. 4th ed. Philadelphia: Lea & Febiger, 1979.

Heinonen, O. P., Slone, D., and Shapiro, S., *Birth Defects and Drugs in Pregnancy*. Littleton, MA: PSG Publishing Co., 1977.

Hollister, Leo E., *Clinical Pharmacology of Psychotherapeutic Drugs*. New York: Churchill Livingstone, 1978.

Huff, Barbara B., ed., *The Physicians' Desk Reference*. 38th ed. Oradell, New Jersey: Medical Economics Company, 1984.

International Drug Therapy Newsletter. Edited by Frank J. Ayd, Jr. Baltimore: Ayd Medical Communications.

Jarvik, M. E., ed., *Psychopharmacology in the Practice of Medicine*. New York: Appleton-Century-Crofts, 1977.

Jefferson, J. W., Greist, J. H., *Primer of Lithium Therapy*. Baltimore: Williams & Wilkins, 1977.

Journal of the American Medical Association. Edited by George D. Lundberg. Chicago: American Medical Association.

Kagan, Benjamin M., *Antimicrobial Therapy*. 2nd ed. Philadelphia: W. B. Saunders Company, 1974.

Kleinfeld, Cynthia, ed., *Handbook of Nonprescription Drugs*. 5th ed. Washington, D. C.: American Pharmaceutical Association, 1977.

Knoben, J. E.; Anderson, P. O.; and Watanabe, A. S., *Handbook of Clinical Drug Data*. Hamilton, Illinois: Drug Intelligence Publications, Inc., 1978.

Kolodny, R. C., Masters, W. H., and Johnson, V. E., *Textbook of Sexual Medicine*. Boston: Little, Brown and Company, 1979.

Lawrence, R. A., *Breast-Feeding*. St. Louis: Mosby, 1980.

Lingeman, Richard R., *Drugs from A to Z*. New York: McGraw-Hill Book Company, 1974.

Martin, Eric W., *Hazards of Medication*. 2nd ed. Philadelphia: J. B. Lippincott Co., 1978.

Martin, E. W., *Drug Interactions Index 1978–1979*. Philadelphia: J. B. Lippincott Co., 1978.

McEvoy, Gerald K., ed., *American Hospital Formulary Service, Drug Informa-*

tion 84. Bethesda, Maryland: American Society of Hospital Pharmacists, 1984.

Mechoulam, R., ed., *Marijuana.* New York: Academic Press, 1973.

The Medical Clinics of North America, *Symposium on Individualization of Drug Therapy.* Vol. 58, No. 5. Philadelphia: W. B. Saunders Company, 1974.

The Medical Letter on Drugs and Therapeutics. Edited by Harold Aaron. New Rochelle, N.Y.: The Medical Letter, Inc.

Melmon, Kenneth L., and Morrelli, Howard F., *Clinical Pharmacology.* 2nd ed. New York: Macmillan, 1978.

Mendelson, W. B.; Gillin, J. C.; and Wyatt, R. J., *Human Sleep and its Disorders.* New York; Plenum Press, 1977.

Meyler, L., and Herxheimer, A., eds., *Side-Effects of Drugs.* Vol. 8. Amsterdam: Excerpta Medica, 1975.

Meyler, L., and Peck, H. M., eds., *Drug-Induced Diseases.* Vol. 4. Amsterdam: Excerpta Medica, 1972.

Miller, Russell R., and Greenblatt, David J., eds., *Drug Effects in Hospitalized Patients.* New York: John Wiley & Sons, 1976.

Modell, Walter, ed., *Drugs of Choice, 1982–83.* St. Louis: The C. V. Mosby Company, 1982.

Modell, Walter; Schild, Heinz O.; and Wilson, Andrew, *Applied Pharmacology.* Philadelphia: W. B. Saunders Company, 1976.

Moss, Arthur J., and Patton, Robert D., *Antiarrhythmic Agents.* Springfield, Illinois: Charles C. Thomas, 1973.

The New England Journal of Medicine. Edited by Arnold S. Relman. Boston: Massachusetts Medical Society.

Nishumura, Hideo, and Tanimura, Takashi, *Clinical Aspects of the Teratogenicity of Drugs.* New York: American Elsevier Publishing Co., Inc., 1976.

The Pediatric Clinics of North America, *Symposium on Pediatric Pharmacology.* Vol. 19. No. 1. Philadelphia: W. B. Saunders Company, 1972.

Public Health Reports. Edited by Marian Priest Tebben. Vol. 92, No. 5. Hyattsville, Maryland: Public Health Service, Department of Health, Education and Welfare, 1977.

Quitkin, F., and Rifkin, A., *Diagnosis and Drug Treatment of Psychiatric Disorders: Adults and Children,* 2nd ed. Baltimore: Williams & Wilkins, 1980.

Reynolds, James E.F., ed., *Martindale, The Extra Pharmacopoeia, 28th ed.* London: The Pharmaceutical Press, 1982.

Schardein, J. L., *Drugs As Teratogens.* Cleveland: CRC Press, 1976.

Shepard, T. H., *Catalog of Teratogenic Agents,* 3rd ed. Baltimore: Johns Hopkins University Press, 1980.

Stockley, Ivan, *Drug Interactions and Their Mechanisms.* London: The Pharmaceutical Press, 1974.

Tuchmann-Duplessis, H., *Drug Effects on the Fetus.* Sydney: ADIS Press, 1975.

The United States Pharmacopeia XX. 20th rev. Rockville, Maryland: United States Pharmacopeial Convention, Inc., 1980.

USAN 1984 and the USP dictionary of drug names. Edited by Mary C. Griffiths. Rockville, Maryland: United States Pharmacopeial Convention, Inc., 1984.

USP Dispensing Information 1984, Vol I, Drug Information for the Health Care Provider. Rockville, Maryland: United States Pharmacopeial Convention, 1984.

Utian, W. H., *Menopause in Modern Perspective.* New York: Appleton-Century-Crofts, 1980.

Wade, O. L., *Adverse Reactions to Drugs.* 2nd ed. London: William Heinemann Medical Books, Ltd., 1976.

Worley, R. J., ed., *Clinical Obstetrics and Gynecology,* Vol. 24, No. 1: *Menopause.* Hagerstown, MD: Harper & Row, 1981.

INDEX

This index combines all the brand and generic drug names included (Section Two) in this book.

Brand names appear in italic type and are capitalized.

Each brand name is followed by the generic name of its Drug Profile in Section Two.

The symbol [CD] indicates that the brand name represents a combination drug that contains the generic drug components listed below it. To be fully familiar with any combination drug [CD], it is necessary to read the Drug Profile of each of the components listed. The brand name of a combination drug *may* or *may not* appear in the brand name list of each Drug Profile that is cited in the index as a component of a particular combination drug. The index listing of component drugs for any combination drug product represents the manufacturer's formulation of that brand at the time this information was compiled for publication.

The designation (Canada) after the brand name of a combination drug indicates that the brand name is used both in the United States and Canada, but that the ingredients in the combination product in each country differ. The Canadian drug is marked with the designation (Canada) to distinguish it from the American drug which has the same name.

A generic name with no page designation indicates an active component of a combination drug for which there is no Profile in Section Two. It is included to alert you to its presence, should you wish to consult your physician regarding its significance.

Index of Brand and Generic Names

A

Accurbron, theophylline, 775
Accutane, isotretinoin, 437
Acet-Am, theophylline, 775
Acet-AM Elixir [CD]
  CONTAINS
  diphenhydramine, 284
  ephedrine, 308
  theophylline, 775
acetaminophen, 29
Acetazolam, acetazolamide, 32
acetazolamide, 32
acetohexamide, 36
Acetophen, aspirin, 75
acetylsalicylic acid. *See* aspirin, 75
Achromycin, tetracycline, 771
Achromycin V, tetracycline, 771
Actidil, triprolidine, 847
Actifed [CD]
  CONTAINS
  pseudoephedrine, 717
  triprolidine, 847
Actifed-A [CD]
  CONTAINS
  acetaminophen, 29
  pseudoephedrine, 717
  triprolidine, 847
Actifed-C Expectorant [CD]
  CONTAINS
  codeine, 212
  pseudoephedrine, 717
  triprolidine, 847
  guaifenesin*
Actifed DM [CD]
  CONTAINS
  dextromethorphan, 250
  pseudoephedrine, 717
  triprolidine, 847
Actifed-Plus [CD]
  CONTAINS
  pseudoephedrine, 717
  triprolidine, 847
  noscapine*
Adalat, nifedipine, 551
Adapin, doxepin, 301
Adrenalin, epinephrine, 313
adrenaline. *See* epinephrine, 313
Advil, ibuprofen, 398
Afrin, oxymetazoline, 590
Afrinol, pseudoephedrine, 717
A-H GEL, antacids, 68
Alconefrin, phenylephrine, 638
Aldactazide [CD]
  CONTAINS
  hydrochlorothiazide, 381
  spironolactone, 742
Aldactone, spironolactone, 742
Aldoclor [CD]
  CONTAINS
  chlorothiazide, 161
  methyldopa, 498
Aldomet, methyldopa, 498

*The symbol [CD] indicates that the brand name given is a combination drug consisting of generic drug components listed below it. If there is no page numbering following the name of the generic drug component, there is no Drug Profile for that ingredient in this book.

Aldoril [CD]
CONTAINS
hydrochlorothiazide, 381
methyldopa, 498
Aldoril-15 [CD]
CONTAINS
hydrochlorothiazide, 381
methyldopa, 498
Aldoril-25 [CD]
CONTAINS
hydrochlorothiazide, 381
methyldopa, 498
Aldoril D30 [CD]
CONTAINS
hydrochlorothiazide, 381
methyldopa, 498
Aldoril D50 [CD]
CONTAINS
hydrochlorothiazide, 381
methyldopa, 498
Algoverine, phenylbutazone, 634
Alka-Seltzer Antacid, [CD]
CONTAINS
antacids, 68
citric acid*
Alka-Seltzer [CD]
CONTAINS
antacids, 68
aspirin, 75
citric acid*
Alka-2, antacids, 68
Alkets, antacids, 69
Allerdryl, diphenhydramine, 284
Allerest [CD]
CONTAINS
chlorpheniramine, 167
phenylpropanolamine, 641
Alloprin, allopurinol, 40
allopurinol, 40
Almocarpine, pilocarpine, 654
Alsimox, antacids, 69
ALternaGEL, antacids, 68
Aludrox, antacids, 69
aluminum hydroxide. *See* antacids,
   68
Alupent, metaproterenol, 479
Alu-Tab, antacids, 68
Ambenyl Expectorant [CD]

CONTAINS
codeine, 212
diphenhydramine, 284
ammonium chloride*
bromodiphenhydramine*
potassium guaiacosulfonate*
Amcill, ampicillin, 59
Amen, medroxyprogesterone, 465
Amersol, ibuprofen, 398
Amesec [CD]
CONTAINS
ephedrine, 308
theophylline, 775
A.M.H. Suspension, antacids, 69
Aminodur, theophylline, 775
aminophylline. *See* theophylline, 775
Amitone, antacids, 68
Amitril, amitriptyline, 43
amitriptyline, 43
amobarbital, 47
Amodrine [CD]
CONTAINS
ephedrine, 308
phenobarbital, 626
theophylline, 775
amoxapine, 51
amoxicillin, 56
Amoxil, amoxicillin, 56
Amphicol, chloramphenicol, 154
Amphojel, antacids, 68
Amphojel 65, antacids, 69
ampicillin, 59
Ampicin, ampicillin, 59
Ampilean, ampicillin, 59
A-M-T, antacids, 69
Amytal, amobarbital, 47
Anacin [CD]
CONTAINS
aspirin, 75
caffeine, 120
Anaprox, naproxen, 544
Ancasal, aspirin, 75
androgens, 62
Android-F, androgens, 62
Android-T, androgens, 62
Android-5, androgens, 62
Android-10, androgens, 62
Android-25, androgens, 62

Angidil, isosorbide dinitrate, 434

Anspor, cephradine, 147

Antabuse, disulfiram, 298

antacids, 68

Antamel, antacids, 69

Antazone, sulfinpyrazone, 755

Antibiopto, chloramphenicol, 154

Anti-B Nasal Spray, phenylephrine, 638

Antivert, meclizine, 462

Antivert [CD]

  CONTAINS

  meclizine, 462

  nicotinic acid, 547

Anturan, sulfinpyrazone, 755

Anturane, sulfinpyrazone, 755

A.P.C. Capsules or Tablets [CD]

  CONTAINS

  aspirin, 75

  caffeine, 120

  phenacetin*

Apo-Acetaminophen, acetaminophen, 29

Apo-Acetazolamide, acetazolamide, 32

Apo-Allopurinol, allopurinol, 40

Apo-Amitriptyline, amitriptyline, 43

Apo-Benztropine, benztropine, 96

Apo-C, vitamin C, 858

Apo-Carbamazepine, carbamazepine, 128

Apo-Chlordiazepoxide, chlordiazepoxide, 157

Apo-Chlorpromazine, chlorpromazine, 170

Apo-Chlorpropamide, chlorpropamide, 175

Apo-Cimetidine, cimetidine, 187

Apo-Diazepam, diazepam, 253

Apo-Dimenhydrinate, dimenhydrinate, 281

Apo-Erythro-S, erythromycin, 328

Apo-Ferrous Gluconate, iron, 414

Apo-Ferrous Sulfate, iron, 414

Apo-Fluphenazine, fluphenazine, 352

Apo-Flurazepam, flurazepam, 356

Apo-Furosemide, furosemide, 360

Apo-Guanethidine, guanethidine, 368

Apo-Haloperidol, haloperidol, 372

Apo-Hydrochlorothiazide, hydrochlorothiazide, 381

Apo-Imipramine, imipramine, 402

Apo-ISDN, isosorbide dinitrate, 434

Apo-Meprobamate, meprobamate, 471

Apo-Methyldopa, methyldopa, 498

Apo-Naproxen, naproxen, 544

Apo-Nitrofurantoin, nitrofurantoin, 554

Apo-Oxazepam, oxazepam, 583

Apo-Perphenazine, perphenazine, 615

Apo-Phenylbutazone, phenylbutazone, 634

Apo-Prednisone, prednisone, 677

Apo-Primidone, primidone, 682

Apo-Propranolol, propranolol, 708

Apo-Sulfamethoxazole, sulfamethoxazole, 746

Apo-Sulfasalazine, sulfasalazine, 750

Apo-Sulfatrim [CD]

  CONTAINS

  sulfamethoxazole, 746

  trimethoprim, 841

Apo-Sulfatrim-DS [CD]

  CONTAINS

  sulfamethoxazole, 746

  trimethoprim, 841

Apo-Sulfinpyrazone, sulfinpyrazone, 755

Apo-Sulfisoxazole, sulfisoxazole, 759

Apo-Thioridazine, thioridazine, 779

Apo-Tolbutamide, tolbutamide, 805

*The symbol [CD] indicates that the brand name given is a combination drug consisting of generic drug components listed below it. If there is no page numbering following the name of the generic drug component, there is no Drug Profile for that ingredient in this book.

Apo-Trifluoparazine, trifluoperazine, 831
A-poxide, chlordiazepoxide, 157
Apresazide [CD]
  CONTAINS
  hydralazine, 376
  hydrochlorothiazide, 381
Apresoline, hydralazine, 376
Apresoline-Esidrix [CD]
  CONTAINS
  hydralazine, 376
  hydrochlorothiazide, 381
Aquachloral, chloral hydrate, 150
Aquatensen, methyclothiazide, 492
Arcoban, meprobamate, 471
Arcum R-S, reserpine, 730
Aristocort, triamcinolone, 822
Aristospan, triamcinolone, 822
Arlidin, nylidrin, 565
Arlidin Forte, nylidrin, 565
Armour Thyroid, thyroid, 787
Arthralgen [CD]
  CONTAINS
  acetaminophen, 29
  salicylamide*
A.S.A. Preparations, aspirin, 75
Ascorbajen, vitamin C, 858
ascorbic acid. *See* vitamin C, 858
Ascorbicap, vitamin C, 858
Ascriptin [CD]
  CONTAINS
  antacids, 68
  aspirin, 75
Asendin, amoxapine, 51
Aspergum, aspirin, 75
aspirin, 75
Aspirjen Jr., aspirin, 75
Astrin, aspirin, 75
Atarax, hydroxyzine, 395
Atasol, acetaminophen, 29
Atasol Forte, acetaminophen, 29
atenolol, 81
Athrombin-K, warfarin, 862
Ativan, lorazepam, 454
Atromid-S, clofibrate, 198
atropine, 86
Aventyl, nortriptyline, 561
Azene, clorazepate, 205

Azo Gantanol [CD]
  CONTAINS
  phenazopyridine, 620
  sulfamethoxazole, 746
Azo Gantrisin [CD]
  CONTAINS
  phenazopyridine, 620
  sulfisoxazole, 759
Azolid, phenylbutazone, 634
Azotrex [CD]
  CONTAINS
  phenazopyridine, 620
  tetracycline, 771
  sulfamethizole*
Azulfidine, sulfasalazine, 750
Azulfidine EN-tabs, sulfasalazine,
  750

B

bacampicillin, 91
Bactocill, oxacillin, 580
Bactopen, cloxacillin, 209
Bactrim [CD]
  CONTAINS
  sulfamethoxazole, 746
  trimethoprim, 841
Bactrim DS [CD]
  CONTAINS
  sulfamethoxazole, 746
  trimethoprim, 841
Balminil D.M. Syrup,
  dextromethorphan, 250
Bamate, meprobamate, 471
Banlin, propantheline, 701
Barazole, sulfisoxazole, 759
Barbidonna [CD]
  CONTAINS
  atropine, 86
  phenobarbital, 626
Barbita, phenobarbital, 626
Bayer Aspirin, aspirin, 75
Bayer Children's Aspirin, aspirin, 75
Bayer Timed-Release Aspirin,
  aspirin, 75
BBS, butabarbital, 112
beclomethasone, 92
Beclovent Inhaler, beclomethasone,
  92

Beconase Nasal Inhaler,
  beclomethasone, 92
Beconase Nasal Spray,
  beclomethasone, 92
Belladenal [CD]
  CONTAINS
  atropine, 86
  phenobarbital, 626
belladonna. *See* atropine, 86
Bell-Ans, antacids, 68
Bellergal [CD]
  CONTAINS
  atropine, 86
  ergotamine, 321
  phenobarbital, 626
Bellergal-S [CD]
  CONTAINS
  atropine, 86
  ergotamine, 321
  phenobarbital, 626
Benacen, probenecid, 686
Benadryl, diphenhydramine, 284
Bendopa, levodopa, 442
Benemid, probenecid, 686
Bensylate, benztropine, 96
Bentyl, dicyclomine, 257
Bentylol, dicyclomine, 257
Benuryl, probenecid, 686
Benylin Cough Syrup,
  diphenhydramine, 284
Benylin Decongestant Cough Syrup
  [CD]
  CONTAINS
  diphenhydramine, 284
  pseudoephedrine, 717
Benylin-DM [CD]
  CONTAINS
  dextromethorphan, 250
  diphenhydramine, 284
  pseudoephedrine, 717
Benylin DM Cough Syrup,
  dextromethorphan, 250
benztropine, 96

Betaloc, metoprolol, 519
Betapen VK, penicillin V, 602
Bicycline, tetracycline, 771
Biphetamine [CD]
  CONTAINS
  dextroamphetamine, 245
  amphetamine*
Biquin Durules, quinidine, 724
BiSoDol Powder, antacids, 68
BiSoDol Tablets, antacids, 69
Blocadren, timolol, 795
Bonamine, meclizine, 462
Bonine, meclizine, 462
Brethine, terbutaline, 767
Brevicon, oral contraceptives, 571
Bricanyl, terbutaline, 767
Brioschi, antacids, 68
Bristamycin, erythromycin, 328
bromocriptine, 100
Bromo-Seltzer, antacids, 68
brompheniramine, 104
Broncho-Grippol-DM,
  dextromethorphan, 250
Brondecon [CD]
  CONTAINS
  theophylline, 775
  guaifenesin*
Bronkaid [CD]
  CONTAINS
  ephedrine, 308
  theophylline, 775
  guaifenesin*
Bronkaid Mistometer, epinephrine,
  313
Bronkodyl, theophylline, 775
Bronkodyl S-R, theophylline, 775
Bronkolixir [CD]
  CONTAINS
  ephedrine, 308
  phenobarbital, 626
  theophylline, 775
  guaifenesin*
Bronkometer, isoetharine, 419

*The symbol [CD] indicates that the brand name given is a combination drug consisting of generic drug components listed below it. If there is no page numbering following the name of the generic drug component, there is no Drug Profile for that ingredient in this book.

Bronkosol, isoetharine, 419
Bronkotabs [CD]
   CONTAINS
   ephedrine, 308
   phenobarbital, 626
   theophylline, 775
   guaifenesin*
Broserpine, reserpine, 730
Brown Mixture [CD]
   CONTAINS
   paregoric, 599
   antimony potassium tartrate*
Bubartal TT, butabarbital, 112
Bufferin [CD]
   CONTAINS
   antacids, 68
   aspirin, 75
bumetanide, 107
Bumex, bumetanide, 107
buphenine. *See* nylidrin, 565
Buta-Barb, butabarbital, 112
butabarbital, 112
butalbital, 116
Butazolidin, phenylbutazone, 634
Butibel [CD]
   CONTAINS
   atropine, 86
   butabarbital, 112
Buticaps, butabarbital, 112
Butisol, butabarbital, 112
Butte, butabarbital, 112

C

Cafecon, caffeine, 120
Cafergot [CD]
   CONTAINS
   caffeine, 120
   ergotamine, 321
Cafergot P-B [CD]
   CONTAINS
   atropine, 86
   caffeine, 120
   ergotamine, 321
   pentobarbital, 611
caffeine, 120
Calan, verapamil, 854
calcium, 125

calcium carbonate. *See* antacids,
   68
Cama Inlay-Tabs [CD]
   CONTAINS
   antacids, 68
   aspirin, 75
Camalox, antacids, 69
Campain, acetaminophen, 29
camphorated tincture of opium. *See*
   paregoric, 599
carbamazepine, 128
carbenicillin, 133
Carbolith, lithium, 450
Cardilate, erythrityl tetranitrate,
   325
Cardioquin, quinidine, 724
Cardizem, diltiazem, 277
carisoprodol, 136
Catapres, clonidine, 202
Ceclor, cefaclor, 139
Cecon, vitamin C, 858
cefaclor, 139
cefadroxil, 142
Cefracycline, tetracycline, 771
Cenafed, pseudoephedrine, 717
Centet, tetracycline, 771
Centrax, prazepam, 664
cephalexin, 145
cephradine, 147
Ceporex, cephalexin, 145
Cerespan, papaverine, 592
C.E.S., estrogen, 332
Cetane, vitamin C, 858
Cevalin, vitamin C, 858
Cevi-Bid, vitamin C, 858
Ce-Vi-Sol, vitamin C, 858
Chardonna-2 [CD]
   CONTAINS
   atropine, 86
   phenobarbital, 626
Chembicarb, antacids, 68
Chemgel, antacids, 68
Chemovag, sulfisoxazole, 759
Cheracol-D [CD]
   CONTAINS
   dextromethorphan, 250
   guaifenesin*

Children's Hold [CD]
  CONTAINS
  dextromethorphan, 250
  phenylpropanolamine, 641
chloral hydrate, 150
chloramphenicol, 154
chlordiazepoxide, 157
Chloromycetin, chloramphenicol,
  154
Chloronase, chlorpropamide, 175
Chloroptic, chloramphenicol, 154
chlorothiazide, 161
Chlorphen, chlorpheniramine, 167
chlorpheniramine, 167
Chlor-Promanyl, chlorpromazine,
  170
chlorpromazine, 170
chlorpropamide, 175
chlorthalidone, 179
Chlor-Trimeton, chlorpheniramine,
  167
Chlor-Trimeton Expectorant [CD]
  CONTAINS
  chlorpheniramine, 167
  phenylephrine, 638
  ammonium chloride*
  guaifenesin*
  sodium citrate*
Chlor-Tripolon, chlorpheniramine,
  167
chlorzoxazone, 185
Choledyl, theophylline, 775
Choledyl SA, theophylline, 775
Cibalith-S, lithium, 450
cimetidine, 187
Cin-Quin, quinidine, 724
Circanol, ergoloid mesylates, 318
Claripex, clofibrate, 198
Cleocin, clindamycin, 195
Cleocin T, clindamycin, 195
clidinium, 191
Climestrone, estrogen, 332

clindamycin, 195
Clinoril, sulindac, 763
Clistin-D [CD]
  CONTAINS
  acetaminophen, 29
  phenylephrine, 638
  carbinoxamine*
clofibrate, 198
clonidine, 202
clorazepate, 205
cloxacillin, 209
Cloxapen, cloxacillin, 209
Cloxilean, cloxacillin, 209
codeine, 212
Cogentin, benztropine, 96
ColBENEMID [CD]
  CONTAINS
  colchicine, 215
  probenecid, 686
colchicine, 215
Colisone, prednisone, 677
Combid [CD]
  CONTAINS
  isopropamide, 426
  prochlorperazine, 693
Combipres [CD]
  CONTAINS
  chlorthalidone, 179
  clonidine, 202
Compazine, prochlorperazine, 693
conjugated estrogens. *See* estrogen,
  332
Contac [CD]
  CONTAINS
  chlorpheniramine, 167
  phenylpropanolamine, 641
Contratuss, dextromethorphan, 250
Cope [CD]
  CONTAINS
  antacids, 68
  aspirin, 75
  caffeine, 120

*The symbol [CD] indicates that the brand name given is a combination drug consisting of generic drug components listed below it. If there is no page numbering following the name of the generic drug component, there is no Drug Profile for that ingredient in this book.

Coprobate, meprobamate, 471
Corgard, nadolol, 533
Coricidin Cough Syrup [CD]
  CONTAINS
  dextromethorphan, 250
  phenylpropanolamine, 641
  guaifenesin*
Coricidin Nasal Mist,
    phenylephrine, 638
Coronex, isosorbide dinitrate, 434
Corutol DH, hydrocodone, 386
Corzide [CD]
  CONTAINS
  nadolol, 533
  bendroflumethiazide*
Cosanyl DM [CD]
  CONTAINS
  dextromethorphan, 250
  pseudoephedrine, 717
CoTylenol [CD]
  CONTAINS
  acetaminophen, 29
  chlorpheniramine, 167
  dextromethorphan, 250
  pseudoephedrine, 717
Coumadin, warfarin, 862
Creamalin, antacids, 69
Crystodigin, digitoxin, 270
Curretab, medroxyprogesterone,
    465
cyclandelate, 219
Cycline-250, tetracycline, 771
cyclobenzaprine, 222
Cyclopar, tetracycline, 771
cyclophosphamide, 226
Cyclospasmol, cyclandelate, 219
cyproheptadine, 230
Cytomel, liothyronine, 446
Cytoxan, cyclophosphamide, 226

D

Dalacin C, clindamycin, 195
Dalmane, flurazepam, 356
Darbid, isopropamide, 426
Darvocet-N [CD]
  CONTAINS

acetaminophen, 29
propoxyphene, 705
Darvon, propoxyphene, 705
Darvon Compound [CD]
  CONTAINS
  aspirin, 75
  caffeine, 120
  propoxyphene, 705
Darvon Compound-65 [CD]
  CONTAINS
  aspirin, 75
  caffeine, 120
  propoxyphene, 705
Darvon-N, propoxyphene, 705
Darvon with ASA [CD]
  CONTAINS
  aspirin, 75
  propoxyphene, 705
Darvon-N with ASA [CD]
  CONTAINS
  aspirin, 75
  propoxyphene, 705
Da-Sed, butabarbital, 112
Datril, acetaminophen, 29
Day-Barb, butabarbital, 112
Deapril-ST, ergoloid mesylates,
    318
Decadron, dexamethasone, 240
Decadron Turbinaire,
    dexamethasone, 240
Declomycin, demeclocycline, 233
Deconamine [CD]
  CONTAINS
  chlorpheniramine, 167
  pseudoephedrine, 717
Delatestryl, androgens, 62
Delcid, antacids, 69
Delestrogen, estrogen, 332
Delta-Cortef, prednisolone, 672
Deltasone, prednisone, 677
Demazin [CD]
  CONTAINS
  chlorpheniramine, 167
  phenylephrine, 638
demeclocycline, 233
Demer-Idine, meperidine, 468
Demerol, meperidine, 468

Demerol APAP [CD]
  CONTAINS
  acetaminophen, 29
  meperidine, 468
Demi-Regroton [CD]
  CONTAINS
  chlorthalidone, 179
  reserpine, 730
Demo-Cineol Antitussive Syrup,
  dextromethorphan, 250
Demulen, oral contraceptives, 571
Demulen 1/35, oral contraceptives,
  571
Depakene, valproic acid, 850
Depakote, valproic acid, 850
Depo-Testosterone, androgens, 62
Deprol [CD]
  CONTAINS
  meprobamate, 471
  benactyzine*
Deronil, dexamethasone, 240
DES. *See* diethylstilbestrol, 263
Desamycin, tetracycline, 771
DeSerpa, reserpine, 730
deserpidine. *See* reserpine, 730
desipramine, 236
Desyrel, trazodone, 819
Detensol, propranolol, 708
dexamethasone, 240
Dexasone, dexamethasone, 240
Dexatrim, phenylpropanolamine,
  641
Dexedrine, dextroamphetamine,
  245
Dexone, dexamethasone, 240
dextroamphetamine, 245
dextromethorphan, 250
Diabinese, chlorpropamide, 175
Diamox, acetazolamide, 32
diazepam, 253
Diban [CD]
  CONTAINS

atropine, 86
paregoric, 599
Dicarbosil, antacids, 68
Dicodid, hydrocodone, 386
dicyclomine, 257
Dietac [CD]
  CONTAINS
  caffeine, 120
  phenylpropanolamine, 641
Dietec, diethylpropion, 260
diethylpropion, 260
diethylstilbestrol, 263
Di-Gel Liquid, antacids, 69
Di-Gel Tablets, antacids, 69
digitoxin, 270
digoxin, 274
Dihycon, phenytoin, 649
dihydrocodeinone. *See* hydrocodone,
  386
Dilantin, phenytoin, 649
Dilantin with Phenobarbital [CD]
  CONTAINS
  phenobarbital, 626
  phenytoin, 649
Dilatrate-SR, isosorbide dinitrate,
  434
diltiazem, 277
Dimacol [CD]
  CONTAINS
  dextromethorphan, 250
  pseudoephedrine, 717
  guaifenesin*
Dimelor, acetohexamide, 36
dimenhydrinate, 281
Dimetane, brompheniramine, 104
Dimetapp [CD]
  CONTAINS
  brompheniramine, 104
  phenylephrine, 638
  phenylpropanolamine, 641
Diovol, antacids, 69
diphenhydramine, 284

*The symbol [CD] indicates that the brand name given is a combination drug consisting of generic drug components listed below it. If there is no page numbering following the name of the generic drug component, there is no Drug Profile for that ingredient in this book.

diphenylhydantoin. *See* phenytoin, 649

diphenoxylate, 288

Diphenylan, phenytoin, 649

dipyridamole, 290

Disipal, orphenadrine, 577

Disophrol [CD]
  CONTAINS
  brompheniramine, 104
  pseudoephedrine, 717

disopyramide, 294

disulfiram, 298

Diucardin, hydroflumethiazide, 390

Diuchlor H, hydrochlorothiazide, 381

Diulo, metolazone, 514

Diupres [CD]
  CONTAINS
  chlorothiazide, 161
  reserpine, 730

Diuril, chlorothiazide, 161

Diutensen [CD]
  CONTAINS
  methyclothiazide, 492
  cryptenamine*

Diutensen-R [CD]
  CONTAINS
  methyclothiazide, 492
  reserpine, 730

Dixarit, clonidine, 202

DM Syrup, dextromethorphan, 250

Dolene, propoxyphene, 705

Dolene AP-65 [CD]
  CONTAINS
  acetaminophen, 29
  propoxyphene, 705

Dolene Compound-65 [CD]
  CONTAINS
  aspirin, 75
  caffeine, 120
  propoxyphene, 705
  phenacetin*

Dolophine, methadone, 483

Donnagel [CD]
  CONTAINS
  atropine, 86
  kaolin*
  pectin*

Donnagel-PG [CD]
  CONTAINS
  atropine, 86
  paregoric, 599
  kaolin*
  pectin*

Donnagel-PG [CD] (Canada)
  CONTAINS
  paregoric, 599
  kaolin*
  pectin*

Donnagel w/Neomycin [CD]
  CONTAINS
  atropine, 86
  kaolin*
  neomycin*
  pectin*

Donnatal [CD]
  CONTAINS
  atropine, 86
  phenobarbital, 626

Donnazyme [CD]
  CONTAINS
  atropine, 86
  phenobarbital, 626
  bile salts*
  pancreatin*
  pepsin*

Dopamet, methyldopa, 498

Dopar, levodopa, 442

doxepin, 301

Doxychel, doxycycline, 305

doxycycline, 305

Dralzine, hydralazine, 376

Dramamine, dimenhydrinate, 281

Dristan Cough Formula [CD]
  CONTAINS
  chlorpheniramine, 167
  dextromethorphan, 250
  phenylephrine, 638
  guaifenesin*
  sodium nitrate*

Drixoral [CD]
  CONTAINS
  brompheniramine, 104
  pseudoephedrine, 717

Duatrol, antacids, 69

Duo-Medihaler [CD]
  CONTAINS
  isoproterenol, 430
  phenylephrine, 638
Duotrate, pentaerythritol
  tetranitrate, 605
Duraquin, quinidine, 724
Duretic, methyclothiazide, 492
Duricef, cefadroxil, 142
Dyazide [CD]
  CONTAINS
  hydrochlorothiazide, 381
  triamterene, 827
Dymelor, acetohexamide, 36
Dyrenium, triamterene, 827
Dysne-Inhal, epinephrine, 313

E

Easprin, aspirin, 75
Econochlor, chloramphenicol, 154
Ecotrin, aspirin, 75
E.E.S., erythromycin, 328
EES-200, erythromycin, 328
EES-400, erythromycin, 328
Elavil, amitriptyline, 43
Elixicon, theophylline, 775
Elixophyllin, theophylline, 775
Elixophyllin SR, theophylline, 775
Elserpine, reserpine, 730
Eltor, pseudoephedrine, 717
Eltroxin, thyroxine, 791
Empirin, aspirin, 75
E-Mycin, erythromycin, 328
Enarax [CD]
  CONTAINS
  hydroxyzine, 395
  oxyphencyclimine*
Endep, amitriptyline, 43
Endotussin-NN [CD]
  CONTAINS
  dextromethorphan, 250
  pyrilamine, 721
  ammonium chloride*

Enduron, methyclothiazide, 492
Enduronyl [CD]
  CONTAINS
  methyclothiazide, 492
  reserpine, 730
Enduronyl Forte [CD]
  CONTAINS
  methyclothiazide, 492
  reserpine, 730
Eno, antacids, 68
Enovid, oral contraceptives, 571
Enovid-E, oral contraceptives, 571
Enovid 5 mg., oral contraceptives,
  571
Enovid 10 mg., oral contraceptives,
  571
Entrophen, aspirin, 75
E-Pam, diazepam, 253
ephedrine, 308
Epifrin, epinephrine, 313
epinephrine, 313
Epitrate, epinephrine, 313
Equagesic [CD]
  CONTAINS
  aspirin, 75
  meprobamate, 471
  ethoheptazine*
Equanil, meprobamate, 471
equilin. *See* estrogen, 332
Ergodryl [CD]
  CONTAINS
  caffeine, 120
  diphenhydramine, 284
  ergotamine, 321
ergoloid mesylates, 318
Ergomar, ergotamine, 321
Ergostat, ergotamine, 321
ergot alkaloids. *See* ergoloid
  mesylates, 318
ergotamine, 321
EryDerm, erythromycin, 328
Erypar, erythromycin, 328
erythrityl tetranitrate, 325

*The symbol [CD] indicates that the brand name given is a combination drug consisting of generic drug components listed below it. If there is no page numbering following the name of the generic drug component, there is no Drug Profile for that ingredient in this book.

Erythrocin, erythromycin, 328
Erythromid, erythromycin, 328
erythromycin, 328
Esidrix, hydrochlorothiazide, 381
Esimil [CD]
  CONTAINS
  guanethidine, 368
  hydrochlorothiazide, 381
Eskalith, lithium, 450
esterified estrogens. *See* estrogen,
  332
Estinyl, estrogen, 332
Estrace, estrogen, 332
Estratab, estrogen, 332
Estratest [CD]
  CONTAINS
  androgens, 62
  estrogen, 332
estrogen, 332
Estromed, estrogen, 332
estrone. *See* estrogen, 332
Estrovis, estrogen, 332
ethchlorvynol, 342
ethosuximide, 346
Ethril, erythromycin, 328
Etrafon [CD]
  CONTAINS
  amitriptyline, 43
  perphenazine, 615
Euthroid [CD]
  CONTAINS
  liothyronine, 446
  thyroxine, 791
Evex, estrogen, 332
Excedrin [CD]
  CONTAINS
  acetaminophen, 29
  aspirin, 75
  caffeine, 120
Exdol, acetaminophen, 29
Expansatol, butabarbital, 112

F

Fastin, phentermine, 630
Fedahist [CD]
  CONTAINS
  chlorpheniramine, 167
  pseudoephedrine, 717

Fedrazil [CD]
  CONTAINS
  pseudoephedrine, 717
  chlorcyclizine*
Feldene, piroxicam, 657
Fellozine, promethazine, 698
Femiron, iron, 414
Femogen, estrogen, 332
Fenicol, chloramphenicol, 154
fenoprofen, 348
Feosol, iron, 414
Ferancee [CD]
  CONTAINS
  iron, 414
  vitamin C, 858
Fergon, iron, 414
Fer-In-Sol, iron, 414
Fernisolone, prednisolone, 672
Fero-Folic-500 [CD]
  CONTAINS
  iron, 414
  vitamin C, 858
  folic acid*
Fero-Grad, iron, 414
Fero-Grad-500 [CD]
  CONTAINS
  iron, 414
  vitamin C, 858
Fero-Gradumet, iron, 414
ferrocholinate. *See* iron, 414
Ferro-Sequels [CD]
  CONTAINS
  iron, 414
  docusate sodium*
Ferrospan, iron, 414
ferrous fumarate. *See* iron, 414
ferrous gluconate. *See* iron,
  414
ferrous sulfate. *See* iron, 414
Fersamal, iron, 414
Fertinic, iron, 414
Fesofor, iron, 414
Fesotyme, iron, 414
Fiorinal [CD]
  CONTAINS
  aspirin, 75
  butalbital, 116
  caffeine, 120

Fiorinal-C 1/2 [CD]
CONTAINS
aspirin, 75
butalbital, 116
caffeine, 120
codeine, 212
Fiorinal-C 1/4 [CD]
CONTAINS
aspirin, 75
butalbital, 116
caffeine, 120
codeine, 212
Fiorinal with Codeine [CD]
CONTAINS
aspirin, 75
butalbital, 116
caffeine, 120
codeine, 212
Fizrin, antacids, 68
Flagyl, metronidazole, 524
Flexeril, cyclobenzaprine, 222
fluoxymesterone. See androgens, 62
fluphenazine, 352
flurazepam, 356
Formula 44-D [CD]
CONTAINS
dextromethorphan, 250
phenylpropanolamine, 641
guaifenesin*
Formulex, dicyclomine, 257
4-Way Cold Tablets [CD]
CONTAINS
aspirin, 75
chlorpheniramine, 167
phenylpropanolamine, 641
4-Way Nasal Spray [CD]
CONTAINS
phenylephrine, 638
pyrilamine, 721
naphazoline*
Fulvicin P/G, griseofulvin, 365
Fulvicin-U/F, griseofulvin, 365
Fumasorb, iron, 414

Furadantin, nitrofurantoin, 554
Furalan, nitrofurantoin, 554
Furaloid, nitrofurantoin, 554
Furantoin, nitrofurantoin, 554
Furatine, nitrofurantoin, 554
furosemide, 360
Furoside, furosemide, 360

G

Ganphen, promethazine, 698
Gantanol, sulfamethoxazole, 746
Gantrisin, sulfisoxazole, 759
Gardenal, phenobarbital, 626
Gaviscon, antacids, 69
Gelusil, antacids, 69
Geocillin, carbenicillin, 133
Geopen, carbenicillin, 133
Geritol Tablets [CD]
CONTAINS
iron, 414
vitamin C, 858
vitamin B complex*
Glaucon, epinephrine, 313
G-Mycin, tetracycline, 771
Gravol, dimenhydrinate, 281
Grifulvin V, griseofulvin, 365
Grisactin, griseofulvin, 365
Grisactin Ultra, griseofulvin, 365
griseofulvin, 365
Grisovin-FP, griseofulvin, 365
Grisowen, griseofulvin, 365
Gris-PEG, griseofulvin, 365
G-Sox, sulfisoxazole, 759
guanethidine, 368
Gustalac, antacids, 68
Gynergen, ergotamine, 321

H

Haldol, haloperidol, 372
Halodrin [CD]
CONTAINS
androgens, 62
estrogen, 332

*The symbol [CD] indicates that the brand name given is a combination drug consisting of generic drug components listed below it. If there is no page numbering following the name of the generic drug component, there is no Drug Profile for that ingredient in this book.

haloperidol, 372
Halotestin, androgens, 62
Hexadrol, dexamethasone, 240
Histanil, promethazine, 698
Histaspan, chlorpheniramine, 167
Hold 4 Hour, dextromethorphan,
   250
Honvol, diethylstilbestrol, 263
Humulin, insulin, 409
Hycodan, hydrocodone, 386
Hycodan [CD]
   CONTAINS
   atropine, 86
   hydrocodone, 386
Hycodan-D [CD]
   CONTAINS
   hydrocodone, 386
   phenylpropanolamine, 641
Hycodan-E [CD]
   CONTAINS
   hydrocodone, 386
   guaifenesin*
Hycomine Compound [CD]
   CONTAINS
   acetaminophen, 29
   caffeine, 120
   chlorpheniramine, 167
   hydrocodone, 386
   phenylephrine, 638
Hycomine Pediatric Syrup [CD]
   CONTAINS
   hydrocodone, 386
   phenylpropanolamine, 641
Hycomine Pediatric Syrup [CD]
   (Canada)
   CONTAINS
   hydrocodone, 386
   phenylephrine, 638
   pyrilamine, 721
   ammonium chloride*
Hycomine Syrup [CD]
   CONTAINS
   hydrocodone, 386
   phenylpropanolamine, 641
Hycomine Syrup [CD] (Canada)
   CONTAINS
   hydrocodone, 386
   phenylephrine, 638

pyrilamine, 721
   ammonium chloride*
Hycotuss Expectorant [CD]
   CONTAINS
   hydrocodone, 386
   guaifenesin*
Hydergine, ergoloid mesylates,
   318
hydralazine, 376
Hydral 25/25 [CD]
   CONTAINS
   hydralazine, 376
   hydrochlorothiazide, 381
hydrochlorothiazide, 381
hydrocodone, 386
HydroDiuril, hydrochlorothiazide,
   381
hydroflumethiazide, 390
Hydro Plus [CD]
   CONTAINS
   hydrochlorothiazide, 381
   reserpine, 730
Hydropres 25 [CD]
   CONTAINS
   hydrochlorothiazide, 381
   reserpine, 730
Hydropres 50 [CD]
   CONTAINS
   hydrochlorothiazide, 381
   reserpine, 730
hydroxyzine, 395
Hydro Z-50, hydrochlorothiazide,
   381
Hygroton, chlorthalidone, 179
hyoscyamine. *See* atropine, 86
Hyperetic, hydrochlorothiazide,
   381
Hyperine, reserpine, 730

I

Iberet [CD]
   CONTAINS
   iron, 414
   multiple vitamins*
Iberet-500 [CD]
   CONTAINS
   iron, 414
   multiple vitamins*

Iberet-Folic-500 [CD]
  CONTAINS
  iron, 414
  folic acid*
  multiple vitamins*
ibuprofen, 398
Iletin Preparations, insulin, 409
Ilosone, erythromycin, 328
Ilotycin, erythromycin, 328
Imavate, imipramine, 402
Imferon, iron, 414
imipramine, 402
Impril, imipramine, 402
Inderal, propranolol, 708
Inderal LA, propranolol, 708
Inderide [CD]
  CONTAINS
  hydrochlorothiazide, 381
  propranolol, 708
Indocid, indomethacin, 405
Indocin, indomethacin, 405
Indocin SR, indomethacin, 405
indomethacin, 405
Inflamase, prednisolone, 672
INH, isoniazid, 423
Insomnal, diphenhydramine, 284
insulin, 409
Insulin Preparations, insulin, 409
Intasedol, butabarbital, 112
Intrabutazone, phenylbutazone, 634
Ionamin, phentermine, 630
iproveratril. *See* verapamil, 854
iron, 414
iron dextran. *See* iron, 414
Ismelin, guanethidine, 368
Ismelin-Esidrix [CD]
  CONTAINS
  guanethidine, 368
  hydrochlorothiazide, 381
Isobec, amobarbital, 47
Isoclor [CD]
  CONTAINS

chlorpheniramine, 167
pseudoephedrine, 717
isoephedrine. *See* pseudoephedrine, 717
isoetharine, 419
isoniazid, 423
Isophrin, phenylephrine, 638
isoprenaline. *See* isoproterenol, 430
isopropamide, 426
isoproterenol, 430
Isoptin, verapamil, 854
Isopto Atropine, atropine, 86
Isopto-Carpine, pilocarpine, 654
Isopto Fenicol, chloramphenicol, 154
Isordil, isosorbide dinitrate, 434
isosorbide dinitrate, 434
Isotamine, isoniazid, 423
isotretinoin, 437
isoxsuprine, 440
Isuprel, isoproterenol, 430
Isuprel Compound Elixir [CD]
  CONTAINS
  ephedrine, 308
  isoproterenol, 430
  phenobarbital, 626
  theophylline, 775
  potassium iodide*
Isuprel-Neo [CD]
  CONTAINS
  isoproterenol, 430
  phenylephrine, 638

J

Janimine, imipramine, 402

K

Kalium Durules, potassium, 660
Kaochlor, potassium, 660
Kaon, potassium, 660
Kay Ciel, potassium, 660
K Cl 5% and 20%, potassium, 660
Keflex, cephalexin, 145
Kelyum, potassium, 660

*The symbol [CD] indicates that the brand name given is a combination drug consisting of generic drug components listed below it. If there is no page numbering following the name of the generic drug component, there is no Drug Profile for that ingredient in this book.

Kenacort, triamcinolone, 822
Kesso-Mycin, erythromycin, 328
Kinesed [CD]
   CONTAINS
   atropine, 86
   phenobarbital, 626
K-Long, potassium, 660
K-Lor, potassium, 660
Klorvess, potassium, 660
Klotrix, potassium, 660
K-Lyte, potassium, 660
Koffex Syrup, dextromethorphan,
   250
Kolantyl, antacids, 69
K-Phen, promethazine, 698
K-Sol, potassium, 660
K-10, potassium, 660

L

LaBID, theophylline, 775
Laniazid, isoniazid, 423
Lanoxicaps, digoxin, 274
Lanoxin, digoxin, 274
Largactil, chlorpromazine, 170
Larodopa, levodopa, 442
Larotid, amoxicillin, 56
Lasix, furosemide, 360
Ledercillin VK, penicillin V, 602
Lemiserp, reserpine, 730
Levate, amitriptyline, 43
levodopa, 442
Levoid, thyroxine, 791
Levothroid, thyroxine, 791
levothyroxine. *See* thyroxine, 791
Librax [CD]
   CONTAINS
   chlordiazepoxide, 157
   clidinium, 191
Libritabs, chlordiazepoxide, 157
Librium, chlordiazepoxide, 157
Limbitrol [CD]
   CONTAINS
   amitriptyline, 43
   chlordiazepoxide, 157
liothyronine, 446
Lipo Gantrisin, sulfisoxazole, 759
Lithane, lithium, 450
lithium, 450
Lithizine, lithium, 450

Lithobid, lithium, 450
Lithonate, lithium, 450
Lithotabs, lithium, 450
Lodrane, theophylline, 775
Loestrin 1.5/30, oral contraceptives,
   571
Loestrin 1/20, oral contraceptives,
   571
Loestrin Fe 1.5/30, oral
   contraceptives, 571
Loestrin Fe 1/20, oral
   contraceptives, 571
Lomine, dicyclomine, 257
Lomotil, diphenoxylate, 288
Lomotil [CD]
   CONTAINS
   atropine, 86
   diphenoxylate, 288
Loniten, minoxidil, 530
Lo/Ovral, oral contraceptives, 571
Lopressor, metoprolol, 519
lorazepam, 454
Lotusate, butalbital, 116
Ludiomil, maprotiline, 457
Luminal, phenobarbital, 626

M

Maalox, antacids, 69
Macrodantin, nitrofurantoin, 554
magaldrate. *See* antacids, 68
Magnatril, antacids, 69
Magnesed, antacids, 69
magnesium carbonate. *See* antacids,
   68
magnesium hydroxide. *See* antacids,
   68
magnesium trisilicate. *See* antacids,
   68
Malogen, androgens, 62
Malogen in Oil, androgens, 62
Malogex, androgens, 62
maprotiline, 457
Marax [CD]
   CONTAINS
   ephedrine, 308
   hydroxyzine, 395
   theophylline, 775
Marblen, antacids, 69
Maxamag, antacids, 69

Maxidex, dexamethasone, 240
Mazepine, carbamazepine, 128
Measurin, aspirin, 75
meclizine, 462
Medarsed, butabarbital, 112
Medicycline, tetracycline, 771
Medihaler-Epi, epinephrine, 313
Medihaler-Ergotamine, ergotamine, 321
Medihaler-Iso, isoproterenol, 430
Medilium, chlordiazepoxide, 157
Medimet-250, methyldopa, 498
Meditran, meprobamate, 471
Medrol, methylprednisolone, 506
medroxyprogesterone, 465
Mellaril, thioridazine, 779
Mellaril-S, thioridazine, 779
Melopa, methyldopa, 498
Menest, estrogen, 332
Menrium [CD]
  CONTAINS
  chlordiazepoxide, 157
  estrogen, 332
meperidine, 468
meprobamate, 471
Meprocon, meprobamate, 471
Meprospan, meprobamate, 471
Meprospan-400, meprobamate, 471
mepyramine. *See* pyrilamine, 721
Meravil, amitriptyline, 43
mesoridazine, 475
Metandren, androgens, 62
Metaprel, metaproterenol, 479
metaproterenol, 479
methadone, 483
methocarbamol, 486
Methotrexate, 489
methotrexate, 489
methyclothiazide, 492
methyldopa, 498
methylphenidate, 502
methylprednisolone, 506
methyltestosterone. *See* androgens, 62

methysergide, 511
Meticortelone, prednisolone, 672
Meticorten, prednisone, 677
metolazone, 514
metoprolol, 519
metronidazole, 524
Meval, diazepam, 253
Mexate, methotrexate, 489
Micro-K Extencaps, potassium, 660
Micronor, oral contraceptives, 571
Micronor 0.35 mg., oral contraceptives, 571
Midol [CD]
  CONTAINS
  aspirin, 75
  caffeine, 120
  cinnamedrine*
Milk of Magnesia, antacids, 68, 69
Milprem [CD]
  CONTAINS
  estrogen, 332
  meprobamate, 471
Miltown, meprobamate, 471
Miltrate [CD]
  CONTAINS
  meprobamate, 471
  pentaerythritol tetranitrate, 605
Minims, chloramphenicol, 154
Minims, pilocarpine, 654
Minipress, prazosin, 668
Minizide [CD]
  CONTAINS
  prazosin, 668
  polythiazide*
Minocin, minocycline, 527
minocycline, 527
Min-Ovral, oral contraceptives, 571
minoxidil, 530
Miocarpine, pilocarpine, 654
Mobenol, tolbutamide, 805
Modecate, fluphenazine, 352
Modicon, oral contraceptives, 571
Moditen, fluphenazine, 352

*The symbol [CD] indicates that the brand name given is a combination drug consisting of generic drug components listed below it. If there is no page numbering following the name of the generic drug component, there is no Drug Profile for that ingredient in this book.

Mol-Iron, iron, 414
Motrin, ibuprofen, 398
Moxilean, amoxicillin, 56
Mudrane [CD]
   CONTAINS
   ephedrine, 308
   phenobarbital, 626
   theophylline, 775
   potassium iodide*
Mychel, chloramphenicol, 154
Mycolog [CD]
   CONTAINS
   nystatin, 568
   triamcinolone, 822
   gramicidin*
   neomycin*
Mycostatin, nystatin, 568
Mylanta, antacids, 69
Mysoline, primidone, 682
Mysteclin-F [CD]
   CONTAINS
   tetracycline, 771
   amphotericin B*

N

nadolol, 533
Nadopen-V, penicillin V, 602
Nadostine, nystatin, 568
Nadozone, phenylbutazone, 634
Nafcil, nafcillin, 538
nafcillin, 538
Nafrine, oxymetazoline, 590
Naldecol [CD]
   CONTAINS
   phenylephrine, 638
   phenylpropanolamine, 641
   phenyltoloxamine, 645
   carbinoxamine*
Naldecon [CD]
   CONTAINS
   chlorpheniramine, 167
   phenylephrine, 638
   phenylpropanolamine, 641
   phenyltoloxamine, 645
Nalfon, fenoprofen, 348
nalidixic acid, 540
Naprosyn, naproxen, 544
naproxen, 544

Natigoxine, digoxin, 274
Natrimax, hydrochlorothiazide, 381
Nauseatol, dimenhydrinate, 281
Navane, thiothixene, 783
Nefrol, hydrochlorothiazide, 381
NegGram, nalidixic acid, 540
Nemasol, para-aminosalicylic acid,
   595
Nembutal, pentobarbital, 611
Neo-Barb, butabarbital, 112
Neo-Calme, diazepam, 253
Neo-Codema, hydrochlorothiazide,
   381
Neo DM, dextromethorphan, 250
Neo-Fer-50, iron, 414
Neo-K, potassium, 660
Neo-Renal, furosemide, 360
Neosar, cyclophosphamide, 226
Neo-Synephrine, oxymetazoline, 590
   phenylephrine, 638
Neo-Synephrinol Day Relief,
   pseudoephedrine, 717
Neo-Tetrine, tetracycline, 771
Neo-Tran, meprobamate, 471
Neo-Tric, metronidazole, 524
Neo-Zoline, phenylbutazone, 634
Nephronex, nitrofurantoin, 554
Nervine Nighttime Sleep-Aid,
   pyrilamine, 721
Neutralca-S, antacids, 69
niacin. *See* nicotinic acid, 547
Nicalex, nicotinic acid, 547
Nicobid, nicotinic acid, 547
Nicolar, nicotinic acid, 547
Nico-Span, nicotinic acid, 547
Nicotinex, nicotinic acid, 547
nicotinic acid, 547
nifedipine, 551
Nifuran, nitrofurantoin, 554
Nilstat, nystatin, 568
Nitrex, nitrofurantoin, 554
Nitro-Bid, nitroglycerin, 557
Nitrodan, nitrofurantoin, 554
Nitrodisc, nitroglycerin, 557
Nitro-Dur, nitroglycerin, 557
nitrofurantoin, 554
nitroglycerin, 557
Nitroglyn, nitroglycerin, 557

Nitrol, nitroglycerin, 557
Nitrong, nitroglycerin, 557
Nitrospan, nitroglycerin, 557
Nitrostabilin, nitroglycerin, 557
Nitrostat, nitroglycerin, 557
Nobesine - 75, diethylpropion, 260
Noctec, chloral hydrate, 150
Nodoz, caffeine, 120
Norflex, orphenadrine, 577
Norgesic [CD]
   CONTAINS
   aspirin, 75
   caffeine, 120
   orphenadrine, 577
Norgesic Forte [CD]
   CONTAINS
   aspirin, 75
   caffeine, 120
   orphenadrine, 577
Norinyl 1+35, oral contraceptives,
   571
Norinyl 1+50, oral contraceptives,
   571
Norinyl 1+80, oral contraceptives,
   571
Norinyl-2, oral contraceptives, 571
Norinyl 2 mg., oral contraceptives,
   571
Norisodrine, isoproterenol, 430
Norlestrin 1/50, oral contraceptives,
   571
Norlestrin 2.5/50, oral
   contraceptives, 571
Norlestrin Fe 1/50, oral
   contraceptives, 571
Norlestrin Fe 2.5/50, oral
   contraceptives, 571
Norpace, disopyramide, 294
Norpanth, propantheline, 701
Norpramin, desipramine, 236
Nor-Q.D., oral contraceptives, 571
Nor-Tet, tetracycline, 771
nortriptyline, 561

Nospaz, dicyclomine, 257
Nostril, phenylephrine, 638
Novafed, pseudoephedrine, 717
Novafed A [CD]
   CONTAINS
   chlorpheniramine, 167
   pseudoephedrine, 717
Novafibrate, clofibrate, 198
Novamobarb, amobarbital, 47
Novamoxin, amoxicillin, 56
Nova-Phenicol, chloramphenicol,
   154
Nova-Pred, prednisolone, 672
Novasen, aspirin, 75
Novo-Ampicillin, ampicillin, 59
Novobutamide, tolbutamide, 805
Novobutazone, phenylbutazone, 634
Novochlorhydrate, chloral hydrate,
   150
Novochlorocap, chloramphenicol, 154
Novochlorpromazine,
   chlorpromazine, 170
Novocimetine, cimetidine, 187
Novocloxin, cloxacillin, 209
Novocolchine, colchicine, 215
Novodigoxin, digoxin, 274
Novodimenate, dimenhydrinate, 281
Novodipam, diazepam, 253
Novodoparil [CD]
   CONTAINS
   hydrochlorothiazide, 381
   methyldopa, 498
Novoferrogluc, iron, 414
Novoferrosulfa, iron, 414
Novoflupam, flurazepam, 356
Novoflurazine, trifluoperazine, 831
Novofumar, iron, 414
Novofuran, nitrofurantoin, 554
Novohydrazide,
   hydrochlorothiazide, 381
Novolexin, cephalexin, 145
Novomedopa, methyldopa, 498
Novomepro, meprobamate, 471

*The symbol [CD] indicates that the brand name given is a combination drug consisting of generic drug components listed below it. If there is no page numbering following the name of the generic drug component, there is no Drug Profile for that ingredient in this book.

Novomethacin, indomethacin, 405
Novonaprox, naproxen, 544
Novoniacin, nicotinic acid, 547
Novonidazol, metronidazole, 524
Novopentobarb, pentobarbital, 611
Novopen-VK, penicillin V, 602
Novopheniram, chlorpheniramine,
    167
Novophenytoin, phenytoin, 649
Novopoxide, chlordiazepoxide, 157
Novopramine, imipramine, 402
Novopranol, propranolol, 708
Novoprednisolone, prednisolone, 672
Novoprednisone, prednisone, 677
Novopropamide, chlorpropamide,
    175
Novopropanthil, propantheline, 701
Novopropoxyn, propoxyphene, 705
Novopurol, allopurinol, 40
Novopyrazone, sulfinpyrazone, 755
Novoridazine, thioridazine, 779
Novorythro, erythromycin, 328
Novosecobarb, secobarbital, 738
Novosemide, furosemide, 360
Novosoxazole, sulfisoxazole, 759
Novotetra, tetracycline, 771
Novothalidone, chlorthalidone, 179
Novotrimel [CD]
    CONTAINS
    sulfamethoxazole, 746
    trimethoprim, 841
Novotrimel DS [CD]
    CONTAINS
    sulfamethoxazole, 746
    trimethoprim, 841
Novotriptyn, amitriptyline, 43
Nuprin, ibuprofen, 398
Nyaderm, nystatin, 568
Nydrazid, isoniazid, 423
nylidrin, 565
Nyquil [CD]
    CONTAINS
    acetaminophen, 29
    dextromethorphan, 250
    ephedrine, 308
    doxylamine*
nystatin, 568

O

Ocuclear, oxymetazoline, 590
Ocusert Pilo-20 and -40,
    pilocarpine, 654
Oestrilin, estrogen, 332
Oestrilin with Methyltestosterone
    [CD]
    CONTAINS
    androgens, 62
    estrogen, 332
Ogen, estrogen, 332
Omnipen, ampicillin, 59
Ophthochlor, chloramphenicol,
    154
Opium Tincture, paregoric,
    599
Oradrate, chloral hydrate, 150
oral contraceptives, 571
Orasone, prednisone, 677
Ora-Testryl, androgens, 62
Orbenin, cloxacillin, 209
orciprenaline. *See* metaproterenol,
    479
Oretic, hydrochlorothiazide,
    381
Oreton, androgens, 62
Oreton Methyl, androgens, 62
Orinase, tolbutamide, 805
Ornade [CD]
    CONTAINS
    chlorpheniramine, 167
    phenylpropanolamine, 641
Ornade-A.F. [CD]
    CONTAINS
    chlorpheniramine, 167
    phenylpropanolamine, 641
Ornade-DM [CD]
    CONTAINS
    chlorpheniramine, 167
    dextromethorphan, 250
    phenylpropanolamine, 641
Ornade Expectorant [CD]
    CONTAINS
    chlorpheniramine, 167
    phenylpropanolamine, 641
    guaifenesin*

Ornex [CD]
  CONTAINS
  acetaminophen, 29
  phenylpropanolamine, 641
orphenadrine, 577
Ortho-Novum 1/35, oral
  contraceptives, 571
Ortho-Novum 1/50, oral
  contraceptives, 571
Ortho-Novum 1/80, oral
  contraceptives, 571
Ortho-Novum 2 mg., oral
  contraceptives, 571
Ortho-Novum 5 mg., oral
  contraceptives, 571
Ortho-Novum 0.5 mg., oral
  contraceptives, 571
Ortho 0.5/35, oral contraceptives,
  571
Ortho 10/11, oral contraceptives,
  571
Ortho 1/35, oral contraceptives,
  571
Os-Cal, calcium, 125
Os-Cal 500 Tablets, calcium, 125
Os-Cal Forte Tablets [CD]
  CONTAINS
  calcium, 125
  iron, 414
  minerals*
  vitamins*
Os-Cal-Gesic-Tablets [CD]
  CONTAINS
  calcium, 125
  saliscylamide*
Os-Cal Plus Tablets [CD]
  CONTAINS
  calcium, 125
  iron, 414
  minerals*
  vitamins*
Os-Cal Tablets [CD]

  CONTAINS
  calcium, 125
  vitamin D*
Ovcon-35, oral contraceptives,
  571
Ovcon-50, oral contraceptives,
  571
Ovral, oral contraceptives, 571
Ovrette, oral contraceptives, 571
O-V Statin, nystatin, 568
Ovulen, oral contraceptives, 571
Ovulen 1 mg., oral contraceptives,
  571
Ovulen 0.5 mg., oral contraceptives,
  571
oxacillin, 580
oxazepam, 583
Oxpam, oxazepam, 583
oxtriphylline. *See* theophylline, 775
oxycodone, 586
oxymetazoline, 590

P

Palafer, iron, 414
Pamelor, nortriptyline, 561
Panadol, acetaminophen, 29
Panectyl, trimeprazine, 835
Panmycin, tetracycline, 771
Panwarfin, warfarin, 862
papaverine, 592
para-aminosalicylic acid, 595
paracetamol. *See* acetaminophen,
  29
Paracort, prednisone, 677
Paraflex, chlorzoxazone, 185
Parafon Forte [CD]
  CONTAINS
  acetaminophen, 29
  chlorzoxazone, 185
Parasal, para-aminosalicylic acid,
  595
paregoric, 599

*The symbol [CD] indicates that the brand name given is a combination drug consisting of generic drug components listed below it. If there is no page numbering following the name of the generic drug component, there is no Drug Profile for that ingredient in this book.

Parepectolin [CD]
  CONTAINS
  paregoric, 599
  kaolin*
  pectin*
Parlodel, bromocriptine, 100
Parnate, tranylcypromine, 813
P.A.S., para-aminosalicylic acid, 595
P.A.S. Acid, para-aminosalicylic acid,
  595
Pasna, para-aminosalicylic acid, 595
Pavabid, papaverine, 592
Pavacap, papaverine, 592
Pavakey, papaverine, 592
Paveral, codeine, 212
Pax 400, meprobamate, 471
PBZ, tripelennamine, 844
PBZ-SR, tripelennamine, 844
Pediamycin, erythromycin, 328
Penamox, amoxicillin, 56
Penapar VK, penicillin V, 602
Penbritin, ampicillin, 59
penicillin V, 602
Penicillin VK, penicillin V, 602
pentaerythritol tetranitrate, 605
Pentamycetin, chloramphenicol, 154
Pentazine, promethazine, 698
pentazocine, 608
pentobarbital, 611
Pentogen, pentobarbital, 611
Pentritol, pentaerythritol
  tetranitrate, 605
Pen-Vee, penicillin V, 602
Pen-Vee K, penicillin V, 602
Pepsogel, antacids, 68
Pepto-Bismol Tablets, antacids, 68
Peptol, cimetidine, 187
Percocet [CD]
  CONTAINS
  acetaminophen, 29
  caffeine, 120
  oxycodone, 586
Percocet-Demi [CD]
  CONTAINS
  acetaminophen, 29
  caffeine, 120
  oxycodone, 586
Percocet-5 [CD]

  CONTAINS
  acetaminophen, 29
  oxycodone, 586
Percodan [CD]
  CONTAINS
  aspirin, 75
  oxycodone, 586
Percodan [CD] (Canada)
  CONTAINS
  aspirin, 75
  caffeine, 120
  oxycodone, 586
Percodan-Demi [CD]
  CONTAINS
  aspirin, 75
  oxycodone, 586
Percodan-Demi [CD] (Canada)
  CONTAINS
  aspirin, 75
  caffeine, 120
  oxycodone, 586
Percogesic [CD]
  CONTAINS
  acetaminophen, 29
  phenyltoloxamine, 645
Periactin, cyproheptadine, 230
Peridol, haloperidol, 372
Peritrate, pentaerythritol
  tetranitrate, 605
Peritrate Forte, pentaerythritol
  tetranitrate, 605
Permitil, fluphenazine, 352
perphenazine, 615
Persantine, dipyridamole, 290
Pertofrane, desipramine, 236
Pertussin [CD]
  CONTAINS
  dextromethorphan, 250
  guaifenesin*
Pervadil, nylidrin, 565
pethidine. *See* meperidine, 468
Pfizer-E, erythromycin, 328
Pfizerpen VK, penicillin V, 602
Phenaphen, acetaminophen, 29
Phenazine, perphenazine, 615
Phenazo, phenazopyridine, 620
phenazopyridine, 620
Phenbuff, phenylbutazone, 634

Phenergan, promethazine, 698
Phenergan Compound [CD]
  CONTAINS
  aspirin, 75
  promethazine, 698
  pseudoephedrine, 717
Phenerhist, promethazine, 698
pheniramine, 622
phenobarbital, 626
phenobarbitone. *See* phenobarbital,
  626
phentermine, 630
phenylbutazone, 634
phenylephrine, 638
phenylpropanolamine, 641
phenyltoloxamine, 645
phenytoin, 649
Pilocar, pilocarpine, 654
pilocarpine, 654
Pilocel, pilocarpine, 654
Pilomiotin, pilocarpine, 654
Piracaps, tetracycline, 771
piroxicam, 657
Placidyl, ethchlorvynol, 342
PMB [CD]
  CONTAINS
  estrogen, 332
  meprobamate, 471
PMB-200 [CD]
  CONTAINS
  estrogen, 332
  meprobamate, 471
PMB-400 [CD]
  CONTAINS
  estrogen, 332
  meprobamate, 471
Polaramine, chlorpheniramine, 167
Polycillin, ampicillin, 59
Polycillin-PRB [CD]
  CONTAINS
  ampicillin, 59
  probenecid, 686
Polymox, amoxicillin, 56

potassium, 660
prazepam, 664
prazosin, 668
prednisolone, 672
prednisone, 677
Prefrin, phenylephrine, 638
Premarin, estrogen, 332
Premarin with Methyltestosterone
  [CD]
  CONTAINS
  androgens, 62
  estrogen, 332
Presamine, imipramine, 402
Primatene Mist, epinephrine, 313
primidone, 682
Principen, ampicillin, 59
Probalan, probenecid, 686
Pro-Banthine, propantheline, 701
probenecid, 686
procainamide, 690
Procan SR, procainamide, 690
Procardia, nifedipine, 551
prochlorperazine, 693
Procytox, cyclophosphamide, 226
Profedrine, pseudoephedrine, 717
Prolixin, fluphenazine, 352
Proloid, thyroid, 787
Prolopa [CD]
  CONTAINS
  levodopa, 442
  benserazide*
Proloprim, trimethoprim, 841
Promachlor, chlorpromazine, 170
Promapar, chlorpromazine, 170
promethazine, 698
Pronestyl, procainamide, 690
Pronestyl-SR, procainamide, 690
Propadrine, phenylpropanolamine,
  641
Propagest, phenylpropanolamine,
  641
Propanthel, propantheline, 701
propantheline, 701

*The symbol [CD] indicates that the brand name given is a combination drug consisting of generic drug components listed below it. If there is no page numbering following the name of the generic drug component, there is no Drug Profile for that ingredient in this book.

Propion, diethylpropion, 260
propoxyphene, 705
propranolol, 708
Prorex, promethazine, 698
Prostaphlin, oxacillin, 580
Protostat, metronidazole, 524
protriptyline, 713
Protylol, dicyclomine, 257
Provera, medroxyprogesterone, 465
Provigan, promethazine, 698
pseudoephedrine, 717
Pseudofrin, pseudoephedrine, 717
Pulmophylline, theophylline, 775
Purified Insulins, insulin, 409
Purinol, allopurinol, 40
Purodigin, digitoxin, 270
P.V. Carpine, pilocarpine, 654
PVF, penicillin V, 602
PVF K, penicillin V, 602
Pyma [CD]
    CONTAINS
    chlorpheniramine, 167
    pheniramine, 623
    phenylephrine, 638
    pyrilamine, 721
Pyopen, carbenicillin, 133
Pyribenzamine, tripelennamine, 844
Pyridium, phenazopyridine, 620
Pyridium Plus [CD]
    CONTAINS
    atropine, 86
    butabarbital, 112
    phenazopyridine, 620
pyrilamine, 721
Pyristan [CD]
    CONTAINS
    chlorpheniramine, 167
    phenylephrine, 638
    phenylpropanolamine, 641
    pyrilamine, 721
Pyronium, phenazopyridine, 620

Q

Quadrinal [CD]
    CONTAINS

ephedrine, 308
phenobarbital, 626
theophylline, 775
potassium iodide*
Quarzan, clidinium, 191
Quelidrine [CD]
    CONTAINS
    chlorpheniramine, 167
    dextromethorphan, 250
    ephedrine, 308
    phenylephrine, 638
    ammonium chloride*
Quibron [CD]
    CONTAINS
    theophylline, 775
    guaifenesin*
Quibron Plus [CD]
    CONTAINS
    butalbital, 116
    ephedrine, 308
    theophylline, 775
    guaifenesin*
Quibron-T, theophylline, 775
Quibron-T Dividose, theophylline, 775
Quibron-T/SR, theophylline, 775
Quibron-T/SR Dividose, theophylline, 775
Quiebar, butabarbital, 112
Quinaglute, quinidine, 724
Quinate, quinidine, 724
Quinidex Extendtabs, quinidine, 724
quinidine, 724
Quinobarb [CD]
    CONTAINS
    quinidine, 724
    phenylethylbarbituate*
Quinora, quinidine, 724

R

ranitidine, 728
Ratio, antacids, 68
Raudixin, reserpine, 730
Rauloydin, reserpine, 730
Rau-Sed, reserpine, 730
Rauserpin, reserpine, 730
rauwolfia. *See* reserpine, 730

Rauzide [CD]
CONTAINS
reserpine, 730
bendroflumethiazide*
Redoxon, vitamin C, 858
Regibon, diethylpropion, 260
Regroton [CD]
CONTAINS
chlorthalidone, 179
reserpine, 730
Reidamine, dimenhydrinate, 281
Rela, carisoprodol, 136
Relium, chlordiazepoxide, 157
Remsed, promethazine, 698
Renbu, butabarbital, 112
Repen-VK, penicillin V, 602
Reserfia, reserpine, 730
Reserpaneed, reserpine, 730
reserpine, 730
Reserpoid, reserpine, 730
Respbid, theophylline, 775
Retet, tetracycline, 771
Rifadin, rifampin, 735
Rifamate [CD]
CONTAINS
isoniazid, 423
rifampin, 735
rifampin, 735
Rifomycin, rifampin, 735
Rimactane, rifampin, 735
Rimactane/INH Dual Pack [CD]
CONTAINS
isoniazid, 423
rifampin, 735
Rimifon, isoniazid, 423
Riopan, antacids, 69
Ritalin, methylphenidate, 502
Ritalin-SR, methylphenidate, 502
Rival, diazepam, 253
Robalate, antacids, 68
Robamate, meprobamate, 471
Robaxin, methocarbamol, 486

Robaxin-750, methocarbamol, 486
Robaxisal [CD]
CONTAINS
aspirin, 75
methocarbamol, 486
Robaxisal-C [CD]
CONTAINS
aspirin, 75
codeine, 212
methocarbamol, 486
Robicillin-VK, penicillin V, 602
Robidex, dextromethorphan, 250
Robidone, hydrocodone, 386
Robidrine, pseudoephedrine, 717
Robigesic, acetaminophen, 29
Robimycin, erythromycin, 328
Robitet, tetracycline, 771
Robitussin-CF [CD]
CONTAINS
dextromethorphan, 250
phenylpropanolamine, 641
guaifenesin*
Robitussin-DM [CD]
CONTAINS
dextromethorphan, 250
guaifenesin*
*Robitussin Night Relief Cold
Formula* [CD]
CONTAINS
acetaminophen, 29
dextromethorphan, 250
phenylephrine, 638
pyrilamine, 721
Rofact, rifampin, 735
Ro-Fedrin, pseudoephedrine, 717
Ro-Hist, tripelennamine, 844
Rolaids, antacids, 69
Rolidrin, nylidrin, 565
Romilar CF 8 Hour Cough Formula,
dextromethorphan, 250
Romilar Children's Cough Syrup,
dextromethorphan, 250

*The symbol [CD] indicates that the brand name given is a combination drug consisting of generic drug components listed below it. If there is no page numbering following the name of the generic drug component, there is no Drug Profile for that ingredient in this book.

Romilar III [CD]
CONTAINS
dextromethorphan, 250
phenylpropanolamine, 641
Roucol, allopurinol, 40
Rounox, acetaminophen, 29
RP-Mycin, erythromycin, 328
Rufen, ibuprofen, 398
Rynatan [CD]
CONTAINS
chlorpheniramine, 167
phenylephrine, 638
pyrilamine, 721
Rythmodan, disopyramide, 294

S

Sal-Adult, aspirin, 75
Salazopyrin, sulfasalazine, 750
Sal-Infant, aspirin, 75
Saluron, hydroflumethiazide,
390
Salutensin [CD]
CONTAINS
hydroflumethiazide, 390
reserpine, 730
Salutensin-Demi [CD]
CONTAINS
hydroflumethiazide, 390
reserpine, 730
Sandril, reserpine, 730
Sansert, methysergide, 511
Sarocycline, tetracycline, 771
Sarodant, nitrofurantoin, 554
Saronil, meprobamate, 471
SAS-500, sulfasalazine, 750
scopolamine. *See* atropine, 86
Scotrex, tetracycline, 771
secobarbital, 738
Secogen, secobarbital, 738
Seconal, secobarbital, 738
Sedadrops, phenobarbital, 626
Sedatuss, dextromethorphan,
250
Septra [CD]
CONTAINS
sulfamethoxazole, 746
trimethoprim, 841

Septra DS [CD]
CONTAINS
sulfamethoxazole, 746
trimethoprim, 841
Seral, secobarbital, 738
Ser-Ap-Es [CD]
CONTAINS
hydralazine, 376
hydrochlorothiazide, 381
reserpine, 730
Serax, oxazepam, 583
Serentil, mesoridazine, 475
Serp, reserpine, 730
Serpalan, reserpine, 730
Serpanray, reserpine, 730
Serpasil, reserpine, 730
Serpasil-Apresoline [CD]
CONTAINS
hydralazine, 376
reserpine, 730
Serpasil Esidrix [CD]
CONTAINS
hydrochlorothiazide, 381
reserpine, 730
Serpate, reserpine, 730
Serpena, reserpine, 730
Sertabs, reserpine, 730
Sertan, primidone, 682
Sertina, reserpine, 730
Sigazine, promethazine, 698
Silain-Gel, antacids, 69
Simron, iron, 414
Sinarest [CD]
CONTAINS
acetaminophen, 29
chlorpheniramine, 167
phenylpropanolamine, 641
Sinarest Nasal Spray,
phenylephrine, 638
Sine-Aid [CD]
CONTAINS
acetaminophen, 29
pseudoephedrine, 717
Sine-Aid [CD] (Canada)
CONTAINS
acetaminophen, 29
phenylpropanolamine, 641

Sinemet [CD]
CONTAINS
levodopa, 442
carbidopa*
Sine-Off [CD]
CONTAINS
aspirin, 75
chlorpheniramine, 167
phenylpropanolamine, 641
Sine-Off Extra Strength [CD]
CONTAINS
acetaminophen, 29
chlorpheniramine, 167
phenylpropanolamine, 641
Sinequan, doxepin, 301
Sinex, phenylephrine, 638
Sinex Long Lasting, oxymetazoline, 590
Singlet [CD]
CONTAINS
acetaminophen, 29
chlorpheniramine, 167
phenylephrine, 638
Sinubid [CD]
CONTAINS
acetaminophen, 29
phenylpropanolamine, 641
phenyltoloxamine, 645
Sinutab [CD]
CONTAINS
acetaminophen, 29
phenylpropanolamine, 641
phenyltoloxamine, 645
642, propoxyphene, 705
SK-Ampicillin, ampicillin, 59
SK-APAP, acetaminophen, 29
SK-Bamate, meprobamate, 471
SK-Chloral Hydrate, chloral hydrate, 150
SK-chlorothiazide, chlorothiazide, 161

SK-Dexamethasone, dexamethasone, 240
SK-Diphenhydramine, diphenhydramine, 284
SK-Diphenoxylate [CD]
CONTAINS
atropine, 86
diphenoxylate, 288
SK-Erythromycin, erythromycin, 328
SK-Furosemide, furosemide, 360
SK Hydrochlorothiazide, hydrochlorothiazide, 381
SK-Lygen, chlordiazepoxide, 157
SK-Penicillin VK, penicillin V, 602
SK-Phenobarbital, phenobarbital, 626
SK-Pramine, imipramine, 402
SK-Prednisone, prednisone, 677
SK-Probenecid, probenecid, 686
SK-Propantheline, propantheline, 701
SK-Quinidine, quinidine, 724
SK-Reserpine, reserpine, 730
SK-65, propoxyphene, 705
SK-65 APAP [CD]
CONTAINS
acetaminophen, 29
propoxyphene, 705
SK-65 Compound [CD]
CONTAINS
aspirin, 75
caffeine, 120
propoxyphene, 705
SK-Soxazole, sulfisoxazole, 759
SK-Tetracycline, tetracycline, 771
SK-Tolbutamide, tolbutamide, 805
Slo-bid Gyrocaps, theophylline, 775
Slo-Phyllin 80, theophylline, 775
Slo-Phyllin Gyrocaps, theophylline, 775
Slo-Pot, potassium, 660

*The symbol [CD] indicates that the brand name given is a combination drug consisting of generic drug components listed below it. If there is no page numbering following the name of the generic drug component, there is no Drug Profile for that ingredient in this book.

Slow-Fe, iron, 414
Slow-K, potassium, 660
SMP Atropine, atropine, 86
Soda Mint, antacids, 68
sodium bicarbonate. *See* antacids,
    68
sodium carbonate. *See* antacids, 68
Solazine, trifluoperazine, 831
Solfoton, phenobarbital, 626
Solium, chlordiazepoxide, 157
Solu-barb, phenobarbital, 626
Soma, carisoprodol, 136
Soma Compound [CD]
    CONTAINS
    aspirin, 75
    carisoprodol, 136
Soma Compound [CD] (Canada)
    CONTAINS
    caffeine, 120
    carisoprodol, 136
    phenacetin*
Soma Compound with Codeine [CD]
    CONTAINS
    aspirin, 75
    carisoprodol, 136
    codeine, 212
Sominex, pyrilamine, 721
Somnifere, diphenhydramine, 284
Somnol, flurazepam, 356
Somophyllin, theophylline, 775
Somophyllin-CRT, theophylline,
    775
Somophyllin-DF, theophylline, 775
Somophyllin-12, theophylline, 775
Somophyllin-T, theophylline, 775
Som-Pam, flurazepam, 356
Sonazine, chlorpromazine, 170
Sopamycetin, chloramphenicol, 154
Sorbitrate, isosorbide dinitrate, 434
Sorquad, isosorbide dinitrate, 434
Sosol, sulfisoxazole, 759
Soxa, sulfisoxazole, 759
S-Pain-65, propoxyphene, 705
Spasmoban, dicyclomine, 257
Spectrobid, bacampicillin, 91
spironolactone, 742
S-P-T, thyroid, 787

Stabinol, chlorpropamide, 175
Stanback, aspirin, 75
Stelazine, trifluoperazine, 831
Stemetil, prochlorperazine, 693
Sterane, prednisolone, 672
Stibilium, diethylstilbestrol, 263
stilbestrol. *See* diethylstilbestrol, 263
Stilphostrol, diethylstilbestrol, 263
St. Joseph Children's Aspirin,
    aspirin, 75
Stress-Pam, diazepam, 253
Sub-Quin, procainamide, 690
Sudafed, pseudoephedrine, 717
Sudafed S.A., pseudoephedrine,
    717
sulfamethoxazole, 746
sulfasalazine, 750
sulfinpyrazone, 755
sulfisoxazole, 759
Sulfium, sulfisoxazole, 759
Sulfizin, sulfisoxazole, 759
sulindac, 763
Sumox, amoxicillin, 56
Sumycin, tetracycline, 771
Supasa, aspirin, 75
Supen, ampicillin, 59
Supeudol, oxycodone, 586
Suprazine, trifluoperazine, 831
Susadrin, nitroglycerin, 557
Sus-Phrine, epinephrine, 313
Sustaire, theophylline, 775
Synalgos [CD]
    CONTAINS
    aspirin, 75
    caffeine, 120
Synalgos-DC [CD]
    CONTAINS
    aspirin, 75
    caffeine, 120
    dihydrocodeine*
Synasal Spray, phenylephrine, 638
Synthroid, thyroxine, 791

T

Tagamet, cimetidine, 187
talbutal. *See* butalbital, 116
Talwin, pentazocine, 608

Talwin Compound [CD]
 CONTAINS
 aspirin, 75
 pentazocine, 608
Talwin Compound-50 [CD]
 CONTAINS
 aspirin, 75
 caffeine, 120
 pentazocine, 608
Talwin Nx [CD]
 CONTAINS
 pentazocine, 608
 naloxone*
Tapar, acetaminophen, 29
Tedral [CD]
 CONTAINS
 ephedrine, 308
 phenobarbital, 626
 theophylline, 775
Teebacin, para-aminosalicylic acid,
 595
Teebaconin, isoniazid, 423
Teebaconin and Vitamin B-6 [CD]
 CONTAINS
 isoniazid, 423
 pyridoxine*
Tegopen, cloxacillin, 209
Tegretol, carbamazepine, 128
Teldrin, chlorpheniramine, 167
Temaril, trimeprazine, 835
Tempra, acetaminophen, 29
Tenax, chlordiazepoxide, 157
Tenormin, atenolol, 81
Tensin, reserpine, 730
Tenuate, diethylpropion, 260
Tenuate Dospan, diethylpropion,
 260
Tepanil, diethylpropion, 260
Tepanil Ten-Tab, diethylpropion,
 260
terbutaline, 767
Terfluzine, trifluoperazine, 831

Tertroxin, liothyronine, 446
testosterone. *See* androgens, 62
testosterone cypionate. *See*
 androgens, 62
testosterone enanthate. *See*
 androgens, 62
testosterone propionate. *See*
 androgens, 62
Testred, androgens, 62
Tet-Cy, tetracycline, 771
Tetra-C, tetracycline, 771
Tetrachel, tetracycline, 771
Tetraclor, tetracycline, 771
Tetra-Co, tetracycline, 771
tetracycline, 771
Tetracyn, tetracycline, 771
Tetralan, tetracycline, 771
Tetralean, tetracycline, 771
Tetram, tetracycline, 771
Tetramax, tetracycline, 771
Tetrastatin [CD]
 CONTAINS
 mystatin, 568
 tetracycline, 771
Tetrex, tetracycline, 771
Thalitone, chlorthalidone, 179
Theobid Duracaps, theophylline,
 775
Theobid Jr. Duracaps, theophylline,
 775
Theo-Dur, theophylline, 775
Theo-Dur Sprinkles, theophylline,
 775
Theogen, estrogen, 332
Theolair, theophylline, 775
Theolair-SR, theophylline, 775
Theolixir, theophylline, 775
Theophyl, theophylline, 775
theophylline, 775
Theophyl-SR, theophylline, 775
Theophyl-225, theophylline, 775
Theovent, theophylline, 775

*The symbol [CD] indicates that the brand name given is a combination drug consisting
of generic drug components listed below it. If there is no page numbering following the
name of the generic drug component, there is no Drug Profile for that ingredient in this
book.

thioridazine, 779
Thioril, thioridazine, 779
Thiosulfil-A [CD]
  CONTAINS
  phenazopyridine, 620
  sulfamethizole*
thiothixene, 783
Thiuretic, hydrochlorothiazide, 381
Thorazine, chlorpromazine, 170
Thyrar, thyroid, 787
Thyrobrom, thyroid, 787
thyroid, 787
Thyrolar [CD]
  CONTAINS
  liothyronine, 446
  thyroxine, 791
thyroxine, 791
Tigan, trimethobenzamide, 838
Timolide [CD]
  CONTAINS
  hydrochlorothiazide, 381
  timolol, 795
timolol, 795
Timoptic, timolol, 795
Titralac, antacids, 68
Tofranil, imipramine, 402
tolazamide, 801
tolbutamide, 805
Tolectin, tolmetin, 809
Tolectin DS, tolmetin, 809
Toleron, iron, 414
Tolinase, tolazamide, 801
tolmetin, 809
Tora, phentermine, 630
Totacillin, ampicillin, 59
Tranmep, meprobamate, 471
Transderm-Nitro, nitroglycerin, 557
Tranxene, clorazepate, 205
Tranxene-SD, clorazepate, 205
tranylcypromine, 813
Travamine, dimenhydrinate, 281
trazodone, 819
Trexin, tetracycline, 771
Trialean, triamcinolone, 822
Triamacort, triamcinolone, 822
triamcinolone, 822
Triaminic [CD]

CONTAINS
pheniramine, 622
phenylpropanolamine, 641
pyrilamine, 721
Triaminic AC [CD]
  CONTAINS
  aspirin, 75
  caffeine, 120
  codeine, 212
  pheniramine, 622
  phenylpropanolamine, 641
  pyrilamine, 721
Triaminic Expectorant [CD]
  CONTAINS
  pheniramine, 622
  phenylpropanolamine, 641
  pyrilamine, 721
  guaifenesin*
Triaminic Expectorant DH [CD]
  CONTAINS
  hydrocodone, 386
  pheniramine, 622
  phenylpropanolamine, 641
  pyrilamine, 721
  guaifenesin*
Triaminic Juvelets [CD]
  CONTAINS
  pheniramine, 622
  phenylpropanolamine, 641
  pyrilamine, 721
Triaminic Oral Infant Drops [CD]
  CONTAINS
  pheniramine, 622
  phenylpropanolamine, 641
  pyrilamine, 721
Triaminicin [CD]
  CONTAINS
  aspirin, 75
  caffeine, 120
  chlorpheniramine, 167
  phenylpropanolamine, 641
Triaminicin [CD] (Canada)
  CONTAINS
  acetaminophen, 29
  caffeine, 120
  pheniramine, 623
  phenylpropanolamine, 641
  pyrilamine, 721

Triaminicin with Codeine [CD]
  CONTAINS
  acetaminophen, 29
  caffeine, 120
  codeine, 212
  pheniramine, 622
  phenylpropanolamine, 641
  pyrilamine, 721
Triaminicol [CD]
  CONTAINS
  chlorpheniramine, 167
  dextromethorphan, 250
  phenylpropanolamine, 641
Triaminicol DM [CD]
  CONTAINS
  dextromethorphan, 250
  pheniramine, 622
  phenylpropanolamine, 641
  pyrilamine, 721
triamterene, 827
Triaphen-10, aspirin, 75
Triavil [CD]
  CONTAINS
  amitriptyline, 43
  perphenazine, 615
Tridil, nitroglycerin, 557
trifluoperazine, 831
Triflurin, trifluoperazine, 831
triiodothyronine. *See* liothyronine,
  446
Trikates, potassium, 660
Trilafon, perphenazine, 615
trimeprazine, 835
trimethobenzamide, 838
trimethoprim, 841
Trimox, amoxicillin, 56
Trimpex, trimethoprim, 841
Trind-DM [CD]
  CONTAINS
  chlorpheniramine, 167
  dextromethorphan, 250
  phenylpropanolamine, 641
Triniad, isoniazid, 423

Trinsicon [CD]
  CONTAINS
  iron, 414
  vitamin B_{12}*
tripelennamine, 844
triprolidine, 847
Triptil, protriptyline, 713
T-Serp, reserpine, 730
T-250, tetracycline, 771
Tuinal [CD]
  CONTAINS
  amobarbital, 47
  secobarbital, 738
Tums, antacids, 68
Tussagesic [CD]
  CONTAINS
  dextromethorphan, 250
  pheniramine, 622
  phenylpropanolamine, 641
  pyrilamine, 721
  terpin hydrate*
Tussend [CD]
  CONTAINS
  hydrocodone, 386
  pseudoephedrine, 717
Tussend Expectorant [CD]
  CONTAINS
  hydrocodone, 386
  pseudoephedrine, 717
  guaifenesin*
Tussionex [CD]
  CONTAINS
  hydrocodone, 386
  phenyltoloxamine, 645
Tuss-Ornade [CD]
  CONTAINS
  phenylpropanolamine, 641
  caramiphen*
Tuss-Ornade [CD] (Canada)
  CONTAINS
  chlorpheniramine, 167
  phenylpropanolamine, 641
  caramiphen*

*The symbol [CD] indicates that the brand name given is a combination drug consisting of generic drug components listed below it. If there is no page numbering following the name of the generic drug component, there is no Drug Profile for that ingredient in this book.

Twin-K-Cl, potassium, 660
Tylenol, acetaminophen, 29
Tylosterone [CD]
  CONTAINS
  androgens, 62
  diethylstilbestrol, 263
Tylox [CD]
  CONTAINS
  acetaminophen, 29
  oxycodone, 586
T-3. *See* liothyronine, 446
T-4. *See* thyroxine, 791

U

Ultracef, cefadroxil, 142
Uniad, isoniazid, 423
Unifast Unicelles, phentermine, 630
Unipen, nafcillin, 538
Unipres [CD]
  CONTAINS
  hydralazine, 376
  hydrochlorothiazide, 381
  reserpine, 730
Univol, antacids, 69
Uridon, chlorthalidone, 179
Urised [CD]
  CONTAINS
  atropine, 86
  benzoic acid*
  methenamine*
  methylene blue*
  phenyl salicylate*
Uritol, furosemide, 360
Urobiotic [CD]
  CONTAINS
  phenazopyridine, 620
  tetracycline, 771
  sulfamethizole*
Urotoin, nitrofurantoin, 554
Urozide, hydrochlorothiazide, 381
Ursinus [CD]
  CONTAINS
  aspirin, 75
  pheniramine, 622
  phenylpropanolamine, 641
  pyrilamine, 721
Uticillin VK, penicillin V, 602
Utimox, amoxicillin, 56

V

Valadol, acetaminophen, 29
Valium, diazepam, 253
valproic acid, 850
Valrelease, diazepam, 253
Vancenase Nasal Inhaler,
  beclomethasone, 92
Vanceril Inhaler, beclomethasone, 92
Vanceril Oral Inhaler,
  beclomethasone, 92
Vanquish [CD]
  CONTAINS
  acetaminophen, 29
  antacids, 68
  aspirin, 75
  caffeine, 120
Vapo-Iso, isoproterenol, 430
Vaponefrin, epinephrine, 313
Vasodilan, isoxsuprine, 440
Vaso-80 Unicelles, pentaerythritol tetranitrate, 605
Vasospan, papaverine, 592
V-Cillin K, penicillin V, 602
VC-K 500, penicillin V, 602
Veetids, penicillin V, 602
Velosef, cephradine, 147
Veltane, brompheniramine, 104
verapamil, 854
Verequad [CD]
  CONTAINS
  ephedrine, 308
  phenobarbital, 626
  theophylline, 775
  guaifenesin*
Vertrol, meclizine, 462
Vibramycin, doxycycline, 305
Vibra Tabs, doxycycline, 305
Vicks Cough Syrup [CD]
  CONTAINS
  dextromethorphan, 250
  guaifenesin*
  sodium citrate*
Vimicon, cyproheptadine, 230
Viscerol, dicyclomine, 257
Vistaril, hydroxyzine, 395

Vistrax [CD]
  CONTAINS
  hydroxyzine, 395
  oxyphencyclimine*
vitamin C, 858
Vitron-C [CD]
  CONTAINS
  iron, 414
  vitamin C, 858
Vivactil, protriptyline, 713
Vivol, diazepam, 253
Voxin-PG [CD]
  CONTAINS
  phenylpropanolamine, 641
  guaifenesin*

W

warfarin, 862
Warfilone, warfarin, 862
Warnerin, warfarin, 862
Wigraine [CD]
  CONTAINS
  caffeine, 120
  ergotamine, 321

Wigraine [CD] (Canada)
  CONTAINS
  atropine, 86
  caffeine, 120
  ergotamine, 321
Win-Gel, antacids, 69
Winpred, prednisone, 677
Wyamycin, erythromycin,
  328
Wygesic [CD]
  CONTAINS
  acetaminophen, 29
  propoxyphene, 705
Wymox, amoxicillin, 56

Z

Zantac, ranitidine, 728
Zarontin, ethosuximide, 346
Zaroxolyn, metolazone, 514
Zide, hydrochlorothiazide,
  381
ZiPan, promethazine, 698
Zyloprim, allopurinol, 40
Zynol, Sulfinpyrazone, 755

*The symbol [CD] indicates that the brand name given is a combination drug consisting of generic drug components listed below it. If there is no page numbering following the name of the generic drug component, there is no Drug Profile for that ingredient in this book.

ABOUT THE AUTHOR

James W. Long, M.D., was born in Allentown, Pennsylvania. He received his pre-medical education from the University of Maryland and his medical degree from the George Washington University School of Medicine in Washington, D.C. For twenty years he was in the private practice of internal medicine in the Washington metropolitan area, and for over thirty-five years he has been a member of the faculty of the George Washington University School of Medicine. He has served with the Food and Drug Administration, the National Library of Medicine, and the Bureau of Health Manpower of the National Institutes of Health. Dr. Long is now director of Health Services for the National Science Foundation in Washington. He lives in Oxford, Maryland.

Dr. Long's involvement in drug information activities includes service on the H.E.W. Task Force on Prescription Drugs, on the F.D.A. Task Force on Adverse Drug Reactions, as a delegate-at-large to the U.S. Pharmacopeial Convention, as Editorial Consultant for *Hospital Formulary,* as a director of the Drug Information Association, and as a member of the Toxicology Information Program Committee of the National Research Council/National Academy of Sciences. He was consultant to the Food and Drug Administration, serving as advisor to their staff on the development of Patient Package Inserts. He is also the author of numerous articles in professional journals. *The Essential Guide to Prescription Drugs* is an outgrowth of his conviction that the general public needs and is entitled to practical drug information which is the equivalent of the professional "package insert." He believes the patient can be reasonably certain of using medications with the least risk and the greatest benefit only when the patient has all the relevant information about the drugs he or she is taking.

Schedules of Controlled Drugs*

Schedule I: Non-medicinal substances with high abuse potential and dependence liability. Used for research purposes only. Examples: heroin, marijuana, LSD. Not legally available for medicinal use by prescription.

Schedule II: Medicinal drugs in current use that have the highest abuse potential and dependence liability. Examples: opium derivatives (morphine, codeine, etc.), meperidine (Demerol), amphetamines (Dexedrine), short-acting barbiturates (Amytal, Nembutal, Seconal). A written prescription is required. Telephoned prescribing is prohibited. No refills are allowed.

Schedule III: Medicinal drugs with abuse potential and dependence liability less than Schedule II drugs but greater than Schedule IV or V drugs. Examples: codeine, hydrocodone and paregoric in combination with one or more non-narcotic drugs, some hypnotics (Doriden, Noludar), some appetite suppressants (Didrex, Tenuate, Sanorex). A telephoned prescription is permitted, to be converted to written form by the dispensing pharmacist. Prescriptions must be renewed every 6 months. Refills are limited to 5.

Schedule IV: Medicinal drugs with less abuse potential and dependence liability than Schedule III drugs. Examples: pentazocine (Talwin), propoxyphene (Darvon), all benzodiazepines (Librium, Valium, etc.), certain hypnotics (Placidyl, Noctec, Valmid, etc.). Prescription requirements are the same as for Schedule III.

Schedule V: Medicinal drugs with the lowest abuse potential and dependence liability. Examples: diphenoxylate (Lomotil), loperamide (Imodium). Drugs requiring a prescription are handled the same as any non-scheduled prescription drug. Some non-prescription drugs can be sold only with approval of the pharmacist; the buyer is required to sign a log of purchase at the time the drug is dispensed. Examples: codeine and hydrocodone in combination with other active, non-narcotic drugs, sold in preparations that contain limited quantities for control of cough and diarrhea.

*Under jurisdiction of the Controlled Substances Act of 1970.